T0210425

FORM AND FUNCTION IN THE BRAIN AND SPINAL CORD

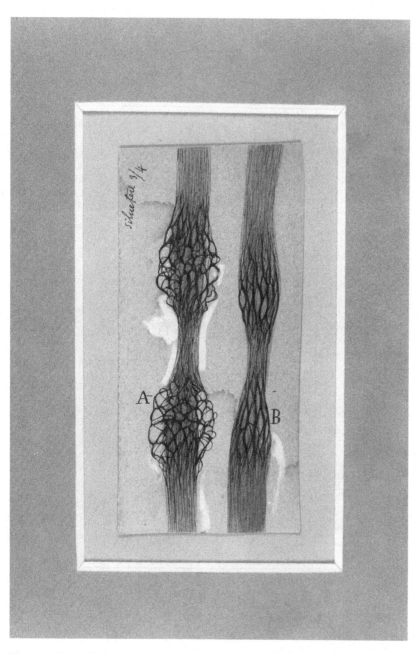

The nerve fiber at the beginning of the twentieth century. Hand-drawn rendering of a node of Ranvier by Ramón y Cajal.

FORM AND FUNCTION IN THE BRAIN AND SPINAL CORD

Perspectives of a Neurologist

Stephen G. Waxman

The MIT Press
Cambridge, Massachusetts
London, England

This book was set in Times New Roman on '3B2' by Asco Typesetters, Hong Kong

Library of Congress Cataloging-in-Publication Data

Waxman, Stephen G.
  Form and function in the brain and spinal cord : perspectives of a neurologist / Stephen G. Waxman.
    p. ;   cm. —
  Includes bibliographical references and index.
  ISBN 978-0-262-23210-4 (hc. : alk. paper) — 978-0-262-73155-3 (pb.)
  1. Central nervous system—Pathophysiology. 2. Central nervous system—Physiology. I. Title. II. Series.
[DNLM: 1. Central Nervous System Diseases—physiopathology—Collected Works. 2. Brain—anatomy & histology—Collected Works. 3. Brain—physiology—Collected Works. 4. Spinal Cord—physiology—Collected Works. WL 300 W356f 2000]
RC360.W39   2000
616.8'047—dc21   00-022476

The MIT Press is pleased to keep this title available in print by manufacturing single copies, on demand, via digital printing technology.

To Merle, Matthew, and David
for teaching me about love and friendship

And to a special circle of friends
for exhorting me to explore the brain and spinal cord
... and for helping me along the way.

Contents

Contents

Foreword

The academic physician has a crucial role to play as investigator, teacher, and practitioner of the art and science of medicine. That role is becoming increasingly difficult to fill as the technical demands of science become ever greater and more and more time must be spent in administration: raising funds to support scientific and clinical work and dealing with the paperwork involved in what should be the straightforward business of caring for the sick. That it is still possible to fill such a role successfully and with distinction is shown by this remarkable volume.

Dr. Waxman has selected from his published works thirty-four papers that have added to our understanding of the form and function of the nervous system and its disorders. The range of the contributions is astonishingly wide. They encompass anatomy and physiology in species as diverse as the Amazonian electric knife fish *Sternarchus* and humans. The analyses have been made from the level of the intact organism to the molecular level, and the techniques used range from observation at the bedside through electrophysiology and electron microscopy to those of molecular biology. The papers gathered here represent original contributions that have become part of the framework of reference for our daily thinking about the problems of clinical and experimental neuroscience. Motivating all the investigations is an underlying curiosity about mechanism.

The questions Dr. Waxman sets himself arise sometimes in the clinic and sometimes in the laboratory. What is striking about the answers contained in the papers in this volume is how, from either starting point, results have been obtained that time and again have been relevant to both. The papers illustrate the importance of choosing the right model with which to explore a problem, and the importance of being creative and flexible in technical approach: it is the question that has dictated the technique, not the technique that has determined the question to be tackled.

Most of the papers are written with Dr. Waxman's colleagues, students, and teachers, and in the linking text he pays generous tribute to the ways in which their ideas and their skills, clinical or laboratory, have enabled the work to move forward. What also emerges from this text is the sense of excitement in investigative work, the sense of being part of the historical continuity of neurological research, of the beauty of the normal structure and function of the nervous system, and of the extraordinary capacity of the nervous system to adapt to the changes imposed by disease.

Although some of the papers are highly technical, the linking text will be readily understood by anyone with even a modest knowledge of biology. To the student this book will be an encouragement through its demonstration of what is possible in a research career focused by clinical relevance; the established investigator will be grateful to have the papers so readily available in the compass of a single volume.

W. I. McDonald

Formerly, Head, Department of Neurology
The National Hospital,
Queen Square, London

Harveian Librarian
Royal College of Physicians

Preface

Over the years, colleagues have occasionally suggested that I write a book encapsulating my experiences as a neurologist and neuroscientist and summarizing my perspectives on form and function in the brain and spinal cord. In response to these suggestions, I prepared a few commentaries describing my experiences and saved them for the day when I would feel ready to put pen seriously to paper. The form that this book was to take crystalized, however, in 1999, when I had the pleasure of being asked to give the Wartenberg Lecture to the American Academy of Neurology. In my lecture I recounted some of my experiences in research and tried to convey my fascination with the beauty and elegance of the nervous system. I also attempted to share my excitement about the rich borderland that brings together the basic and clinical neurosciences and about the opportunities that we will have to help people with disorders of the brain, spinal cord and nerves if we mine this borderland productively.

Following my talk, several individuals suggested that these perspectives might have more general interest and should be published, either as a series of articles or as a book. Discussions with Michael Rutter of MIT Press convinced me that this should take the form of a book, but that the format should not be one of a narrative written entirely *de novo*. Rather, this book was planned as an annotated compendium including about thirty of my previously published papers and chapters, each illustrating an aspect of neuroscience or neurology, or of *being a neuroscientist or neurologist*, that I found especially illustrative or exciting. The articles and chapters that are reproduced in this book were, in fact, chosen in this way. They are introduced by commentaries which place them in scientific and/or historical context.

The papers that have been reproduced in this book are grouped together by topic, and the topics are presented in chronological order, that is, in the order in which I became interested in them. Although this may appear to introduce some arbitrariness with respect to the order of the various papers, it reflects the sequence of emergence and interactions of various themes within my career, an evolution that I hope will be of interest to some readers.

I hope that this book will provide readers with a sense of how one individual has navigated through the rich terrain of a rapidly advancing field. Neuroscience is in an incredibly vibrant state. At a minimum, I hope that this book will give the reader a sense of the elegant interrelatedness of form and function in the brain and spinal cord—both in the healthy state and in disease—and that it will communicate, especially to those just beginning their careers, my excitement not only about neurology and neuroscience, but also about being a neurologist and neuroscientist.

Acknowledgments

Scientists do not work alone. I have not, and I owe a debt of gratitude to the organizations, institutions, and people who have helped me.

Each one of us has benefited from interactions with mentors and teachers. I have been especially fortunate in this respect. I owe special thanks to George P. Sellmer, Howard T. Hermann, J. David Robertson, J. Z. Young, Ruth Bellairs, Dominick P. Purpura, George D. Pappas, Michael V. L. Bennett, Patrick D. Wall, Norman Geschwind, Thomas D. Sabin, and Jerry Lettvin.

My research over the years has been supported by an invaluable group of organizations and friends. Notable among these have been the Medical Research Service and the Rehabilitation Research Service of the Department of Veterans Affairs, the National Institutes of Health, and the National Multiple Sclerosis Society.

I owe a very special debt of gratitude to the Paralyzed Veterans of America and the Eastern Paralyzed Veterans Association. Their members and leadership are too numerous to list, but I extend special thanks to James J. Peters, Vivian Beyda, Gerard Kelly, Gordon Mansfield and John Bollinger. Their vision has made the PVA/EPVA Neuroscience Research Center a reality. I am also grateful to the many other individuals with special interests in diseases of the nervous system whom I have met, as patients, as friends, or as both. Some of them helped to support my research, most of them taught me important lessons, and each has been a continuing source of inspiration.

I am of course deeply appreciative for the collaboration of my coworkers. I have learned something from each one of them, and they have made science fun. Thirty-four previously published papers and chapters constitute the kernel of this book. My coauthors deserve special thanks, and if any credit is given for the research summarized in this book, it should go to them. The work presented in these publications represents the crystals from their sweat, and I am most grateful to them.

Introduction: Growing up in Neuroscience

I always wanted to be a scientist, and, even in high school, I benefited from some role models including family doctors, teachers, and professors at local colleges who encouraged me. It was not, however, until I left home for Harvard College that I was able to get an in-depth feel for science. There I was mentored by Howard Hermann, a family friend and professor of psychiatry who worked on photo-receptors in the tail of the crayfish, and J. David Robertson, a biophysicist who had discovered the bilayer structure of the "unit membrane" that surrounds all cells. Monoclonal antibodies and patch-clamping had not yet been invented, and MR scanning and confocal microscopes did not yet exist. But working in their laboratories, on evenings and weekends, gave me a glimpse of the beauty of the nervous system. It also gave me an opportunity to see scientists at work using the tools that were available, and provided a taste of what science was like.

As part of my experience in the Robertson laboratory I was invited, along with the other students, postdocs, and staff, to what seemed to be a flurry of parties and picnics. It was at one of these that David Robertson's daughter Twissy told me about University College London, where the Robertson family had lived while David was a visiting faculty member, and she urged me to try to work there. I was intrigued by this idea, and persuaded Harvard's registrar to let me spend a semester doing independent study abroad.

J. Z. Young was Professor of Anatomy at University College at the time. He was a dynamic teacher —his books *The Life of Mammals* and *A Model of the Brain* had helped to attract many students, including me, to biology—and he captivated me with his enthusiasm. Among other things, he had discovered the giant nerve fiber of the squid, large enough for physiologists to impale with micro-electrodes so they could listen to the electrical impulses it produced. Young's fascination with nerve fibers, their structure and their function, left a lasting impression. Years later, at a meeting on glial cells held at Cambridge University in 1990, I was asked to introduce "Prof," as he was called. I recalled him as a giant, both physically—he was well over six feet tall—and intellectually. Tea times in the departmental library (which were mandatory) were filled with animated discussion, often about the nervous system. Although the word "neuroscience" had not yet been coined, neuroscience already existed as a discipline at University College London. The facilities were antiquated, but University College was rich in people. One cluster of workers, focusing on the structure of the nervous system and its design principles, was led by Prof in Anatomy. Another cluster worked on cell excitability next door in Physiology and included Andrew Huxley, whose prescient analysis (with Alan Hodgkin) had revealed the ionic basis for impulse conduction in nerve fibers. And still a third cluster was unraveling the mysteries of synaptic function within a vibrant Department of Biophysics led by Bernard Katz, who was to win the Nobel Prize a few years later. I was seduced by the excitement of studying the brain and spinal cord.

As I approached the end of college I considered graduate school, but, even though I was still aimed toward a career in basic science, I opted for a combined M.D.-Ph.D. program. Alfred Gilman, the codiscoverer of mustard gas derivatives that became the first anticancer drugs and the author of the definitive textbook of pharmacology, was the director of the M.D.-Ph.D. program at Albert Einstein College of Medicine, a relatively new medical school located in the Bronx. He introduced me to the triad of neuroscientists—Dominick Purpura, George Pappas, and Michael Bennett—who had recently moved from Columbia, and I was attracted by the idea of being at a young, growing institution, and by their emphasis on "morphophysiology" of the nervous system.

Working in the laboratories with George Pappas and Mike Bennett, I initially participated in studies on the organization of the oculomotor nucleus, a relatively small group of cells that controls, with great precision, the movements of the eyes. One of the problems that the nucleus must solve has to do with synchrony—how to insure that the neurons controlling eye movement in a particular direction fire together, so as to produce a rapid, "saccadic" flick of the eye. This became the topic of my Ph.D. thesis. I also finished a number of studies on synaptic organization of other parts of the brain, under George's aegis. My major interest at the time, however, was in the structure and function of nerve fibers which, from my point of view, were the information highways of the spinal cord and brain. These were my first self-driven research studies, and I was very excited about them. Mike Bennett, who had a penetrating mind, introduced me to the pivotal work of Rushton. While going through Rushton's work, I found that his analysis of the requirements for "optimization" of nerve fibers, in order for them to conduct impulses as rapidly as possible, was quantitatively incorrect. I redid the analysis, which yielded some interesting conclusions, and wrote several drafts of the paper, which Mike said needed improvement. Unable to write a draft that was judged to be acceptable, I finally became impatient and without waiting for Mike's further changes, I sent the manuscript to Rushton—who by then was a very senior scientist—for suggestions. Mike made it clear that he was not pleased, and I trembled in his presence for the next few weeks. However, I finally received a letter from Rushton that began, "Thank you for your kindness in sending a copy of your nice manuscript, so crisp and to the point." The paper was published shortly afterward in *Nature,* and Mike forgave me for my oversight. This episode taught me that even a young, inexperienced scientist, if pointed in the right direction, can make a contribution; and I have learned this lesson again on several occasions, by watching and listening to my students.

My years at Einstein included summers at Woods Hole on Cape Cod, arranged for and paid by George Pappas, who took all of his students. The Marine Biological Laboratories at that time were a very popular place for trainees, and I had the chance to mix, both in the laboratories and at Stony Beach, with the likes of Sir John Eccles, Rodolfo Llinás, John Dowling, and John Nicholls. The "Tuesday night fights" featured some of the notables of neuroscience, who presented and critiqued each other's work. It was an important socializing experience, as well as a scientific one.

While I was a student at Einstein, I applied to the Epilepsy Foundation and received a fellowship that helped me to make another sojourn to University College London, this time to work with Patrick Wall and to attend lectures at the Institute of Neurology in Queen Square, a few blocks away. Pat tended to take one student or visiting scientist at a time, so during our experiments—aimed at characterizing the acute barrage of impulses that is triggered by nerve injury—I enjoyed a running, one-on-one dialog with him. He served as another important role model and introduced me to the injured nervous system, an interest that has endured to the present.

It was not until I was nearly finished with medical school that I realized that I liked clinical medicine. At that time, M.D.-Ph.D. students tended to crowd their clinical clerkships into the last eighteen months of medical school. So it was a belated surprise when I realized how rich the experience of a clinician could be. The medical school registrar's office had scheduled me to rotate through clerkships in internal medicine, then psychiatry, then surgery, and finally neurology. My initial instinct, having taken psychiatry, was to apply for residencies in that subspecialty, and I did so. Several months later, I was accepted into several psychiatry residencies just as I rotated through neurology and realized that I really wanted to be a neurologist. After a few anxious nights, I called the psychiatry program directors and explained that I had made a mistake. They were gracious in understanding. By this time, it was too late to apply for neurology residencies through the usual channels, since the deadline had passed.

Having been well trained in basic science, I wanted a neurology residency that was leveraged toward clinical scholarship. My first choice was the program run by Norman Geschwind—widely respected as a uniquely incisive clinical scholar—at the Harvard Neurology Unit, which was located at Boston City

Hospital. Although all of his slots were filled, Geschwind made an exception and accepted me. The arrangement was that I would be an "extra" resident, unpaid unless he could find a salary. Fortunately, another candidate chose the "Berry Plan" and enlisted in the army as a physician rather than take his chances in the draft. Thus I was given a paid position, as a house officer in neurology.

Boston City Hospital, at the time, was the quintessential teaching hospital, a maze of twenty-six red brick buildings connected by tunnels. I wondered at the abundance of the inpatient material as I walked through the tunnels, until I realized that some of these "patients" had long since been discharged and helped to run the hospital—the former chief of neurology, Derek Denny-Brown, had arranged for some of his favorite patients to be hired as workers (our elevator operator, for example, had myotonic dystrophy). "City," at that time, was shared by the three Boston medical schools, Harvard, Boston University, and Tufts. There was a remarkable sense of camaraderie, together with a healthy competition. There were three sets of medical and surgical wards, three surgical teams, and three medical and three surgical intensive care units. But there was only one neurology service.

The neurology faculty at Boston City Hospital was a small one, centered on Norman Geschwind and the second-in-command, Tom Sabin, who also was a superb clinician. Professors rounds with Geschwind were held every Tuesday morning and were challenging and uplifting experiences. They began in the neurology library. The room itself had an informal yet somewhat imposing atmosphere, its walls covered by the photographs of the many neurological luminaries who had trained at this institution. Having been involved in a spinal tap, I arrived late for my first set of professors rounds and took the only available chair, at the head of the conference table. A few minutes later, Norman Geschwind walked in, puffed on his pipe, and said softly, "That's my chair." I never sat *there* again.

Geschwind's engaging demeanor and lively teaching style dominated at these rounds. He had a gift for making every medical student, every clerk, every house officer feel as if their opinions were important. Geschwind was a master at asking innocent-seeming but probing questions, shifting the dialogue from medical student, to house officer, then again to medical student, at each juncture injecting his own incisive views. Rounds usually continued on the ward. Modern neuroimaging—CT scanning and MR imaging—was not yet available when I began my residency. Accurate diagnosis thus depended on bedside clinical acumen. Geschwind had balletlike grace in the neurological examination, and he managed to find something interesting and instructive in every patient.

One of the keystones of neurology is the *localizationist* approach to neurology. Geschwind's influence on this way of thinking about the nervous system is apparent in my first two clinical papers, written during my time at Boston City Hospital, on the interictal behavior syndrome of temporal lobe epilepsy with Geschwind, and on confusional states associated with right hemisphere lesions with Marsel Mesulam (who was also a resident at the time), Geschwind, and Sabin. The latter paper is notable in including CT scans made on one of the first scanners in Boston. These papers are still quoted— a testament to the standard of clinical scholarship at Boston City Hospital—and they are included in this book.

Toward the end of my residency Geschwind urged me to join the faculty at Harvard Medical School as assistant professor in his department. By this time, the city of Boston had decided that it could not afford to continue to have three medical schools share the hospital, and the Neurological Unit moved from Boston City to Beth Israel Hospital. Laboratory facilities there were limited, however, and there was no space for me. In lieu of my own laboratory, Norman introduced me to Jerry Lettvin, who was at that time professor of biology and electrical engineering at MIT. Lettvin was widely acknowledged as brilliant—his paper entitled "What the frog's eye tells the frog's brain" had been a milestone—and he was also a bit eccentric, a popular and near-theatrical lecturer. Jerry had two sets of laboratories, a

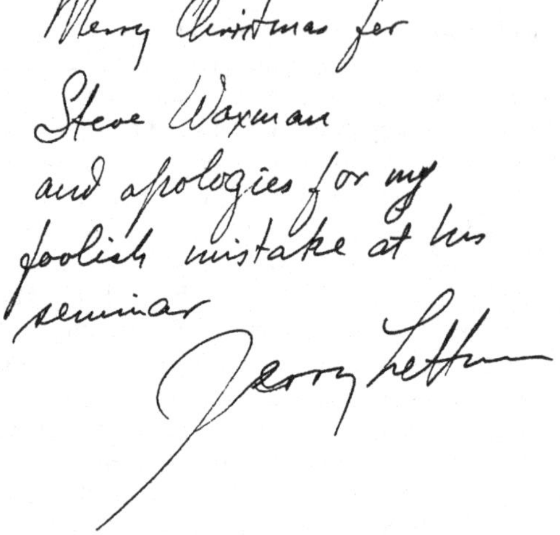

Figure I.1
From Jerry Lettvin's gift in December 1974.

new suite of modern laboratories on the top floor of building 36 (the new Research Laboratory of Electronics), and a much older, cavernous and frankly shabby office-laboratory in the basement of building 20, which had been hastily built to house additional labs for MIT during World War II. Lettvin preferred the latter, and he generously offered to share his newer laboratory suite with me.

As part of the arrangement I agreed to help teach graduate students, and I was appointed as visiting assistant professor of biology on the MIT faculty. When he heard about my appointment, Marshall Devor, who was at the time a graduate student in the Department of Psychology, arranged for me to give an inaugural lecture just before Christmas. The lecture room was a relatively large one and was nearly full. I presented my first four or five slides and, as I began to explain the next one, Lettvin— weighing three hundred-plus pounds, wearing an open-collared shirt—stood, walked to the front of the room, and, with his usual lack of inhibition, began writing on the blackboard. He drew a diagram of the series capacitance in the electromotor neurons in *Sternarchus* and said, "You've got it wrong, but go on with your talk." I was flabbergasted, and, although I knew he had misunderstood, I didn't know what to say. I went on with my lecture, but I thought it was ruined.

As I walked back to building 36 afterward, I was joined by Lettvin. He was silent, clearly thinking. Suddenly he fell to his knees. At first I thought he was sick, but then I saw that he was using his finger to write in the snow. A few moments later he said, "Oh my God! I made a mistake—the series capacitance is on the anterior end, not the posterior!" Two weeks later, he gave me a gift. It was an exquisite, leatherbound copy of the *Handbook of Neurology*. His inscription is shown in figure I.1. I learned from this brilliant teacher that, in addition to taking pride in being right, true scientists can also admit when they are wrong.

While working at Harvard and MIT, I edited a book, *The Physiology and Pathobiology of Axons*. In putting this volume together I wanted to underscore explicitly the importance of pathobiology, the principles underlying diseases of axons. I felt that neuroscience should try to attract the *best* researchers to disease-oriented investigations—if a squid's axon, or a frog's, could be interesting, surely a human axon under assault could be. Geschwind was enthusiastic about this book from the outset. Lettvin was a bit reserved, since he felt that we could not understand diseased axons until healthy axons were more fully understood; nevertheless, while in the hospital recovering from surgery, he generously wrote a provocative chapter on information processing within the axonal tree. The book, I believe, helped to attract interest to axons and disorders that affect them such as multiple sclerosis and peripheral neuropathies and, in a more general sense, to the neurobiology of disease.

Jerry's generosity included an open invitation to the iconoclastic, stimulating world that existed in his laboratories. John Moore, an expert on the squid giant axon from Duke, joined us on sabbatical and became a friend. He taught me about the intricacies of voltage-clamping and computer simulations of excitable membranes. Jerry was surrounded by a flock of adoring students, and his presence helped me to attract a string of energetic postdoctoral fellows. The first three were Don Quick, Harvey Swadlow, and Jeff Kocsis. They were all excellent scientists, and they helped me to launch my research program, which at that time used primarily morphological methods, extracellular recording, and computer simulations to study the functional organization of normal and pathological axons. Jeff, clearly about to embark on a meteoric career, moved with me to Stanford University in 1978.

Shortly after moving to Stanford I attended a meeting at Dartmouth College, organized around the theme of abnormal nerves and muscles as impulse generators. At this meeting Tom Sears, from the Institute of Neurology in London, showed longitudinal current recordings that demonstrated the presence of an outward current in the "internodal" portion of the nerve fiber's membrane that was located beneath the myelin. This suggested that K^+ channels might be located within this part of the nerve fiber membrane. Sears, Murdoch Ritchie (who was at that time chairman of the Department of Pharmacology at Yale), and I decided to search for the "hidden" K^+ channels in nerve fibers. Less than three months later Murdoch mailed me copies of his recordings, which showed that, if one destroyed the myelin, one could see that there were K^+ channels in the internodal part of the membrane. He had beat us to the punch, but it was hard not to smile and be impressed with the beauty of his results. Ritchie had taught me that one can share—and still succeed—in science. Years later I had the pleasure of collaborating with him on several studies.

Stanford University Medical School was relatively new and glistening when I arrived there in 1978, a palace compared to some of the older buildings in Boston. David Prince was chairman of neurology and had a knack for recruiting gifted faculty. I made a number of lifelong friendships at Stanford, including Dennis Choi, Arnold Kriegstein, and Bruce Ransom. Stanford presented the opportunity for me, then thirty-three years old, to run an academic unit, the Neurological Unit at the Palo Alto Veterans Administration Hospital, and to expand my research program.

Our research laboratories were located in the same building as the neurology ward, which was very convenient. Joel Black, a skilled cell biologist who had already made important contributions to the study of cell membranes outside of the nervous system, joined my research group shortly after we set up the new laboratories and rapidly emerged as an insightful neuroscientist and long-term collaborator. He was followed by a series of energetic research fellows and visiting scientists. We continued our ultrastructural studies, focusing now on glial cells as well as neurons, and we added intra-axonal recording methods, pioneered by Jeff Kocsis, to our armamenterium. I also became interested in spinal cord injury at this time, and studied it both in mammalian model systems and in the knife fish *Sternarchus,* which, remarkably, regenerates caudal segments of its spinal cord after they are amputated.

In 1985, I was asked to consider becoming chairman of neurology at Yale. Jeff, Joel, and I talked about it and realized that together we had a research program that was stronger than three separate ones. It was clear that if I were to move to Yale, the entire group would have to relocate. Yale, having little unoccupied space and being a "soft-money" institution, did not have laboratories for us, and in any event we wanted to stay within the Veterans Administration system, which, like its counterparts in other countries, is interested in disorders of the nervous system. The Veterans Administration, within the federal bureaucracy, was not in a position to build new laboratories quickly. So I approached the Paralyzed Veterans of America and the Eastern Paralyzed Veterans Association, on whose advisory boards I had served, and asked whether they might provide funds for a small research building. To my surprise, they sent a delegation, including their research director Vivian Beyda, for a site visit, and they said they would consider the idea. The result was the establishment of the PVA/EPVA Center for Neuroscience and Regeneration Research of Yale University, which we built at the VA Medical Center, West Haven, Connecticut.[1] Our goal was to incorporate molecular biology and molecular pharmacology into our research program, along with cell biology and electrophysiology. The long name of this research center reflects its scientific focus—recovery of function after injury to the nervous system—and its cooperative nature—PVA, EPVA, Yale, and the VA collaborated in giving birth to it. PVA and EPVA have continued to support research in the center, and have been partners in our battle against disorders that affect the brain and spinal cord.

Just after moving to Yale, I was pleasantly surprised to be asked to give the Denny-Brown lecture in Boston. By way of introduction, I was able to trace at least two lineages from my research program back to Denny-Brown. One went through Norman Geschwind, who had been Denny-Brown's successor at Boston City Hospital. And a second passed through Jeff Kocsis, a scientific grandson of John Eccles (Kocsis did his Ph.D. thesis with Steve Kitai, who had worked with Eccles) who had worked together with Denny-Brown under the tutelage of Sir Charles Sherrington. It is amazing how rich the network of associations in science can be.

One of my top priorities after arriving at Yale was to strengthen its Department of Neurology. I was fortunate in being able to recruit a cohort of talented colleagues, mostly at junior faculty levels, who brought a self-reinforcing "can do" ethic that was embraced by the entire faculty, new and old. A few years later, I was able to persuade Bruce Ransom—one of the leading experts in the world on glial cells and their function—to join us at Yale, where he remained for a decade before taking up the chairmanship of neurology at the University of Washington. And I had the good fortune to be joined by creative colleagues in the laboratory, including Harry Sontheimer, Peter Stys, Sulayman Dib-Hajj, and Ted Cummins.

Beginning on my first day, I found Yale to be a stimulating, challenging, and intellectually vibrant receptor site. Like many great medical schools, Yale Medical School was relatively poor in resources— money and space were in short supply. In their place I found a wonderful intellectual orientation, a culture based on collegiality, and a tradition of exploration and academic freedom. A few years after I moved to Yale Leon Rosenberg, the dean who recruited me, asked if I had enough time in the laboratory. "There's never enough time," I told him. "Then make it," he replied. "That's why you are here." Although my maturation as an investigator probably contributed to my productivity at Yale, the contributions of its institutional culture and terrain, and of its expectations, have been immense. Nineteen of the papers reprinted in this book include work that was done at Yale.

Some readers may wonder why, in an essay called "Growing up in Neuroscience," I have described an evolution spanning half a century—surely we grow up more quickly than that. Not so, I would

---

1. The building opened in 1988—in part due to the suggestion, by some friends at PVA/EPVA, that it be designated as a "temporary" structure so that approvals would not take too long.

argue. The professional growth of the scientist can continue throughout a lifetime, since science continues to present fresh challenges, additional chances to learn, and new opportunities for exploration, decade after decade. Around me, neuroscience has grown at an exponential rate, and is generating an avalanche of new information, new concepts, and new questions to be answered. These are some of the reasons that science is so captivating.

The chapters that make up this book span my evolution thus far as a scientist and document some of my explorations. I hope they will give the reader a lens, through which to view neuroscience and its development as seen by one individual. Equally important, I hope they will provide the reader with a glimpse, not only of science per se, but also of what scientists do, of how scientists think and, finally, of the excitement of being a scientist.

I BUILDING A SMART NERVE FIBER

One of the beautiful things about the nervous system is its elegance of design. Within the brain and spinal cord, structure serves function. Although there are subtle variations, each cell has an overall form (size, shape, branching pattern) that allows it to fulfill a specific role in the immense computer that we call our "nervous system."

Some nerve fibers within mammals are covered with a lipid-rich sheath, called myelin, which acts as an insulator. The myelin is periodically interrupted by small gaps (called "nodes of Ranvier") where it is not insulated. The nerve impulse jumps from node to node, in what has been called a "saltatory" manner. In a classic paper, Rushton (1951) examined the structure-functional relationships that determine the speed at which the impulse travels during saltatory conduction in myelinated axons. He noted that the conduction velocity of these nerve fibers is linearly correlated with their diameter and proposed that, at any given overall diameter of the fiber and its myelin, there is a particular myelin thickness that maximizes conduction velocity. For myelin that is too thick or too thin, conduction velocity will fall from this maximum.

Conduction velocity is also dependent on the distance between the nodes of Ranvier. For a fiber with a fixed diameter, the relationship between the internode distance and conduction velocity has the shape of an inverted U with a broad maximum. The conduction velocity is less-than-maximal for axons with short internode distances in which, as a result of the large number of nodes, the impulse must make a large number of saltatory jumps; and conduction speed is also reduced in nerve fibers with long internode distances, which tax the impulse-generating capability of the nerve fiber. Rushton observed that, for most axons within peripheral nerves, the myelin thickness and internode distance correspond to the predicted optima, and concluded that, as a result of natural selection, these axons are constructed "optimally" so as to maximize conduction velocity.

As an undergraduate, I had spent time as a fledging research student working in the laboratory of J. Z. Young at University College London, where he had established one of the first neuroscience units in the world. One of Prof's interests was in the design of the nervous system, and he urged me to think about the brain and spinal cord in engineering terms, always keeping function in mind. In the Waxman and Bennett (1972) paper I returned, together with my Ph.D. mentor Michael Bennett, to this theme and examined another aspect of "smart" design of myelinated nerve fibers. Rushton had argued that on theoretical grounds myelin should only increase conduction velocity when it occurs along axons whose diameter is larger than a "critical" value. Our theoretical analysis showed that this critical value should be close to 0.2 µm. Using the electron microscope to examine the brain and spinal cord, we found that, as predicted for nerve fibers that are designed to maximize conduction velocity, myelin is only produced when the diameter is larger than this critical size. Although Rushton had incorrectly estimated the critical value, he was right in predicting that in most types of nerve fibers myelination is designed to maximize the speed of impulse conduction. Structure serves function.

A rapid speed of impulse conduction clearly has adaptive value for certain neural systems—one can imagine, for example, that saving a few thousandths of a second can have substantial adaptive value when one is running away from a saber-toothed tiger. Thus, it was not surprising when we confirmed that the structure-function relations for most myelinated axons within the brain and spinal cord are such as to maximize conduction velocity.

Maximization of conduction speed is not, however, always good, and "optimization" of nerve fiber function does not always entail maximizing conduction velocity. In some neural systems there is a need for precise timing—not necessarily maximization of speed—of impulse conduction along the axon. One particularly well-studied example is provided by the "electromotor" systems in fish in which specialized electrocytes (electricity-generating cells), located along the entire length of the fish's body, discharge synchronously in order to generate a coherent electrical discharge. In these electromotor systems, the electrocytes fire in response to excitatory messages that they receive from a command nucleus located in the brain (Bennett 1970). The location of the various electrocytes, at different distances from the command nucleus, poses a design problem: the nerve fibers that carry commands to electrocytes in the front half of the fish, close to the brain, must deliver their messages and trigger electrical discharge at the same time as messages carried by longer axons that project to electrocytes in the back half of the fish, much farther away. The problem is solved by having the axons act as "delay lines." Diameters, myelin thickness and internode distance are adjusted so that the message arrives at each electrocyte at the same time, within a few thousandths of a second (Waxman 1975).

Axons that carry information to Purkinje cells, which constitute major computational elements within the cerebellum, offer another example of precisely timed conduction velocities. The cerebellum serves a crucial role in coordinating movements and, in order for it to do so, Purkinje cells in different parts of the cerebellum must be excited in precise sequence, with the messages arriving with an accuracy of thousandths of a second; this requires, again, that some axons act as delay lines (Sugihara, Lang, and Llinas 1993). A third example is provided by the ganglion cells within the retina. In order to convey a coherent picture of the visual world, these cells must send their messages to the brain so that they all arrive at the same time; because different ganglion cells are located at different eccentricities within the retina, and therefore are located at different distances from the brain, the conduction speeds of their axons must be adjusted so that differences in conduction times are minimized (Stanford 1987).

In each of these cases, "optimization" of nerve fiber function involves tuning the axon so that conduction velocity is matched to a precise value, not necessarily a maximum. This is accomplished by adjusting axon size, myelin thickness, and internode distance so that they meet functional requirements (Waxman 1997). Once again, structure serves function.

We are only beginning to understand how myelinated fibers develop with a structure that permits them to maximize or otherwise tune their conduction velocity to meet functional needs. A variety of molecular cues appear to provide a basis for a detailed "conversation" between the axon and myelin-forming cells (Waxman and Sims 1984, see chapter 9; Kaplan et al. 1997; Salzer 1997). But we do not yet understand the details of this conversation. The need for maximizing conduction velocity in some nerve fibers, and for precisely timing impulse conduction in others, imposes a requirement for milli-second precision in the design of myelinated fibers, and suggests that the development of these fibers may have to be guided by functional feedback. This raises the possibility (Waxman 1997) that, during development and afterward, the nervous system "listens" to its own output, monitoring it in an ongoing manner and modifying the structure of nerve cells and glial cells to meet functional requirements.

Compared to the awesome complexity of networks containing millions of neurons and billions of synapses the nerve fiber seems, at first glance, to be a straightforward research target, easy to dissect and easy to understand. In fact, the nerve fiber may be simple, but it is anything but dumb. Even the nerve fiber is "smart," and the principles underlying its design have much to teach us.

References

Bennett, M. V. L. Electric organs. *Annu. Rev. Physiol.* 32: 471–528, 1970.

Kaplan, M. R., Meyer-Franklin, A., Lambert, S., Bennett, V., Duncan, I. D., Levinson, S. R., Barres, B. A. Induction of sodium channel clustering by oligodendrocytes. *Nature* 386: 724–728, 1997.

Rushton, W. A. H. A theory of the effects of fibre size in medullated nerve. *J. Physiol. (Lond.)* 115: 101–122, 1951.

Salzer, J. L. Clustering sodium channels at the node of Ranvier: close encounters of the axon-glia kind. *Neuron* 18: 843–846, 1997.

Stanford, L. R. Conduction velocity variations minimize conduction time differences among retinal ganglion cell axons. *Science* 238: 358–360, 1987.

Sugihara, I., Lang, E. J., Llinás, R. Uniform olivocerebellar conduction time underlies Purkinje cell complex spike synchronicity in the rat cerebellum. *J. Physiol. (Lond.)* 470: 243–271, 1993.

Waxman, S. G. Integrative properties and design principles of axons. *Internat. Rev. Neurobiol.* 18: 1–40, 1975.

Waxman, S. G. Axon-glia interactions: Building a smart nerve fiber. *Curr. Biol.* 7: R406–R410, 1997.

Waxman, S. G., and Bennett, M. V. L. Relative conduction velocities of small myelinated and non-myelinated fibers in the central nervous system. *Nature New Biol.* 238: 217–219, 1972.

Waxman, S. G., and Sims, T. J. Specificity in central myelination: evidence for local regulation of myelin thickness. *Brain Res.* 292: 179–185, 1984.

1 Relative Conduction Velocities of Small Myelinated and Non-myelinated Fibres in the Central Nervous System

S. G. Waxman and M. V. L. Bennett

In peripheral nerve, most axons with diameters of less than 1 μm do not have myelin sheaths, while most fibres more than 1 μm in diameter are myelinated.[1,2] In the central nervous system, axons as small as 0.2 μm in diameter may be myelinated.[2-5] In his paper on the effects of myelin on conduction velocity, Rushton[6] concluded that 1 μm is the "critical diameter" above which "myelin increases conduction velocity" and below which "conduction is faster without myelination." This conclusion is referred to widely (see, for example, refs. 7–9). In this communication we demonstrate that the analysis leading to this conclusion is based on morphological data[10] which do not apply either to central or to peripheral fibres, so that myelinated fibres considerably smaller than 1 μm might be expected to conduct more rapidly than non-myelinated fibres of similar size.

Rushton derived the relations that must hold between myelinated fibres of different sizes if one is to make predictions about their behaviour from size alone. These relations are that the fibres have the same specific membrane properties and are "dimensionally similar." The latter, put in somewhat simplified form, requires that nodal length be constant and that internodal length be proportional to overall diameter. Rushton adduced evidence that dimensional similarity did hold, and inferred that conduction velocity would be nearly proportional to fibre diameter. He showed that, in contrast, conduction velocity of non-myelinated fibres (of uniform specific membrane properties) is proportional to the square root of fibre diameter and concluded that "a very small fibre must conduct faster if it is non-myelinated than if it is myelinated."

The diameter at which myelination first increases conduction velocity was estimated in

Reprinted with permission from *Nature New Biology* 238: 217–219, 1972.

Rushton's figure 5 (see our figure 1.1), in which derived relationships between conduction velocity and fibre diameter for myelinated and non-myelinated fibres were superimposed. The two curves intersect at a point corresponding to a fibre diameter of approximately 1 μm, suggesting that 1 μm is the critical diameter below which "conduction is faster without myelination."[6] In addition, extrapolation of the relationship for myelinated fibres leads to intersection with the abscissa at a diameter of 0.6 μm, suggesting that fibres with diameters of 0.6 μm or less should not conduct impulses at all.

Rushton obtained the diameter–velocity relation for non-myelinated fibres from Gasser's measurements[11] of diameter (1.1 μm) and conduction velocity (2.3 ms^{-1}) of the largest C fibres. Rushton drew a parabola based on the proportionality of the velocity to the square root of diameter through this point perpendicular to the ordinate at the origin (solid line in figure 1.1). The diameter–velocity relation for myelinated fibres was obtained from two sets of empirical data, Sanders's measurements[10] of the ratio g, defined as axon diameter divided by overall fibre diameter (figure 1.3, crosses), and Hursh's measurements[12] of conduction velocity and fibre diameter (figure 1.2, dots and open circles).

If specific membrane properties are constant, and dimensional similarity holds for myelinated fibres, conduction velocity V is related to fibre diameter D and g as follows:

$$V \propto Dg\sqrt{-\log_e g} \qquad (1.1)$$

Rushton used Sanders's measurements to compute the left side of the equation and then chose a constant of proportionality to fit the resulting curve to Hursh's data (figure 1.2, solid line with Rushton's extrapolation indicated by dashes). It is the extrapolated region of this curve that is shown on an expanded scale in figure 1.1 (dashed line). According to Sanders's measurements g

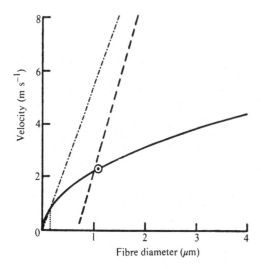

Figure 1.1
Relations between conduction velocity and fibre diameter for small myelinated and non-myelinated fibres. Modified from Rushton's[6] fig. 5 as indicated in the text. The circled point represents Gasser's measurements[11] for the largest C fibres. The linear relation for myelinated fibres intersects the parabolic relation for non-myelinated fibres at a point corresponding to a diameter of about 0.2 μm. –·–·, Linear relation for myelinated fibres; – – –, Rushton's relation for myelinated fibres; ——, parabolic relation for non-myelinated fibres.

decreases rapidly for small fibres. Although Rushton does not give the values he obtained from Sanders's paper, evidently he extrapolated g to zero for a diameter of about 0.6 μm (see figure 1.3). This would account for the predicted failure of conduction at this diameter, since core resistance is infinite when $g = 0$.

The value of g has more recently been shown to remain nearly constant as fibre diameter decreases[13–16]. For the smallest fibres studied g ranged from 0.5 to 0.7 for peripheral nerve, and from 0.5 to 0.9 for central tracts. The finding that g for small fibres remains in this range is teleologically satisfying, for, as Rushton showed from equation 1, conduction velocity has a

broad maximum around $g = 0.6$. It has been suggested that use of light microscopy accounts for Sanders's observation that g decreases for small fibres, since light microscopic measurements give a relation similar to that of Sanders, while electron microscopic measurements on the same nerves show that g remains constant as diameter decreases.[16] Our own electron microscopic measurements of myelinated fibres in the teleost central nervous system show the smallest to be about 0.4 μm in diameter with values of g usually between 0.5 and 0.7.[17] A similar result for neuropil of the oculomotor nucleus of the lizard *Anolis carolinensis* is illustrated by the filled circles in figure 1.3.

If g is constant, equation 1.1 predicts that conduction velocity is proportional to diameter and that the velocity–diameter relation intersects the origin. Figure 1.2 shows the revised, linear relation between conduction velocity and diameter together with Hursh's data and Rushton's relation. The slope of the line was fitted by eye and is 5.5 ms⁻¹ μm⁻¹. The overall closeness of fit is comparable for the linear relation and Rushton's computed curve. (Neither relation fits the points for small diameter axons particularly well, although the fit by Rushton's curve is somewhat better. A linear relation intersecting the origin and with a slightly smaller slope could be drawn for the smaller fibres to give a somewhat better fit in this region. Hursh[12] calculated the slope of the regression line for his data as 6.0 ms⁻¹ μm⁻¹ and stated that velocity in ms⁻¹ could be obtained by multiplying the diameter in μm by this factor. His statement is slightly in error because his regression line does not quite intersect the origin. The slope of our line differs from that of Hursh, because we have drawn it through the origin.) In figure 1.1 we show the revised, linear relation between conduction velocity and diameter, together with Rushton's curves for myelinated and non-myelinated axons. The revised relation for myelinated fibres intersects the relation for non-myelinated fibres at a point corresponding to a diameter of about 0.2 μm. This

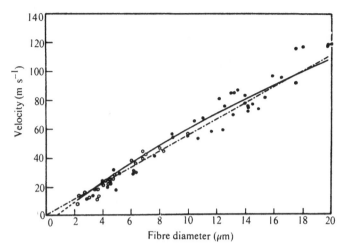

Figure 1.2
Relations between conduction velocity and fibre diameter for myelinated axons. Open circles and dots represent Hursh's observations[12] on fibres from kittens and cats respectively. Rushton's relation computed using Sanders's measurements of g (the ratio of axon diameter to overall fibre diameter) is indicated by the solid curve with dashed extrapolation for small diameters. The linear relation assuming constant g is shown (—·—·—); its slope is 5.5 ms^{-1} μm^{-1}. Modified from Rushton's fig. 3 (ref. 6).

argument suggests that this is the critical diameter above which myelinated fibres conduct more rapidly than non-myelinated fibres of the same size.

It should be pointed out that this diameter is not necessarily one below which (as Rushton[6] argued) "conduction is faster without myelination". We cannot conclude from the results shown in our figure 1.1 that a myelinated fibre below 0.2 μm in diameter would conduct more slowly than a non-myelinated fibre of the same size made up of membrane like that at nodes of Ranvier. Arguments from dimensional similarity expressly do not apply to comparisons between such fibres, for it is "only possible to argue from one nerve to another ... if they are dimensionally similar"[6] and a non-myelinated fibre is not dimensionally similar to a myelinated one. Furthermore, the nodal membrane is probably not like that of non-myelinated fibres. For ex-

ample, the resistivity of nodal membrane is markedly lower than that of most other excitable membranes that have been studied, including invertebrate non-myelinated fibres.[18] Direct measurements have not been made on C fibres, but the non-myelinated terminal at the frog neuromuscular junction, which is of comparable diameter, appears to have a considerably higher resistivity than nodal membrane.[19]

Recent data seem to contradict the assumption that specific membrane properties are constant for myelinated fibres of different diameter. It has been found that the rise time of the spike is greater in small diameter myelinated fibres[20] and, as follows from this result, conduction time per internode is greater in small fibres.[21] We are indebted to Professor A. F. Huxley who drew our attention to these data and the similar trend in Hursh's data (figure 1.2). If it is assumed that a fibre of a given diameter is differentiated for

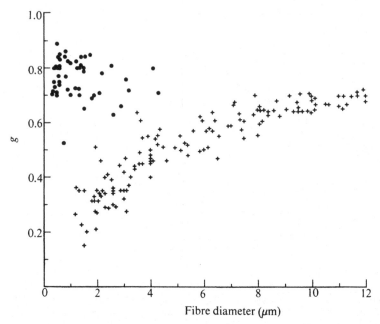

Figure 1.3
Values of *g* as a function of myelinated fibre diameter. Sanders's data[10] for rabbit fibres (+) are taken from his fig. 3. With his light microscopic techniques, *g* seems to decrease markedly for small fibres. Fifty fibres from the oculomotor nucleus of the lizard *Anolis carolinensis* are shown (●). Data were obtained by electron microscopy of OsO_4 fixed material[5]; axons in the dorsolateral nucleus were chosen at random and *D* and *g* were measured along the minor axis of cross sections with axial ratios of less than 1.25. Twenty-four of the fifty fibres have diameters under 1 μm; *g* is independent of diameter and ranges between 0.54 and 0.88 with a mean of 0.77.

maximum conduction velocity, the absence of peripheral myelinated fibres smaller than 1 μm may be accounted for on these grounds.

Hille[22] pointed out that the conductance of individual excitable channels imposes a limit on fibre size that may be related to these data. For reliable operation, resting input conductance should be large compared with the conductance of individual channels. Yet if specific membrane properties were the same in small as in large fibres, this limitation would be approached by 1 μm diameter fibres, both myelinated and unmyelinated.

Morphological considerations make it unlikely that myelinated fibres much smaller than 0.2 μm

will be found. The minimum sheath, consisting of a single layer of myelin, would be about 200 Å thick, implying a minimum fibre diameter of about 0.1 μm if the optimum *g* of 0.6 obtains. The thinnest myelin sheaths we have observed in *Anolis* and in teleosts[17] are two layers thick (that is, have two major dense lines), corresponding to a fibre diameter of 0.2 μm for a *g* of 0.6. Actually these fibres were somewhat larger in diameter because *g* generally exceeds its optimum value.

The properties of small diameter fibres require further investigation. Data obtained by voltage clamping and modern techniques of computation should allow comparisons between fibres that are not dimensionally similar. Precise predictions about conduction velocity will depend on specification of membrane properties and fibre morphology.[23] The dimensional arguments presented here suggest that myelinated fibres with diameters in the range of 0.2 μm to 1 μm, which are commonly found in the central nervous system, conduct more rapidly than non-myelinated fibres of the same diameter. Empirical data may prove otherwise, as is suggested for peripheral fibres. In either case, maximization of conduction velocity for a given fibre diameter need not be the only criterion of design, particularly for central fibres.[24,25]

This work was supported by grants from the US National Institutes of Health. S. G. W. is a postdoctoral fellow in the Medical Science Training Program. M. V. L. B. is a Kennedy scholar.

References

1. Vizoso, A. D., and Young, J. Z., *J. Anat.*, 82, 110 (1948).

2. Matthews, M. A., *Anat. Rec.*, 161, 337 (1968).

3. Bishop, G. H., and Smith, J. M., *Exp. Neurol.*, 9, 483 (1964).

4. Adinolfi, A., and Pappas, G. D., *J. Comp. Neurol.*, 133, 167 (1968).

5. Waxman, S. G., and Pappas, G. D., *J. Comp. Neurol.*, 143, 41 (1971).

6. Rushton, W. A. H., *J. Physiol.*, 115, 101 (1951).

7. Eccles, J. C., *The Neurophysiological Basis of Mind* (Oxford University Press, Oxford, 1953).

8. Davson, H., and Eggleton, M. E., *Principles of Human Physiology* (J. and A. Churchill, London, 1966).

9. Cole, K. S., *Membranes, Ions, and Impulses* (University of California Press, Berkeley, 1968).

10. Sanders, F. K., *Proc. Roy. Soc.*, B, 135, 323 (1948).

11. Gasser, H. S., *J. Gen. Physiol.*, 127, 393 (1950).

12. Hursh, J. B., *Amer. J. Physiol.*, 127, 131 (1939).

13. Schwarzacher, H. von, *Acta Anat.*, 21, 26 (1954).

14. Friede, R. L., and Samorjski, T., *J. Comp. Neurol.*, 130, 223 (1967).

15. Bishop, G. H., Clare, M. H., and Landau, W. M., *Intern. J. Neurosci.*, 2, 69 (1971).

16. Schnepp, P., and Schnepp, G., *Z. Zellforsch.*, 119, 99 (1971).

17. Waxman, S. G., and Bennett, M. V. L., *J. Cell Biol.*, 47, 22A (1970).

18. Tasaki, I., and Freygang, jun., W. H., *J. Gen. Physiol.*, 39, 211 (1955).

19. Katz, B., and Miledi, R., *Proc. Roy. Soc.*, B, 161, 453 (1965).

20. Paintal, A. S., *J. Physiol.*, 184, 791 (1966).

21. Coppin, C. M. L., and Jack, J. J. B., *J. Physiol.*, 222, 91P (1972).

22. Hille, B., *Progr. Biophys. Mol. Biol.*, 21, 1 (1970).

23. Waxman, S. G., *Nature*, 227, 283 (1970).

24. Bennett, M. V. L., in *The Central Nervous System and Fish Behavior* (edit. by Ingle, D. J.), 147 (University of Chicago Press, Chicago, 1968).

25. Waxman, S. G., *Brain Res.*, 27, 189 (1971).

II THE BAUHAUS IN THE BRAIN

The brain and spinal cord, like many other complex systems, operate within a world of principles and rules. One rule has to do with efficiency: efficiency is good, so be efficient. Another rule has to do with simplicity: a machine with a lot of moving parts is more likely to break than a machine with few moving parts—hence, Keep It Simple. A third rule mandates elegance of design: in this context, elegance means that an engineer, analyzing the system, would say, "I wish I had thought of that." Natural selection, operating over millions of years, seems to have incorporated these rules into the design of the brain and spinal cord.

Waxman, Pappas, and Bennett (1972) describes a piece of the nervous system, in a "lower" species, which exemplifies efficiency, simplicity, and elegance. *Sternarchus*[1] is an eel from the gymnotid family, which lives in the muddy waters of the Amazon delta. It spends its time foraging for food, mostly near the river floor or in the poorly lit crevasses between rocks. Like "cave fish," *Sternarchus* has a poorly developed sense of sight. It has, however, another sensory system that makes up for its poor vision.

Sternarchus is an "electric fish," but unlike its cousin, the electric eel, *Sternarchus* does not use electricity to stun prey. Rather, it uses electricity to navigate. *Sternarchus* possesses an *electromotor* system, which generates a small electric field in its vicinity. The field consists of tiny electric waves (which first make the electric field that surrounds *Sternarchus* positive near its head and negative toward its tail, then reversing so that the head is negative and tail positive). *Sternarchus* "listens" to the humming of the electricity that it produces, with an *electrosensory* system consisting of specialized electroreceptor cells located along the length of its body. The electroreceptors sense the oscillations of the electric field and report on them to the brain. When an external object (such as a rock or predator) is present within the electric field generated by *Sternarchus*, the object distorts the oscillations; the electrosensory cells, being finely tuned to respond to the electric field and its oscillations, detect the distortion and report to the brain. Thus, even in the absence of visual information, *Sternarchus* "knows" when something approaches it.

Most electric fish use modified muscle cells to generate electricity in their electric organs (Bennett 1971). This is the case in the electric eel, which possesses an "electric organ" that is made up of modified muscle cells. These "myogenic" (muscle-derived) electrocytes (electricity-generating cells) in the electric eel are lined up in stacks, like rolls of coins, and this architecture permits the electric fields produced by the individual electrocytes to summate, adding up in the aggregate to a large shock. In the electric eel, of course, the electric organ is used only intermittently, when there is a need to disable its prey.

Sternarchus, in contrast to the electric eel, does not need a large electrical field, but it does need ongoing information about its environment, and it therefore must produce its head-positive, then head-negative electric field constantly. The need to generate these high-frequency electrical discharges, throughout its life, poses an important design problem for *Sternarchus*: how can it do so, most reliably and efficiently, with the least metabolic cost? Waxman, Pappas, and Bennett (1972) is an analysis that demonstrates that *Sternarchus* accomplishes this by utilizing some of the nerve cells in its spinal cord in an ingenious way. Its electric organ is not made up of muscle cells. Natural selection appears to have resulted in elimination of the muscle cell in the electromotor system of *Sternarchus* without compromising its function. In the electric eel, nerve fibers project from the spinal cord to the myogenic electric organ, sending it a command to fire. *Sternarchus* saves a synapse by using these nerve fibers, instead of the target muscle cells, to generate its discharge. The electric organ of *Sternarchus* thus consists of specialized nerve fibers which, unlike most conventional nerve fibers, are not designed to

---

1. In some recent textbooks and papers, *Sternarchus* is referred to as *Apteronotus*.

carry information from one nerve cell to another, or to a target cell such as a muscle cell. Nerve cells within the spinal cord have become modified and give rise to these specialized nerve fibers which have taken over the responsibility for generating the electrical fields that, in the aggregate, constitute *Sternarchus'* electric discharge.

The electrocyte nerve fibers in *Sternarchus* have a remarkable structure which reflects their unique role. The axons making up these fibers, and the surrounding Schwann cells, embrace each other in a stereotyped pattern not seen in other nervous systems, and ideally designed for the generation of these electrical fields. Certain parts of the axons, which actively generate nerve impulses, are covered with myelin insulation in a normal fashion and contain sodium channels which function as molecular batteries, while other areas, which do not actively produce impulses, are naked and lack sodium channels. The membranes of these nerve fibers in these naked areas, where there is an increased surface area, are folded and ruffled so that they can act as electrical capacitors, passively storing electrical charge for the next oscillation. Adding to the design of the nerve fibers making up *Sternarchus'* electric organ, these fibers run complex courses, first traveling headward as they exit from the spinal cord, then making a hairpin loop and traveling toward the tail before they end blindly; this complex course provides a basis for the head-positive, head-negative aspect of *Sternarchus'* electric discharge.

Living organisms, and the cell systems that comprise them, provide many examples of elegant design, but there is probably no part of the body that provides as many examples as the nervous system. The *Sternarchus* electromotor system, which I studied early in my career, provides a graphic example of this: *Sternarchus* navigates effectively in its dark and muddy environment, even in the absence of visual cues, using its ingeniously designed electrocytes. By virtue of its clever design, the electric organ of *Sternarchus* utilizes modified nerve cells and their nerve fibers and operates with one less cell, and one less synapse, than its counterpart in the electric eel. It is efficient, simple, and elegant. Even "lower" species can design and use their nervous systems wisely.

References

Bennett, M. V. L. Electric organs. In J. S. Hoar and D. J. Randall (eds.), *Fish Physiology*, Vol. 5, Academic Press, New York, pp. 347–491, 1971.

Waxman, S. G., Pappas, G. D., and Bennett, M. V. L. Morphological correlates of functional differentiation of nodes of Ranvier along single fibers in the neurogenic electric organ of the knife fish *Sternarchus*. *J. Cell Biol.* 53: 210–224, 1972.

2 Morphological Correlates of Functional Differentiation of Nodes of Ranvier along Single Fibers in the Neurogenic Electric Organ of the Knife Fish *Sternarchus*

S. G. Waxman, G. D. Pappas, and M. V. L. Bennett

Abstract Electric organs in Sternarchidae are of neural origin, in contrast to electric organs in other fish, which are derived from muscle. The electric organ in *Sternarchus* is composed of modified axons of spinal neurons. Fibers comprising the electric organ were studied by dissection and by light- and electron microscopy of sectioned material. The spinal electrocytes descend to the electric organ where they run anteriorly for several segments, turn sharply, and run posteriorly to end blindly at approximately the level where they enter the organ. At the level of entry into the organ, and where they turn around, the axons are about 20 μ in diameter; the nodes of Ranvier have a typical appearance with a gap of approximately 1 μ in the myelin. Anteriorly and posteriorly running parts of the fibers dilate to a diameter of approximately 100 μ, and then taper again. In proximal and central regions of anteriorly and posteriorly running parts, nodal gaps measure approximately 1 μ along the axon. In distal regions of anteriorly and posteriorly running parts are three to five large nodes with gaps measuring more than 50 μ along the fiber axis. Nodes with narrow and with wide gaps are distinguishable ultrastructurally; the first type has a typical structure, whereas the second type represents a new nodal morphology. At the typical nodes a dense cytoplasmic material is associated with the axon membrane. At large nodes, the unmyelinated axon membrane is elaborated to form a closely packed layer of irregular polypoid processes without a dense cytoplasmic undercoating. Electrophysiological data indicate that typical nodes in proximal regions of anteriorly and posteriorly running segments actively generate spikes, whereas large distal nodes are inactive and act as a series capacity. Increased membrane surface area provides a morphological correlate for this capacity. This electric organ comprises a unique neural system in which axons have evolved so as to generate external signals, an adaptation involving a functionally significant structural differentiation of nodes of Ranvier along single nerve fibers.

Reprinted with permission from *The Journal of Cell Biology* 53: 210–224, 1972.

Introduction

In the Sternarchidae, a South American family of weakly electric gymnotids or knife fish, the electric organs are derived from peripheral nerve. This neurogenic origin contrasts with that of other electric organs, which are derived from muscle. Comparison to other gymnotids suggests that a myogenic electric organ was originally present, but that its function was taken over by its motor nerves in the course of evolution (Bennett, 1971a). In this respect it is interesting that the sternarchids discharge at frequencies much higher than do other electric fish, the rate varying from 700 to at least 1500 per second. The evidence for neural origin is based on light microscope examination of sections and dissection of the organ (Couceiro et al., 1955; de Oliveira Castro, 1955; Bennett, 1966, 1970, 1971a). Single axons can be followed from the spinal cord into the organ, and are seen to comprise the entire organ, except for connective tissue and blood vessels (Bennett, 1971a). Furthermore, curare, which blocks neuromuscular transmission and transmission from nerve to electrocyte in all other electric fish, has no effect on sternarchid organ discharge although it does block neuromuscular transmission in this group (Bennett, 1966, 1970, 1971a).

Light microscope examination reveals characteristic changes in the nodes of Ranvier along the nerve fibers in this electric organ. We describe here two classes of nodes on the basis of differences in fine structure; one of these classes represents a new nodal morphology. The morphological differentiation of nodes is consistent with physiological data indicating functional differences along the fibers.

Materials and Methods

Whole Fibers

For examination of single dissected fibers, fish were perfused through the conus arteriosus with a 2.5% solution of glutaraldehyde in Sorensen's phosphate buffer at pH 7.3. After perfusion, the electric organ was exposed or dissected out, and left in a 1% solution of OsO_4 in phosphate buffer for 10–25 min. Single fibers were isolated with watchmaker's forceps. They were mounted in distilled water on glass slides under cover slips, where they were examined and photographed with conventional bright-field optics. Some fibers were stained with dilute solutions of toluidine blue (0.1–0.5% in 0.5% borax), which preferentially stains nodes of Ranvier (Hess and Young, 1952).

Sectioned Material for Light and Electron Microscopy

Two fixation procedures yielded generally similar results: (a) topical application of 1% OsO_4 in Millonig's buffer (pH 7.3) to the exposed electric organ, which was removed and left in this fixative for a total of 1 hr; (b) perfusion through the conus arteriosus with 2.5% glutaraldehyde in Sorensen's buffer (pH 7.3) for 15 min, followed by removal of the organ and immersion in this solution for a total of 2 hr, washing for 12 hr in fresh buffer, and postfixation in 1% OsO_4 in Sorensen's buffer for 45 min to 1 hr. All tissue was dehydrated in graded ethanol solutions and embedded in Epon 812. The pieces of electric organ removed for study included short lengths of the efferent spinal nerves, and they were embedded so that sections could be cut along all three major axes. The efferent nerves from some segments were embedded separately. Thick sections (1 μ) for light microscopy were cut from all blocks on Porter-Blum MT-2 and LKB ultramicrotomes and were stained with 1% toluidine

blue in 0.5% borax. Thin sections for electron microscopy were cut with glass and diamond knives, and were stained with lead citrate for 2–5 min, followed by 20% uranyl acetate in absolute methanol for 10–15 min. These sections were examined and photographed with a Philips 200 electron microscope operating at 60 kv.

Results

The electric organ consists of paired midline structures, located ventral to, and running parallel with, the spinal cord from the small caudal fin to just behind the head (figure 2.1). In the abdominal region, the organs lie separated just medial to the rib cage. Caudal to the abdominal cavity, the medial surfaces of the two halves of the electric organ are closely apposed, separated only by a thin connective tissue septum, ventral spinous processes, and segmental nerves running to ventral muscles and skin. The organs are covered by a connective tissue sheath and are distinctly separate from the neighboring muscle, which lies dorsally, ventrally, and laterally.

Isolated Fibers

The cell bodies of the electrocytes are located in the spinal cord. Axons descend vertically from the cord to the electric organ, where they run anteriorly for several segments (5–10 mm in a fish 15 cm long). They then turn sharply around, and run posteriorly to end blindly at about the same level at which they entered the organ or somewhat anteriorly (figure 2.1; Bennett, 1971a). The morphology of the fibers changes characteristically along their course in the organ, as may be seen from the single dissected fiber shown in figure 2.2. At the level of entry into the organ from the spinal cord, the axon is about 20 μ in diameter, and the nodes of Ranvier have the appearance of nodes normally observed in peripheral nerve. The gap in the myelin appears about

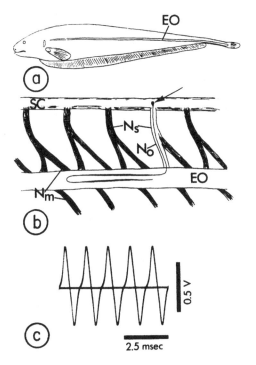

Figure 2.1
Anatomy and discharge of the *Sternarchus* electric organ. (*a*) Position of the organ (*EO*) in the fish. (*b*) Diagram of the spinal cord (*SC*) and electric organ. The ventral branch of the segmental spinal nerve (N_s) sends a branch to the organ (N_o) and a mixed sensory and motor branch (N_m) to more ventral structures. A single electrocyte is shown, with its cell body in the spinal cord (arrow) and its axon running into the organ. (*c*) Electric organ discharge of *Sternarchus*, recorded differentially between head and tail. The high frequency discharge is diphasic, consisting of a head-positive phase followed by a head-negative phase (head positivity upward). The horizontal line represents the zero level, and there is little or no DC component in the discharge. This recording was made after curarization of the fish, which had no effect on the discharge.

1 μ long, and the axon is slightly constricted at the node (figure 2.2*a*). The distance between nodes is 150–200 μ. As the fiber runs anteriorly, it becomes dilated to 100 μ or more in diameter, and then tapers again to 10–20 μ where the fiber turns around. In the proximal, expanding region and in the central region of the anteriorly running portion, the gap at the nodes is narrow (figure 2.2*b*). Internode distances increase to 400–500 μ in the thickest part of the fiber. In the distal tapering region (figures 2.2*c*, 2.4), there are three to five nodes that are long, up to 50 μ or more measured along the axis of the fiber. The axons do not appear constricted at these large nodes. The nodes become normal again where the fiber becomes thin (less than 20 μ in diameter) and turns around. The sequence is repeated in the caudally running segment of the fiber. Anteriorly the axon is about 20 μ in diameter, with nodes about 1 μ long (figure 2.2*d*). As the fiber continues to run caudally, it expands to a diameter of about 100 μ, and the nodes remain narrow. In the most caudal region, the nodes are very large (figures 2.2*f*, 2.3) and the fiber tapers and ends blindly. A thin connective tissue strand runs somewhat farther (figure 2.5) and often ends in the sheath of the organ. Oval creaselike depressions in the myelin, with their long axes parallel to the axis of the fiber, are present in the paranodal regions at all of the nodal types described above. A fibrous sheath can be seen surrounding the axon at nodes (figure 2.4) and in internodal areas.

Visualization of large nodes in dissected fibers is enhanced by staining with dilute solutions of toluidine blue (cf. Hess and Young, 1952). Over a period of 5–10 min, the axon at the node becomes deeply stained, in contrast to myelinated regions, which take up the stain only faintly. In these preparations, nodes stand out as dense transverse bands around the axon. Figure 2.3 shows part of a fiber before and after staining with toluidine blue (see also figure 2.5).

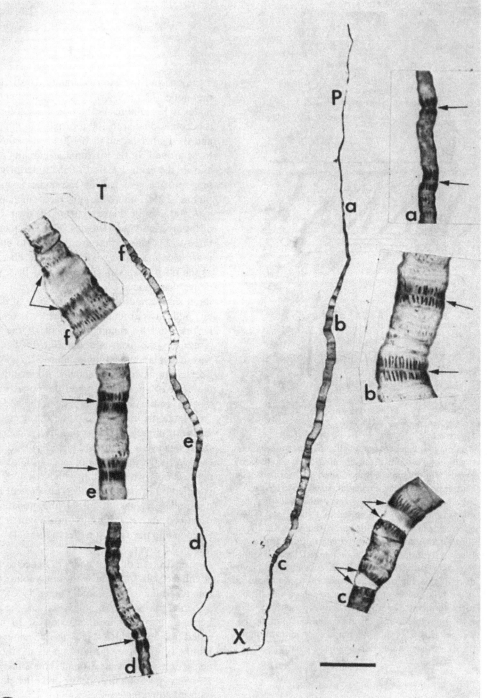

Sectioned Material

Examination of sectioned material of *Sternarchus* electric organ with the light- and electron microscopes reveals that the nodes fall into two classes corresponding to the two types of nodes seen in isolated fibers. The first, those with narrow gaps, resemble typical nodes of peripheral nerve. The second, those with large gaps, exhibit a distinctive morphology involving a great elaboration of the nodal surface.

Nodes with Narrow Gaps   The first type of node is found in both small diameter and dilated regions of the fibers. Fibers entering the organ were identified from their small diameter (*circa* 20 μ), orientation, and medial position with respect to the organ (figure 2.6*a*). They were also examined in isolated efferent nerves. Similar fibers are also present in sections through the body of the organ. Some of these fibers are oriented at approximately right angles to the large longitudinally running fibers, which indicates that they are fibers which have become thin and are turning around (figure 2.6*b*). Where the fibers enter the organ and where they turn around, light micrographs show the nodes as gaps of about 1 μ in the myelin, associated with constriction of the axon (figures 2.6*a*, *b*). The myelin in these regions is about 1 μ thick, which is somewhat greater than elsewhere along the fiber. The longitudinally oriented depressions in the myelin seen in isolated fibers near nodes frequently appear in section as deep indentations or isolated ovals.

In both regions where the fibers are of small diameter, electron micrographs show the nodes as abrupt interruptions in the myelin sheath (figure 2.7). The paranodal region (the region in which the myelin lamellae terminate) usually extends for less than 3 μ along the axis of the fiber on either side of the node. The paranodal Schwann cell cytoplasm contains mitochondria and microtubules which run circumferentially around the axon (cf. figure 2.8, inset). The axon is usually constricted slightly at the node. Stacked desmosomes are sometimes present (cf. Harkin, 1964). The axon membrane is in direct contact with the extracellular space at these nodes. The gap in the myelin at the node measures about 0.5 μ along the length of the fiber, but the extracellular channel is somewhat narrower because it is lined with the outermost layer of paranodal Schwann cytoplasm (figure 2.7, arrow). Small microvillous processes may be present within the extracellular channel, and in some sections these can be seen to originate from the Schwann cell (cf. Robertson, 1959; Elfvin, 1961). The axon membrane at the node has an irregular contour and occasionally bulges outward. Associated with the axon membrane at the node is a dense layer of cytoplasmic undercoating less than 300 A wide (figure 2.7, inset; cf. Elfvin, 1961; Peters, 1966). Elements of a tubular reticulum and some vesicles are usually present in the nodal axoplasm. A basement lamina of inter-

Figure 2.2
Photomontage of a single fiber from the electric organ of *Sternarchus*, isolated under a dissecting microscope and mounted under a cover slip. The most proximal part of the fiber, near its site of entry into the organ, is marked *P*. The anteriorly running portion extends from *P* to *X*, where the fiber turns around. The posteriorly running portion extends from *X* to *T*, where the fiber terminates. Nodal morphology changes characteristically along the course of the fiber. Nodes from different parts of the fiber are enlarged in the insets; in each case, the nodal gap in the myelin is indicated by arrows. In the thin regions near the site of entry into the organ (*a*) and near the point at which the fiber turns around (*d*) the nodal gap is small. Nodes exhibit a similarly small gap in the proximal and central part of the dilated anteriorly running segment (*b*) and in the proximal and central part of the dilated posteriorly running segment (*e*). Distal nodes of the anteriorly running segment (*c*) and distal nodes in the posteriorly running segment (*f*) are large. The fiber ends in a tapering, apparently collagenous filament (*T*). The bar represents 1 mm for the fiber and 150 μ for the insets. ×15; insets, ×100.

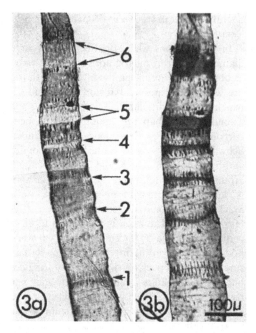

Figure 2.3
Effect of staining on nodes of Ranvier in an isolated fiber from *Sternarchus* electric organ. (*a*) shows the distal region of the posteriorly running part of an unstained dissected fiber. The morphology of the nodes changes in a characteristic manner. The most proximal node (*1*) measures about 1 μ along the axis of the fiber. Gaps in the myelin at the node appear as light areas. The nodes increase in size (*2–6*) along the course of the fiber, the largest nodes (*5, 6*) being located in the most distal portion (at the upper part of the figure). (*b*) shows the same region from the same fiber, after staining with 0.25% toluidine blue for 5 min. The nodes appear as densely stained transverse bands on the fiber; internodal regions stain only lightly. The fiber was rotated and flattened somewhat during the staining procedure, so that it appears to have a slightly increased diameter. ×100.

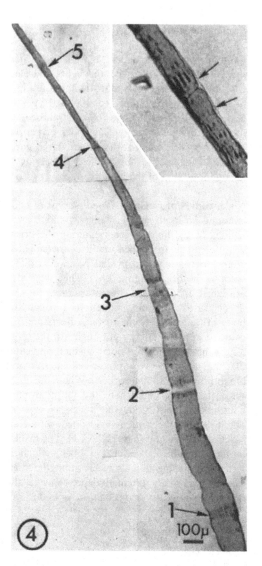

Figure 2.4
The distal part of the anteriorly running segment of an isolated fiber from *Sternarchus* electric organ. Five nodes of Ranvier are present (*1–5*). Node *1* has a narrow gap; nodes *2–4* are large; node *5*, from the region where the fiber becomes thin and turns around, is narrow. Node *5* is enlarged in the inset. The connective tissue sheath surrounding the fiber can be seen over the node and adjacent myelinated regions (arrows). Photomontage, ×55; inset, ×175.

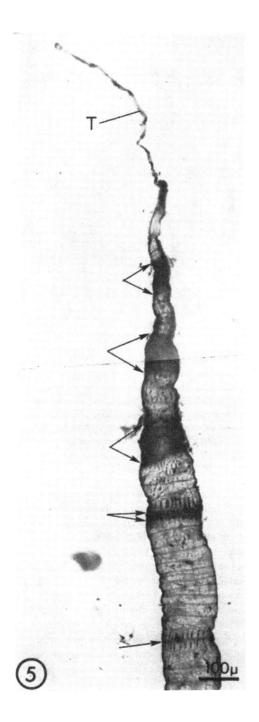

mediate density extends over the nodal gap. Collagen fibers and occasionally fibroblasts are located outside the basement lamina.

Both light- and electron micrographs show the nodes with narrow gaps in dilated portions of the axons to be of similar morphology to the other narrow nodes (figure 2.6c, figure 2.8). The narrow nodes in dilated regions must include ones from both anteriorly and posteriorly running segments of the fibers, as they comprise a single class found in all parts of the organ. The myelin is usually about 0.5 µ thick, somewhat thinner than in the small diameter regions of the fibers. Constriction of the axon at the narrow nodes is more marked in dilated parts of the fibers, and the myelin can give the appearance of abruptly indenting the axon in the paranodal region. Indentations or ovals from sectioning of the longitudinal depressions in the paranodal myelin are a common feature. As at the nodes in small diameter regions, a distinct channel from the axon membrane to the extracellular space is always present (figure 2.8, arrow).

Nodes with Large Gaps and Surface Elaborations A second type of node is present in sections of dilated regions of the fibers; these correspond to the large nodes seen in isolated fibers. Again, the distribution indicates that these nodes are from both anteriorly and posteriorly running segments of the fibers. In light micrographs the axonal surface exhibits a thick layer of denser staining with poorly defined striations perpendicular to the axis of the fiber (figure 2.6d). In electron micrographs this layer is

Figure 2.5
Photomontage of the terminal part of an isolated fiber from *Sternarchus* electric organ. This preparation has been stained with toluidine blue. The most proximal node (bottom arrow) is narrow. Subsequent nodes (double arrows) are enlarged, measuring from 20 µ to about 100 µ along the axis of the fiber. The fiber tapers and ends in an extension of its connective tissue sheath (*T*). ×100.

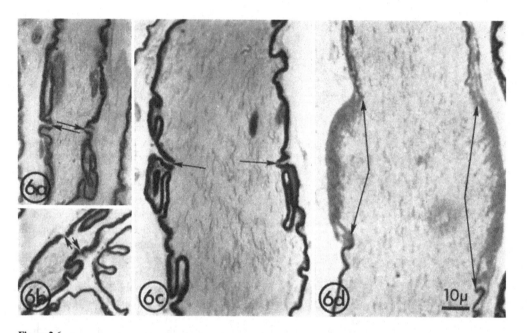

Figure 2.6
Light micrographs of thick (1 μ) sections through several types of nodes of Ranvier in *Sternarchus* electric organ. All figures show the nodes in longitudinal section. (*a*) A fiber at its site of entry into the electric organ. The nodal gap in the myelin extends for about 1 μ (arrows). (*b*) Part of a thin fiber within the body of the organ. Because the fiber runs perpendicular to the other fibers in the organ, one can conclude that the section is from the region in which the fiber narrows and turns around. The arrows indicate the nodal gap. (*c*) A typical node with a narrow gap in a dilated part of the fiber (arrow). Note the folds in the paranodal myelin. (*d*) A large node, with an unmyelinated region extending for more than 40 μ, as indicated by the arrows. The surface region of the axon at the node is diffusely stained, with a suggestion of a striated appearance. ×700.

revealed as a striking proliferation of the axon membrane, which is elaborated to form a large number of irregular polypoid processes over the entire unmyelinated nodal surface (figures 2.9, 2.10). In cross-section these processes are roughly circular in outline and between 800 A and 5000 A in diameter. Examination of serial sections indicates that each process is in continuity with the axon. Although the protrusions themselves run irregular courses, they are separated from each other by narrow regions of extracellular space, and form a discrete layer, usually less than 5 μ thick. Parts of the outer layer of axonal processes are covered by a basement lamina, and some of this material extends into the spaces between the processes. Fibroblasts and collagen fibers in turn surround the outer margin of the basement lamina.

The myelin is thinner near the large nodes than in other regions of the fiber. The paranodal regions can extend relatively great distances, at least as far as 40 μ (figure 2.9). A further specialization at these nodes is the increased frequency with which mitochondria are present in the axoplasm immediately subjacent to the nodal elaborations. The core of the axon at the

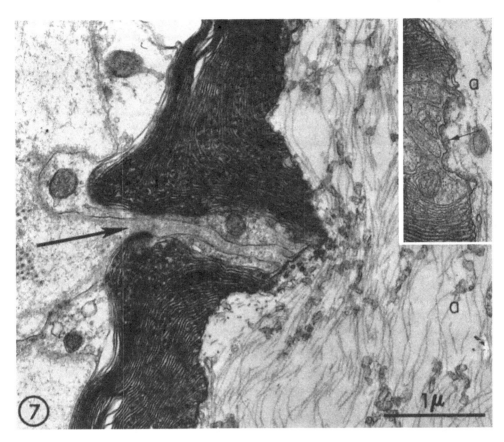

Figure 2.7
Electron micrograph of a section through a node of Ranvier, from a 15 μ diameter fiber in the efferent nerve to the electric organ. In this and all subsequent micrographs, the axis of the fiber runs vertically from top to bottom of the page. The axoplasm (*a*) contains neurofilaments, vesicles, and elements of a tubular reticulum. Associated with the axon surface at the node is a dense cytoplasmic layer about 200 A thick. A distinct extracellular channel, less than 0.5 μ wide, runs to the axon membrane (arrow). The inset shows the axon membrane at a node from a larger fiber within the electric organ. Note the dense cytoplasmic undercoating associated with the axon membrane at the node (arrow) Glutaraldehyde-OsO₄, ×27,000; inset, ×42,000.

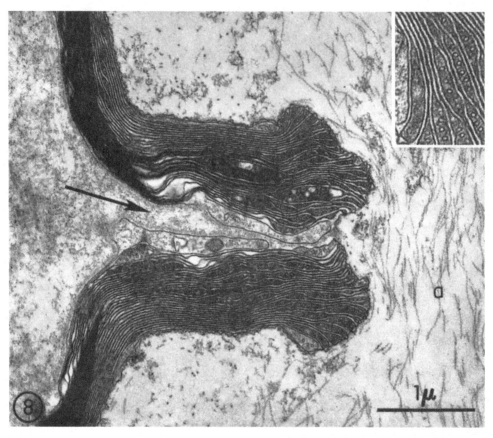

Figure 2.8
Electron micrograph of a section through a node of Ranvier from a dilated (60 μ) part of a fiber within the electric organ. The axoplasm at this node (*a*) contains neurofilaments oriented parallel to the axis of the fiber. Microtubules within the paranodal Schwann cell cytoplasm (enlarged in inset) run circumferentially around the axon. The arrow indicates the extracellular gap at the node. Glutaraldehyde-OsO$_4$, ×27,000; inset, ×52,000.

node contains numerous longitudinally oriented neurofilaments, mitochondria with a similar orientation, and elements of a tubular reticulum. This reticulum is more prominent in nodal than in internodal axoplasm. Occasional clear membrane-bounded vesicles, 400–800 A in diameter, are also present in the nodal axoplasm. While mitochondria within the core of the axon are oriented parallel to the axis of the fiber, mitochondria subjacent to the nodal surface have no simple orientation. The irregular axonal processes contain electron-lucent cytoplasm. Rarely, the profiles of small mitochondria or multivesticular bodies are present within the axonal processes. The dense cytoplasmic material associated with the axon membrane at narrow nodes is not present at the enlarged nodes after fixation with either osmium tetroxide or glutaraldehyde, although its presence can be demonstrated in the same specimens at the nodes with narrow gaps.

Discussion

The present study demonstrates a structural variation in nodes of Ranvier along single fibers from *Sternarchus* electric organ. Two types of nodes may be distinguished on the basis of fine structure; one of these represents a new nodal morphology. The structural differentiation of nodes is consistent with physiological differences that will be described below.

The fibers described in this report comprise a neurogenic electric organ. The fine structural studies confirm and extend earlier light microscope data indicating that the fibers are modified axons which end blindly (Bennett, 1970, 1971a). Although we have not studied the morphology of the blind endings in a definitive manner, we have encountered, in studies of sections through the organ, processes which appear to be the terminations of these fibers. We have also seen bundles of collagen fibers that apparently represent the connective tissue strands extending beyond the blind tips of the axons (figures 2.2, 2.5). The structure of these unique nerve endings will be the subject of a future report.

As in other electric fish, the electric signal from *Sternarchus* represents the summated activity of many electrocytes which discharge synchronously. The discharge in *Sternarchus* consists of diphasic pulses (initially head-positive). Physiological data indicate that impulses propagate to involve both anteriorly and posteriorly running segments of the axons, the first generating the head-positive phase and the second generating the head-negative phase of the discharge (Bennett, 1971a).

The conclusions from microelectrode studies are summarized in figure 2.11a. Intracellular recordings are diagrammed in the center column as they would be obtained at the sites indicated in the diagram of the electrocyte on the left. The directions of current flow during the two successive phases are indicated for the electrocyte drawn on the right, the light areas of which represent nodes of Ranvier. A single cycle of externally recorded organ discharge is shown in the uppermost trace of the center column. During the head-positive phase the narrow nodes at the posterior of the anteriorly running segment become active, and pass inward current. Large nodes at the anterior of this segment are inexcitable and pass only outward current (arrows on left part of the right diagram). During this phase a large action potential is recorded in the proximal region of the anteriorly running segment and the potential becomes markedly smaller and somewhat delayed more anteriorly. Thus, during this phase current runs anteriorly through the core of this segment of the electrocyte and from head to tail in the external circuit, thereby generating head positivity. The reduced spike at the anterior end of the anteriorly running segment is able to excite ordinary narrow nodes in this region and the impulse propagates around to invade the posteriorly running segment of the fiber. The head-negative phase is then generated in the same manner as the head-positive phase. Active

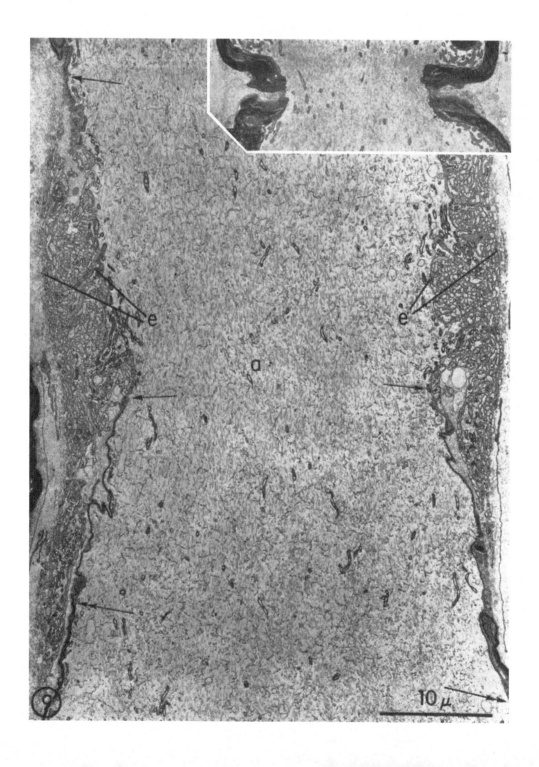

narrow nodes at the anterior of the posteriorly running segment pass inward current and the inexcitable large nodes at the posterior pass outward current. The action potential is large at the proximal end of the posteriorly running segment and decrements markedly in reaching the distal end. Current flows caudally in the fiber core and from tail to head in the external medium to generate the head-negative phase. (During each phase some "external" current flows back through the segment which is inactive during that phase; the external potentials are small enough that these currents have no effect on organ function and they constitute only a small fraction of the total current.)

As would be expected the space constant is quite large in the dilated regions of the fibers, which must increase the generation of external fields. It is not clear whether narrow nodes in the dilated regions become active. The reduction in spike amplitude moving distally along each segment could represent loading by the large area of the inexcitable nodes as well as decrement in passive propagation from active nodes restricted to the proximal regions. In the earlier light microscope studies, it appeared that nodes in the proximal portion of the anteriorly running and posteriorly running segments were somewhat larger (Bennett, 1971a). Although there may be some differentiation of nodal regions in these parts of the fibers, gap width is not markedly greater. Gap width varies somewhat at single nodes and it is still possible that there is a modest difference in area at these nodes. However, narrow nodes in the large diameter regions certainly have a considerably greater area than narrow nodes in small diameter regions.

A number of data indicate that the inactive large nodes act as a series capacity. The evidence is essentially that there is no net current flow averaged over a single discharge cycle. How a series capacity prevents net current flow may be understood with reference to the equivalent circuit in figure 2.11b. During the initial part of an action potential current enters the fiber at active nodes, flows axially along the axon, leaves the fiber through the series capacity, and returns through the low resistance of the external medium across which the external potential is recorded. During this period the charge on the series capacity becomes more positive. At some point on the falling phase of the action potential, the charge on the capacity exceeds the potential generated by the active membrane and current begins to flow in the opposite direction. During firing at a steady frequency the capacity cannot continue to accumulate or lose net charge. Thus, in the steady state the integrated current flows during head-positive and head-negative phases of a discharge must be equal, and when the potential recorded across the external resistance is averaged over a complete discharge cycle, the result is zero (figure 2.1).

A diphasic discharge without net current flow can also result from two successive monophasic discharges that are oppositely oriented. In this mechanism each phase is generated as in figure 2.11 except that one surface of the electrocyte behaves as a series resistance instead of a series capacity. It was initially thought that this mechanism might be found in *Sternarchus*, anteriorly and posteriorly running segments generating the two phases. However, when propagation between the two segments is blocked by anoxia, the

Figure 2.9
Electron micrograph of a large node with surface elaborations. Numerous polypoid processes from the axon surface (*a*) form a layer about 5 μ thick around the unmyelinated region at the node (*e*). The terminations of the myelin sheath are indicated by arrows. The paranodal region (in which the myelin terminates layer by layer) extends to the double-headed arrows. The unmyelinated area extends for approximately 30 μ along the axis of the fiber. The inset shows, for comparison, a node of Ranvier from a fiber near its site of entry into the organ, at the same magnification. The gap in the myelin measures less than 1 μ along the axis of the fiber. OsO₄; ×3000.

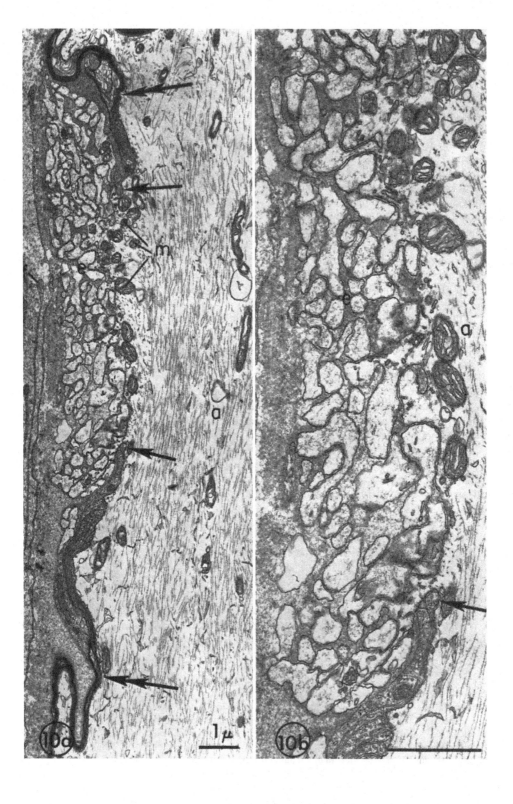

m

e

a

1 μ

10a

e

a

10b

discharge still exhibits no net current flow, and thus the output of each segment must exhibit no net current flow. Furthermore, in other sternarchid species in which the anteriorly running segments of the electrocytes are reduced or absent, the active head-negative phase of the discharge is reduced or absent, but there is still no net current flow (Bennett, 1971*a*).

The proposal that one surface of the electrocytes acts as a series capacity is supported by data from the African electric fish *Gymnarchus* (Bennett, 1971*a*). This species has myogenic electrocytes which are more accessible for microelectrode studies, and one surface of the cell has been directly shown to act as a series capacity.

The large nodes located in the distal parts of the dilated anteriorly running and posteriorly running segments have an extraordinarily large surface. The large area provided by the diameter and length of the unmyelinated region at the node (which can exceed 50 µ along the axis of the fiber) is markedly augmented by the polypoid elaborations of the axon membrane. This extensive area provides a morphological basis for the series capacity indicated by physiological and comparative data. On the reasonable assumption that the capacity per unit area of this membrane is similar to that of other cell membranes (1 µF/cm^2; cf. Bennett, 1970, 1971*a*), the capacity of these nodes is greatly increased. For them to act as a series capacity, it is necessary that the membrane time constant be long compared to the duration of the action potential. This

requires the membrane resistivity to be high compared to that of ordinary nodes of Ranvier (but not necessarily higher than that of many other membranes). This requirement is not contradicted by the morphological data.

Membranes acting as a series capacity occur in receptor cells of certain electroreceptors and in at least the one electrocyte noted above (Bennett, 1970, 1971*a*, 1971*b*). In both electrocytes (Schwartz, 1968; Schwartz and Pappas, 1968) and receptor cells (cf. Bennett, 1971*b*), the membranes are greatly elaborated as in the *Sternarchus* electrocytes. In fine structural studies of eight different teleost electric organs derived from muscle, it was found that membrane invaginations increased the surface area of all electrocytes, but that the increase in surface area was most marked for electrically inexcitable regions of the cells, those which have a low resistivity and act as a series resistance as well as those which have a high resistivity and act as a series capacity (Schwartz, 1968; Schwartz and Pappas, 1968). Similar findings apply to membranes acting as a series resistance in strongly electric organs (cf. Bennett, 1971*a*). The morphological techniques available do not yet distinguish between membranes of high and low resistivity.

The role of nodes of Ranvier in saltatory conduction is firmly established. Rushton (1951) has argued that myelinated fibers of ordinary peripheral nerve are "designed" so as to maximize conduction velocity for fibers of any given diameter. However, it is probable that the functions of some nerve fibers require different

Figure 2.10

(*a*) The gap in the myelin at an elaborated node. The axis of the fiber runs vertically, from top to bottom of the page. The paranodal region begins at the double-headed arrows, and the nodal bare area extends between the single-headed arrows. The axon surface is elaborated to form a layer of irregular processes (*e*). The axon (*a*) contains numerous neurofilaments, as well as mitochondria (*m*) which are especially common subjacent to the surface elaborations. Attenuated processes of fibroblasts (*f*) surround the network of processes at the node. The bar indicates 1 µ. Glutaraldehyde-OsO$_4$; ×12,000. (*b*) Part of the node shown in (*a*), at the same magnification as figs. 2.7 and 2.8. The polypoid processes contain electron-lucent cytoplasm with few organelles. There is no dense undercoating of the axon (*a*) membranes in this region. ×27,000.

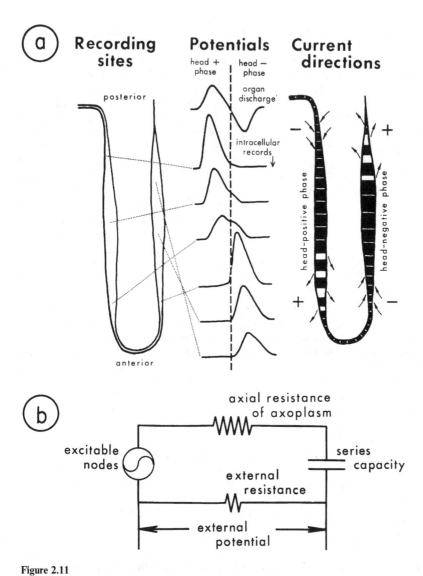

Figure 2.11

Electrocyte function during organ discharge. (*a*) Diagrams of intracellular potentials and directions of current flow during electrocyte activity generating the head-positive and head-negative phases of organ discharge. The central column represents organ discharge on the upper line and intracellular recordings on the lower lines at the sites indicated in the diagram of an electrocyte on the left. The directions of current flow during the two phases are indicated on the right diagram. (Modified from Bennett, 1971 *a*). (*b*) Equivalent circuit of an electrocyte segment to illustrate the effect of a series capacity.

characteristics. Morphological studies of neuropil from the teleost (Waxman, 1970; Waxman and Bennett, 1970) and mammalian central nervous system (Waxman and Melker, 1971) have demonstrated that the pattern of myelination of preterminal fibers differs from the pattern in peripheral nerve, in that the nodes of Ranvier are closely spaced. Nodal surface area in preterminal fibers may also be somewhat increased, and it has been suggested that variations in patterns of myelination and nodal structure could modulate spatiotemporal patterning of impulses (Waxman, 1971). There is evidence that at some nodes, conduction is blocked at specific frequencies (Wall et al., 1956) and there are some physiological data which suggest that more complex filtering of spike trains occurs at regions of low safety factor, i.e., nodes or branch points (Chung et al., 1970). Axons act as delay lines for synchronization of firing of the electric organ in the electric eel (Bennett, 1971*a*); in this case the fibers are not myelinated in the manner required for maximal conduction velocity in that the ratios of myelin thickness and internode distance to fiber diameter are too small (Meszler and Bennett, 1972). These ratios of myelin thickness and internode distance to fiber diameter are also considerably smaller along the *Sternarchus* electrocytes than previously reported for most nerves, including teleost lateral line nerves (Thomas and Young, 1949). The function of the electrocytes is quite different from that of ordinary nerve fibers, and apparently does not require maximization of conduction velocity.

The *Sternarchus* electric organ provides an example of a unique neural system in which myelinated nerve fibers act so as to transform action potentials into diphasic external signals, and in which nodes of Ranvier are structurally differentiated in a manner referable to physiological specializations. It also presents interesting problems in developmental neurobiology, particularly with respect to the relations between neurons and glia and the specificity of regional differentiation of the axonal surface.

Acknowledgments

This work was supported in part by grants from the United States Public Health Service (NB-07512, 5T5-GM-1674, and HD-04248) and the Alfred P. Sloane Foundation.

References

Bennett, M. V. L. 1966. An electric organ of neural origin. *Fed. Proc.* 25: 569. (Abstr.)

Bennett, M. V. L. 1970. Comparative physiology: electric organs. *Annu. Rev. Physiol.* 32: 471.

Bennett, M. V. L. 1971*a*. Electric organs. *In* Fish Physiology. W. S. Hoar and D. J. Randall, editors. Academic Press Inc., New York. 5: 347.

Bennett, M. V. L. 1971*b*. Electroreception. *In* Fish Physiology. W. S. Hoar and D. J. Randall, editors. Academic Press Inc., New York. 5: 493.

Chung, S. H., S. A. Raymond, and J. Y. Lettvin. 1970. Multiple meaning in single visual units. *Brain Behav. Evol.* 3: 72.

Couceiro, A., A. A. P. Leao, and G. de Oliveira Castro. 1995. Some data on the structure of the electric organ of the itui (*Sternarchus albifrons, Linn.*). *Ann. Acad. Brasil. Cien.* 5: 323.

Elfvin, L. G. 1961. The ultrastructure of nodes of Ranvier in cat sympathetic nerve fibers. *J. Ultrastruct. Res.* 5: 374.

Harkin, J. C. 1964. A series of desmosomal attachments in the Schwann sheath of myelinated mammalian nerves. *Z. Zellforsch. Mikrosk. Anat.* 64: 189.

Hess, A., and J. Z. Young. 1952. The nodes of Ranvier. *Proc. Roy. Soc. Ser. B.* 140: 301.

Meszler, R. M., and M. V. L. Bennett. 1972. Morphology of the spinal nucleus innervating the electric organ of the electric eel. *Electrophorus electricus. Anat. Rec.* In press. (Abstr.)

Oliveira Castro, G. de. 1955. Differentiated nervous fibers that constitute the electric organ of *Sternarchus alfibrons Linn. Ann. Acad. Brasil. Cien.* 4: 557.

Peters, A. 1966. The node of Ranvier in the central nervous system. *Quart. J. Exp. Physiol. Cog. Med. Sci.* 51: 229.

Robertson, J. D. 1959. Preliminary observations on the ultrastructure of nodes of Ranvier. *Z. Zellforsch. Mikrosk. Anat.* 50: 553.

Rushton, W. A. H. 1951. A theory of the effects of fibre size in medullated nerve. *J. Physiol.* (*London*). 115: 101.

Schwartz, I. R., 1968. The fine structure of electroplaques in eight species of weakly electric teleosts. Doctoral dissertation. Yale University, New Haven.

Schwartz, I. R., and G. D. Pappas. 1968. The fine structure of electroplaques in some weakly electric fish. *Anat. Rec.* 160: 424. (Abstr.)

Thomas, P. K., and J. Z. Young. 1949. Internode lengths in the nerves of fishes. *J. Anat.* 83: 336.

Wall, P. D., J. Y. Lettvin, W. S. McCulloch, and W. H. Pitts. 1956. Factors limiting the maximum impulse transmitting ability of an afferent system of nerve fibers. *In* Information Theory. C. Cherry, editor. Third London Symposium, London.

Waxman, S. G. 1970. Closely spaced nodes of Ranvier in the teleost brain. *Nature* (*London*). 227: 283.

Waxman, S. G. 1971. An ultrastructural study of the pattern of myelination of preterminal fibers in teleost oculomotor nuclei, electromotor nuclei, and spinal cord. *Brain Res.* 27: 189.

Waxman, S. G., and M. V. L. Bennett, 1970. An analysis of the pattern of myelination of some preterminal fibers in the teleost central nervous system. *J. Cell Biol.* 47 (2, Pt. 2): 222 a. (Abstr.)

Waxman, S. G., and R. J. Melker. 1971. Closely spaced nodes of Ranvier in mammalian brain. *Brain Res.* 32: 445.

III WHAT IS IT? WHERE IS IT?

Each of us has at some time been to the doctor and, while being examined, watched the doctor tap close to the kneecap with a rubber hammer, testing the reflexes. The testing of reflexes is part of a systematic and detailed ritual called the neurological examination. In its complete form, the neurological examination includes the testing not only of reflexes, but also of various aspects of motor activity, coordination, sensory function, and mental state. Why are these functions tested? What does the doctor learn from these tests about our brains, spinal cord, and nerves?

In 1994 I was surprised to be asked to take over the authorship of the textbook *Correlative Neuroanatomy*; the previous authors, Jack de Groot and Joseph Chusid, were retiring. Although I had not thought about authoring a neuroanatomy text, this challenge struck a chord—the *Correlative* in the title meant *clinical* and *functional*—that resonated with my interest in structure-function relations within the nervous system. The following chapter (Waxman 1996), which I wrote for *Correlative Neuroanatomy*, discusses what neuroanatomy can teach us about neurology and what the doctor can learn from the neurological examination.

At the beginning of the twentieth century some scientists believed that the nervous system operates via a principle of mass action. According to this principle, neurons distributed throughout the brain contribute to any given function, and few if any functions depend on localized groups of neurons within a single, well-demarcated part of the brain or spinal cord. If the brain and spinal cord were, in fact, organized according to the principle of mass action, an injury to any region of the central nervous system would be expected to impair many functions, and few, if any, functions would be lost as a result of a localized injury affecting a single part of the brain or spinal cord.

We now understand that, with respect to many functions, the principle of mass action is incorrect. Different parts of the brain and spinal cord have distinctly different functions. Thus, some groups of neurons, and some nerve tracts, encode and/or carry sensory information about tactile stimuli of particular types (for example, about pain, or touch, or temperature of stimuli impinging on the body). Other parts of the nervous system subserve visual function, and still other regions control motor activity. The brain and spinal cord also contain a number of "maps" of the outside world. Within the cerebral cortex, for example, there is a motor map (which has the form of a small man, and is therefore called a homunculus), within the primary motor cortex of the frontal lobe; stimulation of the "arm" area evokes movement of the arm while stimulation of the leg area elicits movement of the leg. There are several sensory maps of the body surface (again, in the form of homunculi) within the sensory cortex. And there are multiple maps of the visual world within the occipital lobes, and within the temporal and parietal lobes of the cortex—these contain information about various aspects (color, movement, etc.) of our visual world and are called "retinotopic" because they preserve the geometrical relationships between objects imaged on the retina, and thus provide spatial representations of the visual environment, within the brain. Because of the presence of these maps, injury to a small region of the cortex does not cause global or diffuse loss of function. Damage to the arm area of the motor cortex, for example, causes weakness of the arm. Injury to part of the visual cortex may cause loss of vision in part of the visual field, for example, inability to recognize objects in the upper right part of the visual world. Damage to deeper parts of the brain produce still other abnormalities (such as tremors and other abnormal movements after injury to the basal ganglia).

Neurologists use the principle of localized function within the nervous system, to infer the part of the brain or spinal cord that is injured ("where is the lesion?") on the basis of a neurological examination which tests the nervous system in specific ways, assaying each of its functions. Because each function depends on the integrity of a specific group of neurons and pathways, it is possible, on the basis of the examination, to tell whether specific parts of the brain and spinal cord are intact, or are damaged.

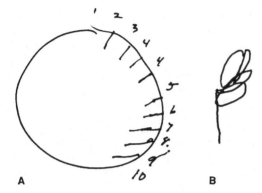

A   **B**

Figure III.1
Drawings made by a patient with damage to the cerebral cortex on the right side, when he was asked to (*A*) fill in the numbers in a clock, and (*B*) draw a flower. This patient neglected the left half of the world.

Other aspects of the patient often provide clues about the disease process that is causing the damage. Thus neurologists use the history and neurological examination to answer two questions: *where* is the lesion? and *what* is the lesion?

Some injuries to the brain produce striking, or even bizarre, abnormalities. An example is provided by the syndrome of "unilateral neglect." This syndrome usually arises as a result of damage to the right side of the brain, particularly a part of the cerebral cortex called the parietal cortex. Patients with unilateral neglect fail to respond to stimuli in the left half of their world. These patients are unaware of and bump into things in the neglected visual field, fail to dress or shave the neglected half of the body, and are unaware of motor or sensory deficits on the neglected side. Figure III.1 shows the response of a patient with unilateral neglect, when asked to fill in the numbers on the face of a clock and to draw a flower.

Neurology presents a panorama of interesting and unusual syndromes. On the basis of a careful description of a patient's behavior, and of an examination of the patient, it is often possible to answer the questions, where is the lesion? what is the lesion? There is, however, more to medicine than just making a diagnosis. Patients are feeling human beings and, as healers, we must not forget this. Most of the idealized case histories in *Correlative Neuroanatomy* illustrate the clinical implications of neuro-anatomy, but Clinical Illustration 3.3, at the end of the following chapter, makes a different point: it reminds medical students that they do not just treat cases or diseases. Our patients teach us that listening, and feeling with and for others, are important parts in the healing process. I hope that as medicine becomes more efficient, computerized, and even driven by "expert systems," this human aspect of medicine will not be lost.

Reference

Waxman, S. G. The relationship between neuroanatomy and neurology. In *Correlative Neuroanatomy*, 23ᵈ edition, pp. 36–44. Appleton and Lange, Stamford, CT, 1996.

3 Introduction to Clinical Thinking: The Relationship between Neuroanatomy and Neurology

S. G. Waxman

Neurology, more than any other specialty, rests on clinicoanatomic correlation. The neurologic clinician attempts, with each patient, to answer two questions: (1) **Where** is (are) the lesion(s)? and (2) **What** is (are) the lesion(s)?

The term **lesion** refers to a zone of localized dysfunction within the CNS or PNS. Lesions can be **anatomic**, with dysfunction resulting from structural damage (examples are provided by stroke, trauma, and brain tumors). Lesions also can be **physiologic**, reflecting physiologic dysfunction in the absence of demonstrable anatomic abnormalities (an example is provided by transient ischemic attacks (TIAs) in which temporary and reversible loss of function of part of the brain occurs without structural damage to neurons or glial cells, as a result of metabolic changes due to vascular insufficiency).

The answers to the previously mentioned questions permit the clinician to define the disease process in a given patient, thus leading to a **diagnosis**. This sequence of events is crucial for the development of an appropriate **treatment plan**. The diagnosis also suggests the patient's **prognosis**. In addition, by arriving at a correct diagnosis and following the patient, the clinician begins to understand the **natural history** of neurologic disease, both in each individual patient and in the population, and can begin to understand the **pathophysiology** of the disorder as well as assess the **efficacy** of various treatments.

This chapter gives a brief overview of clinical thinking in neurology and emphasizes the relationship between neuroanatomy and neurology. It is not meant as a comprehensive or even introductory primer in neurology (a number of excellent neurology texts are available and are listed in the references at the end of this chapter). On the contrary, it has been included to help the

Reprinted with permission from *Correlative Neuroanatomy*, Appleton and Lange, 1996.

reader to begin to think as the clinician does and, thus, to place neuroanatomy, as outlined in the subsequent chapters, in a patient-oriented framework. Together with the Clinical Illustrations and Cases placed throughout this book, the information in this chapter provides a clinical perspective on neuroanatomy.

Symptoms and Signs of Neurologic Diseases

Neurologic diagnosis depends on a careful **history** obtained from the patient, the patient's family, and colleagues and on the **neurologic examination**, which tests the function of each part of the nervous system. The information obtained is synthesized using a knowledge of the relevant neuroanatomy to arrive at a provisional diagnosis. This diagnosis may be confirmed or refined via a variety of **laboratory tests** and **neuroimaging**.

In taking a history and examining the patient, the neurologic clinician elicits both **symptoms** and **signs**. Symptoms are subjective sensations resulting from the disorder (ie, "I have a headache"; "The vision in my right eye became blurry for two or three days a month ago"). Signs are objective abnormalities detected on examination or via laboratory tests (eg, a hyperactive reflex or abnormal eye movements).

The clinician usually obtains a history first. The history may provide crucial information about diagnosis. For example, a patient was admitted to the hospital in a coma. His wife told the admitting physician: "My husband has high blood pressure but doesn't like to take his medicine. This morning he complained of the worst headache in his life. Then he passed out." On the basis of this history and a brief (but careful) examination, the physician rapidly reached a tentative diagnosis of subarachnoid hemorrhage (bleeding from an aneurism, ie, a defect in a cerebral artery into the subarachnoid space). He confirmed this diagnostic impression with appropriate (but focused) laboratory tests and instituted appropriate therapy.

The astute clinical observer may be able to detect signs of neurologic disease by carefully observing the patients' spontaneous behavior as they walk into the room and tell their story; thus, for example, even prior to touching the patient, the clinician may observe the "festinating" (shuffling, small-stepped) gait of Parkinson's disease, hemiparesis (weakness of one side of the body) owing to a hemispheric lesion such as a stroke, or a third nerve palsy suggesting an intracranial mass. The **way** patients tell their story also may be informative, eg, it may reveal aphasia (difficulty with language), confusion, or impaired memory. A carefully taken history can provide very important information about the patient's illness and is essential. Details of history taking and the neurologic examination are included in Appendix A.

In synthesizing the information obtained from the history and examination, the clinician usually keeps asking the questions, "Where is the lesion? What is the lesion?" Several points should be kept in mind while going through the diagnostic process.

Neurologic Signs and Symptoms Often Reflect Focal Pathology of the Nervous System

At the beginning of this century, some investigators believed that the nervous system operates via a principle of *mass action*. According to the principle of mass action, neurons distributed widely throughout the brain contribute to any given function, and few if any functions depend on localized groups of neurons within a single, demarcated part of the brain. If the brain were, in fact, organized according to the principle of mass action, a lesion affecting any region of the brain would be expected to impair many functions, and few, if any, functions would be lost as a result of a well-circumscribed, localized lesion affecting a single part of the brain.

We now know that, with respect to many functions, the principle of mass action is incorrect. Different parts of the nervous system subserve distinctly different functions. In turn, in many parts of the brain or spinal cord, even relatively small well-circumscribed lesions produce loss or severe impairment of a specific function. This reflects the principle of **localized function** within the nervous system.

There are numerous examples of localized function. (1) Aphasia (difficulty producing or understanding language) often results from damage to well-localized *speech areas* within the left cerebral hemisphere. (2) Control of fine movements of each hand is dependent on signals sent from a *hand area* within the *motor cortex* in the contralateral cerebral hemisphere; the motor cortex is organized in the form of a map, or "homunculus," reflecting the fact that different parts of the motor cortex control movements of different parts of the body (see Chapter 10, especially Fig 10–14). A lesion affecting the hand area or the highly circumscribed pathways that descend from it to the spinal cord can result in loss of skilled movements or even paralysis of the hand. (3) At a more basic level, many simple and complex reflexes, which are tested as part of the neurologic examination, depend on circuits that run through particular parts of the nervous system. For example, the patellar reflex (knee jerk) depends on afferent and efferent nerve fibers in the femoral nerve and L3 and L4 spinal roots and the L3 and L4 spinal segments, where afferent IA axons synapse with motor neurons that subserve the reflex. Damage to any of the parts of this circuit (nerve, spinal roots, or L3 or L4 spinal segments) can interfere with the reflex.

As a corollary of the principle of localized function, it is often possible to predict, from neurologic signs and symptoms, which parts of the nervous system are involved. By obtaining an accurate history and carrying out a careful examination, the clinician can obtain important clues about the localization of dysfunction in the nervous system.

Manifestations of Neurologic Disease May Be Negative or Positive

Negative manifestations result from **loss of function**, eg, hemiparesis, weakness of an eye muscle, impaired sensation, or loss of memory. Negative manifestations of neurologic disease may reflect damage to neurons (eg, in Parkinson's disease, where there is degeneration of neurons in the substantia nigra) or to glial cells or myelin (eg, in multiple sclerosis in which there is inflammatory damage to myelin). **Positive** abnormalities result from inappropriate excitation. These include, for example, seizures (caused by abnormal cortical discharge) and spasticity (from the loss of inhibition of motor neurons). Another example is provided by Lhermitte's sign, in which the patient experiences tingling paresthesias extending into the legs, triggered by flexion of the neck; this phenomenon is seen when there is pathology in or near the cervical spinal cord and is a result of abnormal mechanosensitivity of sensory axons in the spinal cord.

Lesions of White and Gray Matter Cause Neurologic Dysfunction

Damage to **gray** or **white matter** (or both) interferes with normal neurologic function. Lesions in gray matter interfere with the function of neuronal cell bodies and synapses, thereby leading to negative or positive abnormalities as previously described. Lesions in white matter, on the other hand, interfere with axonal conduction and produce **disconnection syndromes**, which usually cause negative manifestations; examples of these syndromes include optic neuritis (demyelination of the optic nerve), which interferes with vision; and infarction affecting pyramidal tract axons, which descend from the motor cortex in regions such as the internal capsule, which can cause "pure motor stroke," figure 3.1).

Some neurologic disorders affect primarily gray matter (eg, amyotrophic lateral sclerosis, a degenerative disease leading to the death of motor neurons in the cerebral cortex and gray mat-

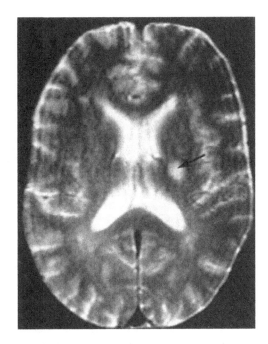

Figure 3.1
Magnetic resonance (MR) image of a 51-year-old hypertensive patient. The patient complained of weakness of the right side of the face and the right arm and leg, which had developed over a 5-h period. There was no sensory loss, and there were no problems with language or cognition. The MR scan revealed a small infarction in the internal capsule (arrow). which destroyed axons descending from the motor cortex, thus causing a "pure motor stroke" in this patient.

ter of the spinal cord). Others primarily affect white matter (eg, multiple sclerosis). Still other disorders affect both gray and white matter, for instance large strokes, which lead to necrosis of the cerebral cortex and underlying white matter.

Neurologic Disease Can Result in Syndromes

A **syndrome** is a constellation of signs and symptoms frequently associated with each other and suggests a common origin. Recognition of a syndrome may point to a specific localization and can suggest a particular diagnosis. An ex-

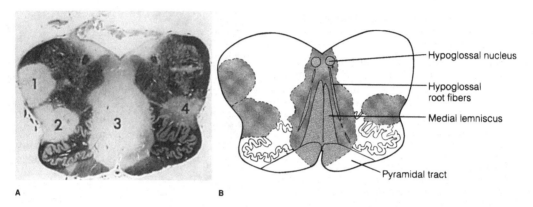

A   **B**

Figure 3.2
(*A*) Section through the medulla, stained for myelin, from a patient with multiple sclerosis. Notice the multiple demyelinated plaques (labeled 1–4) that are disseminated throughout the CNS. (*B*) Even a single lesion can interfere with function in multiple neighboring parts of the CNS. Notice that plaque 3 involves the hypoglossal root (producing weakness of the tongue) and the medial lemnisci (causing an impairment of vibratory and touch pressure sense).

ample is **Wallenberg's syndrome**, which is characterized by vertigo, nausea, hoarseness, and dysphagia (difficulty swallowing). Other signs and symptoms include ipsilateral ataxia, ptosis, and meiosis, impairment of all sensory modalities over the ipsilateral face, and loss of pain and temperature sensitivity over the contralateral torso and limbs. This syndrome results from dysfunction of a group of clustered nuclei and tracts in the **lateral medulla** and is usually due to infarction resulting from occlusion of the posterior inferior cerebellar artery, which irrigates these neighboring structures.

Neighborhood Signs May Help to Localize the Lesion

The brain and spinal cord are highly complex structures and contain many tracts and nuclei that are intimately associated with each other. Particularly in the brain stem and spinal cord, where there is not much room in the transverse plane, there is crowding of nuclei and fiber tracts. Many pathologic processes result in

lesions that are larger than any single nucleus or tract. **Combinations of signs and symptoms** may help to localize the lesion. Figure 3.2 shows a section through the medulla of a patient with multiple sclerosis. The patient had a long-standing history of sensory loss in the legs (impaired touch-pressure sense and position sense) and also had weakness of the tongue. As an alternative to positing the presence of two separate lesions to account for these two abnormalities, the clinician should pose the question "Might a *single* lesion account for both abnormalities?" In this case, knowledge of brain stem neuroanatomy allowed the clinician to predict the presence of a lesion located in the medial part of the medulla—a hypothesis that was confirmed at postmortem examination.

Dysfunction of the Nervous System Can Be Due to Destruction or Compression of Neural Tissue, or Compromise of the Ventricles or Vasculature

Several types of structural pathology can lead to dysfunction of the nervous system (table 3.1).

Table 3.1
Mechanisms leading to dysfunction in typical neurologic diseases

Mechanism	Disease example	Target	Comments
Destruction	Stroke	Neurons (often cortical)	Acute destruction, within hours of loss of blood flow
Destruction	Parkinson's disease	Neurons (subcortical)	Chronic degeneration of neurons in substantia nigra
Destruction	Spinal cord injury	Ascending and descending axons	Injury to fiber tracts due to trauma
Destruction	Multiple sclerosis	Myelin	Inflammatory damage to myelin sheaths in CNS
Compression	Subdural hematoma	Cerebral hemisphere	Expanding blood clot injures underlying brain tissue
Compromise of ventricular pathways	Cerebellar tumor	Fourth ventricle	Expanding mass compresses ventricle, impairs CSF outflow

Destruction of neurons (or associated glial cells) accounts for the clinical abnormalities in disorders, such as stroke (in which neurons are acutely injured as a result of vascular compromise producing ischemia) and Parkinson's disease (in which chronic degeneration of neurons occurs in one particular region of the brain stem, the substantia nigra). Destruction of axons secondary to trauma causes much of the dysfunction in spinal cord injury, and destruction of myelin as a result of inflammatory processes leads to the abnormal function in multiple sclerosis.

Compression of the nervous system can also cause dysfunction, without the invasion of the brain and spinal cord per se. This occurs, for example, in subdural hematoma, when an expanding blood clot, contained by the skull vault, compresses the adjacent brain, initially causing reversible dysfunction, prior to triggering the death of neural tissue. Early recognition of this disorder and surgical drainage of the clot can lead to full recovery of function.

Finally, **compromise of ventricular pathways** or of the **vasculature** can lead to neurologic signs and symptoms. For example, a small cerebellar astrocytoma, critically located above the fourth ventricle, may compress the ventricle and obstruct the outflow of cerebrospinal fluid. Even if the tumor has not produced symptoms, it may lead to obstructive hydrocephalus with widespread destructive effects on both cerebral hemispheres. In this case, a small, critically placed mass produces widespread neural dysfunction as a result of its effect on the outflow tracts for cerebrospinal fluid. Critically placed vascular lesions can also produce devastating effects on the nervous system. For example, occlusion of the carotid artery, owing to atherosclerosis in the neck, can lead to infarction in the cerebral hemisphere, which it supplies.

Where Is the Lesion?

Processes Causing Neurologic Disease

Focal Process Focal pathology causes signs and symptoms on the basis of a single, geographically contiguous lesion. The most common example is stroke, which occurs when ischemia within the territory of a particular artery leads to infarction of neural tissue in a well-defined area (figure 3.3). Another example is provided by

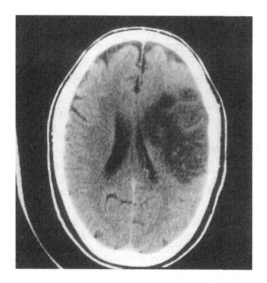

Figure 3.3
Computed tomographic (CT) scan showing a stroke in
the territory of the middle cerebral artery.

solitary brain tumors. In thinking about the
patient, the physician should ask, "Is there a
single lesion that can account for the signs and
symptoms?"

Multifocal Process   Multifocal pathology results
in damage to the nervous system at numerous,
separate sites. In multiple sclerosis, for example,
lesions are disseminated throughout the nervous
system in the spatial domain as well as over time
(ie, the lesions do not develop at once). Figure
3.2 shows the multifocal nature of the pathology
in a patient with multiple sclerosis. Another example is provided by leptomeningeal seeding of a
tumor. As a result of dissemination throughout
the subarachnoid space, tumor deposits can affect
numerous spinal and cranial nerve roots distributed along the entire neuraxis and can also block
CSF outflow, thereby producing hydrocephalus.

Diffuse Process   Diffuse dysfunction of the nervous system can be produced by a number of

toxins and metabolic abnormalities. In arriving
at a diagnosis, the clinician must ask, "Is there a
systemic disorder than can account for the
patient's signs and symptoms?" Metabolic or
toxic coma, for instance, can result in abnormal
function of neurons throughout the nervous
system.

Rostrocaudal Localization

In determining the rostrocaudal localization of
the lesion, it is important to determine the nuclei
and fiber tracts that are affected and to consider
the *constellation* of structures that is involved.
Each of the major motor (descending) and sensory (ascending) pathways decussates (ie, crosses
from one side of the neuraxis to the other) at a
specific level. The levels of decussation of three
major pathways are briefly summarized in figure
3.4 and are discussed in Chapter 5. By examining
the constellation of deficits in a given patient and
relating them to appropriate tracts and nuclei, it
is often possible to place the lesion at the appropriate level along the rostrocaudal axis.

For example, consider a patient with weakness
of the left leg. This could be caused by a lesion
involving the nerves innervating the leg or by a
lesion affecting the corticospinal pathway at any
level from the cortex, through the midbrain, and
down to the lumbar spinal cord. If the patient
also had loss of vibratory and position sense of
the left leg (indicating dysfunction in the dorsal
column pathway) and loss of pain and temperature sensation over the *right* leg (indicating
impaired function of the spinothalamic pathway), the clinician would then think about dysfunction of the left half of the spinal cord, above
the decussation of the spinothalamic fibers
(which decussate within the spinal cord, close to
the level where they enter the cord) but *below* the
medullary-cervical spinal cord junction where
the corticospinal tract decussates. Furthermore,
normal function in the arms and trunk suggests
normal function in cervical and thoracic parts of
the spinal cord (which carry fibers for the arm

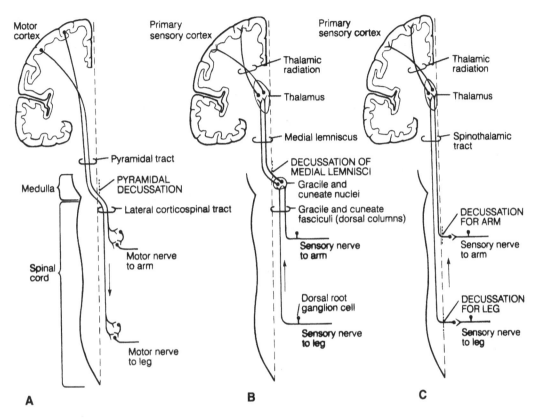

Figure 3.4
(*A*) Pyramidal tract. (*B*) Dorsal column system. (*C*) Spinothalamic system.

and trunk). The combination of deficits could, in fact, be parsimoniously explained by a *single* lesion, located in the left side of the spinal cord.

Transverse Localization

In localizing the lesion, the clinician must also consider its placement in the transverse plane, ie, within the cross section of the brain or spinal cord. Here again, neighborhood signs are important. In the previously described patient with a spinal cord lesion, the dorsal and lateral white matter columns in the spinal cord must be

involved because the dorsal column pathway and corticospinal tract are involved. Moreover, the clinician can predict that the lesion is centered in the left half of the spinal cord because there is no evidence of dysfunction of the corticospinal tract, dorsal column system, or spinothalamic tract on the right side in this patient.

By carefully considering the tracts and nuclei involved and their relationships along the rostrocaudal axis and in the transverse plane, it is often possible to identify, with a high degree of probability, the site(s) of the nervous system that are involved in a given patient.

What Is the Lesion?

In considering the pathologic nature of a lesion, the neurologic clinician uses information derived from both the examination and the history. The **age** of the patient must be considered. Cerebrovascular disease, for example, is more common in individuals over the age of 50; in contrast, multiple sclerosis is a disease of the second and third decades and rarely presents in elderly individuals.

The **gender** of the patient may provide important information. **Duchenne's muscular dystrophy**, for instance, is a sex-linked disorder that occurs only in males. Carcinoma of the prostate (a male disease) and of the breast (predominantly a female disease) commonly metastasize to the vertebral column, and these metastases can cause spinal cord compression.

The **general medical context** also provides an important cortex: Is the patient a smoker? Has the patient lost weight? Lung and breast tumors, for example, commonly metastasize to the nervous system. The development of hemiparesis in an otherwise healthy, nonsmoking 75-year-old is most likely the result of cerebrovascular disease. In a smoker with a lesion on chest x-ray, on the other hand, hemiparesis may result from a metastasis in the brain. The neurologic examination and history *must* be interpreted in the context of a patient's general medical status.

Time Course of the Illness

The **time course** of the illness may provide invaluable information about its nature. Brief episodes of dysfunction lasting minutes to hours, occurring throughout the life of the patient, may represent seizures or migraine attacks (figure 3.5A). A **recent-onset cluster of brief episodes** or a **crescendo pattern** of neurologic dysfunction, on the other hand, may represent nonstable evolving disease. For example, **transient ischemic attacks** (TIA) [brief episodes of neurologic dysfunction followed by full recovery, resulting from reversible ischemia] are the harbingers of stroke in some patients. A pattern of recent-onset headaches on wakening, increasing in intensity, may be caused by the presence of an expanding brain tumor (figure 3.5B). A **relapsing-remitting** course, in which the patient experiences bouts of dysfunction lasting days to weeks followed by functional recovery, is characteristic of multiple sclerosis (figure 3.5C). **Sudden onset** of a fixed deficit is characteristic of cerebrovascular disease, which includes ischemic stroke and intracerebral hemorrhage (figure 3.5D). **Slowly progressive dysfunction** evolves over years and is suggestive of neurodegenerative diseases, such as Alzheimer's and Parkinson's (figure 3.5E). **Subacutely progressive dysfunction**, which advances over weeks to months, is often seen with brain tumors (figure 3.5F). Although the time and course of the illness does not permit a definitive diagnosis, it can provide helpful information.

The Role of Neuroimaging and Laboratory Investigations

A careful synthesis of the clinical data permits the clinician to arrive, with a high degree of accuracy, at a differential diagnosis (ie, a list of diagnostic possibilities that fit, in a positive way, with the patient's clinical picture). Armed with a good working knowledge of correlative neuroanatomy, the clinician should not have to blindly "rule out" a multitude of diseases. On the contrary, by focusing on the questions "Where is the lesion?" and "What is the lesion?", it is usually possible to identify a limited field of diagnostic choices that have a high probability of explaining the patient's clinical picture. This field of possibilities can be further delimited, and the diagnosis refined, by the use of neuroimaging methods. Recent progress in neuroimaging has provided a number of important new diagnostic techniques that permit rapid, precise, and in many cases, noninvasive visualization of the

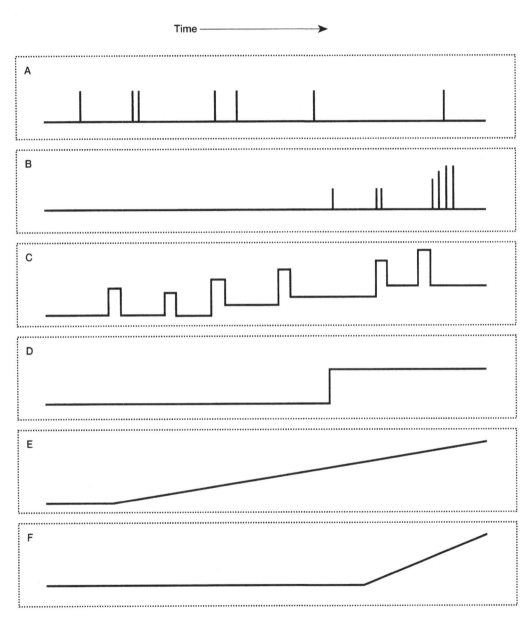

Figure 3.5
Characteristic time-courses for various neurologic disorders.

brain, spinal cord, and surrounding structures, such as the skull and vertebral column.

Neuroimaging investigations include plain x-rays; dye studies, such as angiography (to visualize cerebral vessels) and myelography (which fills and outlines the subarachnoid space surrounding the spinal cord); CT scanning; and MRI scans. Neuroimaging can provide invaluable information in terms of confirming the location of a lesion within the CSN. In addition, neuroimaging studies can help define the size of the lesion and sometimes provide information about the nature of the lesion. For example, some brain tumors can be differentiated from cerebral abscesses on the basis of their radiographic appearance.

In obtaining neuroimaging studies, the radiologist is usually guided by clinical information. This helps in choosing the most appropriate imaging procedure and in "targeting" the imaging studies on the right part of the nervous system.

Although neuroimaging procedures represent an extremely powerful set of tools, they do not always, in and of themselves, provide the correct diagnosis. The results of neuroimaging studies must be interpreted in the light of history and clinical examination and interpreted in terms of neuroanatomy. Examples are provided by Clinical Illustrations 3.1 and 3.2.

Clinical Illustration 3.1

A 52-year-old accountant weighing 320 pounds saw his physician with the complaints of back pain and weakness in his legs. A neurologic consultant found moderate weakness in both legs associated with hyperactive reflexes, Babinski's reflexes, and sensory loss below the umbilicus. There was focal tenderness over the spine at the T5 level.

The weakness of the legs, associated with signs of upper-motor-neuron dysfunction (hyperactive reflexes and Babinski's responses), suggested the possibility of a lesion affecting the spinal cord

and the sensory loss, which extended to the T10 level, indicated that the lesion was located above this level. Because of the patient's focal back pain, the neurologist suspected that there was a mass compressing the spinal cord, close to the T5 level of the spinal column. Because the patient would not fit in the MR scanner at the hospital, he was sent to another clinic, 60 miles away, where an older MR scanner with a wider bore could accommodate him. The neurologist's report, outlining his findings and requesting an MR scan of the entire spine including thoracic regions, was lost in transit. The radiologist, who had not examined the patient, noted his history of leg weakness and obtained MR scans of the lumbar spinal cord. No lesion was seen.

Despite the report of a "normal" MR scan, the neurologist reasoned there was a lesion, compressing the spinal cord in the midthoracic region. He ordered a myelogram that revealed a meningioma at the T4 level. Following surgery, the patient's strength improved.

This case illustrates several points. First, a careful history and examination, together with knowledge of neuroanatomy, provides crucial information to guide the neuroradiologist so the proper regions of the nervous system are examined. In this case, the neurologist's guidance might have focused the radiologist's attention on the appropriate part of the spinal column. Second, clinical intuition can be as good as, or in some cases better than, imaging. "Normal" radiologic results most commonly reflect normal anatomy but can also result from technical difficulties, improper patient positioning, or imaging methodology. In situations in which imaging results are not consistent with the history and examination, a repeat examination, together with a reexamination of the questions, "Where is the lesion? What is the lesion?" can be helpful.

Clinical Illustration 3.2

A 45-year-old Latin teacher was evaluated by her family doctor after she complained of pain in her left arm. Because of weakness, he suspected a herniated intervertebral disk and ordered cervical spine x-rays that revealed an intervertebral disk protrusion at the C6–C7 level, which was confirmed by CT scans. The pain progressed over several weeks, and surgery (excision of the protruded disk) was considered.

As part of her work-up, the patient was seen by a neurologist. Careful examination revealed sensory loss in the distribution of the C6, C7, and C8 dermatomes. There was a pattern of weakness that did not conform to any single nerve root, but rather suggested involvement of the lower brachial plexus. Chest x-ray demonstrated a small-cell carcinoma located in the apex of the lung, which had invaded the brachial plexus. The patient was immediately referred for chemotherapy.

This case illustrates that radiographic studies can, in some patients, reveal structural abnormalities that are not relevant to the patient's disease. In this case, the patient's herniated cervical disk had not caused symptoms. The family physician had not appreciated all of these findings and could not correlate the full clinical picture with the radiographic images. Therefore, he ascribed the patient's pain to the wrong lesion (the asymptomatic herniated intervertebral disk), and was lulled into a false sense of security so that he missed the relevant pathology, ie—the patient's tumor.

A more complete examination coupled with the question "Where is the lesion?", would have led to the conclusion that the brachial plexus was involved. Once this localization was appreciated, the radiologist obtained apical views of the lungs to examine the possibility of a tumor that had spread to the brachial plexus. As illustrated by this case, abnormal neuroimaging studies do not necessarily lead to a definitive diagnosis. A careful examination of the patient with appropriate emphasis on neuroanatomy must be correlated with the neuroimaging studies.

A number of other laboratory tests can provide additional information about the patient's illness. The **lumbar puncture**, or **spinal tap**, for instance, provides cerebrospinal fluid (CSF). Lumbar puncture is further discussed in Chapter 25. Analysis of the CSF (measurement of its protein, glucose, and immunoglobulin content, along with its cell count) can provide a definitive diagnosis of infections (such as bacterial meningitis) and can help to confirm the diagnosis in such disorders as multiple sclerosis and brain tumor. Chapter 25 provides a discussion of CSF analysis.

Electrophysiologic tests permit the measurement of electrical activity from the brain, spinal cord, and peripheral nerves and can provide important information. These tests include the **electroencephalogram (EEG), evoked potentials, electromyography (EMG),** and **nerve conduction studies.** Like CSF analysis, the results of electrophysiologic studies should be interpreted in the context of the history and physical examination. These tests are discussed further in Chapter 24.

The Treatment of Patients with Neurologic Disease

In collecting a history, performing an examination, and implementing treatment, the clinician is "acting" not only as doctor to patient, but as care giver to another human being. It is essential to remember this and to keep in mind the important role that sensitivity and caring can have. The effective clinician can play a crucial role in helping the patient cope with neurologic disease. Listening is very important. Neurologic clinicians do not just treat cases or diseases; they treat people. An example is provided in Clinical Illustration 3.3.

Clinical Illustration 3.3

A neurologic consultant was asked to evaluate a patient who was known to have a malignant melanoma. The patient had been in the hospital for 10 days, and the nursing staff noticed that he did not dress himself properly, tended to get lost while walking on the ward, and bumped into things.

Although the patient had no complaints, his wife recalled that, beginning several months earlier, he had developed difficulty putting on his clothes properly. He had been fired after working for 30 years as a truck driver because he had developed difficulty reading a map.

Careful examination revealed a hemiinattention syndrome. The patient tended to neglect the left half of the world. When asked to draw a clock, he squeezed all of the numbers in the right-hand half. He drew only the right half of a flower and tended to eat only off the right half of his plate. When asked to put on his hospital robe, he wrapped it around his waist, but was unable to properly put it on. Careful examination of the motor system revealed that, in addition, the patient had a mild left hemiparesis.

"Hemiinattention" syndrome usually occurs as a result of lesions in the nondominant (right) cerebral hemisphere, most commonly the parietal lobe. Lesions in this area can also cause difficulty dressing ("dressing apraxia"). The presence of a hemiinattention syndrome and dressing apraxia, together with a mild left hemiparesis, strongly suggested the presence of a lesion in the right cerebral hemisphere, most likely in the right parietal lobe, and the history suggested metastatic melanoma. Subsequent imaging confirmed the diagnosis.

Following the examination, the neurologic consultant asked the patient and his wife whether they had any questions. His wife replied, "We know that my husband has metastatic cancer and that he will die. He has been in the hospital for 10 days, but nobody has explained what will happen. Will my husband have pain? Will he need to be sedated? Will he be able to make out a will? As he gets worse, will he be able to recognize the children?"

In this instance, the patient's physician had correctly diagnosed and managed the primary melanoma. However, he did not have a strong knowledge of neuroanatomy, and during the neurologic examination he had failed to recognize the presence of metastasis in the brain. Equally important, the treating physician had focused his attention on the patient's *disease*, and not met his needs as a *person*. An open, relaxed discussion ("How do you feel about your disease? What frightens you the most? Do you have any questions?") is an essential part of the physician's role.

References

Adams RE, Victor M: *Principles of Neurology*, 5th ed. McGraw-Hill, 1993.

Aminoff MF, Greenberg DA, Simon RP: *Clinical Neurology,* 3rd ed. Appleton & Lange, 1993.

Bradley WG, Daroff RB, Fenichel GM, Marsden CD: *Neurology in Clinical Practice*, 2nd ed. Butterworth-Heinemann, 1996.

Brazis PW, Masdeu JC, Biller J: *Localization in Clinical Neurology*, Little Brown and Co., 1990.

Haymaker W: *Bing's Local Diagnosis in Neurological Disease.* 15th ed. CW Mosby, 1969.

Menkes JH: *Textbook of Child Neurology.* 3rd ed. Lea & Febiger, 1985.

Plum F, Posner JB: *The Diagnosis of Stupor and Coma.* 3rd ed. FA Davis, 1980.

Rowland LP: *Merritt's Textbook of Neurology.* 8th ed. Lea & Febiger, 1989.

IV SEEING THE BRAIN: THE IMPACTS OF MODERN BRAIN IMAGING

The following paper (Mesulam et al. 1976) provided an early glimpse of the importance of the right cerebral hemisphere in the process of attention. By describing three patients who had a common problem—an inability to focus their attention—and by demonstrating that these patients all suffered from strokes affecting particular regions of the right cerebral hemisphere, this paper demonstrated the importance of this part of the brain for the maintenance of a coherent, goal-directed sequence of behavior. This was the first of a series of beautiful studies by Mesulam that have examined the brain structures, and processes, involved in maintaining selective attention (see, e.g., Mesulam 1998, 1999).

This study was carried out at the beginning of the era of modern brain imaging. Figure 4.1D, made with one of the first CT scanners to be installed in Boston, displays a resolution of approximately one centimeter, about tenfold less fine-grained than the CT scanners that are currently in use. The images provided by this machine nevertheless revealed previously unseen aspects of the nervous system that were extremely exciting. Imaging of this type permitted us, and others, to visualize the brain non-invasively for the first time.

Brain imaging has developed with dizzying speed since the advent of these first CT scanners. CT scanning has been supplanted, in part, by the introduction of magnetic resonance imaging, which provides exquisitely detailed pictures of the brain. More recently, magnetic resonance techniques and positron emission tomography (PET) scanning have been refined so as to provide methods for "functional brain imaging." These modern methods provide pictures of the brain in which it is possible to identify regions with increased metabolic activity. Because increased metabolic activity is thought to correlate with increased electrical activity of nerve cells, it is possible to use these new imaging techniques to infer which parts of the brain are involved in a particular task. For example, it is possible to use functional brain imaging to identify the parts of the brain that are active when one squeezes on a rubber ball using one hand, or when one does mental arithmetic, reads a poem, or imagines a pleasant activity. Neuroanatomy, previously based on the study of the structure and of the connections between groups of neurons, is being redefined: functional imaging now permits the brain to be mapped in terms of *function*. The results of functional imaging studies will undoubtedly take us a long way toward an understanding of how the brain works.

Functional brain imaging may also have important societal consequences. Functional imaging studies have identified parts of the brain that are involved in the retrieval of memories. In one recent study (Schachter et al. 1996), functional brain imagers asked, "What parts of the brain are involved when one remembers incorrectly?" and were able to identify several brain regions that seemed to be linked to accurately remembering and other regions that were linked to making mistakes. In another study (Castro-Caldas et al. 1998), brain imagers examined the hypothesis that learning during childhood affects the functional organization of the brain. They did this by using functional imaging to study brain activity in literate individuals, and in individuals who were illiterate because, for social reasons, they had never entered school. These investigators found that, in trying to read, these two groups of individuals activated different parts of their brain—an elegant demonstration of how our surroundings and social situations can help to shape the development of our brains.

It seems inevitable that, sooner or later, someone will ask, "What parts of the brain are activated when one lies?" Or someone may ask whether it is possible to study children at various stages in the educational process, distinguishing those who are "learning" well, as opposed to those who are not. When that happens, we may have to face the specter of technologies that permit the visualization of brain activity that is putatively related to various behaviors, social actions, or intervention strategies. One can imagine a variety of uses—or abuses—of these methodologies. It will be important for us, as a society, to carefully consider whether, and how, to use brain imaging techniques for constructive purposes, outside of the research domain, within our diverse society.

References

Castro-Caldas, A., Petersson, K. M., Reis, A., Stone-Elander, S., and Ingvar, M. The illiterate brain. Learning to read and write during childhood influences the functional organization of the adult brain. *Brain* 121: 1053–1063, 1998.

Mesulam, M-M. From sensation to cognition. *Brain* 121: 1013–1052, 1998.

Mesulam, M-M. Spatial attention and neglect: parietal, frontal, and cingulate contributions to the mental representation and attentional targeting of salient extrapersonal events. *Phil. Trans. Roy. Soc. (Lond). B.* 354: 1325–1346, 1999.

Mesulam, M. M., Waxman, S. G., Geschwind, N., and Sabin, T. D. Acute confusional states with right middle cerebral artery infarctions. *J. Neurol. Neurosurg. Psychiat.* 39: 84–90, 1976.

Schachter, D. L., Reiman, E., Curran, T., et al. Neuroanatomical correlates of veridical and illusory recognition memory: evidence from positron emission tomography. *Neuron* 17: 267–274, 1996.

4 Acute Confusional States with Right Middle Cerebral Artery Infarctions

Marek-Marsel Mesulam, Stephen G. Waxman, Norman Geschwind, and Thomas D. Sabin

Synopsis Three patients presenting predominantly with acute confusional states (ACS) are shown to have infarctions in the distribution of the right middle cerebral artery. It is suggested that the main deficit in ACS is in the function of selective attention. On the basis of cortical connections of homologous areas in the monkey brain, it is argued that this deficit arises from lesions in convergence areas for association cortex.

We would like to report three patients whose clinical presentation was dominated by acute confusional states (ACS), and who were shown to have infarcts in the distribution of branches of the middle cerebral artery in the right cerebral hemisphere.[1] In clinical practice, the vast majority of ACS result from metabolic encephalopathies, intoxications, withdrawal states, infections, head trauma, or post-ictal states (Cohen, 1953; Engel and Romano, 1959; Lipowski, 1967; Adams and Victor, 1974). ACS have occasionally been reported as dominating the clinical presentation of infarcts in the distribution of the posterior (Horenstein et al., 1967; Medina et al., 1974) or of the anterior (Hyland, 1933; Amyes and Nielsen, 1955) cerebral arteries. However, except for a brief description by Pearce and Miller (1973), of confusion resulting from right parietal lesions. ACS are not recognized as major sequellae of infarcts in the distribution of the middle cerebral artery. Furthermore, since the target in the central nervous system of most insults causing ACS cannot be specified, it has not been possible to localize the responsible lesion. Our purpose in this communication is, therefore, twofold: first, to alert the clinician to another cerebro-vascular cause of ACS; and, secondly, to advance some preliminary thoughts on the anatomy of cerebral dysfunction in ACS.

Reprinted with permission from *Journal of Neurology, Neurosurgery, and Psychiatry* 39: 84–89, 1976.

Case 1

A 61 year old, right-handed man was admitted because of the sudden onset of agitated confusion. He was living alone and effectively taking care of his shopping and cooking until the day before admission when he was discovered by his landlady in a disoriented, incoherent and agitated state, banging on the doors and shouting in the middle of the night. At admission, the vital signs were unremarkable and the general physical examination was within normal limits except for a systolic ejection murmur. The neurological examination found the patient to be awake but to have a severely diminished attention span, being able to repeat only two numbers forward. Minor and irrelevant stimuli elicited dramatic orienting responses and resulted in extreme distractibility. The stream of thought was incoherent; the ability to grasp environmental cues and to react accordingly was severely compromised. There was no concern for this incapacitating change in mental status. The quantity of activity varied from sluggishness to agitation for which the patient required physical restraints. Several examiners thought that auditory hallucinations were present. The patient was disoriented in all spheres. He had difficulty in naming objects presented in the visual, auditory, or tactile modes and his speech contained paraphasias and circumlocutions. He could read but could not write. Extreme distractibility rendered the remainder of the mental status examination unreliable. The gait was retropulsive and unsteady. There was minimal reaction to visual stimuli in the left hemifield but the differentiation could not be made between inattention and hemianopsia. No other abnormalities of cranial nerves, sensori-motor function, or plantar responses could be detected. The patient was incontinent, unkempt, and would not use utensils for eating.

In the next few days, the agitation disappeared completely and the patient became amiable and placid. In the next month, the anomic aphasia also improved considerably; however, the attention span remained severely compromised and there was no ability to maintain a coherent stream of thought. Routine laboratory investigations were unremarkable. A technetium brain scan, which was normal at admission, revealed an area of increased uptake in the right parieto-occipital region 10 days later (figure 4.1A). A four-vessel arteriogram showed the right angular branch of the middle cerebral artery to be occluded. A pneumoencephalogram was consistent with mild cerebral atrophy.

Case 2

A 65 year old, right-handed alcoholic man was brought to the accident floor by his landlord who reported the onset of confusion and incoherent speech four days previously. Before that time, the patient had been entirely self sufficient. The general medical examination was essentially unremarkable. The patient was fully awake but extremely inattentive and easily distractible. Neither a coherent stream of thought nor a coherent sequence of goal-directed behaviour could be maintained. He was initially agitated but this rapidly subsided into a state of placidity. Disorientation was noted in all spheres. Knowledge of remote and current world events, the ability to memorize, calculate, and abstract were all severely impaired. There was a mild naming difficulty and also dysgraphia in the absence of alexia, finger agnosia, or left–right confusion. Constructions were poorly performed. He showed severe deficits in his ability to make use of such common objects as matches or eating utensils. The gait was unsteady and retropulsive and urinary incontinence was occasionally present. The patient showed no concern for his predicament. Neglect of visual stimuli as well as minor deficits of graphaesthesia and stereognosis

could intermittently be demonstrated on the left. No elementary deficits in cranial nerve or in sensorimotor functions could be demonstrated. Laboratory investigations were essentially normal. A technetium scan of the brain revealed an area of increased isotope uptake in the right parietotemporal region (figure 4.1B); this abnormality disappeared 16 days after admission. The patient was unchanged at discharge, one month after the onset of his illness.

Case 3

A 74 year old right-handed male was admitted because of a sudden mental deterioration. He had been managing his personal and financial affairs successfully until the day of admission when he was discovered by his son in a disoriented and incoherent state, wearing nothing more than a necktie and a bed sheet. On admission, vital signs were unremarkable except for occasional premature ventricular contractions. The general examination showed signs of cardiomegaly and iridectomy. The mental status examination revealed minimal drowsiness, moderate inattentiveness, and agitation. The stream of thought was incoherent. His answers to questions were irrelevant and facetious. Disorientation was noted in all spheres. Details of a simple story could not be recalled five minutes later. Paraphasic errors as well as left–right confusion were noted. Cranial nerves and all sensorimotor functions, including the plantar response, were normal. There was no concern for this illness, despite the additional retropulsive gait and incontinence. Abnormal laboratory findings consisted of a blood urea nitrogen of 12.1 mmol/l, blood glucose of 16.3 mmol/l, bilirubin of 23.9 µmol/l. On the third hospital day, a brain scan showed an area of increased uptake in the right inferior frontal gyrus (figure 4.1C, D); this area was not present on a repeat brain scan six months later. A right carotid arteriogram was negative. A computerized axial tomography of

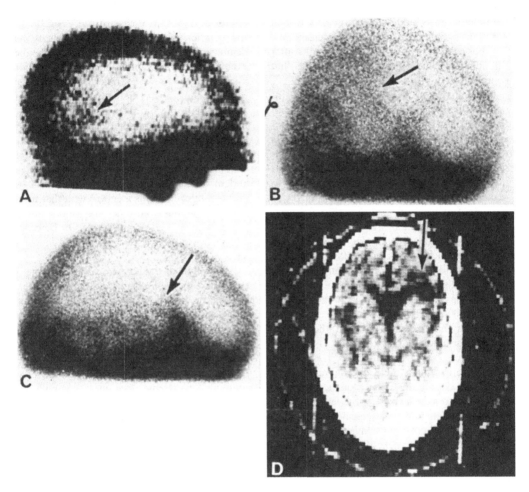

Figure 4.1

(*A*, *B*, and *C*) are right lateral radioisotope scans. The anterior part of the brain is to the right. (*A*) case 1; (*B*) case 2; (*C*) case 3. (*D*) is a computerized axial tomography picture of case 3. Arrows point towards the site of abnormality.

the brain localized an area in the inferior frontal gyrus of the right hemisphere with a density profile consistent with infarction. Six months after this admission, the patient was less confused but continued to display irritable sluggishness.

In summary, we have described three right-handed elderly male patients who presented with the acute onset of a confusional state. The salient and common symptoms included inattentiveness to relevant stimuli, distractibility by irrelevant stimuli, inability to grasp the immediate situation so as to react to it appropriately, inability to maintain either a coherent stream of thought or a coherent sequence of goal directed behaviour, disorientation, anomia, dysgraphia, abnormal gait, incontinence, difficulty in using common objects, and lack of concern for the illness. The level of arousal was never significantly depressed and the initial agitation rapidly resolved into a state of sluggishness. The deficits in memorizing and in intellectual functions which were also elicited may have been secondary to the inattentiveness during the testing situation. The lateralizing neurological signs were unimpressive and, indeed, were demonstrable intermittently, consisting of deficits in visual function, graphaesthesia, and stereognosis on the left. All three of these patients had radiological findings consistent with a recent right hemisphere infarct in the distribution of branches of the middle cerebral artery, two of these being situated in the general area of the inferior parietal lobule and one in the region of the inferior frontal gyrus.

Discussion

Clinical Considerations

The problem which brought each of these patients to the hospital consisted exclusively of behavioural abnormalities. In fact, the lateralizing neurological findings were so unimpressive that ACS secondary to toxic or metabolic encephalopathy was the diagnostic impression at admission in all three cases. Even when the initial agitation subsided, the left-sided deficits were demonstrable only intermittently. More detailed examination of perceptual and motor functions might well have revealed other left-sided deficits but the characteristic inattentiveness of the confused patients precluded such testing. In terms of the behavioural abnormality, moreover, the diagnosis of ACS was fully justified, since the impairments of mental status (agitation, inattentiveness, incoherent thought, cognitive deficits) and of higher cortical functions (anomia, dysgraphia, dyscalculia) is identical with that found in ACS resulting from other and more common causes (Engel and Romano, 1959; Lipowski, 1967; Chédru and Geschwind, 1972; Adams and Victor, 1974).

In addition to these cases with infarctions in the distribution of the middle cerebral artery, ACS have also been reported with occlusions of the posterior or anterior cerebral arteries (Hyland, 1933; Amyes and Nielsen, 1955; Horenstein et al., 1967; Medina et al., 1974). Our cases differ from these, since they displayed neither the persistent and extreme agitation, forced shouting, or extreme reaction to stimuli which have been noted in ACS resulting from occlusions of the posterior cerebral artery (Horenstein et al., 1967) nor the sexually inappropriate or markedly irrational behaviour described in occlusions of the anterior cerebral artery with softening in the medial frontal lobes (Hyland, 1933, case 1; Amyes and Nielsen, 1955, cases 3 and 4).

The small infarcts which our three patients suffered may be rather rare causes of ACS. In a busy neurological service, we have been able to find three definite and three other possible examples of this syndrome in a period of two years, while, during the same time, we have seen many dozens of ACS due to toxic, metabolic, traumatic, infectious, or post-ictal encephalopathies. It is conceivable that a significant number of such cases elude detection, since the paucity of elementary sensorimotor deficits in the presence of a very abnormal mental status may dissuade the primary physician from pursuing the possibility of focal neurological disease. The accurate diagnosis of these cases depends on a careful clinical assessment of focal deficits and on such laboratory investigations as the electroencephalogram, brain scan, and computerized axial tomography of the brain. Of course, each patient with an acute confusional state requires a meticulous medical assessment as well as laboratory evaluations of cerebrospinal fluid, blood, and urine, since most of these patients will suffer from a reversible toxic, metabolic, or infectious disorder which may become irreversible or fatal if not recognized and treated promptly.

Anatomical Considerations

The confusional state consists of a complex pattern of deficits in mental status. Attempts at reducing this syndrome into a disorder of one fundamental function will undoubtedly meet with objections. Nevertheless, the concept that the basic abnormality in ACS is a reduction and erratic shifting of attention (Chédru and Geschwind, 1972) is consistent with our clinical observations.

Although the definition of "attention" is fraught with controversy (Meldman, 1970), it is generally accepted that this construct denotes at least two distinct processes. One of these is *tonic* and regulates the threshold which a stimulus must exceed before gaining access to consciousness; the second is *phasic* (selective attention) and selects, from among the many stimuli which exceed this threshold, those which will occupy the centre of awareness. The *tonic* process of attention is closely related to the concept of 'arousal' and, in man, this component is severely impaired with focal infarcts in the dimesencephalic junction (Segarra, 1970). In our patients, this aspect of attention was relatively well preserved. On the other hand, the proper exercise of selective attention is a far more complicated task which requires the rapid and continuous integration of environmental cues and of internal stimuli with past experiences, present needs, and expectations about the future. Furthermore, an intact capacity for selective attention would be necessary for the production of a coherent stream of thought and for the maintenance of a coherent sequence of goal-directed behaviour. It is to be expected, therefore, that selective attention is coordinated, at least in part, at a cortical level and that the cortical areas in question are association regions of the highest order where information from many other areas of the brain converges. It is this function of selective attention which seemed preferentially impaired in our three cases.

Although pathological examination is not available, we infer, from radiological investigations, that the lesions primarily involve the inferior frontal gyrus (case 3) and the inferior parietal lobule (cases 1 and 2). Experimental data on the connections of cortex in primates is most readily available for the rhesus monkey, in which areas 45 and 46 of Walker (1940) and the banks of the caudal superior temporal sulcus may be homologous in man to the inferior frontal gyrus and inferior parietal lobule, respectively. Analysis of corticocortical connections of these areas in the monkey brain reveals that they constitute nodal sites for the convergence of afferent fibres from secondary and tertiary association cortices in the visual, somaesthetic, and auditory modalities (Pandya and Kuypers, 1969; Pandya and Vignolo, 1969; 1970; Jones and Powell, 1970; Van Hoesen et al., 1972; Chavis and Pandya, 1974). As a possible consequence of similar convergence of neocortical afferent pathways in man, the inferior frontal gyrus (Broca's area) and the inferior parietal lobule (angular and supramarginal gyri) in the left cerebral hemisphere have crucial roles in language functions (Geschwind, 1965) but ACS do not usually result when these areas are infarcted. It is tempting to speculate, on the basis of the present cases, that the same regions in the right hemisphere are indispensable for the complex integrative processes required for the effective execution of selective attention. The notion that right hemisphere mechanisms are particularly important in maintaining selective attention is further supported by studies showing that evoked responses to visual and somatosensory stimuli have greater amplitude in the right hemisphere of normal individuals (Schenkenbery et al., 1971). There is reasonable evidence to suggest that the amplitude of such evoked responses is an index of attention (Haider et al., 1964; Sakai et al., 1966).

The confusional states associated with anterior or with posterior cerebral artery occlusions may be analysed in similar fashion since, in the monkey, the cingulate gyrus which is irrigated by the anterior cerebral artery and the inferomedial temporal cortex supplied by the posterior cerebral artery also contain convergence areas for afferents from various high order association cortices (Van Hoesen et al., 1972). Furthermore, these regions also provide direct neocortical input into such limbic structures as the amygdala (Whitlock and Nauta, 1956; Pandya et al., 1973), presubiculum (Pandya et al., 1972), and the entorhinal cortex (Van Hoesen et al., 1972; Van Hoesen and Pandya, 1975). Whereas the deficit in selective attention in these cases of ACS may result from the involvement of corticocortical convergence areas, the additional features of extreme agitation or apathy and the psychosis-like inappropriate behaviour may be conceptualized as resulting from a disconnection of limbic structures from essential neocortical input. In contrast, the agitation in our three cases with infarctions in the inferior frontal gyrus or in the inferior parietal lobule, neither of which has direct connections with the limbic brain, was mild and transient; and psychosis-like behaviour was not observed.

On the basis of these observations, several locations in the human nervous system may be designated where focal lesions interfere with the process of attention. One such site is the dimesencephalic junction where an infarct will se-

verely impair "arousal" and the related function of *tonic* attention. On the other hand, lesions in the inferior parietal lobule, inferior frontal gyrus, medial frontal lobe and inferomedial temporal lobe will cause ACS with a global deficit in selective attention. By analogy with the connections of homologous areas in the monkey brain, each one of these cortical regions may be considered as a nodal convergence site for afferent fibres from association cortex. At this point, we could not exclude the possibility that circumscribed infarctions in still other cortical sites may produce ACS. Such sites would be likely, however, to have similar corticocortical connectivity patterns for the convergence of afferent fibres from multiple association cortices in order to have an influence on the process of selective attention. In turn, the differences in clinical manifestations would be expected to reflect the unique anatomical relationships of the involved region. Furthermore, lesions in still other convergence sites in the human brain could result in *unilateral* trimodal neglect as suggested by Heilman and Valenstein (1972). It could be argued that such lesions would involve areas where the thalamic input predominates over the callosal; whereas, in the regions implicated in the aetiology of ACS the converse may be true. The dominance of thalamic influence would favour a unilateral deficit, whereas powerful callosal input would explain the global nature of the resultant symptomatology. If unilateral neglect is considered a subset of impaired selective attention, then this explanation would be consistent with the previous discussion.

These anatomical speculations must remain tentative since, in the absence of pathological examination, we cannot exclude the possibility either of antecedent lesions or of simultaneous involvement of subcortical grey matter. However, neither the past medical history of our patients nor the known territories of the implicated arterial branches support these possibilities. Furthermore, there may exist significant misgivings about the possibility of localizing, indeed of identifying, as complex a process as 'selective attention'. The heuristic value of assuming that such a unitary function exists, and that it may be localized on the basis of anatomical connectivity patterns may be evaluated only in the light of future cases.

Acknowledgments

This work was supported in part by grants NB 06209 from the National Institute of Neurological Disease and Blindness, and NS 12307 and NS-00010 from the National Institute of Health.

We express our gratitude to Dr R. Duffield, Director of Nuclear Medicine at Boston City Hospital, for his gracious help in interpreting and making available the brain scans.

References

Adams, R. D., and Victor, M. (1974). Delirium and other confusional states. In *Principles of Internal Medicine*, pp. 149–156. Edited by M. M. Wintrobe, G. W. Thorn, R. D. Adams, E. Braunwald, K. J. Isselbacher, and R. G. Petersdorf. McGraw-Hill: New York.

Amyes, E. W., and Nielsen, J. M. (1955). Clinicopathologic study of vascular lesions of the anterior cingulate region. *Bulletin of the Los Angeles Neurological Society*, 20: 112–130.

Chavis, D., and Pandya, D. N. (1974). Frontal lobe projections of the cortical sensory association areas of the rhesus monkey. *Transactions of the American Neurological Association*, 99: 29–32.

Chédru, F., and Geschwind, N. (1972). Disorders of higher cortical functions in acute confusional states. *Cortex*, 8: 395–411.

Cohen, S. (1953). The toxic psychoses and allied states. *American Journal of Medicine*, 15: 813–828.

Engel, G. L., and Romano, J. (1959). Delirium, a syndrome of cerebral insufficiency. *Journal of Chronic Diseases*, 9: 260–277.

Geschwind, N. (1965). Disconnexion syndromes in animals and man. Part 1. *Brain*, 88: 237–294.

Haider, M., Spong, P., and Lindsley, D. B. (1964). Attention, vigilance, and cortical evoked potentials in humans. *Science*, 145: 180–182.

Heilman, K. M., and Valenstein, E. (1972). Frontal lobe neglect in man. *Neurology (Minneap.)*, 22: 660–664.

Horenstein, S., Chamberlain, W., and Conomy, J. (1967). Infarction of the fusiform and calcarine regions: agitated delirium and hemianopia. *Transactions of the American Neurological Association*, 92: 85–89.

Hyland, H. H. (1933). Thrombosis of intracranial arteries. *Archives of Neurology and Psychiatry (Chic.)*, 30: 342–356.

Jones, E. G., and Powell, T. P. S. (1970). An anatomical study of converging sensory pathways within the cerebral cortex of the monkey. *Brain*, 93: 793–820.

Lipowski, Z. J. (1967). Delirium, clouding of consciousness and confusion. *The Journal of Nervous and Mental Disease*, 145: 227–253.

Medina, J. L., Rubino, F. A., and Ross, A. (1974). Agitated delirium caused by infarction of the hippocampal formation and fusiform and lingual gyri: a case report. *Neurology (Minneap.)*, 24: 1181–1183.

Meldman, M. J. (1970). *Diseases of Attention and Perception*, Pergamon: London.

Pandya, D. N., Domesick, V. B., Van Hoesen, G. W., and Mesulam, M. (1972). Projection of the cingulate gyrus and cingulum in the rhesus monkey. *Anatomical Records*, 172: 379.

Pandya, D. N., and Kuypers, H. G. J. M. (1969). Cortico-cortical connections in the rhesus monkey. *Brain Research*, 13: 13–36.

Pandya, D. N., Van Hoesen, G. W., and Domesick, V. B. (1973). A cingulo-amygdaloid projection in the rhesus monkey. *Brain Research*, 61: 369–373.

Pandya, D. N., and Vignolo, L. A. (1969). Interhemispheric projections of the parietal lobe in the rhesus monkey. *Brain Research*, 15: 49–65.

Pandya, D. N., and Vignolo, L. A. (1970). Intra- and interhemispheric projections of the parietal, premotor and arcuate areas in the rhesus monkey. *Brain Research*, 26: 217–233.

Pearce, J., and Miller, E. (1973). *Clinical Aspects of Dementia*, p. 41. Baillière Tindall: London.

Sakai, M., Gindy, K., and Dustman, R. (1966). Amplitude change of components of the visually evoked response as related to mental state. *Proceedings of the American Psychological Association*, 2: 139–140.

Schenkenberg, T., Dustman, R. E., and Beck, E. C. (1971). Changes in evoked responses related to age, hemisphere and sex. *Electroencephalography and Clinical Neurophysiology*, 30: 163.

Segarra, J. M. (1970). Cerebral vascular disease and behavior. *Archives of Neurology*, 22: 408–418.

Van Hoesen, G. W., and Pandya, D. N. (1975). Some connections of the entorhinal (area 28) and perirhinal (area 35) cortices of the rhesus monkey. 1. Temporal lobe afferents. *Brain Research*, 95: 1–24.

Van Hoesen, G. W., Pandya, D. N., and Butters, N. (1972). Cortical afferents to the entorhinal cortex of the rhesus monkey. *Science*, 175: 1471–1473.

Walker, A. E. (1940). A cytoarchitectural study of the prefrontal area of the macaque monkey. *Journal of Comparative Neurology*, 73: 59–86.

Whitlock, D. G., and Nauta, W. J. H. (1956). Subcortical projections from the temporal neocortex in *Macaca mulatta. Journal of Comparative Neurology*, 104: 183–212.

V NOVELS, POEMS, AND COSMIC MURALS

Where does the brain end, and the mind begin? How does activity within the brain contribute to our experience of the external world? The following paper, derived from work I did as a resident with Norman Geschwind, explores this topic.

Temporal lobe epilepsy (also called "limbic" epilepsy) arises from a region of the brain called the temporal lobe. This is part of the "emotional" or limbic part of the cerebral cortex, whose activity contributes to the preservation of the individual and the continuation of the species. Activities in the limbic cortex contribute to feeding behavior, "fight-or-flight" responses, aggression, and sexual behavior. The limbic system is ancient, having evolved much earlier than other parts of the cortex and it is well developed even in species much more primitive than mammals. Parts of the limbic system are devoted to olfaction (the sense of smell) and taste, the oldest senses from an evolutionary point of view. Because of its important role in controlling self-serving and emotionally charged behaviors, one neuroanatomist termed the limbic system "a suburb of hell within the brain."

Seizures arising from the temporal lobe, within the limbic system, occur in only a small proportion of patients with epilepsy. Reflecting the close association of the limbic system with the older parts of the brain that are devoted to taste and smell, these "temporal lobe" or "limbic" seizures often begin with an "aura" in which the patient experiences an unusual, and sometimes unpleasant, sensation. Temporal lobe seizures frequently include other features, for example, lip-smacking, that reflect the limbic system's role in behaviors such as feeding. There is usually a loss of consciousness, but convulsive, shaking movements may not be present. Notably, temporal lobe seizures often include an "affective" component, that is, a profound sensation of fear, dread, or pleasure.

In the majority of patients with epilepsy, seizures are the only manifestation of a disorder of the nervous system. Between seizures (in the "interictal" periods), these individuals are no different than anyone else and there is nothing special about their behavior. Norman Geschwind, the director of the Harvard Neurology Service at Boston City Hospital, however, had noted a very different situation in patients with temporal lobe epilepsy. Geschwind described striking behavioral changes in these patients: a tendency to write incessantly and to produce voluminous writings, an unusual need to deal with things in great detail, and a preoccupation with deep philosophical thoughts. He talked about this frequently on his teaching rounds, and I first heard about it while I worked with and learned from him as a resident in 1972. My entreaty for a reference about the subject was met with a puff on his pipe and a shrug of his shoulders: "It's not in the literature, Steve, but these patients are a dime a dozen."

Being trained as a scientist, my first instinct was to ask myself if these changes in fact were present. Because of this, I modified the way in which I took case histories and began systematically to ask my patients about their behavior between seizures (an unusual step for a neurologist because seizures were considered to be important, but not the periods between them). I could not discern any unusual patterns of behavior in patients with epilepsy that did not involve the limbic parts of the brain. But in patients with temporal lobe epilepsy, the answers were as predicted by Geschwind. These patients displayed profound changes in behavior, associated with dysfunction in a specific part of the brain. When asked whether she ever wrote, one patient brought a shopping bag full of her handwritten notes to the hospital; this was especially striking because she had not finished high school. Some patients wrote poetry, and in some cases they wrote dozens of poems each day. Others kept notebooks, often many volumes in length. One patient brought us a multivolume diary, with other typewritten notebooks including "addenda" and "special incidents" that were cross-referenced to it. Several patients had written novels—not yet published, and, judging from the samples I saw, unlikely to be published. And one had hired a stenographer because he could not write fast enough to keep up with his thoughts. Several patients wrote in mirror writing to conceal their very private thoughts, another repeatedly drew pictures of scenes that had special meaning for her, and one drew "cosmic murals" because words could not connote the depth of his feelings.

The preoccupation with detail in these patients was evident both from interviews (which often took hours because of their need to describe events and feelings in great detail, a characteristic called "stickiness" in the psychiatric literature) and from their writings: "For this month of March I have had ten (10) sexual non-fearing five (5) second seizures." The philosophical concerns of these patients were evident in their behavior and in their writings. One patient had interrupted a sermon at his church, where he mounted the pulpit to debate his pastor's liturgical teachings; he had to be escorted out. Another brought typed copies of two sermons that he had delivered at his church at his own request; the first was called "The meaning within" and the second "The meaning Deeper within." A third patient had written a novel on "Good and Evil, Man's Place in the World."

Geschwind and I believed, and I still believe, that this syndrome may be able to teach us some important lessons about the brain and its role in experiential behavior. In describing this syndrome, we tried to indicate that it was not necessarily an "abnormality" and explicitly noted that "we have described this syndrome as one of behavioral change in temporal lobe epilepsy rather than as a syndrome of behavioral disorder.... The changes are not necessarily maladaptive" (Waxman and Geschwind 1975).

Our description of this syndrome was, and still is, widely quoted. But despite our efforts to be accurate and nonjudgmental, this work remains controversial, probably the most controversial that I have published. Other investigators carried out studies on large numbers of patients (Bear and Fedio 1977) which provided additional evidence for the existence of the interictal syndrome and it is widely accepted within the psychiatric literature, but many neurologists have remained skeptical.

Because some researchers suggested that the "interictal syndrome" was not truly associated with temporal lobe epilepsy, but was a random occurrence that we had inappropriately tied to temporal lobe epilepsy, we did a follow-up study eight years later. This study (Sachdev and Waxman 1981) was meant to be a writer's Rorschach test. We sent a letter to all patients who had been discharged from the hospital with the diagnosis of epilepsy and asked them to "describe to the best of your ability, your present state of health, understanding of your seizure disorder, and the changes in your life resulting from it. You may choose to write as much as you wish, in any form, on any kind of paper." We enclosed a return, stamped envelope. Among the patients who responded, the results were striking: out of seventeen patients who replied to our letter, nine had temporal lobe epilepsy. In contrast, out of thirty-three patients who did not reply, only seven had temporal lobe epilepsy. Two patients sent us unusually long responses (5540 words and 4200 words long, respectively), and both of them had temporal lobe epilepsy. Three other patients sent responses of more than four hundred words, and all of them had temporal lobe epilepsy. Only patients with temporal lobe epilepsy, therefore, had taken the time to write more than four hundred words. We blindly (without knowledge of the type of epilepsy) scored the responses and here, too, the results were dramatic. Three of the responses referred to philosophical or religious themes, and one to "waves from flying saucers controlling my thoughts," and all of these were sent by patients with temporal lobe epilepsy.

How profoundly can the interictal syndrome affect behavior? Geschwind argued that Dostoyevsky suffered from temporal lobe epilepsy (Geschwind 1984). Prince Myshkin's descriptions of his seizures in *The Idiot* include detailed documentation of the subjective experience of temporal lobe epilepsy; they far exceed anything that was available in the medical literature of the time and were almost certainly written by a person who had experienced temporal lobe seizures. Geschwind argued that the depth of Dostoyevsky's feelings arose (at least in part) from his temporal lobe epilepsy. Dostoyevsky referred, in fact, to his "nervous disturbances" and suggested that "in such a state I could write much more and much better than usual" (Dostoyevsky 1915; Devinsky 1991).

A parallel may be present in the work and life of the O. Henry Award-winning writer Thom Jones. Speaking about his own temporal lobe epilepsy, he noted "before my injury, I wasn't . . . obsessed with God and the meaning of life. . . . Ever since this happened to me I've been . . . more introspective, constantly reading philosophy, studying world religions and then having a fever, literally a fever to write" (Angier 1993).

Can temporal lobe epilepsy contribute to the creativity of the artist? It has been suggested that the artist Van Gogh suffered from temporal lobe epilepsy (Koshbin 1986). This artistic genius, according to Khoshbin, displayed all the characteristics of the interictal syndrome. I have seen several patients who, interestingly, also expressed themselves by drawing rather than writing; none of them, however, were Van Goghs.

We can never know, for sure, whether Dostoyevsky's genius and Van Gogh's unique talents arose from their temporal lobe epilepsy. Certainly, experience must have shaped part of their talent. But, on the other hand, their innate and unique behavior, resting in part on the function of their brains, contributed to their creativeness. The interictal syndrome of temporal lobe epilepsy, and the questions that it raises, exemplify the complexity, ambiguity, and importance of the borderland between neurology and psychiatry, and the richness of the mind-brain problem.

References

Angier, N. In the temporal lobes, seizures and creativity. *New York Times*, October 18, 1993.

Bear D. M., and Fedio, P. Quantitative analysis of interictal behavior in temporal lobe epilepsy. *Arch. Neurol* 34: 454–467, 1977.

Dostoyevsky, F. M. "Letters to His Family and Friends." E. C. Mayne, translator. New York: Macmillan, 1915.

Devinsky, O. Interictal behavioral changes in epilepsy. pp 1–21 in O. Devinsky and W. H. Theodore (eds.), *Epilepsy and Behavior*, Wiley-Liss, New York, 1991.

Geschwind, N. Dostoyevsky's epilepsy. In D. Blumer (ed.), *Psychiatric Aspects of Epilepsy.* Washington, D.C.: American Psychiatric Press, 325–334, 1984.

Khoshbin, S. Van Gogh's malady and other cases of Geschwind's syndrome. *Neurology* 36 (Suppl. 1), 213, 1986.

Sachdev, H. S., and Waxman, S. G. Frequency of hypergraphia in temporal lobe epilepsy: an index of interictal behavior syndrome. *J. Neurol. Neurosurg. Psychiat.* 44: 358–360, 1981.

Sacks, O. *An Anthropologist on Mars.* New York: Alfred A. Knopf, 1995.

Waxman, S. G., and Geschwind, N. Hypergraphia in temporal lobe epilepsy. *Neurology* 14: 629–637, 1974.

Waxman, S. G., and Geschwind, N. The interictal behavior syndrome of temporal lobe epilepsy. *Arch. Gen. Psychiat.* 32: 1580–1586, 1975.

5 Hypergraphia in Temporal Lobe Epilepsy

Stephen G. Waxman and Norman Geschwind

Article abstract   The phenomenon of hypergraphia, or the tendency toward extensive and, in some cases, compulsive writing in temporal lobe epilepsy is described in seven patients, in each of whom there was electroencephalographic demonstration of a temporal lobe focus. Unusually detailed and strikingly copious writing was evidenced in each patient. Six patients provided documentation of their extensive writing, which often was concerned with religious or moral issues. A seventh patient claimed to have written extensively, but refused to exhibit his writings. Aggressiveness, religiosity, and changes in sexual behavior in temporal lobe disorders have been described previously. The hypergraphia of temporal lobe epilepsy appears to be part of a specific behavioral syndrome of special interest because of its association with dysfunction at specific anatomic loci.

There is general agreement that specific personality changes are not seen in all forms of epilepsy. Several authors, however, have described certain distinctive personality traits that may be found in patients with temporal lobe epilepsy. Previous reports have dealt with aggressiveness,[1-3] changes in sexual behavior,[4-6] and religiosity[7] associated with temporal lobe disorders. These findings suggest that the behavioral changes in temporal lobe epilepsy do not represent a nonspecific "chronic brain syndrome," but rather represent a distinct behavioral syndrome in which affective response is deepened in the presence of relatively preserved intellectual function. We believe that characterization of this syndrome is of importance, not only in terms of understanding the psychiatric implications of epilepsy, but also as an example of a human behavioral disorder associated with damage at specific sites in the central nervous system. The present paper describes still another characteristic of the interictal behavior of patients with temporal lobe disorders, hypergraphia, or the tendency toward extensive and, in some cases, compulsive writing.

In this paper we present seven case histories that illustrate the phenomenon of hypergraphia in temporal lobe epilepsy. In six cases (cases 1 to 6), the patients provided striking documentation of their unusual writing. The seventh patient (case 7) volunteered that he wrote extensively but, as was true of several patients we have seen, was reluctant to exhibit his writings.

Reprinted with permission from *Neurology* 24: 629–637, 1974. Copyright 1974, by The New York Times Media Company, Inc.

Case 1

This 24-year-old right-handed woman began to have seizures at age 10 and to exhibit behavioral disturbances at age 15. Her father and paternal aunt were reported to have epilepsy, but her siblings apparently were well. At the age of 10, the patient began to have generalized seizures, often beginning with focal twitching of the left arm and face, on some occasions associated with lip-smacking or chewing movements, and followed by urinary incontinence and tongue biting. Neurologic examination, lumbar puncture, skull films, and brain scan were reportedly normal, but electroencephalogram (EEG) showed a right anterior temporal spike focus. She was treated with various anticonvulsants but continued to have seizures at a frequency of about one per month. At the age of 15, the patient was admitted to a hospital after slashing her wrist. In the following year, her grades in school deteriorated. When she was 17 years old, the patient again was admitted to a hospital because of confused and agitated behavior following two brief left-sided seizures. There was no history of ingestion of drugs, toxins, or hallucinogens. She was noted to be "agitated, crying, incoherent ... (with) peculiar posturing," and she asked if she were on a spaceship or being controlled by radio.

Neurologic examination at that time revealed slight left facial weakness and slightly greater deep tendon reflexes on the left side. Skull x-rays were normal. A sonar scan was suggestive of some enlargement of the trigone of the left lateral ventricle. EEG showed slow waves and spikes bitemporally, more pronounced on the left. The patient was diagnosed as having an acute schizophrenic psychosis and was treated for several months with trifluoperazine hydrochloride. She was discharged on primidone, diphenylhydantoin, and phenobarbital.

In the ensuing four years, she continued to have seizures several times a month. During this period, the patient became devoutly religious and experienced at least five religious conversions, each of which she felt was of major importance. She also began to experience déjà vu feelings. An EEG at the age of 20 revealed a spike focus in the right anterior temporal lobe.

The patient was admitted to hospitals twice at the age of 21 because of seizures; on both occasions she had failed to take her anticonvulsant medication. She described an aura consisting of a sensation of epigastric distress and a feeling of fear before her seizures. She now admitted to visual hallucinations of blue-green flashing lights moving from left to right in the right visual field. The hallucinations often, but not always, were followed by seizures. The patient professed great interest in mystical issues and in particular in the meaning of her existence and in the fate of the universe. She also complained of having no interest in sexual activities.

Neurologic examination revealed no focal deficits. All language performances were normal; constructions were fairly well done, calculations were performed reasonably well, and memory was normal. Results of hemogram, urinalysis, and routine blood chemistries were normal. Serum thyroxin, cortisol, and B_{12} levels were normal, and serology gave negative results. A chest x-ray and skull x-rays were unremarkable. Results of lumbar puncture were normal. An EEG revealed prominent sharp waves over both hemispheres.

When questioned about writing, the patient stated that she usually spent at least several hours per day writing things down. She dated the onset of this behavior at age 15, and felt that it was nearly coincident with the development of her interest in religion. She stated that she often wrote things down because "I want to be sure of what I do." She carried several tablets of writing paper with her at all times. She often recorded, in her writing pads or scraps of paper, what she had done in the preceding few hours "especially if I believe a seizure is coming on so I couldn't memorize it." She described in detail her seizures, hallucinations, and feelings of déjà vu. She often made lists, and produced catalogs of her records, or songs her father could play on the harmonica, of items of furniture in her apartment, of her relatives ("so I will know how many there are") and of her "likes" and "dislikes." She also often wrote poetry, usually with a moral or philosophical theme. She had the impression that the act of writing might abort her seizures, but did not feel that the content of what she wrote was important in this regard. Usually, she did not interrupt other activities to write, but she did recount having written at least several hundred times the words of a song she had learned at 17, using whatever was available (scraps of paper, napkins) and, in several cases, interrupting other activities to do so. She also reported sometimes feeling compelled to write a word over and over or to copy, once or several times, the printed labels on items she purchased. Some of her writing was reversed (mirror writing) (figure 5.1). The patient stated that she had never written in the reversed manner before development of her seizures. She denied other compulsive or ritualistic actions but did describe herself as very meticulous. She claimed to read only rarely.

Case 2

This right-handed man began at age five to have "staring spells" lasting about 30 seconds. His father reportedly had had three seizures when he

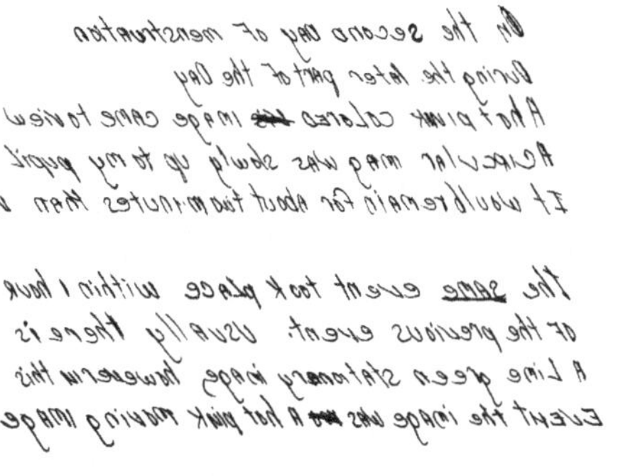

[The following text appears in mirror-reversed writing in the figure:]

In the second day of menstruation during the later part of the day. After a pink colored image came to view. A vascular map was shown up to my eyes. It would remain for about two minutes. Then vanish.

The same event took place within I hour of the previous event. Usually there is a time green stationary image, however this event the image was a hot pink moving image

Figure 5.1
Reversed writing of patient 1 describes visual hallucinations. The description may be read by holding the page up to a mirror.

was 20 years old, but his mother and his 12 siblings had no history of neurologic disorder. Petit mal epilepsy was diagnosed initially and was treated with phenobarbital for about two years. The staring spells abated at age six and the patient was well until age 18, when on two occasions he assaulted siblings, claiming afterwards to have no recollection of the assaultive behavior. Between the ages of 18 and 23, he experienced almost daily seizures, consisting of staring spells and stiffening of the body, during which he was aware of his surroundings but was unable to respond; these episodes were preceded by an aura in which the patient experienced a sensation of profound fear and sexual pleasure. He also exhibited occasional psychomotor automatisms, during which he behaved inappropriately with no awareness of his behavior. Surface and depth electrode EEGs revealed bilateral anterior and midtemporal spike activity that in some recordings predominated on the left.

The patient responded poorly to treatment with anticonvulsant medications. At age 23 he underwent a left temporal lobectomy. Pathologic examination revealed a cystic cavity of the temporal white matter with hypertrophy of astrocytes in the neighboring cortex and white matter. After the lobectomy, he was relieved of his star-

ing spells, although he continued to experience episodic sensations of fear and sexual excitement similar to his previous auras. No further psychomotor episodes occurred. Postoperatively, neurologic examination showed a homonymous right upper visual field deficit, and a mild impairment of recent and remote memory (Memory Quotient, Wechsler Memory Scale 103 preoperatively, 86 postoperatively; Wechsler Adult Intelligence Scale (WAIS) Full Scale IQ 90 preoperatively, 99 postoperatively) that did not interfere with his performance as a truck loader. The patient was married, but has experienced difficulty in deriving pleasure from sexual intercourse with his wife.

The patient has kept copious notes on his disorder. At age 23, several months before his lobectomy, the patient's notes contain entries primarily on the days of seizures, and the descriptions are of the form: "_____ said I had another seizure in my sleep. Matches on night table gone in morning. I found empty match pack by bed. I had to have touched them in my sleep," or "I had a seizure while sitting on the toilet." There are also some lists with dates, followed either by the word "seizure" and the time of day it occurred, or by the word "OK" if there was no seizure. One year after surgery (age 24) the lists appear more ritualized and have clear religious overtones. Thus, each day of the month is listed on a separate line, followed either by the time of the seizures (which occurred less than 10 times per month) or by the carefully and stereotypically written phrase "Thank "GOD"— none." The words on each line are in nearly perfect register with the words of the lines above and below. Each page is signed by the patient. Each month's list is followed by a total "_____ seizures" and by a summary, e.g., "For this month of _____ I have had only one (1) sexual fear seizure which only lastted five (5) seconds. . . ." [parentheses and misspellings as in the patient's original notes]. One year later (figure 5.2) the references to days without seizures are still ritualized but more elaborate: "I thank

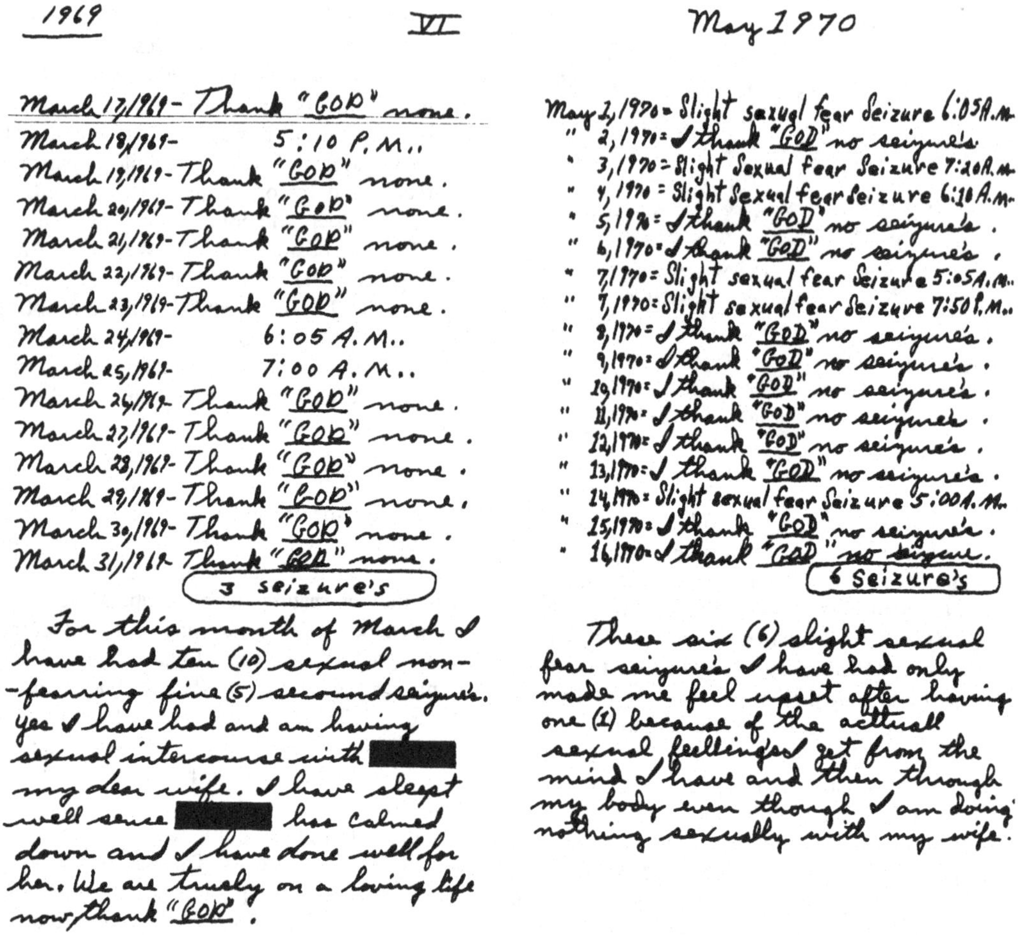

1969   VI   May 1970

March 17/1969- Thank "GOD" none.

May 1, 1970= Slight sexual fear Seizure 6:05 A.M.

March 18/1969-   5:10 P.M..

" 2, 1970= I thank "GOD" no seizure's

March 19/1969- Thank "GOD" none.

" 3, 1970= Slight Sexual fear Seizure 7:20 A.M.

March 20/1969- Thank "GOD" none.

" 4, 1970 = Slight sexual fear Seizure 6:30 A.M.

March 21/1969- Thank "GOD" none.

" 5, 197= I thank "GOD" no seizure's.

March 22/1969- Thank "GOD" none.

" 6, 1970= I thank "GOD" no seizure's.

March 23/1969- Thank "GOD" none.

" 7, 1970= Slight sexual fear Seizure 5:05 A.M.

March 24/1969-   6:05 A.M..

" 7, 1970= Slight sexual fear Seizure 7:50 P.M..

March 25/1969-   7:00 A.M..

" 8, 1970= I thank "GOD" no seizure's

March 26/1969- Thank "GOD" none.

" 9, 1970= I thank "GOD" no seizure's

March 27/1969- Thank "GOD" none.

" 10, 1970= I thank "GOD" no seizure's.

March 28/1969- Thank "GOD" none.

" 11, 197= I thank "GOD" no seizure's.

March 29/1969- Thank "GOD" none.

" 12, 197= I thank "GOD" no seizure's.

March 30/1969- Thank "GOD" none.

" 13, 1970= I thank "GOD" no seizure's.

March 31/1969- Thank "GOD" none.

" 14, 197= Slight sexual fear Seizure 5:00 A.M.

(3 Seizure's)

" 15, 197= I thank "GOD" no seizure's

" 16, 197= I thank "GOD" no seizure.

(6 Seizure's)

For this month of March I have had ten (10) sexual non-fearing five (5) second seizure's. Yes I have had and am having sexual intercourse with ▮▮▮ my dear wife. I have slept well sence ▮▮▮ has calmed down and I have done well for her. We are truely on a loving life now, thank "GOD".

These six (6) slight sexual fear seizure's I have had only made me feel upset after having one (1) because of the actuall sexual feellings I get from the mind I have and then through my body even though I am doing nothing sexually with my wife.

Figure 5.2
Two pages from the extensive notes kept by patient 2. The page on the left was written at age 24, one year after temporal lobectomy. The page on the right was written one year later. Note the more elaborate entries in the latter record.

"GOD" no seizures." There are now elaborate addenda to each month's record, with frequent use of underlined words, and words written entirely in capital letters or in red so as to stand out from the remainder of the text. Five years after the operation, the diary is much the same, although the daily entries ("I do thank dear "GOD" above, no seizures") are slightly more elaborate.

Case 3

This right-handed man suffered from grand mal and psychomotor seizures beginning at age 13. A cousin had a history of epilepsy. EEGs revealed a spike focus in the right temporal tip with lesser spike activity in the right posterior temporal area. Seizures were not adequately controlled with anticonvulsant medication, and a right temporal lobectomy was performed at the age of 40. Postoperatively, the EEGs showed spike activity over the right low central area. Grand mal seizures no longer occur, but psychomotor seizures occur nocturnally once every 7 to 10 days. The patient has been followed psychiatrically by Dr. D. Blumer for a period of eight years beginning seven years after the operation. The patient volunteered a log of his daily events, and was noted to be "verbose but at the same time highly circumspect and meticulous in his statements. Thus, when he was asked what he would do if he saw a fire in a theater ... he answered with good judgment but made sure he had pinned down all the possibilities, such as ... whether the fire was large or small, had just begun or had been going on for some time." (Blumer, 1974)

Examination of this patient's daily notes showed them to be highly meticulous, with great attention to detail. Each sheet records in carefully typed text, a day-by-day account of the patient's experiences. For example: "It was cool last night so I opened the windows and left the air conditioner off. I had a very bad night. I was awake about every two hours. I hung three pictures today on three 3/4 screws I put in the wall. It made me so weak I had to lay down. I slept for two hours." Some phrases are underlined or typed in red for emphasis. As in case number 2, there is frequent use of parenthetical expressions to qualify or clarify the meaning of words; thus, "On weekends (Sat. and Sun.) I don't go walking." The single-spaced, typed record of daily events is 1,000 to 2,000 words in length for most months and often has pencilled notes following it. In addition, typed addenda to each month's record, in many cases 450–500 words long, describe in greater detail the patient's dreams. There are also lengthy, detailed accounts of experiences or "incidents" that the patient felt were of specific importance. At the end of each month's day-by-day account, a summary includes detailed "generalizations" (figure 5.3).

Case 4

This right-handed man began to have seizures at age 18, several months after being struck on the head with a heavy metal object. One brother died shortly after birth; there were no other siblings, and neither of the parents had epilepsy.

The patient had a history of numerous assaultive episodes for which he had spent several years in prison. The patient's seizures, which were generalized and included tongue-biting and incontinence, were preceded by either a "rising" or "fluttering" epigastric sensation or by a tingling sensation over the lips and face, sometimes associated with a feeling of derealization or falling or rising off the ground. Lip-smacking was observed during some seizures. The patient often experienced feelings of déjà vu but denied olfactory or gustatory hallucinations. There had been one episode of auditory hallucinations, thought to be due to acute alcohol withdrawal. The patient was treated with diphenylhydantoin and chlordiazepoxide. His seizures occurred up to two times per month.

June 5 - I have taken Valeum as perscribed. one morning and one evening. I slowly became
less irritible and less nervous. ▓▓▓▓ noticed the change also. The pain in my
right chest almost gone. Only slightly sore when pressed on. My legs still
quiver when I lay down.

June 9 - I took a walk this morning (8:30 to 9:30) when the sun was weak. This afternoon
I had to take a nap for an hour (1:00 to 2:00) I was too sleepy to stay awake
I will be glad when I can stop taking this valeum. It makes me awful sleepy
and tired. I will be glad when I can stop taking it.

June 11 - This is the last night I am to take Valeum. Only one at 8:00 A.M. untill my next
visit. I am glad . They make me feel sleepy and slow. The slowness I can fight
off. The pain in my chest is gone and I feel much better,more quiet and a lot
less irritible.

June 12 - This morning I woke with a slight pain in my right chest (center and bottom)
and a slight morning pain in my heart. As I became fully awake and had breakfast
the pains left.(Valeum at 8:00). I also rember Post nasel drip in my sleep.

June 13 - No pain in my chest this morning. Doing fine on one pill at 8:00 A.M.

June 14 - The sun is rising earler each day giving me less time to go out in the morning
Today I was out too long (8:30 to 11:00). Then I came in I ate lunch and went
to bed. I slept for two hours. I felt better wner I woke. At bedtime my face
and head felt hot (like sunburn).

June 15 - Today was a cloudy and cool day. A beautiful day for a walk. This afternoon
the sun came out. By the time I got home , then met ▓▓▓▓ (in the shade of
a big tree). I was tired when I got home and went to bed for 1½ hours.My chest
cavity and lungs quivered. I had suppersed rested in bed . By bed time (9:30)
most of the quivering was gone and I was tired.

June 21 - This morning it was 9/10 cloudy and looked like rain. I dresses and caught the
9:20 bus and went to the Post Office.The sun came out as I was waiting for the
buss to come home. I stood in a doorway out of the sun and cought the buss. I
got home at 11:20, had lunch at 12:00 and worked on stamps in my bedroom all
afternoon . I met ▓▓▓▓ at 5:15 and we came home. I felt fair.

June 22 - I woke at 3:00 A.M. I felt slept out. Just a very slight quiver in my legs.
I fell back to sleep for a few naps and got up at 6:15. I stayed in today
(sunny). The air conditioner did so much good yesterday I have it on this
afternoon again. I took a nap after supper and slept untill 11:00 wher
▓▓▓▓ woke me for pills (ehich I forgot). I turned the conditioner off then
went back to sleep untill 3:00 A,M. then cat naped untill 6:1".

June 23 - Another cloudy day which I took advantage of. Walked from 9:30 untill noon.
then had lunch andafter a little rest walking again untill 2:00 when the sun
came out. I came in and had a short nap (1 hour) with the air conditioner
cooling things off.At bedtime the quivering in my legs was almost gone leaving
them feeling thick and week.

Genelerisation

The sunshine makes me week in general and the nervs in my limbs, mostly legs,
quiver. The severity depending upon exposer to sun (length of time and strength
of the suns rays) .A nap in a rather cool air conditioned room will bring
back my strength. The quivering of the nervs takes longer to stop. Very graduall
becoming weeker. This takes two or three days depending upon severity.My skin
also feels like sunburn even where not exposed (mid section of body) when the
quivering lets uo I t leaves my limbs feeling week espicially my hands if exposed
   The days are getting longer and the sun stronger. This gives me less time
for walking or going outside at all.

   The pains in my chest are gone and I am not as irritible. Only a very slight
warning pain in my heart when I wake after recovery from a sun exposure.
        Please look at eyeye.

Figure 5.3

One of the monthly records produced by patient 3. The patient kept several copies of each page. Note the frequent
use of parenthetical expressions. Following the day-by-day account is a set of "generalisations."

At the age of 31, normal results on cranial nerve, motor, and sensory examinations were recorded. There was mild dysmetria on finger-nose testing bilaterally. Lumbar puncture and skull x-rays were normal. An EEG showed bilateral slow waves, with sharp waves over the right anterior temporal region.

A brain scan four years later was normal. Neurologic examination showed intact cranial nerves, motor and sensory function. The patient's speech and memory were normal. Calculations were performed fairly well and constructions were done well. Moderate concreteness was noted in the interpretation of proverbs and in the judgment of similarities. The patient had attended art school for several years. At age 19, he was married and later had two children, but he was divorced five years later. He became deeply interested in "black magic," but limited his participation in this because he believed occult practices might cause "funny things to happen." The patient stated that he began writing extensively at the age of 17 or 18, keeping a diary and writing songs and poems. One of the songs, he stated, had been "taken" from him and published by a friend. Subsequently, he concealed most of his writings in various locations in his home. He often wrote aphorisms, on some occasions writing for several hours at a time and filling one of more sheets of paper (figure 5.4); he stated "once I start, I can't stop." He usually kept a pencil and paper with him, and reported having written the sentences "Why Can't A Man Live Before He Dies?" and "God Bless The Child That Has Its Own" many hundreds of times, on several occasions on newspapers or on the pages of books when blank paper was not available. He was unable to explain why he wrote these sentences, but stated that he felt they concerned "basic questions of life" that had interested him for many years. He denied ever having written anything during his seizures, but did report finding, in various hiding places in his home, notes that he did not recall having written.

Case 5

This ambidextrous man was well until he was 34 years old, when he developed headache, nausea, vomiting, and a right hemiparesis; he underwent multiple craniotomies for excision of a left temporoparietal brain abscess. Postoperatively he exhibited a right hemiparesis and sensory loss, right homonymous hemianopia, and a global aphasia. EEGs revealed left-sided theta activity; over the left anterior temporal leads, there was a marked delta-theta focus. He was treated initially with diphenylhydantoin and later phenobarbital. Three years after surgery, he was noted to have a mild right hemiparesis and sensory loss, with persistence of the right homonymous hemianopia. He exhibited an anomic aphasia, with difficulties with simple calculations and recognition of fingers, mild confusion between left and right, and dysgraphic writing. At this time, his hospital records noted that "he now expresses interest in religion and possibly in becoming a minister, and hopes to increase his 'use of good words' toward that end." He initially had occasional grand mal seizures, but beginning seven years postoperatively had episodes in which he was "dazed" and unaware of his surroundings, with tremors of the right face, arm, and, to a lesser degree, leg, without loss of consciousness. At this time he also reported seeing "multicolors," especially green and purple flashes, over the entire visual field. He denied visceral, gustatory, or olfactory hallucinations. The patient complained to his physicians of loss of interest in sexual activities. One year later the patient was still unemployed but was spending many hours per day in volunteer work for religious organizations, where he was involved primarily in making charts and graphs. He subsequently at his own suggestion delivered several sermons at his church. He spontaneously volunteered typed copies of the texts of these sermons to his physician. The sermons concerned

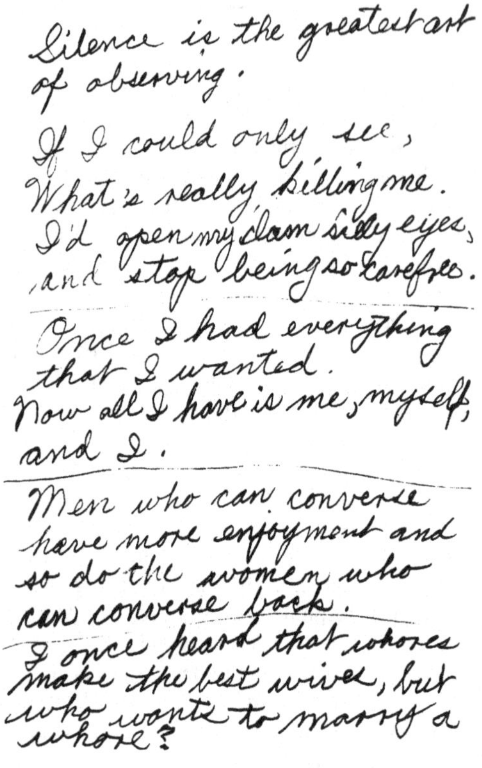

*Silence is the greatest art
of observing.*

*If I could only see,
What's really killing me.
I'd open my dam silly eyes,
and stop being so carefree.*

*Once I had everything
that I wanted.
Now all I have is me, myself,
and I.*

*Men who can converse
have more enjoyment and
so do the women who
can converse back.
I once heard that whores
make the best wives, but
who wants to marry a
whore?*

Figure 5.4

A page containing aphorisms, written by patient 4 while in the hospital. This patient produced many such pages, often spending hours at a time doing so, as well as recurrently writing certain sentences.

highly moral issues, which were dealt with in highly circumstantial and meticulous detail.

Specific reference is made in his writings to an "inner meaning" for certain events. Some words are underlined for emphasis, and others are written entirely in capitals. The meaning of words is emphasized and detailed, with frequent use of qualifying expressions in parentheses and with frequent digressions along secondary themes, which are often concerned with precise definitions or qualifications.

Case 6

This right-handed man with unilateral temporal lobe atrophy had episodic behavior disturbances. No family history of neurologic or psychiatric disease was elicited. The patient performed well in school until the age of 11, when his grades deteriorated. One year later, there was an episode of fuguelike state in which the patient walked 150 yards across a field, then pedaled his bicycle for a distance of four blocks with no awareness of his surroundings.

From the age of 11, he did poorly in school until age 17, at which time he enlisted in the armed services. He did well during his first three years, but at age 20 became involved in several altercations and subsequently was discharged. After his discharge, he began to experience episodes in which he was unaware of his behavior. During one of these episodes, without apparent aggravation, the patient continuously struck his head and fists against a brick wall for between three and five minutes. Shortly thereafter, he began to exhibit easily provoked rage. He was arrested on several occasions, charged with assaulting an officer and with causing considerable property damage. He was subsequently admitted to several psychiatric institutions, where he was treated with thioridazine and perphenazine. At age 24, he was evaluated neurologically. Cranial nerves and deep tendon reflexes were normal. Motor and sensory examination were unremarkable. Cerebellar function was thought to be normal but the patient deviated slightly to the left in tandem gait. The full scale WAIS IQ estimate was 109. A brain scan and skull x-rays were normal. A pneumoencephalogram with satisfactory ventricular filling showed enlargement of the lateral recess of the left temporal horn (10 mm in width anteriorly and posteriorly), while the remaining portions of the lateral ventricles, the third and fourth ventricles, and the cerebral gyri appeared normal. EEG recordings from sphenoidal electrodes revealed moderate to high amplitude sharp and spike discharges persistently from right and left temporal regions. The patient was treated with diphenylhydantoin and primidone, 750 mg per day, with only slight improvement, but following treatment with primidone 1,500 mg per day he has experienced a markedly decreased frequency in his seizures. He has had no further episodes of rage, but remains very sensitive to environmental stress.

At age 27 the patient recorded his subjective impressions of his illness. This was done by dictating to a public stenographer, "because I couldn't write fast enough." He dictated for a period of 17 hours beginning at 5 P.M. without stopping to eat and with only several brief intermissions of several minutes' duration. The result was a 56 page typed account, in meticulous and deeply emotional detail, of the patient's military service and subsequent hospitalizations. The patient reports having been fully aware of his behavior while dictating and denies any relation to a seizure. He reports having specifically omitted profanity from his account because the stenographer was a female. There have been no other episodes similar to the foregoing, but the patient claims to keep detailed lists of things he must do, and often makes written records of telephone calls.

Case 7

This right-handed man was well until age six, when he reportedly had a meningitis secondary to sinusitis, during which he had at least one convulsion. There was some question as to whether he may have had some minor spells of speech arrest for several months after this illness. The patient then remained in good health until age 14, when he contracted poliomyelitis with paralysis of his legs lasting two months, which resolved without neurologic sequelae. He received formal education in law and accountancy and as a clergyman.

At age 21 he was beaten around the head and rendered unconscious. Five years later, the patient began to have minor motor seizures, characterized by an absence spell preceded by an aura of a "vision of light." These spells occurred several times per week. Sometimes they were associated with a feeling of fear or sadness. A year later he began to have grand mal seizures, which occurred about once a month. Findings on general physical and neurologic examinations were normal. Skull x-rays suggested atrophy or hypoplasia of the left frontotemporal region. Electroencephalography initially showed bilateral temporal discharges, predominant on the right. A subsequent EEG with nasopharyngeal and sphenoidal leads revealed an active right anterior spike focus, and intravenous pentylenetetrazol (200 mg) resulted in a verbal report of the patient's visual aura, followed by an absence seizure during which the patient raised his trunk, rubbed the examiner's arm, and made chewing motions, with EEG activation in right sphenoidal electrodes. The patient's seizures were poorly controlled with medication, and at age 37 a right anterior temporal lobectomy was performed. Postoperatively, the patient no longer had major motor seizures, but did have occasional minor spells generally without aura, consisting usually of a brief absence seizure or, in some cases, of automatisms (on one occasion the patient disrobed in public). After the lobectomy, the patient showed markedly decreased interest in his law practice, and spent much of his time at home reading magazines and prayer books and listening to records. The patient was hospitalized one year later because of "paranoid outbursts" and "bizarre behavior." In the following four years, he was investigated at several hospitals because of a "generalized slowing down" and "less initiative." EEG revealed residual epileptic activity over the right midtemporal region. Five years after the operation, psychometric testing revealed a WAIS full-scale IQ of 109 (verbal 112; performance 104; memory quotient 114), normal performance on the Bender-Gestalt test, and a T-score of 79 on the Hunt-Minnesota Test for organic brain damage. Neurologic examination showed a slightly widened left palpebral fissure, mild left-sided hyperreflexia, and slight downward drift of the extended left arm. When asked to write a sentence about the weather, the patient wrote "Today's weather seems to be the epitome of 'April showers bring May's flowers,' with rain and nasty weather all day." When asked about writing, the patient showed his physician a copy of an outline for a novel. He refused, however, to discuss this further or to show a copy of the manuscript to his physician, stating that a previous novel he had written had been plagiarized by the faculty of a foreign university.

Discussion

The case histories summarized above are striking in that in each case there was an unusual tendency for the patient to write extensively, typically in a meticulous manner. Each of the authors has observed many other patients besides these seven in whom there was evidence for a temporal lobe disorder and who also wrote to an unusual degree. The literature contains numerous references to the circumstantial and pedantic character of the speech of temporal lobe epileptics. In describing a patient with psychomotor seizures, Kraepelin,[8] in 1906, noted that the patient "gives a connected, though very long-winded account of his condition." Similarly, Beard,[9] in his description of the schizophrenia-like psychoses in epilepsy, noted the speech of his patients to be "ponderous, circumstantial, pedantic, long-winded." Glaser,[10] in describing the performance of 37 patients with psychomotor temporal lobe epilepsy on a battery of psychologic tests, noted a pattern of striking similarities in the manner in which the patients responded to and performed the various tests, rather than a characteristic pattern of scores. Thus, Glaser notes that "many of the patients

were concerned with clarity of their thinking, and made significant efforts to control, restrict, or contain emotions and actions in order to become clear, accurate, and realistic." However, with the exception of a report by Blumer,[11] which includes examples of the written material produced by the patient described in case 3 above, we are aware of no studies that document the extensive writing of patients with temporal lobe disorders.

There is now a strong body of evidence indicating the existence of a striking syndrome of interictal personality changes characteristically occurring in temporal lobe epilepsy. Gibbs[12] reported an incidence of 49 percent of psychiatric disorders (32 percent "severe personality disorders," 17 percent "psychosis") among 163 patients with anterior temporal epileptic foci; psychiatric symptoms were three times more common than in patients with foci in other areas. Beard,[9] in a study of epileptics in whom schizophrenia-like psychoses had developed, noted a disproportionately high number of patients with temporal lobe disorders (48 of 69 patients exhibited electrographic evidence of temporal lobe foci). Other authors have questioned the presence of distinct personality changes in temporal lobe epileptics as compared with "non-psychomotor"[13] or "grand mal-petit mal" epileptics.[14] However, even in the study of Guerrant and associates,[15] which questions the presence of personality alterations in patients with temporal lobe epilepsy as compared with a nonepileptic hospital population, results show a striking difference between the psychologic "profiles" of temporal lobe epileptics and controls (Minnesota Multiphasic Personality Inventory profiles were judged as psychotic in 23 percent of the temporal lobe patients, as opposed to 4 percent of the controls).

The interictal personality changes often become manifest some years after the onset of seizures. Slater and Beard[16] reported a latency of 12.8 to 15.6 years (14.1 years average) between the onset of epilepsy and the onset of overt psychiatric symptoms. Glaser[10] reported a latency of six years. The behavioral alterations appear to reflect changes in affective or experiential function and specifically changes in the depth of emotional experience. Thus, a number of studies have reported changes in sexual function,[4–6,17] the frequent presence of religiosity,[7,18] and often a deepened interest in moral and ethical issues.[3] In addition, evidence for an unusual degree of aggressiveness exists in the interictal behavior of some patients with temporal lobe foci.[1,2,19] In this regard, it is interesting that the behavior of these patients is often remarkably well tolerated by their families, a fact that may reflect the capacity of these patients for striking emotional warmth as another aspect of their deepened emotional responses.

The extensive writing we have observed in temporal lobe patients may be explained, in part, on the basis of the above. The writings of four of the patients described have clear moral or religious overtones. The striking preoccupation with detail appears to reflect the importance accorded by the writer to his material. Little room is left for error. Thus, three of the patients (cases 2, 3, and 5) commonly use parenthetical expressions ("On weekends [Sat and Sun]...," or "five [5] seconds") to make the meaning of words absolutely clear. Words are defined, and sometimes redefined, several times. Underlining or writing in all capitals or red for emphasis is common in the material produced by three of the patients. Even minute details (for instance, the number and size of screws used to hang a picture) are accorded importance.

There is a compulsive quality to much of the written material we have examined. Patient 1 wrote down the words to a single song at least several hundred times. Similarly, patient 4 wrote two sentences repetitively. Patient 2 recorded, in a highly ritualized and compulsive fashion, the dates of his seizures. In the context of highly moralistic and/or religious beliefs in these patients, such compulsive acts are not unexpected. In this regard, it is interesting that one

patient (case 4) concealed many of his writings, and another (case 7) was reluctant to show his writings to his physicians.

A number of studies indicate the presence of memory deficits in patients with temporal lobe damage. This has been noted not only when bilateral lesions are present[20–22] but also has been seen after unilateral temporal lobectomies[23–25] and proven unilateral temporal infraction.[26] It might be argued that the extensive writings of our patients represent a compensatory mechanism for deficits in memory. This theory, however, does not explain the *content* (for instance, recurrently written words to songs) or the *form* ("I do thank dear "GOD" above, no seizures") of the writing. In addition, we have not observed extensive or compulsive writing in patients with other types of memory disorder.

We believe that the extensive and in some cases compulsive writing we have observed in temporal lobe epileptic patients reflects the previously documented deepening of emotional response in the presence of relatively preserved intellectual function. In this context, it is not surprising that, in speech, some temporal lobe epileptics are described as circumstantial or pedantic or as exhibiting "stickiness" or "viscosity."

The constellation of interictal behavioral changes in temporal lobe epilepsy is of interest for several reasons. Documentation of interictal changes may be as relevant to an understanding of epilepsy as a description of the seizures themselves. The occurrence of a well-defined syndrome of interictal personality changes in many cases of temporal lobe epilepsy suggests that the assessment of behavior itself may be of great value in diagnosis. In addition, the behavioral changes are of considerable theoretical interest, because they occur in association with disorders at *specific anatomic loci*. Similar changes commonly occur in patients with functional psychiatric disorders, particularly in schizophrenia. Indeed, a number of patients subsequently found to have temporal lobe disorders have been initially diagnosed as exhibiting "functional psychoses[27] (see also cases 1 and 6 above). Our understanding of the pathogenesis of the functional psychoses, and of schizophrenia in particular, is very incomplete at the present time. We believe that it is not unreasonable to expect that further clinical studies on temporal lobe epilepsy may yield information relevant to a fuller understanding of the mechanisms involved in some of the functional psychoses.

Acknowledgments

We wish to thank Drs. D. Blumer and V. Mark for making available case records on their patients.

Supported in part by NINDS grants NS 06209 and NS 5074.

References

1. Davidson GA: Psychomotor epilepsy. Can Med Assoc J 53: 410–414, 1947

2. Serafetinides EA: Aggressiveness in temporal lobe epileptics and its relation to cerebral dysfunction and environmental factors. Epilepsia 6: 33–42, 1963

3. Geschwind N: The clinical setting of aggression in temporal lobe epilepsy. In Fields WS, Sweet WH (Editors): The Neurobiology of Violence. St. Louis, Warren H. Green, 1974

4. Mitchell W. Falconer MA, Hill D: Epilepsy with fetishism relieved by temporal lobectomy. Lancet 2: 626–629, 1954

5. Davies BM, Morgenstern FS: A case of cysticercosis, temporal lobe epilepsy, and transvestism. J Neurol Neurosurg Psychiatry 23: 247–249, 1960

6. Blumer D: Hypersexual episodes in temporal lobe epilepsy. Am J Psychiatry 126: 1099–1106, 1970

7. Dewhurst K, Beard AW: Sudden religious conversions in temporal lobe epilepsy. Br J Psychiatry 117: 497–507, 1970

8. Kraepelin E: In Johnstone T (Editor): Lectures in Clinical Psychiatry. New York, William Wood and Co., 1906

9. Beard AW: The schizophrenia-like psychoses of epilepsy. II. Physical aspects. Br J Psychiatry 109: 113–130, 1963

10. Glaser GH: The problem of psychosis in psychomotor temporal lobe epileptics. Epilepsia 5: 271–278, 1964

11. Blumer D: Organic personality disorder. In Lion J (Editor): Severe Personality Disorders. Baltimore, The Williams & Wilkins Company, 1974

12. Gibbs FA: Ictal and non-ictal psychiatric disorders in temporal lobe epilepsy. J Nerv Ment Dis 113: 522–528, 1951

13. Mignone RJ, Donnelly EF, Sadorosky D: Psychological and neurological comparisons of psychomotor and non-psychomotor epileptic patients. Epilepsia 11: 345–359, 1970

14. Stevens JR: Psychiatric implications of psychomotor epilepsy. Arch Gen Psychiatry 14: 461–471, 1966

15. Guerrant J, Anderson WW, Fischer A, et al: Personality in Epilepsy. Springfield, IL, Charles C Thomas, 1962

16. Slater E, Beard AW: The schizophrenia-like psychoses of epilepsy. I. Psychiatric aspects. Br J Psychiatry 109: 95–112, 1963

17. Hierons R, Saunders M: Impotence in patients with temporal lobe epilepsy. Lancet 2: 761–764, 1966

18. Geschwind N: Effects of temporal lobe surgery on behavior. N Engl J Med 289: 480–481, 1973

19. Taylor DC: Aggression and epilepsy. J Psychosom Res 13: 229–236, 1969

20. Scoville WB, Milner B: Loss of recent memory after bilateral hippocampal lesions. J Neurol Neurosurg Psychiatry 20: 11–21, 1957

21. Victor M, Angevine JB, Mancall EL, et al: Memory loss with lesions in hippocampal formation. Arch Neurol 5: 244–263, 1961

22. DeJong RN, Itabashi HH, Olson JR: Memory loss due to hippocampal lesions. Arch Neurol 20: 339–348, 1969

23. Walker EA: Recent memory impairment in unilateral temporal lobectomies. Arch Neurol Psychiatry 78: 543–552, 1957

24. Serafetinides EA, Falconer MA: Some observations on memory impairment after temporal lobectomy

for epilepsy. J Neurol Neurosurg Psychiatry 25: 251–255, 1962

25. Dinsdale H, Logue V, Piercy M: A case of persisting impairment of recent memory following temporal lobectomy. Neuropsychologia 1: 287–298, 1964

26. Geschwind N, Fusillo M: Color-naming defects in association with alexia. Arch Neurol 15: 137–146, 1966

27. Malamud N: Psychiatric disorder with intracranial disorders of limbic system. Arch Neurol 17: 113–123, 1967

VI STOCKINGS, GLOVES, AND MEANINGLESS CHANTS

Every medical student learns that, to diagnose peripheral nerve disease, one looks for "stocking-glove" deficits: numbness, tingling, or insensitivity to stimulation in the parts of the legs and arms farthest from the trunk, that is, in the territory covered by stockings and gloves. Like all medical students, I had learned this lesson, but it was not until I worked with Tom Sabin and Norman Geschwind, at the Boston City Hospital, that I saw that there was more to the story. Our peripheral nerves act as information highways carrying sensory messages from our body surfaces to the spinal cord, which then relays them to the brain. Sabin had become interested in the pattern of sensory loss in peripheral nerve diseases while he worked at the U.S. Public Service Hospital in Carville, Louisiana, a facility devoted to the care of people with leprosy (the term Hansen's disease is preferred by individuals who have this disorder).

Hansen's disease is characterized by injury to peripheral nerves as a result of the proliferation of the leprosy bacilli, *Mycobacterium leprae*, within them. This sensory loss is manifested by, for example, numbness and failure to appreciate the pain of a pinprick in the skin that is innervated by the affected nerves. While working at Carville, Sabin meticulously mapped the sensory changes within patients with Hansen's disease, and observed a previously unappreciated and unique pattern of sensory loss: early in the course of the disease, sensation is lost over the ears, nose, cheekbones, and in other regions where nerves course closest to the surface of the skin, all regions where the body temperature is lowest. Sabin, a neurologist, was seeing an interesting reflection of the biology of leprosy. Only in these relatively cool regions of the body could the *Mycobacterium leprae* survive; at higher temperatures closer to the body's core, the bacilli are unable to proliferate. Later in the course of the disease, as the infection progresses, more proximal (and warmer) parts of the body are affected, and finally, sensation is lost over the entire surface of the body except in the warmest parts, (e.g., the armpits, creases behind the knees, etc.) where sensation is preserved.

As an outgrowth of his interest in the pattern of sensory loss in peripheral nerve disease, Sabin also carefully mapped the pattern of sensory deficit in patients with other diseases of peripheral nerves, such as diabetes. In Sabin et al. (1978) we pointed out that the sensory loss in these "symmetrical polyneuropathies" does not simply affect the hands and feet. Sensory nerve fibers lose function according to their length, regardless of the peripheral nerve in which they run. Thus, if one measures the length of preserved fibers, by placing one end of the tape measure at the proximal border of the sensory loss and the other end at the level of the spinal cord from which sensory nerves arise, the measurements coincide within centimeters. It is as if all of the nerves, to all four extremities, follow the same rules of engagement in their battle with the disease process.

With progression of peripheral nerve disease, the impairment of sensation becomes more and more severe, and finally is not limited to the limbs. When the sensory loss has progressed to involve the most proximal portions of the limbs, the next longest population of nerve fibers to be affected are those traversing the body wall. These fibers originate in the spinal cord, and course with the ribs downward along the thorax. Thus, as diabetes worsens, there can be loss of sensation over the anterior part of the trunk, that is, over the abdomen and lower chest. Again there is invariance of the distance from the spinal cord, along the nerves, to the border of sensory loss. We thought this was important from an experimental point of view, for an understanding of the pathophysiology of peripheral nerve disease; and also clinically, partly because, as the sensory loss progresses and invades the torso, the stocking-glove pattern of involvement is blurred. Sensory loss over the trunk from peripheral nerve disease can be confused (especially in patients with weakness and numbness in the legs as can occur in diabetes) with spinal cord compression, so it is important to diagnose it correctly. We described this syndrome of "diabetic truncal neuropathy" in the paper that follows (Waxman and Sabin 1981).

But why does sensory loss occur in a stocking-glove pattern in peripheral nerve disease? The catechism at the time was that distal sensory loss implies distal pathology, that is, that the most distant parts of the longest nerve fibers were affected first, in a "dying-back" manner. But Sabin suggested another possibility, that the stocking-glove pattern of sensory deficit might be explained by a random scattering of lesions, along the entire course of nerve fibers within a nerve. If the lesions were placed randomly, a longer nerve fiber would be more likely to be injured somewhere along its course.

Because I had become interested in demyelination and axonal injury, this idea intrigued me. To test the hypothesis, I used computer simulations to examine probabilistic models of peripheral nerve dysfunction, together with Mike Brill, a graduate student at MIT. Our simulations confirmed that a random scattering of hits, distributed along the course of a nerve fiber, could interfere with impulse transmission, thereby producing distal sensory loss because the longest fibers lose function at the earliest stages of disease (Waxman et al. 1976). Stated differently, loss of function in a damaged nerve can result from failure of the weakest link, and does not necessarily imply damage to the link closest to the end. The longest fibers, according to their schema, were most likely to be affected because they contained the most links. Distal pathology was not a prerequisite for distal sensory loss.

We were also interested in the question of why some patients with peripheral nerve disease experienced paraesthesia, i.e., a tingling pins-and-needles sensation within their hands and feet. These abnormal sensations are disturbing to many patients and, in some, are so unpleasant that any contact with the hands and feet is avoided. We predicted that weak interactions between nerve fibers could produce a situation in which small increments or decrements in membrane potential could bring a given fiber closer to, or farther from, threshold. We further suggested that this might produce interactions between axons that were similar to the weak coupling between nonlinear oscillators described a century ago by Huyghens, who observed the entrainment of the pendulums of the clocks on the wall of a watchmaker's shop. Our colleague Jerry Lettvin, who at that time was professor of biology at MIT, added a graphic description of the proposed physiological events to the final manuscript: "One imagines that an impulse, coming to a partial block, either halts there or is aided in passage by an impulse in the neighboring fiber. If it is so aided, the two fibers carry impulses in phase and will be even more effective with respect to a block in some third fiber a little farther up the path. In this way, a coherent front forms, subverting the information available from the fibers separately into the meaningless chant of a group in lock-step … similar to the 'pins-and-needles' of paraesthesia" (Waxman et al. 1976).

A few years later, Jeff Kocsis and I used microelectrodes to study electrical activity in peripheral nerves as the axons regenerated following injury. To our surprise, we found that, although the regenerated nerve fibers could conduct impulses, they also showed some instability; this poised them to fire erratically, a factor that could contribute to paraesthesia after nerve injury (Kocsis and Waxman 1983). During a sabbatical in our laboratory a few years later, Claes Hildebrand, who was on the faculty of the Karolinska Institute in Stockholm, examined regenerating nerve fibers in the microscope and provided a hint as to why this might occur: during normal development, Schwann cells enwrap the entire length of growing nerve fibers prior to forming myelin, and they compete for space along the length of the fiber. Some Schwann cells win the competition and crowd out others during a period of "remodeling." This occurs as the animal (and its limbs) are growing, and eventually the nerve becomes long enough to accommodate all of the remaining Schwann cells, so the remodeling stops. In nerve fibers that are regenerating after injury, the situation is different. Schwann cell remodeling occurs after nerve injury and as in normal development, there is a competition for space along the nerve fibers. But if the nerve injury has occurred in adulthood the limbs are no longer growing, so the Schwann cell competition persists as an ongoing process. We hypothesized that persistent Schwann cell remodeling interferes with the establishment of mature, tight Schwann cell-axon junctions necessary for effective insulation of the axon by myelin. Together with a persistent or "slow" sodium channel, whose presence we had inferred from microelectrode recordings in injured nerves (Kocsis, Ruiz, and Waxman 1983; Kocsis and Waxman 1987), this would be expected to result in abnormal hyperexcitability and bursting (Hildebrand et al. 1985; Hildebrand, Mustafa, and Waxman 1986).

Learning about the nervous system does not always require a microelectrode or an electron microscope. Tom Sabin taught us that with a tool as simple as a pin a careful observer can glean some important lessons about the nervous system and how it is organized. This was the topic of a chapter we wrote more than twenty years ago (Sabin, Geschwind, and Waxman 1978) which is still widely quoted. We still do not, however, definitively know what causes "positive" abnormalities such as tingling in the hands and feet of patients with peripheral nerve disease. Our research suggests that abnormal expression of sodium channels may be involved. One day, we will use the knowledge collected at the bedside with our pins and in the laboratory with our microelectrodes and electron microscopes to understand more fully the basis for loss of sensation and tingling in peripheral nerve disease. When that happens we may be in a position to develop therapies that will alleviate the numbness and the meaningless chant of injured nerves.

References

Hildebrand, C., Kocsis, J. D., Berglund, S., and Waxman, S. G. Myelin sheath remodeling in regenerated rat sciatic nerve. *Brain Res.* 358: 163–170, 1985.

Hildebrand, C., Mustafa, G. Y., and Waxman, S. G. Remodeling of internodes in regenerated rat sciatic nerve: electron microscopic observations. *J. Neurocytol.* 15: 681–692, 1986.

Kocsis, J. D., and Waxman, S. G. Long-term regenerated nerve fibers retain sensitivity to potassium channel blocking agents. *Nature* 304: 640–642, 1983.

Kocsis, J. D., and Waxman, S. G. Ionic channel organization of normal and regenerating mammalian axons. *Progress in Brain Research*, Vol. 71, *Neural Regeneration.* Seil, F. J., Herbert, E., and Carlson, B. (eds.), pp. 89–102, 1987.

Kocsis, J. D., Ruiz, J. A., and Waxman, S. G. Maturation of mammalian myelinated fibers: changes in action potential characteristics following 4-aminopyridine application. *J. Neurophysiol.* 50: 449–463, 1983.

Sabin, T. D., Geschwind, N., and Waxman, S. G. Patterns of clinical deficits in peripheral nerve disease. In *Physiology and Pathobiology of Axons*, Waxman, S. G. (ed.), Raven Press, New York, pp. 431–439, 1978.

Waxman, S. G., Brill, M. H., Geschwind, N., Sabin, T. D., and Lettvin, J. Y. Probability of conduction deficit as related to fiber length in random-distribution models of peripheral neuropathies. *J. Neurol. Sci.* 29: 39–53, 1976.

Waxman, S. G., and Sabin, T. D. Diabetic truncal polyneuropathy. *Arch. Neurol.* 38: 46–47, 1981.

6 Diabetic Truncal Polyneuropathy

Stephen G. Waxman and Thomas D. Sabin

Abstract Diabetic truncal polyneuropathy is a clinical entity characterized by sensory deficit in the distribution of the thoracic intercostal nerves. The sensory loss is relatively symmetric and involves multiple thoracic dermatomes, beginning close to the anterior midline. Diabetic truncal polyneuropathy occurs in patients with advanced distal polyneuropathy involving the limbs. This entity is important because it can be confused with myelopathies that produce sensory levels over the torso. Moreover, recognition of diabetic truncal polyneuropathy is important since this disorder is associated with autonomic neuropathy.

While a polyneuropathy affecting the limbs, usually in a distal or "stocking-glove" distribution, has long been recognized in diabetes mellitus,[1–3] involvement of the nerves of the trunk has received less attention. Ellenberg[4] has presented an important description of diabetic truncal mononeuropathy, in which involvement of individual intercostal nerves and/or spinal roots is manifested by sensory abnormalities in a single thoracic root distribution. The purpose of our report is to separate this monoradicular truncal syndrome from a second, distinct, neuropathic syndrome with involvement of the thoracic intercostal nerves and/or roots—diabetic truncal polyneuropathy—as part of the diabetic nerve involvement. This syndrome is of interest for two reasons. First, it can, unless recognized and properly diagnosed, present a confusing clinical picture that may obscure proper diagnosis and management of diabetic polyneuropathy. Second, it has important implications in terms of suggesting possible pathophysiologic mechanisms in diabetic neuropathy. The entity has a distinct clinical picture, which is illustrated by the following two patients.

Reprinted with permission from the *Archives of Neurology* 38: 46–47, 1981. Copyright 1981, American Medical Association.

Patients

Figures 6.1 and 6.2 show representative sensory maps from two patients with this entity. Figure 6.1 shows a sensory map from a 67-year-old man with an 18-year history of diabetes mellitus. There was sensory loss in a distal (stocking-glove) distribution in the arms and legs. Hyperesthesia was present at the proximal border of sensory loss in the legs. There was also a relatively symmetric band of sensory loss along the anterior trunk, extending from the T-2 level to below the umbilicus and extending approximately 5 cm to either side of the anterior midline over the abdomen. The patient gave a history of urinary retention, impotence, nocturnal diarrhea, and orthostatic light-headedness.

The sensory map of a second patient, who had a more advanced picture of neuropathic involvement,[5] is shown in figure 6.2. The patient was a 35-year-old juvenile diabetic with a long-standing history of peripheral neuropathy and retinopathy. Sensory signs in the limbs extended nearly to the inguinal crease and axilla, and there was a large and nearly symmetric area of sensory loss over the anterior trunk. Sensation on the back appeared normal. There was also sensory loss over the most distal portion of the trigeminal nerve. Postural hypotension, nocturnal diarrhea, and irregular pupils with a sluggish response to light were present.

It is not unusual for patients with advanced diabetic polyneuropathy to exhibit truncal polyneuropathy. One patient, a 62-year-old, obese woman with adult onset of diabetes and a severe polyneuropathy exhibited anterior truncal sensory loss extending to the midaxillary line. There was also postural hypotension and nocturnal diarrhea. The "sensory level" on the anterior torso resulted in an erroneous initial impression of a spinal cord syndrome, but this patient in fact

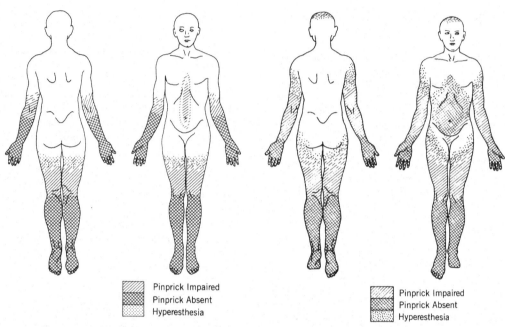

Pinprick Impaired
Pinprick Absent
Hyperesthesia

Pinprick Impaired
Pinprick Absent
Hyperesthesia

Figure 6.1
Sensory map from 67-year-old man with 18-year history of diabetes mellitus. There is sensory loss in distal ("stocking-glove") distribution in limbs and in band over anterior trunk. Autonomic dysfunction was also present.

Figure 6.2
Sensory map from 35-year-old patient with juvenile-onset diabetes and with long-standing peripheral neuropathy. In addition to sensory loss over limbs extending nearly to inguinal crease and axilla, note symmetric sensory loss over anterior trunk in distal part of distribution of intercostal nerves (modified from Sabin et al.).

exhibited truncal sensory loss on the basis of diabetic polyneuropathy.

The clinical course in these patients usually parallels that of the distal polyneuropathy, though, as noted by Sabin et al,[5] truncal signs often appear late in the course of the disease. The syndrome is rare in young diabetics, appears as the polyneuropathy becomes severe, and is usually accompanied by signs of autonomic involvement. In a series of 55 patients referred from a diabetic clinic for neurologic evaluation, five showed sensory loss over the anterior torso. The average duration of diabetes in these patients was 24 years, while the average for the whole group was only eight years. All five patients have serious problems with proximal

autonomic dysfunction (eg, postural hypotension, impotence, nocturnal diarrhea, gastric crises, urinary bladder distention, and pupillary changes). Progression does not appear to be favorably modified by control of the diabetes, though definitive studies here, as in limb polyneuropathy, are not, to our knowledge, available.

Comment

As just illustrated, truncal involvement, beginning close to the anterior thoracic midline, represents a readily recognized feature of symmetric diabetic polyneuropathy. Truncal neuropathy in diabetes has previously received little attention. Ellenberg[4] described the syndrome of diabetic truncal mononeuropathy. The latter condition is characterized by sensory abnormalities in a unilateral root distribution over the thorax; the disorder is usually associated with a classic diabetic neuropathy and has a good prognosis, with the majority of cases exhibiting a notable degree of recovery in about three months. Longstreth and Newcomer[6] described abdominal pain caused by diabetic radiculopathy. Pain occurred in the upper abdomen, the lower chest, or the region of the thoracic spinal column and was unilateral in three of four patients. Three of four patients with this syndrome had other signs of a peripheral neuropathy. Pain resolved in six to 20 months.

In the case of diabetic truncal polyneuropathy, sensory loss involves a number of thoracic intercostal nerves, is relatively symmetric, and does not exhibit recovery. There are usually associated autonomic disturbances. In early cases (eg, figure 6.1) the pattern of sensory loss, as indicated by the width of the region of sensory loss, is somewhat greater in the lower thoracic dermatomes; as noted below, this may reflect the fact that the lower thoracic intercostal nerves course downward as well as anteriorly and thus traverse a greater distance than do the upper thoracic nerves.[7] The increasing obliquity and thus length of the nerves traversing the body wall of the abdomen often results in a "teardrop" configuration to the sensory loss on the anterior torso.

In our experience, diabetic truncal polyneuropathy always occurs in association with a symmetric distal polyneuropathy involving the limbs in a stocking-glove distribution. We have previously noted that this pattern of sensory loss reflects a relative invariance of the distance, along each dermatome, along which sensation is preserved; measurements of the length of preserved sensation in the limbs and trunk, from the proximal border of sensory loss to the appropriate spinal level, are often within centimeters of

each other.[5] Thus, symmetric sensory loss over the anterior trunk does not occur until sensory loss in the limbs has progressed to the thighs and elbows (figure 6.1).

It should be noted that this pattern of sensory loss is not unique to diabetic patients but can occur as a more general accompaniment of the symmetric distal polyneuropathies, eg, ethanolic-nutritional polyneuropathy, the symmetric polyneuropathy of dominantly inherited amyloidosis, and hereditary sensory neuropathy.[5]

The pathologic changes of diabetic symmetric polyneuropathy in man remain in question; axonal degeneration, segmental demyelination, thickening of the basement membrane, and vascular changes have all been indicted,[3] but as noted by Ellenberg,[2] a number of changes may occur independently and/or in combination.

Of note in diabetic symmetric polyneuropathy is the relative invariance of the length of preserved sensation along the four limbs and the trunk.[5] One possible substrate for such a pattern of clinical deficit is provided by a "dying-back" or distal axonopathy; such a process has been elegantly demonstrated in the case of some toxic neuropathies.[8] Another possible explanation is that all nerve fibers are subject to affection along their entire length, with pathologic changes occurring at random; such a model is, in fact, consistent with a distal pattern of clinical deficit.[9] Evidence for multiple lesions scattered at random along both proximal and distal regions of nerve fibers has been adduced in the case of alcoholic and uremic polyneuropathies,[10] in experimental lead neuropathy,[11] and in the Landry-Guillain-Barré syndrome.[12] In diabetic polyneuropathy, Kimura et al[13] suggested, on the basis of M response and F-wave studies, that motor conduction abnormalities are diffuse over the total length of the nerve but are more intense in the distal than proximal segment.

Finally, it should be emphasized that in most patients with diabetic truncal polyneuropathy, there is notable proximal autonomic neuropathy.[2] This is extremely important to recognize from a clinical point of view since patients may not complain explicitly of the associated symptoms. Thus, any patient with diabetic truncal polyneuropathy should be examined for signs of autonomic neuropathy, and appropriate treatment should be instituted.

Acknowledgments

This work was supported in part by the Medical Research Service, Veterans Administration, and by a grant from the Kroc Foundation.

References

1. Mulder DW, Lambert EH, Bastron JA, et al: The neuropathies associated with diabetes mellitus: A clinical and electrophysiological study of 103 unselected patients. *Neurology* 11: 275–290, 1961.

2. Ellenberg M: Diabetic neuropathy: Clinical aspects. *Metabolism* 25: 1627–1655, 1976.

3. Thomas PK, Eliasson SG: Diabetic neuropathy, in Dyck PJ, Thomas PK, Lambert EH (eds): *Peripheral Neuropathy*. Philadelphia, WB Saunders Co, 1975, pp 956–981.

4. Ellenberg M: Diabetic truncal mononeuropathy: A new clinical syndrome. *Diabetes Care* 1: 10–13, 1978.

5. Sabin TD, Geschwind N, Waxman SG: Patterns of clinical deficits in peripheral nerve disease, in Waxman SG (ed): *Physiology and Pathobiology of Axons*. New York, Raven Press, 1978, pp 431–438.

6. Longstreth GF, Newcomer AD: Abdominal pain caused by diabetic radiculopathy. *Ann Intern Med* 86: 166–168, 1977.

7. Gardner E: Gross anatomy of the peripheral nervous system, in Dyck PJ, Thomas PK, Lambert EH (eds): *Peripheral Neuropathy*. Philadelphia, WB Saunders Co, 1975, pp 9–36.

8. Spencer PS, Schaumburg HH: Central-peripheral distal axonopathy: The pathology of dying-back polyneuropathies. *Prog Neuropathol* 3: 253–295, 1976.

9. Waxman SG, Brill MH, Geschwind N, et al: Probability of conduction deficit as related to fiber length in random-distribution models of peripheral neuropathies. *J Neurol Sci* 29: 39–53, 1976.

10. Guiheneuc P, Bathien N: Two patterns of results in polyneuropathies investigated with the H reflex: Correlation between proximal and distal conduction velocities. *J Neurol Sci* 30: 83–94, 1976.

11. Dyck PJ, O'Brien PC, Ohnishi A: Lead neuropathy: 2. Random distribution of segmental demyelination among 'old internodes' of myelinated fibers. *J Neuropathol Exp Neurol* 36: 570–575, 1977.

12. Kimura J: Proximal versus distal slowing of motor nerve conduction velocity in the Guillain-Barre syndrome. *Ann Neurol* 3: 344–350, 1978.

13. Kimura J, Yamada T, Stevland NP: Distal slowing of motor nerve conduction velocity in diabetic polyneuropathy. *J Neurol Sci* 42: 291–302, 1979.

VII SELF-REPAIR IN THE NERVOUS SYSTEM

Neurology has always been an intellectually beautiful discipline. Traditionally, it focused on the diagnosis of diseases of the brain and spinal cord, a meticulous exercise in which every deficit and every abnormal reflex carries important information. But until the relatively recent past, neurology was a therapeutically nihilistic specialty. Because there was little to offer to patients in the way of effective therapy, neurologists classically would make a diagnosis and then walk away.[1]

Multiple sclerosis is a disorder that is commonly encountered by neurologists. It is important for several reasons. The first has to do with its incidence. More than 250,000 individuals in the United States alone carry the diagnosis of multiple sclerosis; the disease usually makes its appearance when its victims are in their twenties and thirties, so that it takes a disproportionately large human toll. The second has to do with the remarkable clinical course of multiple sclerosis. Patients with multiple sclerosis tend to experience relapses—in which they lose functions such as vision or ability to walk—but many patients also have remissions, in which they recover and regain these lost functions. Multiple sclerosis may thus provide an example, in humans, which challenges the classical dictum that, following injury to the brain and spinal cord, there is little or no functional recovery. In this sense, multiple sclerosis can serve as a model disease, teaching us about the nervous system's ability to respond adaptively to injury; hopefully, careful study of multiple sclerosis can provide us with clues, about how to induce functional recovery after injury to the brain and spinal cord. The following four papers are part of a series, in which my colleagues and I have tried to address the questions: how do remissions occur in multiple sclerosis? What are the cellular and molecular mechanisms that are responsible for recovery of function in this disorder?

Many of the nerve fibers within the brain and spinal cord are covered by a substance called myelin which acts as an insulator, increasing the speed and efficiency of impulse conduction. It has been known, since the earliest descriptions of multiple sclerosis, that the myelin is damaged in this disorder. Loss of the myelin insulation was classically considered to be the mechanism underlying loss of function in multiple sclerosis. Moreover, once the myelin is destroyed within the brain and spinal cord, it is not replaced. How, in the absence of remyelination, could remissions occur?

In Waxman (1977) I summarized early studies from my laboratory carried out with my first postdoc, Don Quick (Quick and Waxman 1977; Waxman and Quick 1977), and from the laboratory of J. Murdoch Ritchie (Ritchie and Rogart 1977), which asked whether there might be more to the design of myelinated fibers, than just a covering of the axon by the insulating myelin sheath. These studies focused on sodium channels, the "molecular batteries" that are necessary for conduction of electrical impulses along nerve fibers. Quick and I used electron microscopy in an effort to determine *where*, along the course of myelinated nerve fibers, the sodium channels were located. Antibodies against sodium channels were not available at this time but Quick had developed a stain (the ferric ion-ferrocyanide stain) which provided a marker, at the electron microscopic level, for regions of the cell membrane with a high density of sodium channels. Ritchie and his colleagues used tetrodotoxin and saxitoxin—toxins produced by pufferfish, and by tiny flagellates which float within the "red tide"—to ask *how many* sodium channels are present along myelinated fibers; these toxins block sodium channels by binding to them, one molecule of toxin attaching to one sodium channel. By tagging saxitoxin and/ or tetrodotoxin with radioactivity, and using the radioactive tag to count the number of toxin molecules that attached to nerve fibers, Ritchie and his colleagues developed a method for counting sodium channels.

---

1. It is rumored that a distinguished neurologist in Boston, as recently as the late 1960s, taught his students that "no neurological examination is complete without a postmortem."

The results from the two laboratories converged on an important conclusion: in the normal myelinated axon, sodium channels are not distributed along the entire length of the nerve fiber. These crucial impulse-producing molecules are clustered in large numbers at the nodes of Ranvier—rings of unmyelinated, excitable membrane that punctuate the myelin sheath and which form the stepping stones along which electrical impulses "jump," in a process called saltatory conduction. Our findings with the electron microscope showed the highly focal distribution of sodium channels that tended to be clustered at the nodes. Ritchie's results also suggested that there is aggregation of sodium channels at the node, and provided an estimate of channel density—several thousand sodium channels per square micron—which made the nerve fiber's membrane at the node the recordholder, with a higher density of sodium channels than any other membrane that had been studied.

These results made functional sense, since they showed that the sodium channels were focused, in normal myelinated fibers, just where they are needed for impulse conduction. They also provided an important clue to the pathophysiology of multiple sclerosis. Following loss of the myelin, the exposed parts of the nerve fiber contained only a few sodium channels, too few to support impulse conduction. We thus learned that demyelination does more than merely deprive the nerve fiber of insulation. It exposes parts of the axon membrane that do not contain the molecular machinery necessary for the generation of electrical impulses.

One of the remarkable things about the nervous system is that it is not static. It changes dramatically during normal development, in response to sensory inputs about the surrounding world, and in response to various injuries. Elegant electrophysiological studies carried out by Bostock and Sears (1976, 1978) at the Institute of Neurology in Queen Square had suggested that some chronically demyelinated nerve fibers regain the capability to conduct impulses in a "continuous" manner, with the impulse crawling along the length of the fiber rather than jumping in a saltatory fashion. How does this remarkable recovery occur? In Foster, Whalen, and Waxman (1980) we used Quick's staining methods and demonstrated that, following loss of the myelin sheath, the denuded axon membrane does not remain passive. We learned that the axon can rebuild itself, acquiring a higher-than-normal number of sodium channels. This result was subsequently confirmed by others using immunocytochemical methods (England et al. 1990, 1991). This plasticity provided an explanation, at the molecular level, of how remissions might occur: self-repair of the demyelinated axons, via the insertion of sodium channels into their membranes.

How many sodium channels are needed, within the demyelinated part of a nerve fiber, in order to restore conduction of impulses? And are there any other changes in the demyelinated fiber that are prerequisites for recovery of impulse conduction? "Computational neuroscience" was not yet a formal discipline, but John Moore, a biophysicist from Duke University, was visiting Cambridge on a sabbatical and shared his programs for simulating the behavior of neurons—and his passion for using them as an experimental tool—with me. Working in the evenings in the laboratory of Jerry Lettvin at MIT, together with Michael Brill, a graduate student, I used Moore's programs in a series of simulations to answer these questions. At the time, the only machine available to us was a PDP LINC-8 computer, which we used for free after 10 P.M. Largely as a result of slow peripherals, our computations, in the mid-1970s, took much longer than they would now (Brill, who smoked at that time, could finish nearly an entire cigarette while we waited for the results of a simulation that would, at the present time, be carried out in a few seconds). In Waxman and Brill (1978) we found that the insertion of even a modest number of sodium channels into the demyelinated nerve fiber—with a density much lower than at the nodes—can under some circumstances be effective in promoting the restoration of conduction. We thus learned that it was not necessary for a demyelinated axon to incorporate sodium channels in the very high density that is present at the node of Ranvier, although some channels must be added.

Years after Brill and I did these computer simulations, my colleagues and I used saxitoxin binding in collaboration with Murdoch Ritchie, to experimentally determine the number of sodium channels necessary to support impulse conduction in nerve fibers lacking myelin (Waxman et al. 1989). We found that in nerve fibers with very small diameters (where "input impedance" is high so there is little current leakage), a surprisingly low density of sodium channels will suffice. We suggested on this basis that a reduction in diameter of demyelinated axons might contribute to restoration of conduction in them, but we still are not sure whether this occurs.

Proximity to engineers at MIT focused our attention on another challenge faced by demyelinated axons in restoring conduction, a problem that electrical engineers call "impedance mismatch." In a demyelinated nerve fiber, an impulse must travel from a normally myelinated region (in which the electrical current necessary for impulse conduction is produced at nodes of Ranvier, which are relatively small gaps in the myelin sheath), to invade large regions of the nerve fiber which are devoid of myelin. Even if sodium channels are present within the demyelinated zone, the small nodes of Ranvier may be unable to generate enough electrical current to stimulate larger demyelinated regions—looked at in a simple way, there is not enough juice. Our experiments showed that there are several biologically tenable solutions to the impedance matching problem in demyelinated nerve fibers. One solution is to reduce the lengths of the transitional myelin segments, located at the junction between the normally myelinated and demyelinated region. Our simulations indicated that if these transitional myelin segments are shorter than usual, the voltage drop along them will be reduced, and nerve impulses will be more likely to invade, and thus travel through, the demyelinated region (Waxman and Brill 1978)

Neuropathologists had, for decades, recognized the existence of short myelinated segments, at the edges of demyelinated lesions in multiple sclerosis. They had interpreted the presence of these short myelin segments as being the result of abortive attempts at remyelination. Our results, however, showed that the reduced length of these transitional myelin segments served a functional purpose, facilitating invasion of nerve impulses into the demyelinated zone. We had glimpsed, once again, the resourcefulness of the nervous system.

Impedance mismatch has now been accepted by physiologists as a significant contributor to conduction failure after demyelination. But this work is less well known to researchers interested in immunology, and there is one aspect of it that, in my opinion, deserves additional attention: if the transitional myelin segments, at the junction between myelinated and demyelinated parts of the nerve fibers, are critical for the conduction of nerve impulses, then any event that disrupts these crucial links should have a significant effect on conduction. Because of their location at the transition zone where demyelination begins, these short myelin segments are located at the edges of the demyelinated lesions (also called plaques) that are present in multiple sclerosis. There is a high level of inflammatory activity at the edges of plaques, and inflammatory cells, poised in a state of readiness, tend to congregate there. If these immune cells were to injure the transitional myelin segments—permanently by physically destroying them, or transiently by secreting toxic cytokines near them—a critical link would be injured, and impulse conduction would be impaired. This focuses attention on inflammatory activity at the edge of the plaque, not just in terms of enlarging the demyelinated lesion, but also as factor than can damage a critical link which can make or break impulse conduction.

We have begun to learn about the endogenous mechanisms, such as molecular plasticity and impedance matching, that the nervous system uses for self-repair following injury. A next step is to build upon this, to develop techniques that trigger or promote self-repair in experimental models after injury to the brain and spinal cord. If we can do this, we may be able to emulate the nervous system's self-reparative capabilities. When we can promote functional recovery in diseases of the brain and spinal cord, we will have a new, restorative neurology and a new, more effective science of rehabilitation. After making a diagnosis of damage to the nervous system, the neurologist will no longer have to walk away.

References

Bostock, H., and Sears, T. A. Continuous conduction in demyelinated mammalian nerve fibres. *Nature* 263: 786–787, 1976.

Bostock, H., and Sears, T. A. The internodal axon membrane: electrical excitability and continuous conduction in segmental demyelination. *J. Physiol. (Lond.)* 280: 273–301, 1978.

England, J. D., Gamboni, F., and Levinson, S. R. Increased numbers of sodium channels form along demyelinated axons. *Brain Res.* 548: 334–337, 1991.

England, J. D., Gamboni, F., Levinson, S. R., and Finger, T. E. Changed distribution of sodium channels along demyelinated axons. *Proc. Natl. Acad. Sci. U.S.A.* 87: 6777–6786, 1990.

Foster, R. E., Whalen, C. C., and Waxman, S. G. Reorganization of the axonal membrane of demyelinated nerve fibers: morphological evidence. *Science* 210: 661–663, 1980.

Quick, D. C., and Waxman, S. G. Specific staining of the axon membrane at nodes of Ranvier with ferric ion and ferrocyanide. *J. Neurol. Sci.* 31: 1–11, 1977.

Ritchie, J. M., and Rogart, R. B. The density of sodium channels in mammalian myelinated nerve fibers and the nature of the axonal membrane under the myelin sheath. *Proc. Natl. Acad. Sci. U.S.A.* 74: 211–215, 1977.

Waxman, S. G. Conduction in myelinated, unmyelinated, and demyelinated fibers. *Arch. Neurol.* 34: 585–590, 1977.

Waxman, S. G., Black, J. A., Kocsis, J. D., and Ritchie, J. M. Low density of sodium channels supports action potential conduction in axons of neonatal rat optic nerve. *Proc. Natl. Acad. Sci. U.S.A.* 86: 1406–1410, 1989.

Waxman, S. G., and Brill, M. H. Conduction through demyelinated plaques in multiple sclerosis: computer simulations of facilitation by short internodes. *J. Neurol. Neurosurg. Psychiat.* 41: 408–417, 1978.

Waxman, S. G., and Quick, D. C. Cytochemical differentiation of the axon membrane in A- and C-fibers. *J. Neurol. Neurosurg. Psychiat.* 40: 379–386, 1977.

7 Conduction in Myelinated, Unmyelinated, and Demyelinated Fibers

Stephen G. Waxman

Abstract Conduction in demyelinated axons is characterized by decreased conduction velocity, temporal dispersion of impulses, and conduction failure. It is not possible to infer the electrical properties of the bared internodal axon membrane in demyelinated fibers from observations of decreased conduction velocity or conduction failure. Cytochemical evidence indicates that there are, in fact, distinct structural differences between nodal and internodal regions of the normal axon membrane. This conclusion is confirmed by freeze-fracture and pharmacological studies. A number of approaches to the development of effective symptomatic therapy in the demyelinating diseases are suggested by recent experimental findings: determination of the membrane properties necessary for conduction across focally demyelinated regions and the identification of agents that would encourage the development of these properties; alterations in the external milieu of demyelinated fibers; and the development of agents that might promote remyelination.

The past decade has seen a reawakening of interest in the biology and pathophysiology of nerve fibers. As part of this development, there has been a remarkable expansion of our understanding of the physiology of the myelinated axon and of the demyelinated axon. It is the purpose of this report to review some recent advances in this area, and, in particular, to summarize recent progress in understanding the functional architecture of the membrane of myelinated and demyelinated fibers. These advances have added substantially to our understanding of the pathophysiology of the demyelinating diseases and suggest the possibility of rational approaches to symptomatic therapy.

Effects of Demyelination on Conduction

A number of abnormalities of conduction occur in the demyelinated, or partially demyelinated,

Reprinted with permission from the *Archives of Neurology* 34: 585–589, 1977. Copyright 1977, American Medical Association.

axon: (1) Decreased conduction velocity has been demonstrated in both peripheral[1-3] and central[4,5] demyelinated axons. Rasminsky and Sears[6] demonstrated internodal conduction times of more than 600 μsec in demyelinated ventral root fibers, compared with 19.7 μsec in control fibers. (2) Temporal dispersion of impulses, as a result of unequal slowing of conduction in the fibers of a given nerve or tract, was suggested by Gilliatt and Willison[7] on the basis of their clinical observation that nerve action potentials were reduced or lost in some diabetic patients with motor conduction velocities close to the lower limit of the normal range. They pointed out that this could account for the early loss of deep tendon reflexes and vibration sensibility in these patients. McDonald[8] suggested that loss of temporal coherence of activity in visual fibers could contribute to the diminished critical flicker fusion frequency in patients with multiple sclerosis. (3) Conduction block has been demonstrated in both peripheral[1,2] and central[4] demyelinated fibers. In general, conduction failure is more likely to occur with high-frequency impulse trains than with low-frequency trains or single impulses.[4,9,10] (4) Finally, as noted by Davis and Schauf,[11] demyelinated fibers, in which the safety factor approaches a value of 1, should be highly susceptible to exogenous influences. It has been suggested that these can include abnormal ephaptic interactions with nearby fibers,[12] and, in fact, pathological transmission of impulses from fiber to fiber has been shown in the abnormally myelinated nerve roots of dystrophic mice.[13]

What are the cellular substrates for the deficits in conduction in demyelinated fibers? This question is of fundamental importance not only for an understanding of the pathophysiology of the demyelinating diseases but also as a basis for rational approaches to symptomatic therapy. One key question concerns the properties of the internodal axon membrane that is under the myelin sheath in the normal fiber, but bared in the demyelinated fiber. Is this membrane excitable, ie, is it capable of sustaining impulse activity? If so, does it share the same intrinsic membrane properties as the membrane at the node of Ranvier, or does it resemble the membrane of normally unmyelinated fibers, which is known to be quite different?[14,15] Does the demyelinated axon membrane exhibit any plasticity in terms of its electrical properties? What are the membrane properties that would optimize conduction in demyelinated fibers, and what agents might encourage the development of these properties?

Membrane Properties of Demyelinated Fibers

It might have been hoped that the membrane properties of demyelinated axons could be inferred from observations of conduction block or decreased conduction velocity. This has not turned out to be the case. Koles and Rasminsky[16] showed that, if the internodal axon membrane were inexcitable, conduction would be slowed along demyelinated fibers and that conduction block would occur at completely demyelinated internodes. Figure 7.1 shows a computer simulation of activity in a fiber totally demyelinated between nodes 7 and 8, in this case under the assumption that the bared internodal axon membrane is excitable, with the same intrinsic properties as the nodal membrane. Conduction fails at the site of demyelination, not because of shunting of current through inexcitable membrane, but rather because of the impedance mismatch between the normally myelinated and demyelinated regions. As shown in figure 7.2, conduction may thus fail in the case of severe focal demyelination, with either excitable or inexcitable membrane in the internodal region. On the other hand, if the fiber were to be *totally* demyelinated, ie, if there were no myelin present along the entire fiber, and if the axon

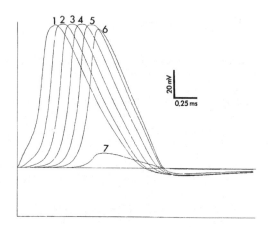

Figure 7.1
Computed action potentials at nodes 1 through 7 for a fiber totally demyelinated at internode 7–8. Computational methods and parameters have been described by Brill et al. It was assumed that demyelinated internodal axon membrane had the same specific membrane properties as nodal membrane. Conduction fails at demyelinated region due to impedance mismatch.

membrane had nodal characteristics in all regions, there would be no impedance mismatch, and conduction would proceed without block, but with conduction velocity decreased to less than 10% of that of the normally myelinated fiber. Thus, as shown in figure 7.2, with either excitable or inexcitable membrane in the internodal region, conduction block would occur at sites of focal demyelination, and slowing of impulse conduction would occur as a result of demyelination. In the fiber represented in figure 7.2, B, however, conduction would proceed, albeit slowly, following total demyelination of the entire fiber, whereas in the fiber represented in figure 7.2, A, conduction would fail.

Huxley and Stämpfli[17] showed in 1949 that conduction in normal myelinated fibers occurs in a saltatory manner, ie, that action currents are confined to the nonmyelinated portion of the axon at the nodes of Ranvier. Their experiments did not, however, answer the question of whether

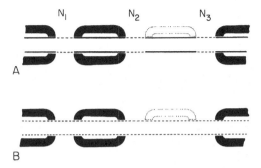

Figure 7.2
Organization of membrane of myelinated fiber. Regions of axon membrane that exhibit nodal membrane properties are represented by broken lines, while regions of axon membrane that exhibit different characteristics are represented by solid lines. Properties of internodal axon membrane are not significant at normally myelinated internodes (eg, between nodes N_1 and N_2), but are highly relevant to function of demyelinated axons (eg, between nodes N_2 and N_3).

the internodal axon membrane is excitable since, even if it were excitable, it might not normally generate action potentials because of the overlying layer of high-resistance myelin.

It was not until approximately two decades later that Rasminsky and Sears[6] examined conduction at the cellular level in demyelinated nerve fibers. They studied undissected rat ventral root fibers demyelinated with diphtheria toxin, using a modification of the Huxley-Stämpfli technique for measuring longitudinal axonal currents. Their results showed marked slowing of conduction, with internodal conduction times increased to over 600 μsec for some internodes, compared with control values of 19.7 ± 4.6 μsec. There was considerable variation in internodal conduction times at successive internodes along single fibers. Most importantly, they showed that impulse conduction remained saltatory to the point of conduction block rather than becoming continuous as in normal myelinated fibers.

A number of recent studies have more directly addressed the question of whether there are structural differences between nodal and internodal domains of the axon membrane. Cytochemical studies using the binding of ferric ion have shown distinct differences in the ion-binding properties of the nodal, as compared with the internodal, axon membrane (figure 7.3). Dense binding of the electron-dense ferric ion occurs at cytoplasmic surfaces of the nodes, but not at the internodes. Ferric ion is not bound to the membranes of C fibers.[18,19] In studies on the specialized electrolyte axons in the eel *Sternarchus*, in which there are both excitable and inexcitable regions of the axon membrane,[20,21] ferric ion was only bound to the excitable regions, suggesting that the binding reaction may provide a marker for normally excitable nodal membrane.[18] A second set of studies has used the freeze fracture technique. Rosenbluth[22] examined central nodes of Ranvier using this method and found an appreciably higher density (approximately 1,200/sq μ) of outer leaflet membrane particles at the nodal membrane than in the internodes. He speculated that these particles may be related to the sodium channels. Kristol et al.[23] examined the specialized *Sternarchus* axons using similar methods and found a higher density of outer leaflet membrane particles at the normally excitable nodes of Ranvier than in the inexcitable nodes, which resembled the internodes.

Ritchie and Rogart[24] have attempted to estimate the density of sodium channels in mammalian myelinated fibers from measurements of the binding of tritiated saxitoxin to rabbit sciatic nerve. Binding to both intact nerve and homogenized nerves was studied. Their results suggest a sodium channel density of approximately 10,000/sq μ at the nodes of Ranvier, compared with a density of less than 25 channels per square micron in the axon membrane under the myelin in the internodes. Nonner et al.,[25] using data derived from voltage clamp experiments, arrived at a value of approximately 5,000 sodium channels per square micron at the node. In contrast, the density of sodium channels in unmyelinated

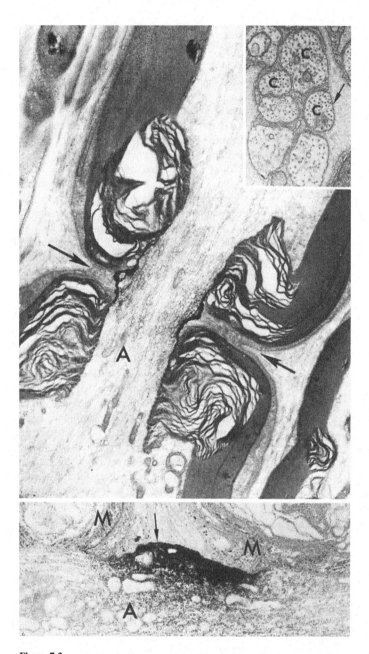

Figure 7.3
Cytochemical differentiation of the axon membrane. (Top) Node of Ranvier in rat sciatic nerve (arrows) sectioned in the longitudinal plane. Ferric ion-ferrocyanide is bound specifically at the nodal axolemma and is not present in internodal regions. A indicates axoplasm (×12,800). (Bottom) Another node at higher magnification. Axon membrane can be resolved (arrow) and stain can be seen to lie on axoplasmic surface of that structure. A indicates axoplasm, and M, terminating myelin loops (×32,000). (Inset) C fibers (C) exposed to similar staining conditions. There is no binding of ferric ion-ferrocyanide to C fiber membranes, even in areas where they are directly exposed to extracellular milieu (arrow) (×21,000) (from Quick and Waxman).

C fibers is approximately 110/sq μ.[26] The cyto-chemical, freeze-fracture, and pharmacological data summarized in the above two paragraphs support the generalization that the normal nodal axolemma is structurally and physiologically different from the internodal axolemma and from the axolemma of unmyelinated fibers (figure 7.2, A).

Yet, the conclusion that the internodal axon membrane is less capable of sustaining impulse conduction than the nodal membrane may not apply in all situations, and indeed the electrical properties of various domains of the axon membrane may not be immutable. Bostock and Sears[27] have recently examined conduction in small (internodal length < 850 μ) demyelinated ventral root fibers and found a number of examples in which the internodal membrane was electrically excitable and supported continuous conduction across a demyelinated internode. They correctly pointed out that this does not necessarily imply that internodal excitability varies with fiber size, but could rather reflect differences in pathology or geometry of small, as compared with large myelinated fibers. Rasminsky and Kearney[28] have recently studied conduction in large diameter (5 to 6 μ) spinal root axons in dystrophic mice, which are either bare or invested with abnormally thin myelin. Using techniques for recording the external longitudinal currents, they found that adjacent portions of the axon membrane in these dysmyelinated fibers are capable of sustaining both saltatory and continuous conduction.

Clinical Implications

What are the implications of these findings? It is well known that the extent of lesions in multiple sclerosis is in many cases far greater than would be anticipated from clinical observations.[29-32] Furthermore, the relatively subtle behavioral defects seen in mouse mutants deficient of myelin[33] stand in direct contrast to the often pro-found deficits seen in acute episodes of clinical demyelination. Ritchie and Rogart[24] have suggested that sodium channel density in axonal membranes may change over time and that, analogous to the spread of acetylcholine receptors in denervated muscle, there may be a spread of sodium channels into the demyelinated internodal region, so that after a time it may support impulse conduction. One approach for further studies would be the determination, using computer simulations, of which membrane properties would be most likely to support conduction across a demyelinated region. Having determined these properties, one could search for agents that would encourage their development.

A somewhat different approach to this problem has been taken by those who have examined the immediate effects of exogenous agents on conduction in demyelinated fibers. It has long been known that clinical symptoms in multiple sclerosis worsen with increasing body temperature.[34,35] This has recently been shown to be due to conduction block.[36,37] Lowering of body temperature, however, has not, in general, proved useful as a mode of therapy. Davis et al.[38] and Becker et al.[39] studied the effect of various procedures designed to lower serum ionized calcium (intravenous sodium bicarbonate, disodium edetate, hyperventilation, and oral phosphate) on visual and oculomotor function in patients with multiple sclerosis. Improvement in clinical deficits was observed, but it was transient (lasting a few minutes to one or two hours) in all cases. Thus, this modality of therapy has not proved to be of practical clinical value to date. Nevertheless, the possibility that alterations in the external milieu could favorably alter the conduction properties of demyelinated axons is an attractive one and should be pursued.

A final approach to symptomatic therapy in the demyelinating diseases is suggested by the computer simulations of Koles and Rasminsky,[16] which indicate that conduction can be facilitated by the presence of myelin sheaths as thin as 2.7% of normal myelin thickness. This suggests that remyelination, even with sheaths much thinner than normal, could be clinically advantageous. While morphological studies indicate that remyelinated myelin segments may be inappropriately thin[40] or short,[41,42] even these morphologically aberrant sheaths may be functionally beneficial, and it might not be unreasonable to search for agents that would promote even a minor degree of remyelination.

This investigation was supported in part by Public Health Service grants NS-12307 and RR-05479 and Career Development Award K04-NS-00010 from the National Institutes of Health, and by grants from the National Multiple Sclerosis Society and from the Health Sciences Fund.

References

1. McDonald WI: The effects of experimental demyelination on conduction in peripheral nerve: A histological and electrophysiological study: II. Electrophysiological observations. *Brain* 86: 501–524, 1963.

2. Mayer RF, Denny-Brown D: Conduction velocity in peripheral nerve during experimental demyelination in the cat. *Neurology* 14: 714–726, 1964.

3. Hall JL: Studies on demyelinated peripheral nerves in guinea pigs with experimental allergic neuritis: A histological and electrophysiological study: II. Electrophysiological observations. *Brain* 90: 313–332, 1967.

4. McDonald WI, Sears TA: The effects of experimental demyelination on conduction in the central nervous system. *Brain* 93: 583–598, 1970.

5. Mayer RF: Conduction velocity in the central nervous system of the cat during experimental demyelination and remyelination. *Int J Neurosci* 1: 287–308, 1971.

6. Rasminsky M, Sears TA: Internodal conduction in undissected demyelinated nerve fibers. *J Physiol* 227: 323–350, 1972.

7. Gilliatt RW, Willison RG: Peripheral nerve conduction in diabetic neuropathy. *J Neurol Neurosurg Psychiatry* 25: 11–18, 1962.

8. McDonald WI: Pathophysiology in multiple sclerosis. *Brain* 97: 179–196, 1974.

9. Davis FA: Impairment of repetitive impulse conduction in experimentally demyelinated and pressure-injured nerves. *J Neurol Neurosurg Psychiatry* 35: 537–544, 1972.

10. Waxman SG: Integrative properties and design principles of axons. *Int Rev Neurobiol* 18: 1–40, 1975.

11. Davis FA, Schauf CL: The pathophysiology of multiple sclerosis: A theoretical model, in Klawans HL (ed): *Models of Human Neurological Diseases.* Amsterdam, Excerpta Medica, 1974.

12. Waxman SG, Brill MH, Geschwind N, et al.: Probability of conduction deficit as related to fiber length in random-distribution models of peripheral neuropathies. *J Neurol Sci* 29: 39–53, 1976.

13. Huizar P, Kuno M, Miyata Y: Electrophysiological properties of spinal motoneurones of normal and dystrophic mice. *J Physiol* 248: 231–246, 1975.

14. Tasaki I, Freygang WH Jr: The parallelism between the action potential, action current, and membrane resistance at a node of Ranvier, *J Gen Physiol* 39: 211–223, 1955.

15. Katz B, Miledi R: Propagation of electric activity in motor nerve terminals. *Proc R Soc Lond (Biol)* 161: 453–482, 1965.

16. Koles ZJ, Rasminsky M: A computer simulation of conduction in demyelinated nerve fibres. *J Physiol* 227: 351–364, 1972.

17. Huxley AF, Stämpfli R: Evidence for saltatory conduction in peripheral myelinated nerve fibres. *J Physiol* 108: 315–339, 1949.

18. Quick DC, Waxman SG: Specific staining of the axon membrane at nodes of Ranvier with ferric ion and ferrocyanide. *J Neurol Sci* 31: 1–11, 1977.

19. Waxman SG, Quick DC: Cytochemical differentiation of the axon membrane in A- and C-fibers. *J Neurol Neurosurg Psychiatry* 40: 379–385, 1977.

20. Bennett MLV: Comparative physiology: Electric organs. *Ann Rev Physiol* 32: 471–528, 1970.

21. Waxman SG, Pappas GD, Bennett MVL: Morphological correlates of functional differentiation of nodes of Ranvier along single fibers in the neurogenic electric organ of the knife fish *Sternarchus. J Cell Biol* 53: 210–224, 1972.

22. Rosenbluth J: Intramembranous particle distribution at the node of Ranvier and adjacent axolemma in myelinated axons of the frog brain. *J Neurocytol* 5: 731–745, 1976.

23. Kristol C, Akert K, Sandri C, et al.: The Ranvier nodes in the neurogenic electric organ of the knifefish *Sternarchus:* A freeze-etching study on the distribution of membrane-associated particles. *Brain Res* 125: 197–212, 1977.

24. Ritchie JM, Rogart RB: The density of sodium channels in mammalian myelinated nerve fibers and the nature of the axonal membrane under the myelin sheath. *Proc Natl Acad Sci USA* 74: 211–215, 1977.

25. Nonner W, Rojas E, Stämpfli R: Gating currents in the node of Ranvier: Voltage and time dependence. *Philos Trans R Soc Lond (Biol)* 270: 483–492, 1975.

26. Ritchie JM, Rogart RB, Strichartz G: A new method for labeling saxitoxin and its binding to non-myelinated fibres of the rabbit vagus, lobster walking, and garfish olfactory nerves. *J Physiol* 261: 477–494, 1976.

27. Bostock H, Sears TA: Continuous conduction in demyelinated mammalian nerve fibres. *Nature* 263: 786–787, 1976.

28. Rasminsky M, Kearney RE: Continuous conduction in large diameter bare axons in spinal roots of dystrophic mice. *Neurology* 26: 367, 1976.

29. MacKay RP, Hirano A: Forms of benign multiple sclerosis: Report of two clinically silent cases discovered at autopsy. *Arch Neurol* 17: 588–600, 1967.

30. Namerow NS, Thompson LR: Plaques, symptoms, and the remitting course of multiple sclerosis. *Neurology* 19: 765–774, 1969.

31. Ghatak NR, Hirano A, Lijtmaer H, et al.: Asymptomatic demyelinated plaque in the spinal cord. *Arch Neurol* 30: 484–486, 1974.

32. Wisniewski H, Oppenheimer D, McDonald WI: Relation between myelination and function in MS and EAE. *J Neuropathol Exp Neurol* 35: 327, 1976.

33. Sidman RL, Green MC, Appel SH: *Catalog of the Neurological Mutants of the Mouse.* Cambridge, Harvard University Press, 1965.

34. Simons DJ: A note on the effect of heat and cold upon certain symptoms of multiple sclerosis. *Bull Neurol Inst NY* 6: 385–386, 1937.

35. Guthrie TC: Visual and motor changes in patients with multiple sclerosis: A result of induced changes in environmental temperature. *Arch Neurol Psychiatry* 65: 437–451, 1951.

36. Davis FA, Jacobson S: Altered thermal sensitivity in injured and demyelinated nerve. *J Neurol Neurosurg Psychiatry* 34: 551–561, 1971.

37. Rasminsky M: The effects of temperature on conduction in demyelinated single nerve fibers. *Arch Neurol* 28: 287–292, 1973.

38. Davis FA, Becker FO, Michael JA, et al.: Effect of intravenous sodium bicarbonate, disodium edetate (Na$_2$EDTA), and hyperventilation on visual and oculomotor signs in multiple sclerosis. *J Neurol Neurosurg Psychiatry* 33: 723–732, 1970.

39. Becker FO, Michael JA, Davis FA: Acute effects of oral phosphate on visual function in multiple sclerosis. *Neurology* 24: 601–607, 1974.

40. Harrison BM, McDonald WI, Ochoa J: Remyelination in the central diphtheria toxin lesion. *J Neurol Sci* 17: 293–302, 1972.

41. Suzuki K, Andrews JM, Waltz JM, et al.: Ultrastructural studies of multiple sclerosis. *Lab Invest* 20: 444–445, 1969.

42. Gledhill RF, Harrison BM, McDonald WI: Pattern of remyelination in the CNS. *Nature* 244: 443–444, 1973.

43. Brill MH, Waxman SG, Moore JW, et al.: Conduction velocity and spike configuration in myelinated fibers: Computed dependence on internode distance. *J Neurol Neurosurg Psychiatry*, to be published.

8 Conduction through Demyelinated Plaques in Multiple Sclerosis: Computer Simulations of Facilitation by Short Internodes

Stephen G. Waxman and Michael H. Brill

Summary Clinical and laboratory observations both suggest that it may be possible for action potentials to traverse, in a continuous manner and without interruption, demyelinated zones along some axons. This continuous mode of conduction requires the presence of sufficient numbers of sodium channels in the demyelinated region. One of the factors which will tend to prevent such conduction is the impedance mismatch at sites of focal demyelination, which may result in a reduction in current density sufficient to cause conduction failure. As part of an effort to examine the conditions which would promote conduction into, and beyond, the demyelinated region, we examined, using computer simulations, the effects of reduction in length of the proximal internodes closest to the demyelinated region. Our results indicate that reduction in length of the two internodes closest to the demyelinated region, to approximately one-third of normal length or less, will facilitate conduction beyond the plaque. The results suggest that reductions in internode length, which have been histologically observed along some demyelinated fibres, may have functional significance in terms of facilitating conduction past focally demyelinated zones.

An important problem in the pathophysiology of multiple sclerosis concerns the prerequisites for axonal conduction through demyelinated plaques. Clinical and experimental observations both suggest that, under some conditions, conduction may proceed without interruption, albeit at a reduced conduction velocity, through regions of total demyelination. Pathological studies, for example, have demonstrated that some demyelinated plaques may be asymptomatic (Ghatak et al., 1974), and that the distribution of plaques may be more widespread than would be predicted from the clinical deficits (Namerow and Thompson, 1969). One implication of these observations is that conduction may be preserved along at least some of the demyeli-

Reprinted with permission from *Journal of Neurology, Neurosurgery, and Psychiatry* 41: 408–416, 1978.

nated axons. Clinical neurophysiological observations are consistent with this hypothesis. Visual evoked potentials, for example, may be delayed by more than 40 ms in multiple sclerosis patients with no history of optic neuritis (Halliday et al., 1973). Finally, it has recently been shown experimentally that impulse conduction may occur in a continuous fashion along demyelinated regions as long as 500 μm in fibres exposed to diphtheria toxin (Bostock and Sears, 1976). These observations bring up an important question in the physiology of demyelinated fibres. Recent data suggest that in normal fibres, sodium channel density at nodes of Ranvier ($12\,000/\mu m^2$) is much higher than in the internodal axon membrane beneath the myelin ($<25/\mu m^2$; Ritchie and Rogart, 1977). On the other hand, the observations of conduction past regions of focal demyelination imply the existence of a sufficient density of sodium channels to support conduction in the demyelinated region of some fibres, and it has been suggested that sodium channel densities may change after demyelination (Ritchie and Rogart, 1977; Waxman, 1977). However, computer simulations (Waxman, 1977) have demonstrated that the presence of a high density of sodium channels in the demyelinated region may not, in itself, ensure conduction past the site of demyelination. For example, conduction failure may occur at a single focally demyelinated internode, even if ionic channel densities are as high in the demyelinated region as at normal nodes of Ranvier, as a result of impedance mismatch between the normal and demyelinated regions. Conduction block will occur as a result of failure of *initiation* of activity in the demyelinated region, if current density in the demyelinated area is sufficiently small because of the increased surface area of bared axonal membrane in the demyelinated zone. Thinning of myelin in areas adjacent to the bared region may contribute to current loss. The situation is similar to that at other regions of impedance mismatch—for example, at sites of axial inhomogeneity in non-myelinated axons (Khodorov et al., 1969; Ramon et al., 1975; Parnas et al., 1976) and at the junction between neuronal cell body and initial segment (Dodge and Cooley, 1973), where safety factor is low and where conduction failure has been experimentally observed.

The elegant studies of Rasminsky and Sears (1972), which have been followed by the investigations of Bostock and Sears (1976) and Rasminsky et al. (1977), have examined the physiology of conduction along abnormally myelinated fibres. The latter two studies provide experimental evidence for continuous conduction along portions of some demyelinated and amyelinated axons. The earlier computer simulation studies of Koles and Rasminsky (1972) were important in delineating some of the biophysical bases of abnormal conduction in demyelinated fibres, and were based on the assumption that membrane excitability remains confined to the nodes in demyelinated axons. As part of a programme to explore further the pathophysiology of multiple sclerosis and of mechanisms which might promote impulse conduction past demyelinated plaques, we have studied, using computer simulations, several possible mechanisms for continuous conduction along focally demyelinated axons. In this paper we present results which suggest that reduction in internode length proximal to a demyelinated region may promote conduction of impulses into, and past, that region. As noted in the Discussion, there is experimental evidence for reductions in internode distance along axons which have been subjected to demyelination.

Methods

Methods used in the present study were adapted from those of Brill et al. (1977) and involve the numerical integration of the equation

$$c(x)\frac{\partial}{\partial_t} V(x, t) = \frac{1}{r_a}\frac{\partial^2}{\partial_{X^2}} V(x, t) - i_m(x, t) \qquad (1)$$

where:

V is the potential across either the nodal membrane or myelin.

r_a is the axial resistance of the fibre per unit length.

$c(x)$ is the capacitance per unit length—that is, trans-myelin capacitance C_M in the internodal region, and the nodal and demyelinated axolemma capacitance C_N at nodes of Ranvier and demyelinated regions.

i_m is the ionic current per unit length of membrane.

In the internodal regions,

$$i_m(x, t) = g_M V(x, t) \qquad (2a)$$

where g_M is the myelin conductance per unit length. At each node j,

$$i_m(x, t) = I_{HH}\,\pi d.\frac{NL}{\Delta_X} + \frac{\Delta_X - NL}{\Delta_X}[V_j.g_M] \qquad (2b)$$

where the current density I_{HH} is given by

$$I_{HH} = \bar{g}_{Na}m_j^3 h_j[V_j - V_{Na}]$$
$$+ \bar{g}_K n_j^4[V_j - V_K] + g_L[V_j - V_L] \qquad (3)$$

where m_j, n_j, and h_j satisfy the usual differential equations in time (Hodgkin and Huxley, 1952; Fitzhugh, 1962).

Equations were integrated numerically by the Crank-Nicholson method implemented on a PDP 9 computer, as described for unmyelinated fibres by Moore et al. (1975) and adapted for the myelinated fibre by R. W. Joyner.

We used an integration time increment $\Delta_t = 5$ μs and a length increment $\Delta_X = 200$ μm. Thus there were 10 spatial lumped-parameter segments per normal internode length ($L = 2000$ μm). We composed each of our simulated fibres out of three kinds of segments (see Table for parameter

Table 8.1

Parameters

Symbol	Explanation	Nodal membrane value	Hodgkin-Huxley membrane value
$\bar{g}_{Na}$	sodium conductance (mho/cm^2)	1.2	0.12
$\bar{g}_K$	potassium conductance (mho/cm^2)	0.09	0.036
g_L	leakage conductance (mho/cm^2)	0.02	0.0003
V_r	resting potential (mV)	0	0
V_{Na}	sodium equilibrium potential[1] (mV)	115	115
V_K	potassium equilibrium potential (mV)	−12	−12
V_L	leakage equilibrium potential (mV)	−.05	10.613
d	axon diameter (inner diameter of myelin sheath) (μm)	10	10
NL	nodal length[2] (μm)	3.183	3.183
r_a	axoplasmic resistance per unit axon length[3] (ohm/cm)	1.26×10^8	1.26×10^8
g_M	myelin conductance per unit length (mho/cm)	5.60×10^{-9}	5.60×10^{-9}
C_M	myelin capacitance per unit axon length (F/cm)	1.87×10^{-11}	1.87×10^{-11}
C_N	nodal and demyelinated axolemma capacitance per unit axon length[4] (F/cm)	3.14×10^{-9}	3.14×10^{-9}
L	internodal distance[5] (μm)	2000	2000

[1] All voltage signs are reversed from those of the original Hodgkin-Huxley formulation.
[2] Calculated from nodal area of 100 μm^2.
[3] Calculated from specific axoplasmic resistance of 100 ohm-cm.
[4] Calculated from capacitance per unit area of 10^{-6} F/cm^2.
[5] Except proximal to demyelinated regions as indicated in text.

values): (i) segments with the electrical properties of normal myelin; (ii) segments containing a node of Ranvier, with lumped electrical parameters from the node and its adjacent myelin; for length increment Δ_X and nodal length NL, the capacitance assigned to a segment containing a node is $C^* = (C_N NL + C_m(\Delta_X - NL))/\Delta_X$; (iii) segments consisting of active membrane with no adjacent myelin. These segments comprise the demyelinated region of the fibre. We allowed the active membrane to be normal nodal membrane (table 8.1; see also Brill et al., 1977) or Hodgkin-Huxley membrane (table 8.1), and observed the effect on conduction of each of these alternatives.

For a normal fibre (without focal demyelination) every tenth segment contains a node (type ii segment), and the rest are myelin (type i). We modelled focal demyelination by replacing the segment containing the fourth node with a myelin segment, and by replacing the following internode and node with 10 type iii segments. This left a region of non-myelinated axon (D_1–D_4) equal in length to one normal internode. Distal to this demyelinated region the fibre was composed of normal internodes and nodes. We designated the three nodes proximal to the demyelinated region "1," "2," and "3," and the nodes distal to the demyelinated region as "4,"

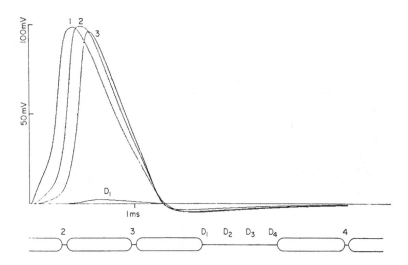

Figure 8.1

Computed action potentials for a fibre focally demyelinated in the region from D_1 to D_4. The axon membrane in the demyelinated region of the fibres represented in figures 8.1 to 8.5 has the same specific membrane properties as nodal axolemma. For the fibre shown in this figure, the internode proximal to the demyelinated region ($3-D_1$) is of normal (2000 μm) length. Despite the assumption of excitable membrane in the demyelinated region, conduction fails at point D_1 as a result of inadequate current density. In this and the following figures, potentials from nodes 1–6 and in the demyelinated region (D_1-D_4) are shown; potentials at nodes 7–11 are omitted for clarity. Schematic diagrams below the traces show fibre geometry in the vicinity of the demyelinated region; internode 1–2 and all internodes distal to node 4 are of normal length.

"5," "6," etc. Simulated fibres were 11 nodes in length, although only the demyelinated region and first six nodes are shown in the figures.

Fibres were examined with either normal nodal membrane in the demyelinated region (figures 8.1–8.5) or with Hodgkin-Huxley membrane in this region (figure 8.6). We examined the conduction properties of each of these fibres by stimulating with a twice-threshold current for 200 μs at the beginning of the internode before node 1. Conduction delays were measured by noting the time differences for the first 50 mV crossings of action potentials at designated points along the fibre. Rate constants were adjusted to 20 °C.

In order to model the effect of interposing short internodes proximal to the demyelinated region, we replaced one of the myelin segments

between node 3 and the demyelinated region (D_1-D_4) with a nodal (type ii) segment. Figure 8.2 shows a representative case: the demyelinated region is made of normal nodal membrane, and the new node partitions the preceding internode into two internodes, one with length 1600 μm and one with length 400 μm. We also examined the effect of replacing, with type ii segments, *two* of the internodal segments between node 3 and the demyelinated region, in order to interpose two short internodes proximal to the demyelinated zone. Representative cases are shown in figures 8.3 to 8.6. In all figures, the new nodes are labelled A and B, and the first, fourth, seventh, and tenth segments of the demyelinated region are labelled D_1-D_4. Internodes were designated by reference to their endpoints: thus, internode 2–3 extends between node 2 and node

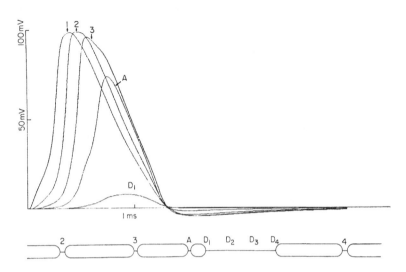

Figure 8.2
Computed action potentials for a fibre similar to that shown in figure 8.1, but with a single short internode (A–D_1; 400 µm) interposed proximal to the demyelinated region. There is conduction failure at point D_1.

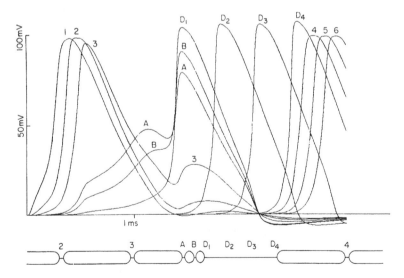

Figure 8.3
Computed action potentials for a fibre similar to that shown in figure 8.1, with two short internodes (A–B, B–D_1; 200 µm) interposed proximal to the demyelinated region. Under these conditions, the impulse invades the demyelinated region, and passes without interruption into the distal part (for example, nodes 4, 5, 6) of the fibre.

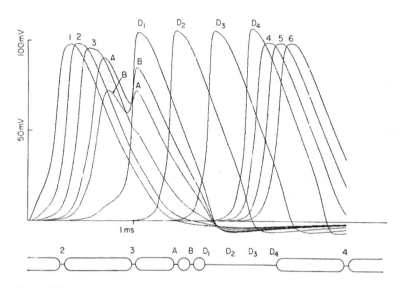

Figure 8.4
Computed action potentials for a fibre with two 400 μm internodes (A–B, B–D₁) proximal to the demyelinated zone. Conduction again proceeds through the demyelinated region, but with a shorter latency that in figure 8.3.

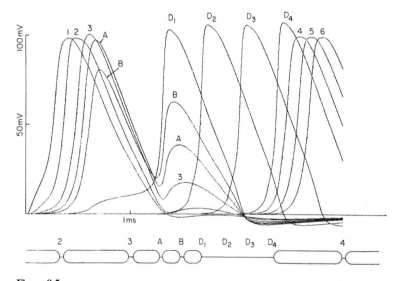

Figure 8.5
Computed action potentials for a fibre with two 600 μm internodes (A–B, B–D₁) proximal to the demyelinated zone. Conduction proceeds through the demyelinated region, but requires longer than for the fibre shown in figure 8.4.

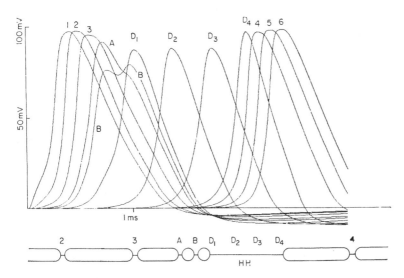

Figure 8.6
Conduction past a demyelinated region (D_1–D_4) in which the axon membrane has the characteristics of Hodgkin-Huxley membrane. Despite the lower sodium channel density than at nodes of Ranvier, conduction into, and beyond, the demyelinated region occurs. However, as in the simulations shown previously, uninterrupted conduction requires the presence of two short (400 μm) internodes proximal to the demyelinated zone.

3, and internode A–D_1 extends between node A and point D_1.

Results

The effect of focal demyelination at a single internode is shown in figure 8.1. In the fibre represented, internodes 1–2 (the internode between 1 and 2), 2–3, 3–D_1, D_4–4, 4–5, 5–6, and all subsequent internodes are normally myelinated (see table 8.1). The internode between points D_1 and D_4 is focally demyelinated, with nodal specific membrane properties throughout the demyelinated region. Internodal conduction time proximal to the site of demyelination was 102 μs (conduction velocity = 19.7 m/s), as in simulations of normally myelinated fibres. Despite the assumption of nodal membrane properties in the demyelinated region, conduction failure

occurs, and the spike does not invade the demyelinated zone. This failure does not reflect inexcitability of the demyelinated axon membrane, but rather reflects the low current density in this region.

Figure 8.2 shows the effect of introducing a single internode, substantially reduced in length (400 μm) just proximal to the site of demyelination. Internode 3–D_1 (originally 2000 μm in length) is now replaced by internode 3–A (1600 μm), node A, and internode A–D_1 (400 μm). Excitation of node A is delayed (internodal conduction time for 3–A is 0.19 ms, compared to a normal internodal conduction time of 0.102 ms), and the impulse does not invade the demyelinated region. A similar simulation, in which internode A–D_1 was made 200 μm long, also resulted in conduction failure.

Figure 8.3 shows the effect of two closely spaced nodes (nodes A, B; internode lengths A–

B and B–D_1 = 200 μm) located immediately proximal to the demyelinated area. In contrast to the simulations shown previously, in this case conduction proceeds through the demyelinated zone. The impulse invades the demyelinated region (D_1–D_4), propagates at a conduction velocity close to the steady-state value of 1.64 m/s observed in simulations of uniform non-myelinated fibres with nodal membrane properties, and then proceeds along the normally myelinated distal part of the fibre (nodes 4, 5, 6, and subsequent nodes) at a normal conduction velocity (19.7 m/s). In this case, nodes A and B and point D_1 fire almost synchronously. The delay from excitation at node 3 to excitation at point D_1 is 0.92 ms.

A focally demyelinated fibre, with two 400 μm internodes interposed before the demyelinated region, is shown in figure 8.4. Conduction again proceeds into and beyond the demyelinated region. In this case, the delay between excitation of node 3 and of point D_1 is 0.51 ms, a value considerably shorter than in the previous simulation. Conduction velocity within the demyelinated region is, as in the previous simulation, approximately 1.64 m/s, and conduction proceeds at a normal conduction velocity in the distal myelinated internodes.

Figure 8.5 shows a still larger spacing of the nodes proximal to the demyelinated area; in this case the two proximal internodes closest to the demyelinated region are 600 μm long. Conduction proceeds into, and past, the demyelinated zone, although invasion time (from excitation of node 3 to point D_1) is increased to 0.82 ms. If length of the two internodes proximal to the demyelinated region is increased to 1000 μm, conduction failure occurs at point D_1. Thus, the optimal value for internode distances proximal to the demyelinated region, in terms of minimising the time required for invasion of the demyelinated region, falls between 200 μm and 600 μm, and internode lengths of more than 1000 μm will not facilitate invasion of the demyelinated zone.

Since it is also possible (see Discussion) that specific membrane properties in demyelinated regions may be different from those at normal nodes, we examined conduction in focally demyelinated fibres, in which the axon membrane in the demyelinated region had properties of Hodgkin-Huxley (1952) membrane (see table 8.1). Despite the much higher resistance than at nodal membrane, conduction again failed when the internodes proximal to the demyelinated region were of normal (2000 μm) length. However, when the proximal internodes closest to the demyelinated region were reduced in length, as shown in figure 8.6, the impulse invaded, and passed, the demyelinated region. In this case, the delay from excitation of node 3 to excitation of point D_1 was 0.42 ms, and conduction velocity in the demyelinated region was approximately equal to that for a uniform fibre with Hodgkin-Huxley membrane properties—that is 1.62 m/s. This simulation demonstrates that (a) impulses can propagate through, and beyond, regions of demyelination at which sodium channel density is significantly lower than at normal nodal membrane, but (b) such propagation may require a mechanism for impedance matching in the demyelinated zone, which in the present simulation was provided by reduction in internode length proximal to the site of demyelination.

Discussion

The present results, like those of earlier studies (Koles and Rasminsky, 1972), indicate that impulse propagation in demyelinated fibres is sensitive to fibre geometry. The present findings further suggest that reduction in internode distance proximal to a demyelinated region may play a role in permitting action potentials to invade, and pass, the demyelinated area. The situation is similar to that described by Revenko et al. (1973) who showed that, because current density is inadequate, an impulse from a myelinated fibre will fail to invade a non-myelinated terminal, unless either the last internode is shorter than the rest, or the terminal has a reduced diameter. In the case of the present simulation, we assumed the presence of a sufficient density of sodium channels in the demyelinated region to support conduction, but nevertheless found that it was necessary to reduce the length of the two proximal internodes closest to the demyelinated region. The two final nodes then exhibited diphasic impulses and fired nearly synchronously, so that current density in the demyelinated region was increased not only as a result of the decreased capacitative and resistive current loss in the shortened internodes, but also as a result of increased current generation. This is similar to the observation by Goldstein and Rall (1974) and by Ramon et al. (1975) that at transitional regions along some inhomogeneous non-myelinated axons close to zones of low safety factor, the action potential may be diphasic and will be generated simultaneously along large regions of the axon. The degree of internodal shortening required for invasion of the demyelinated region in our simulations was relatively modest, with reduction to approximately one-third of normal or less being required for propagation into and beyond the demyelinated region. Since safety factor is dependent on temperature (Davis and Jacobson, 1971; Rasminsky, 1973), it should be noted that the present simulations, like those of Koles and Rasminsky (1972), were carried out at 20°C. Our simulations, like those of earlier workers (Koles and Rasminsky, 1972; Schauf and Davis, 1974), are based on the assumption that mammalian nodes of Ranvier exhibit specific membrane properties similar to those in amphibian nerve fibres. As noted by Koles and Rasminsky (1972), the available data suggest that this is not unreasonable. Our own studies (Moore et al., 1978) indicate that conduction velocity in myelinated fibres is far more sensitive to internodal parameters than to the nodal description. Nevertheless, it should be noted that the precise degree of internodal shortening required will, of course, depend

on the exact description of the myelin and of the membrane properties in the nodes and demyelinated area.

Our results are similar to those of Revenko et al. (1973) in indicating that increasing the resistivity of the demyelinated axon membrane did not effectively promote conduction into the demyelinated region. As in normal fibres (Moore et al., 1978), conduction properties in demyelinated fibres appear to be quite sensitive to internodal structure.

Internode distances are reduced, compared to those in peripheral fibres, in some preterminal fibres in the normal central nervous system (Waxman, 1970, 1975). At these sites, the changes in internode distances may permit axons to function as delay lines (Waxman, 1975) or may function so as to modulate invasion of axonal terminals (Waxman, 1972; Revenko et al., 1973).

Several ultrastructural studies have shown that internode distances may also be substantially reduced along central remyelinated axons (Suzuki et al., 1969; Gledhill et al., 1973). The present results suggest that the reduced internode distances might function so as to facilitate conduction past focally demyelinated regions. It should be emphasised in this context that several lines of evidence suggest that, in normal fibres, sodium channels are present at higher density at the nodes of Ranvier than in the internodes (Ritchie and Rogart, 1977; Waxman, 1977). An explicit assumption of the simulations shown in figures 8.1 to 8.5 is that normal nodal sodium channel densities develop at the newly formed nodes and over demyelinated regions of the axolemma. While there is, at present, little evidence directly bearing on the question of sodium channel density at newly formed nodes, there is some evidence for normal or near normal physiological function of newly formed nodes in remyelinated fibres (see Rasminsky, 1978). It should be noted, however, that invasion of a demyelinated region with lower values of sodium conductance than at normal nodes is also possible if there is a reduction in length of the proximal internodes (see figure 8.6). Cytochemical studies in dystrophic mice suggest, in fact, that ionic channel densities along the amyelinated regions of ventral root axons may be lower than at normal nodes of Ranvier (Waxman et al., 1978).

Longitudinal current analyses, which show a transition from saltatory to continuous conduction along some ventral root fibres demyelinated with diphtheria toxin (Bostock and Sears, 1976), and along some amyelinated ventral root fibres in dystrophic mice (Rasminsky et al., 1977), have not, to date, resolved the question of whether there are short internodes at the transitional zones along these axons. As noted by Rasminsky et al. (1977), resolution of the recording techniques was such that shorter internodes would not be detected. It is possible that some other mechanism facilitates invasion of non-myelinated zones in these axons, or, as suggested by figure 8.5, that only small changes in fibre geometry are required. However, reduced internode distances were observed histologically in the amyelinated axons (Rasminsky et al., 1977).

Our previous studies (Brill et al., 1977) showed that substantial reductions in internode distance are associated with decreased axonal conduction velocity. Several authors, however, have suggested that clinical deficits in multiple sclerosis may be primarily related to conduction failure, rather than to slowing of conduction (see, for example, Rasminsky, 1973; Halliday and McDonald, 1977). It has been suggested that the demyelinated axon membrane may exhibit structural plasticity (Ritchie and Rogart, 1977; Waxman, 1977). If this is the case, reduction in internode distances along remyelinated fibres might play a role in promoting functional recovery as a result of facilitation of uninterrupted transmission along affected axons, despite the prolonged conduction time. As in the normal central nervous system (Waxman, 1975), matching of internode distances to functional require-

ments may be of considerable importance. This conclusion may be relevant to the search for agents which initiate, and control, remyelination in multiple sclerosis.

Acknowledgments

This work was supported in part by grants from the US National Multiple Sclerosis Society (RG-1133-A-1), the National Institute of Health (NS-12307, RR-05479), and the Health Sciences Fund (78-10). Dr Waxman is the recipient of a Research Career Development Award (K04-NS-00010) from the National Institute of Neurological and Communicative Disorders and Stroke. We thank Professor J. Y. Lettvin for helpful discussions.

References

Bostock, H., and Sears, T. A. (1976). Continuous conduction in demyelinated mammalian nerve fibres. *Nature*, 263: 786–787.

Brill, M. H., Waxman, S. G., Moore, J. W., and Joyner, R. W. (1977). Conduction velocity and spike configuration in myelinated fibres: computed dependence of internode distance. *Journal of Neurology, Neurosurgery, and Psychiatry*, 40: 769–774.

Davis, F. A., and Jacobson S. (1971). Altered thermal sensitivity in injured and demyelinated nerve. *Journal of Neurology, Neurosurgery, and Psychiatry*, 34: 551–561.

Dodge, F. A., and Cooley, J. W. (1973). Action potential of the motoneuron. *IBM Journal of Research and Development*, 17: 219–229.

FitzHugh, R. (1962). Computation of impulse initiation and saltatory conduction in a myelinated nerve fiber. *Biophysical Journal*, 2: 11–21.

Ghatak, N. R., Hirano, A., Lijtmaer, H., and Zimmerman, H. M. (1974). Asymptomatic demyelinated plaque in the spinal cord. *Archives of Neurology (Chicago)*, 30: 484–486.

Gledhill, R. F., Harrison, B. M., and McDonald, W. I. (1973). Pattern of remyelination in the CNS. *Nature*, 244: 443–444.

Goldstein, S. S., and Rall, W. (1974). Changes of action potential shape and velocity for changing core conductor geometry. *Biophysical Journal*, 14: 731–757.

Halliday, A. M., and McDonald, W. I. (1977). Pathophysiology of demyelinating disease. *British Medical Bulletin*, 33: 21–27.

Halliday, A. M., McDonald, W. I., and Mushin, J. (1973). Visual evoked response in diagnosis of multiple sclerosis. *British Medical Journal*, 4: 661–664.

Hodgkin, A. L., and Huxley, A. F. (1952). A quantitative description of membrane current and its application to conduction and excitation in nerve. *Journal of Physiology* (*London*), 117: 500–544.

Khodorov, B. I., Timin, Y. N., Vilenkins S. Y., and Gulko, F. B. (1969). Theoretical analysis of the mechanisms of conduction of nerve impulse over an inhomogeneous axon: conduction through a portion with increased diameter. *Biofizika*, 14: 304–315.

Koles, Z. J., and Rasminsky, M. (1972). A computer simulation of conduction in demyelinated nerve fibres. *Journal of Physiology*, 227: 351–364.

Moore, J. W., Ramon, F., and Joyner, R. W. (1975). Axon voltage-clamp simulations I. Methods and tests. *Biophysical Journal*, 15: 11–24.

Moore, J. W., Joyner, R. W., Brill, M. H., Waxman, S. G., and Najar-Joa, M. (1978). Simulations of conduction in myelinated fibres: relative sensitivity to changes in nodal and internodal parameters. *Biophysical Journal*, 21: 147–160.

Namerow, N. S., and Thompson, L. R. (1969). Plaques, symptoms, and the remitting course of multiple sclerosis. *Neurology* (*Minneapolis*), 19: 765–774.

Parnas, I., Hochstein, S., and Parnas, H. (1976). Theoretical analysis of parameters leading to frequency modulation along an inhomogeneous axon. *Journal of Neurophysiology*, 39: 909–923.

Ramon, F., Joyner, R. W., and Moore, J. W. (1975). Propagation of action potentials in inhomogeneous axon regions. *Federation Proceedings*, 34: 1357–1363.

Rasminsky, M. (1973). The effects of temperature on conduction in demyelinated single nerve fibers. *Archives of Neurology* (*Chicago*), 28: 287–292.

Rasminsky, M. (1978). Physiology of conduction in demyelinated axons. In *Physiology and Pathobiology of Axons*, pp. 361–376. Edited by S. G. Waxman. Raven Press: New York.

Rasminsky, M., and Sears, T. A. (1972). Internodal conduction in undissected demyelinated nerve fibres. *Journal of Physiology*, 227: 323–350.

Rasminsky, M., Kearney, R. E., Aguayo, A. J., and Bray, G. M. (1977). Conduction of nervous impulses in spinal roots and peripheral nerves of dystrophic mice. *Brain Research*. In press.

Revenko, S. V., Timin, Ye. N., and Khodorov, B. I. (1973). Special features of the conduction of nerve impulses from the myelinized part of the axon into the non-myelinated terminal. *Biofizika*, 18: 1074–1078.

Ritchie, J. M., and Rogart, R. B. (1977). The density of sodium channels in mammalian myelinated nerve fibres and the nature of the axonal membrane under the myelin sheath. *Proceedings of the National Academy of Sciences*, 74: 211–215.

Schauf, C. L., and Davis, F. A. (1974). Impulse conduction in multiple sclerosis: a theoretical basis for modification by temperature and pharmacological agents. *Journal of Neurology, Neurosurgery, and Psychiatry*, 37: 152–161.

Suzuki, K., Andrews, J. M., Waltz, J. M., and Terry, R. D. (1969). Ultrastructural studies of multiple sclerosis. *Laboratory Investigation*, 20: 444–454.

Waxman, S. G. (1970). Closely spaced nodes of Ranvier in the teleost brain. *Nature*, 227: 283–284.

Waxman, S. G. (1972). Regional differentiation of the axon: a review with special reference to the concept of the multiplex neuron. *Brain Research*, 47: 269–288.

Waxman, S. G. (1975). Integrative properties and design principles of axons. *International Review of Neurobiology*, 18: 1–40.

Waxman, S. G. (1977). Conduction in myelinated, unmyelinated, and demyelinated fibres. *Archives of Neurology* (*Chicago*), 34: 585–589.

Waxman, S. G., Bradley, W. G., and Hartwieg, E. A. (1978). Organization of the axolemma in amyelinated axons: a cytochemical study in dy/dy dystrophic mice. *Proceedings of the Royal Society. Series B*. 201: 301–308.

9 Reorganization of the Axon Membrane in Demyelinated Peripheral Nerve Fibers: Morphological Evidence

Robert E. Foster, Christopher C. Whalen, and Stephen G. Waxman

Abstract Cytochemical staining of demyelinated peripheral axons revealed two types of axon membrane organization, one of which suggests that the demyelinated axolemma acquires a high density of sodium channels. Ferric ion-ferrocyanide stain was confined to a restricted region of axon membrane at the beginning of a demyelinated segment or was distributed throughout the demyelinated segment of axon. The latter pattern represents one possible morphological correlate of continuous conduction through a demyelinated segment and suggests a reorganization of the axolemma after demyelination.

At least three responses have been demonstrated when an action potential arrives at a demyelinated segment of an axon. Conduction block may occur if the demyelinated axolemma is inexcitable (*1, 2*) or as a result of impedance mismatch (*3, 4*). Slowed saltation of action potentials between nodes of Ranvier results when passive internodal properties are altered due to loss of myelin (*5*). Finally, continuous conduction can occur across demyelinated internodal membranes that possess electrical excitability (*6, 7*).

In normal myelinated fibers, Na^+ channels are concentrated at the nodes of Ranvier; in the internodal axolemma their density is lower than that necessary to sustain conduction (*2*). It has been suggested that demyelinated axonal regions develop electrical excitability, much as denervated muscle develops hypersensitivity (*2*). Electrophysiological observations of continuous conduction in demyelinated axons (*6, 7*) indicate that internodal membranes undergo reorganization resulting in the development of electrical excitability. The physiological observations (*6, 7*) suggest that (i) Na^+ channels and associated structures remain aggregated in clusters that be-

Reprinted with permission from *Science* 210: 661–663, 1980. Copyright © 1980 by the American Association for the Advancement of Science.

come distributed along the length of the axon, (ii) reorganization of the axon membrane occurs such that individual Na^+ channels are dispersed through the demyelinated internodal membrane, and/or (iii) new channels are added to the demyelinated axon membrane.

Although the structural heterogeneity (*8*) of the axolemma of normally myelinated axons is clearly established (*2, 9–11*), sufficient anatomical evidence has yet to be presented to illustrate the morphological basis of abnormal modes of conduction in demyelinated fibers or to demonstrate structural modification of the axon membrane. This report provides morphological evidence showing that in some demyelinated fibers the axolemma reorganizes into a configuration that can sustain continuous conduction.

Fibers from the peroneal nerve of adult male Wistar rats, demyelinated by crushing (*12*), were examined. Seven to 30 days after the sciatic nerve was crushed, the peroneal nerve distal to the crushed area was excised, immersed in fixative for 3 hours, and stained by the ferric ion-ferrocyanide (FeFCN) cytochemical technique (*13*). We previously summarized evidence indicating that this staining technique provides a cytochemical marker for regions of high Na^+ channel density (*14*).

Figure 9.1 shows electron micrographs of demyelinated peroneal nerve fibers 16 days after the sciatic nerve was crushed for 30 seconds with watchmaker's forceps. This interval offers examples of demyelination, remyelination, and regeneration. Figure 9.1A illustrates the pattern of FeFCN staining in a heminode, one of the common stages of demyelination observed after this survival period. The axon (*a*) is myelinated (*m*, myelin) on one side of the stained area (left of the bracket) and is demyelinated on the other side (right of the bracket). A Schwann cell (*s*) has established a one-to-one relationship with the demyelinated segment, suggesting that remyeli-

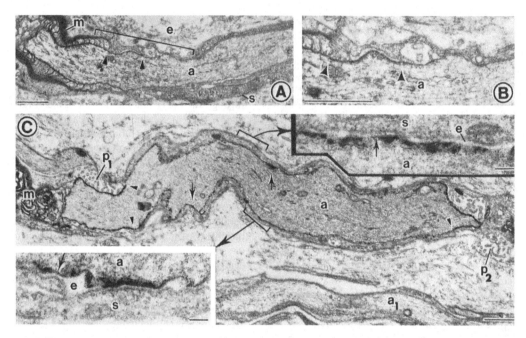

Figure 9.1
Electron micrographs of demyelinated nerve fibers stained by the ferric ion-ferrocyanide technique. Scale bars: (*A*), (*B*), and (*C*), 1 μM; insets, 0.1 μm.

nation is imminent for that segment (*e*, extracellular space). The region of the axon shown in figure 9.1B (from the bracketed region in figure 9.1A) has accumulated only a moderate amount of FeFCN stain (between arrows) and this is confined to the axoplasmic side of the axolemma for a 1-μm region (the length of a normal node of Ranvier) adjacent to the last terminal loop of the myelinated side. Axoplasm in the region beneath the stained axolemma is more electron-dense than contiguous axoplasm or internodal axoplasm of neighboring axons. This pattern of staining resembles the pattern observed at normal nodes of Ranvier (*2, 10, 11*), in that the length of the zone of FeFCN staining in the demyelinated fiber is restricted to ∼1 μm. No apparent Schwann cell specializations form the right boundary of the stained region.

In contrast, the axon shown in figure 9.1C (a photomontage of electron micrographs of the same tissue as in figure 9.1, A and B) has a demyelinated region 12 μm long and is characterized by dense staining distributed throughout the demyelinated zone on the cytoplasmic surface of the axolemma. This stained demyelinated zone retains two well-defined areas of very dense stain (arrowheads mark the inner boundary) adjacent to degenerating myelin and networks of fingerlike processes (p_1, p_2). Distinct subaxolemmal aggregates of stain (insets in figure 9.1C) are distributed throughout the demyelinated region (*15*). While the FeFCN staining appears to be uneven in the demyelinated zone, its distribution throughout this region is relatively continuous. Adjacent regenerating axons (such as a_1), with or without myelin sheaths in the same section, are not stained beneath the axolemma. However, in this material there were many examples of normally stained nodes with the stain present at the nodal axolemma, as in normal tissue. Examination of serial sections revealed that the axolemma of axon *a* (figure 9.1C) is densely stained in the demyelinated region, in contrast to axolemma wrapped by compact myelin, which is not stained.

The neurophysiological data for demyelinated fibers are consistent with several patterns of distribution of Na^+ channels and associated structures. For example, the channels can be concentrated in patches at separate nodal regions so as to allow for distinct zones of inward current, thereby causing slowed saltation (5) and conduction block. Alternatively, the distribution of the channels can be relatively continuous, allowing for spatially continuous inward current (6, 7) and continuous conduction along the demyelinated region.

Our results suggest morphological correlates for both predicted patterns of organization of the axolemma in peripheral demyelinated axons. Figure 9.1, A and B, presents the anatomical correlate of the type of axonal membrane that might conduct with slowed saltation or exhibit conduction blocking. When an action potential reaches the demyelinated zone from the myelinated portion of the fiber, conduction may be blocked because of reduced excitability of the demyelinated membrane (1, 2) or impedance mismatch at the junction of the myelinated and demyelinated regions (3, 4). Saltation may continue, although slowed because of changes in passive properties of the internodal membrane, namely an increase in internodal capacitance and a decrease in internodal transverse resistance (5).

The electron micrograph in figure 9.1C presents a possible morphological correlate of continuous conduction. The spatial distribution of FeFCN stain that we have described suggests a high density of Na^+ channels along the demyelinated (former paranodal or internodal) region. This pattern of staining offers one morphological correlate for the physiological observation of spatially continuous inward current associated with continuous conduction along the demyelinated axon. In this case the demyelinated axolemma, which presumably contained a low density (2) of Na^+ channels prior to demyelination, reorganized by redistributing channels or by acquiring new ones.

These data concerning reorganization of the axon membrane after demyelination are of interest not only in terms of understanding the pathophysiology of demyelinated fibers, but also with respect to the mechanisms that mediate subsequent recovery of conduction. Future studies incorporating freeze-fracture or pharmacological methods should provide further information about this phenomenon.

References and Notes

1. Z. J. Koles and M. Rasminsky, *J. Physiol.* (*London*) 227, 351 (1972).

2. J. M. Ritchie and R. B. Rogart, *Proc. Natl. Acad. Sci. U.S.A.* 74, 211 (1977).

3. S. G. Waxman, *Neurology* 28, 27 (1978).

4. T. A. Sears, H. Bostock, M. Sherratt, *ibid.*, p. 21; H. Bostock, R. M. Sherratt, T. A. Sears, *Nature* (*London*) 274, 385 (1978).

5. M. Rasminsky and T. A. Sears, *J. Physiol.* (*London*) 227, 323 (1972).

6. H. Bostock and T. A. Sears, *Nature* (*London*) 263, 786 (1976).

7. ———, *J. Physiol.* (*London*) 280, 273 (1978).

8. Using ^3H-labeled saxitoxin, Ritchie and Rogart (2) showed that in the normally myelinated axon, Na^+ channels are concentrated in nodal axolemma and are present at a very low density in the internodal axolemma. Likewise, a high density of external-face intramembranous particles (9) and a specific pattern of FeFCN staining (10, 11) are found at the node, indicating specialization of the nodal membrane.

9. J. Rosenbluth, *J. Neurocytol.* 5, 731 (1976); C. Kristol, K. Akert, C. Sandri, U. Wyss, M. V. L. Bennett, H. Moor, *Brain Res.* 125, 197 (1977); C. Kristol, C. Sandri, K. Akert, *ibid.* 142, 391 (1978).

10. D. C. Quick and S. G. Waxman, *J. Neurol. Sci.* 31, 1 (1977); S. G. Waxman, W. G. Bradley, E. A. Hartwieg, *Proc. R. Soc. London Ser. B* 201, 301 (1978).

11. S. G. Waxman and D. C. Quick, *J. Neurol. Neurosurg. Psychiatry* 40, 379 (1977).

12. D. Denny-Brown and C. Brenner, *Arch. Neurol. Psychiatry* 52, 1 (1944); J. Ochoa, T. J. Fowler, R. W. Gilliatt, *J. Anat.* 113, 433 (1972). The results described are not due to crushing per se, since we made similar observations using the JHM model of virus-induced demyelination [R. E. Foster, C. C. Whalen, S. G. Waxman, L. P. Weiner, *J. Cell Biol.* 87, 68a (1980)].

13. The tissue was fixed for 3 hours in cold 5 percent glutaraldehyde buffered with $0.2M$ sodium cacodylate (pH 7.4; 360 mOsm), washed three times in fresh $0.2M$ cacodylate buffer, postfixed for $1\frac{1}{2}$ hours in 2 percent OsO_4, washed in distilled water three times at 5 minutes per wash, and stained by the FeFCN technique. For this the tissue sample was placed in $0.01M$ ferric chloride, washed three times in distilled water (5 minutes per wash), placed in 1 percent potassium ferrocyanide, and washed two more times in distilled water. The sample was then dehydrated and embedded in Epon-Araldite (*11*). Thick (3 μm) serial sections were examined by light microscopy, and selected thick sections were reembedded. Ultrathin sections were cut from these, stained on a grid with aqueous uranyl acetate and Reynold's lead citrate, and examined with a JEOL 100 CX electron microscope.

14. In normal mammalian peripheral nerve, the FeFCN technique stains the cytoplasmic surface of the axon membrane at nodes of Ranvier but not at internodal regions of the same fibers. Absence of internodal membrane staining was shown not to be due to lack of ability of the stain to reach these areas (*10, 11*). Specific staining of initial segment membrane rather than soma or dendritic membrane is consistent with the hypothesis that this stain is specific to regions densely supplied with Na^+ channels [S. G. Waxman and D. C. Quick, in *Physiology and Pathobiology of Axons*, S. G. Waxman, Ed. (Raven, New York, 1978), pp. 125–130]. In the electrocyte axons of *Sternarchus albifrons*, in which there are both excitable and inexcitable nodes [M. V. L. Bennett, in *Fish Physiology*, W. S. Hoar and D. J. Randall, Eds. (Academic Press, New York, 1971), pp. 374–491; S. G. Waxman, G. D. Pappas, M. V. L. Bennett, *J. Cell Biol.* 53, 210 (1972)], the excitable nodes stain densely with FeFCN while inexcitable

nodes along the same fiber do not (*10*). It should be emphasized that absence of staining with FeFCN does not necessarily imply membrane inexcitability, since C fibers are not stained with this technique (*11*). Sodium channel density for C fibers, estimated from measurements of the binding of ^{3}H-labeled saxitoxin, is approximately 110 per square micrometer [J. M. Ritchie, R. B. Rogart, G. R. Strichartz, *J. Physiol.* (*London*) 261, 477 (1976)]. Axolemma staining with FeFCN thus appears to reflect quantitative differences in membrane structure.

15. This staining is not due to preferential accessibility of the demyelinated membrane to the extracellular milieu, since C fibers do not stain even when directly exposed to the extracellular space (*11*), and since the inexcitable type II nodes in *S. albifrons* (*14*) also do not stain.

16. Supported in part by NIH grant NS-15320, National Multiple Sclerosis Society grant RG-1231, and by the Medical Research Service of the Veterans Administration. We thank S. Cameron and M. Smith for technical assistance.

Current Concepts in Neurology: Membranes, Myelin, and the Pathophysiology of Multiple Sclerosis

Stephen G. Waxman

Demyelination, or the loss of myelin, characterizes a number of common neurologic diseases. The most common of these is multiple sclerosis. At any given time, there are approximately 250,000 patients with the diagnosis of multiple sclerosis in the United States alone. Moreover, multiple sclerosis may serve as a model disease, since in its classic form its course includes remissions in the presence of apparently fixed histologic abnormalities.

This article will briefly review the pathophysiology of nerve-impulse conduction in demyelinated fibers. In particular, it will focus on three major questions: What is the physiology of conduction in normal myelinated fibers? What electrophysiologic factors contribute to abnormal conduction in demyelinated nerve fibers? How does recovery of function occur in demyelinated nerve fibers, and how might we attempt to restore relatively normal function in demyelinated nerve fibers? These questions are briefly reviewed here. More complete reviews are available.[1-4] This article will focus on changes in axonal conduction that lead to clinical abnormalities in the "negative" jacksonian sense, i.e., in which normal function is diminished or lost. Conduction changes that lead to clinical abnormalities in the "positive" jacksonian sense (e.g., trigeminal neuralgia, tonic flexion spasms, and Lher-mitte's sign) have been discussed elsewhere.[4,5]

The Myelin Sheath

Myelin is a compact spiral of closely apposed glial-cell membranes surrounding the axon (figure 10.1) (glial-cell membranes making up the myelin are produced by the Schwann cell in the peripheral nervous system and by the oligoden-

Reprinted with permission from the *New England Journal of Medicine* 306: 1529–1533, 1982.

droglial cell in the central nervous system). The myelin sheath is characterized by high electrical resistance and low capacitance, which permit it to function essentially as an electrical insulator. The myelin sheath is periodically interrupted at axonal regions approximately 1 μm long and devoid of myelin, which are designated the nodes of Ranvier.

Myelinated fibers conduct action potentials in a saltatory manner, with the impulse jumping discontinuously from node to node rather than progressing continuously along the axon, as in unmyelinated fibers. Impulse conduction occurs at a greater velocity in myelinated fibers than in nonmyelinated fibers of the same size.[6] In addition, myelinated fibers can conduct impulses at higher frequencies and consume less energy per impulse than nonmyelinated fibers.[7]

The Pathophysiology of Conduction in Demyelinated Axons

Demyelinated fibers have a spectrum of conduction abnormalities. In moderately demyelinated fibers, there is decreased conduction velocity.[8,9] As a corollary, there can be temporal dispersion of impulse conduction (i.e., the loss of synchrony of impulses carried by the fibers within a tract), which is due to different degrees of slowing, reflecting differential pathologic involvement in the constituent fibers in a bundle or tract. This mechanism has been invoked as an explanation for the early loss of deep tendon reflexes and vibratory sensibility in patients with diabetic neuropathy, in whom nerve-conduction velocities (reflecting the conduction velocity of the population as a whole) are in the low-normal range.[10] In more severely affected fibers, conduction block occurs. This can be related to frequency, with low-frequency impulse trains conducting relatively reliably and high-frequency

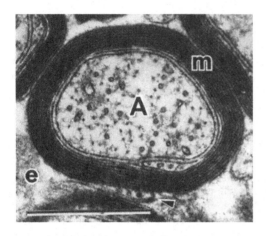

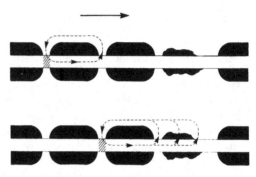

Figure 10.1
Electron micrograph showing transverse section through myelinated axon (A) from rabbit corpus callosum. The myelin sheath (m) consists of a nearly compact spiral of glial-cell membranes. A thin tongue of cytoplasm (arrowhead) connects the myelin to its oligodendroglial cell of origin. The bar indicates 0.5 μm, and e denotes extracellular space.

Figure 10.2
Schematic diagram of impulse conduction in normal (upper panel) and demyelinated (lower panel) regions of a nerve fiber. The solid arrow indicates the direction of impulse conduction; the shaded area indicates the region occupied by the impulse. Current flow is indicated by the broken arrows. In normally myelinated regions (upper panel), the high-resistance, low-capacitance myelin shunts the majority of action current to the next node of Ranvier. In contrast, in demyelinated regions (lower panel), action current is lost through the damaged myelin sheath or denuded regions of the axon.

impulse trains failing to propagate. Conduction can also be totally blocked.[8,9]

In demyelinated fibers, the high-resistance, low-capacitance myelin is damaged or lost. Thus, when an impulse approaches a demyelinated region, the density of action current is reduced as a result of capacitative and resistive shunting (figure 10.2). Therefore, either it takes longer for the demyelinated region to reach the threshold, in which case conduction velocity is decreased, or the threshold is not reached at all, in which case conduction is blocked. The loss of myelin over the previously myelinated region (designated the internode) leads to an important question concerning axonal-membrane organization (figure 10.3). Is the internodal axon membrane excitable—i.e., can it conduct impulses—or does it lack the capability for spike electrogenesis? This question is not especially germane to conduction in normal myelinated fibers, in which little voltage drop occurs across

the internodal axon membrane as a result of the properties of the overlying myelin sheath. However, it is crucial to an understanding of conduction in demyelinated axons, in which the insulating myelin sheath is damaged or lost.

The first systematic attempts to answer this question were made by Rasminsky and Sears,[9] who used a longitudinal current-analysis technique in demyelinated ventral-root fibers. Although the resolution of the technique was not sufficient to answer this question unequivocally, their study was of seminal importance, since it focused attention explicitly on this important problem.

Organization of the Axon Membrane

Several years later, morphologic studies provided clear evidence of structural differences

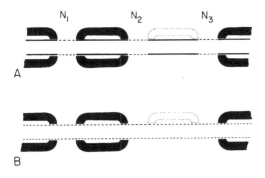

Figure 10.3
Alternative models of organization of the membrane in myelinated axons. Regions of the axon membrane that have nodal properties are represented by broken lines, and regions that have different properties are represented by solid lines. Thus, (A) represents a fiber in which nodal and internodal membranes have different properties, and (B) represents a fiber in which nodal and internodal membranes have similar properties. The properties of the internodal axon membrane are not important for conduction in normally myelinated internodes (e.g., between nodes N_1 and N_2) but are highly relevant to the function of demyelinated axons (e.g., between N_2 and N_3).

between nodal and internodal regions of the axon membrane. Cytochemical studies indicated distinct differences between the nodal and internodal axon membrane and suggested a higher density of sodium channels at the nodes than in the internodal membrane.[11,12] Freeze-fracture investigations revealed a high density of external-face intramembranous particles in the axon membrane at the nodes, and it was suggested that these might be related to sodium channels.[13] Quantitative data were provided by studies of the binding of ^{3}H-saxitoxin, a ligand that binds to sodium channels. These studies indicated a high sodium-channel density (approximately 10,000 channels per square micrometer) in the axon membrane at the nodes, in contrast to a very low density (<25 per square micrometer, which is too low to support impulse conduction)

in the internodes.[14] Thus, the model outlined in figure 10.3A appeared to be correct.

Subsequent voltage-clamp studies provided evidence that the Hodgkin–Huxley[15] model of nerve-membrane excitation might not apply to myelinated fibers in mammalian peripheral nerve. These recent studies suggest that sodium channels are responsible for the depolarization phase of the action potential, but that potassium conductance (which contributes substantially to repolarization in the classical Hodgkin–Huxley formulation) is attenuated or lacking in some mammalian myelinated axons, with repolarization occurring by rapid sodium inactivation or large leakage currents or both.[16,17] These results have been extended by intra-axonal recording to myelinated axons in the dorsal columns of the mammalian spinal cord.[18]

Further studies suggest a complementary distribution of sodium and potassium channels in some mammalian myelinated fibers, with sodium channels clustered in the axon membrane at the node of Ranvier and potassium channels located in the internodal axon membrane under the myelin. The primary evidence for this concept came from voltage-clamp studies by Chiu and Ritchie,[19] who showed the appearance of potassium conductances in mammalian nerve fibers after the acute disruption of myelin. Developmental studies[3] showed that before myelination both sodium and potassium channels contributed to action-potential waveform, but that after myelination in some fibers the contribution of potassium conductance to action-potential waveform was attenuated. Again, the data were consistent with the hypothesis that potassium channels might be located in the internodal axon membrane, but that they contributed minimally to repolarization because they were covered by the myelin sheath. A schematic representation of this current working model of the myelinated fiber is presented in figure 10.4. It must be emphasized that there may be differences in the detailed architecture of fibers of different sizes or types. Nevertheless, the

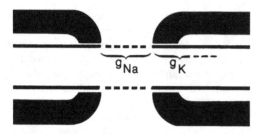

g_{Na} g_K

Figure 10.4
Current working model of the myelinated fiber. A node of Ranvier, bounded on either side by the paranodal portion of the myelin sheath, is shown schematically in longitudinal section. Sodium channels (g_{Na}) are clustered in a high concentration in the axon membrane at the node but are present in a low density or are absent in the internodal axon membrane. Potassium channels (g_K) are located beneath the myelin sheath in paranodal and internodal regions.

concept that nodal and internodal sections of axon membrane are structurally and functionally distinct is well established.

The model shown in figure 10.4 has important implications for the pathophysiology of conduction in demyelinated fibers. After the acute loss of myelin, the density of sodium channels in the demyelinated area is probably too low to support impulse conduction; the demyelinated axon membrane is thus essentially electrically inexcitable. In addition, the presence of potassium channels in the denuded axon membrane will tend to "clamp" the demyelinated axon membrane close to its resting potential and thus further prevent conduction.[20]

Mechanisms of Conduction in Demyelinated Axons

At this point, it is worth considering the time course of diseases such as multiple sclerosis, which in their classic form are characterized by exacerbations and remissions. It is a common finding that remyelination in the central-nervous-system plaques of multiple sclerosis is not brisk and in many cases does not occur at all. Thus, there can be recovery of function (clinical remission) in the absence of a strict recapitulation of prepathologic structure. What accounts for the recovery of function in clinical remissions of multiple sclerosis? The important possibility that recovery is due to alterations in levels of circulating ("blocking") factors has been reviewed elsewhere.[21,22] There is also some experimental evidence that resolution of edema may have a role,[23] and in some cases the clinical course is consistent with this mechanism. However, the effects of edema on conduction are not well understood. Moreover, the time course of remission suggests that in certain instances other factors are important. In some cases, conduction through alternative pathways, or synaptic alterations, can be invoked as a mechanism for recovery. Yet in other cases, such as demyelination of the optic nerve, there must be recovery of conduction through demyelinated axons.[24] The recent studies of Bostock and Sears,[25] in fact, have shown the development of "continuous" conduction across demyelinated regions of some damaged fibers; this suggests the capacity for spike electrogenesis (and thus the development of a density of sodium channels sufficient for impulse propagation) in certain demyelinated areas. Conduction block due to increased threshold, or impedance mismatch due to inadequate current density at the junction between normally myelinated and demyelinated axon regions, must be overcome, but small changes in fiber geometry may subserve this function.[25,26] Furthermore, there is recent morphologic evidence of reorganization of the demyelinated axon membrane, with the acquisition of increased numbers of sodium channels in the demyelinated region.[27] It is not yet clear whether this involves the redistribution of preexisting sodium channels or the production of new ones. In either case, the available data suggest that plasticity at the subcellular (membrane) level may be involved in the response to demyelination and possibly the recovery from it.

Possible Pharmacologic Approaches

How might conduction through demyelinated axon regions be facilitated? It was suggested as early as 1974 by Schauf and Davis[28] that modification of the kinetics of sodium and potassium channels to provide increased current density in demyelinated fibers might promote conduction across previously demyelinated regions. Davis et al.[29] had shown that lowering serum ionized calcium, which increases axonal excitability, could facilitate conduction in demyelinated fibers and lead to transient improvement in the clinical status of patients with multiple sclerosis. The results were transitory, lasting for minutes to hours, and thus were not of practical clinical value. But they were of considerable theoretical importance, indicating that the pharmacologic manipulation of axonal excitability might be relevant to the development of symptomatic therapies in the demyelinating diseases. Bostock et al.[30] demonstrated the reversible abolition of conduction block in demyelinated fibers with the application of *Leiurus quinquestriatus* toxin, which blocks the closing of sodium channels and thereby increases the amount of action current available. More recently, Sherratt et al.[31] showed an improvement in conduction block in demyelinated fibers after the application of 4-aminopyridine, an agent that blocks potassium channels. Again, the mechanism presumably involves the generation of increased amounts of action current. Yet agents such as 4-aminopyridine affect normal as well as abnormal elements in the white matter and neuropil, in addition to altering the conduction properties of demyelinated nerve fibers.[32] In fact, pilot clinical trials using 4-aminopyridine in patients with longstanding multiple sclerosis have shown unacceptable side effects, emphasizing the caution necessary with this pharmacologic approach.[33] Nevertheless, as Davis and Schauf[34] have pointed out, the possibility of developing pharmacologic agents to promote conduction through demyelinated or otherwise damaged nerve fibers has a firm theoretical basis, and the search for clinically effective agents appears practical and worthy of a sustained and organized effort.

It should be noted in this context that demyelinated fibers are highly sensitive to temperature, with the reliability of impulse conduction falling as the temperature is raised.[28,35] This is probably due to the decreased amount (time integral) of current generated at higher temperatures,[35] and it may explain (at least in part) the fact that clinical symptoms in some patients with multiple sclerosis worsen as body temperature is raised.[36] It is entirely possible that other changes in the exogenous milieu may alter the conduction properties of demyelinated fibers. Structure-function relations in nerve fibers are not static; on the contrary, they are dynamic, and they may reflect changes in temperature or in metabolic or immunologic status. Such changes could account for the transitory symptoms reported by other patients.

Finally, it should be noted that newly formed nodes in remyelinated fibers may develop relatively normal morphologic and physiologic characteristics,[37,38] and that even a small degree of remyelination may facilitate conduction in previously demyelinated nerve fibers.[26,39,40] Although remyelination after episodes of myelin loss is not nearly as brisk in the central nervous system as in the peripheral nervous system, the development of agents that might promote even a minor degree of remyelination is a promising area, and is being carefully pursued.

Acknowledgments

Supported by the Medical Research Service, Veterans Administration, and by grants from the National Multiple Sclerosis Society, the National Institutes of Health, and the Kroc Foundation.

References

1. McDonald WI. Pathophysiology in multiple sclerosis. Brain. 1974; 97: 179–96.

2. Rasminsky M. Physiology of conduction in demyelinated axons. In: Waxman SG, ed. Physiology and pathobiology of axons. New York: Raven Press, 1978: 361–76.

3. Waxman SG, Foster RE. Ionic channel distribution and heterogeneity of the axon membrane in myelinated fibers. Brain Res Rev. 1980; 2: 205–34.

4. Waxman SG. Clinicopathological correlations in multiple sclerosis and related diseases. In: Waxman SG, Ritchie JM, eds. Demyelinating disease: basic and clinical electrophysiology. New York: Raven Press, 1981: 169–82.

5. Rasminsky M. Hyperexcitability of pathologically myelinated axons and positive symptoms in multiple sclerosis. In: Waxman SG, Ritchie JM, eds. Demyelinating disease: basic and clinical electrophysiology. New York: Raven Press, 1981: 289–97.

6. Waxman SG, Bennett MVL. Relative conduction velocities of small myelinated and non-myelinated fibres in the central nervous system. Nature (New Biol). 1972; 238: 217–9.

7. Hodgkin AL. The conduction of the nervous impulse. Springfield, Ill.: Charles C Thomas, 1964.

8. McDonald WI, Sears TA. The effects of experimental demyelination on conduction in the central nervous system. Brain. 1970; 93: 583–98.

9. Rasminsky M, Sears TA. Internodal conduction in undissected demyelinated nerve fibres. J Physiol (Lond). 1972; 227: 323–50.

10. Gilliatt RW, Willison RG. Peripheral nerve conduction in diabetic neuropathy. J Neurol Neurosurg Psychiatry. 1962; 25: 11–8.

11. Quick DC, Waxman SG. Specific staining of the axon membrane at nodes of Ranvier with ferric ion and ferrocyanide. J Neurol Sci. 1977; 31: 1–11.

12. Waxman SG, Quick DC. Cytochemical differentiation of the axon membrane in A- and C-fibres. J Neurol Neurosurg Psychiatry. 1977; 40: 379–85.

13. Rosenbluth J. Intramembranous particle distribution at the node of Ranvier and adjacent axolemma in myelinated axons of the frog brain. J Neurocytol. 1976; 5: 731–45.

14. Ritchie JM, Rogart RB. Density of sodium channels in mammalian myelinated nerve fibers and nature of the axonal membrane under the myelin sheath. Proc Natl Acad Sci USA. 1977; 74: 211–5.

15. Hodgkin AL, Huxley AF. A quantitative description of membrane current and its application to conduction and excitation in nerve. J Physiol (Lond). 1952; 117: 500–44.

16. Chiu SY, Ritchie JM, Rogart RB, Stagg D. A quantitative description of membrane currents in rabbit myelinated nerve. J Physiol (Lond). 1979; 292: 149–66.

17. Brismar T. Potential clamp analysis of membrane currents in rat myelinated nerve fibres. J Physiol (Lond). 1980; 298: 171–84.

18. Kocsis JD, Waxman SG. Absence of potassium conductance in central myelinated axons. Nature. 1980; 287: 348–9.

19. Chiu SY, Ritchie JM. Potassium channels in nodal and internodal axonal membrane of mammalian myelinated fibres. Nature. 1980; 284: 170–1.

20. Ritchie JM, Chiu SY. Distribution of sodium and potassium channels in mammalian myelinated nerve. In: Waxman SG, Ritchie JM, eds. Demyelinating disease: basic and clinical electrophysiology. New York: Raven Press, 1981: 329–42.

21. Seil FJ. Tissue culture studies of neuroelectric blocking factors. In: Waxman SG, Ritchie JM, eds. Demyelinating disease: basic and clinical electrophysiology. New York: Raven Press, 1981: 281–8.

22. Schauf CL, Davis FA. Circulating toxic factors in multiple sclerosis: a perspective. In: Waxman SG, Ritchie JM, eds. Demyelinating disease: basic and clinical electrophysiology. New York: Raven Press, 1981: 287–90.

23. Arnason BGW, Chelmicka-Szorc E. Peripheral nerve segmental demyelination induced by intraneural diphtheria toxin injection. I. Effect of hydrocortisone as measured by muscle twitch tension. Arch Neurol. 1974; 30: 157–62.

24. Wisniewski HM, Oppenheimer D, McDonald WI. Relation between myelination and function in MS and EAE. J Neuropathol Exp Neurol. 1976; 35: 327. abstract.

25. Bostock H, Sears TA. The internodal axon membrane: electrical excitability and continuous conduction in segmental demyelination. J Physiol (Lond). 1978; 280: 273–301.

26. Waxman SG, Brill MH. Conduction through demyelinated plaques in multiple sclerosis: computer simulations of facilitation by short internodes. J Neurol Neurosurg Psychiatry. 1978; 41: 408–16.

27. Foster RE, Whalen CC, Waxman SG. Reorganization of the axon membrane in demyelinated peripheral nerve fibers: morphological evidence. Science. 1980; 210: 661–3.

28. Schauf CL, Davis FA. Impulse conduction in multiple sclerosis: a theoretical basis for modification by temperature and pharmacological agents. J Neurol Neurosurg Psychiatry. 1974; 37: 152–61.

29. Davis FA, Becker FO, Michael JA, Sorensen E. Effect of intravenous sodium bicarbonate, disodium edetate (Na_2EDTA), and hyperventilation on visual and oculomotor signs in multiple sclerosis. J Neurol Neurosurg Psychiatry. 1970; 33: 723–32.

30. Bostock H, Sherratt RM, Sears TA. Overcoming conduction failure in demyelinated nerve fibres by prolonging action potentials. Nature. 1978; 274: 385–7.

31. Sherratt RM, Bostock H, Sears TA. Effects of 4-aminopyridine on normal and demyelinated mammalian nerve fibres. Nature. 1980; 283: 570–2.

32. Kocsis JD, Malenka RC, Waxman SG. Enhanced parallel fiber frequency-following after reduction of postsynaptic activity. Brain Res. 1981; 207: 321–31.

33. Sears TA, Bostock H. Conduction failure in demyelination: is it inevitable? In: Waxman SG, Ritchie JM, eds. Demyelinating disease: basic and clinical electrophysiology. New York: Raven Press, 1981: 357–75.

34. Davis FA, Schauf CL. Approaches to the development of pharmacological interventions in multiple sclerosis. In: Waxman SG, Ritchie JM, eds. Demyelinating disease: basic and clinical electrophysiology. New York: Raven Press, 1981: 505–10.

35. Rasminsky M. The effects of temperature on conduction in demyelinated single nerve fibers. Arch Neurol. 1973; 28: 287–92.

36. Watson CW. Effects of lowering body temperature on the symptoms and signs of multiple sclerosis. N Engl J Med. 1959; 261: 1252–9.

37. Weiner LP, Waxman SG, Stohlman SA, Kwan A. Remyelination following virus-induced demyelination: ferric ion-ferrocyanide staining of nodes of Ranvier within the CNS. Ann Neurol. 1980; 8: 580–3.

38. Ritchie JM, Rang HP, Pellegrino R. Sodium and potassium channels in demyelinated and remyelinated mammalian nerve. Nature. 1981; 294: 257–9.

39. Koles ZJ, Rasminsky M. A computer simulation of conduction in demyelinated nerve fibres. J Physiol (Lond). 1972; 227: 351–64.

40. Smith KJ, Blakemore WF, McDonald WI. The restoration of conduction by central remyelination. Brain. 1981; 104: 383–404.

VIII SILENT DAMAGE

Self-repair of the nervous system is an important concept and, as illustrated in the previous part (part VII), it can be readily demonstrated in the laboratory. But how often does self-repair occur in the human brain or spinal cord? As discussed in part III, the nervous system contains localized groups of nerve cells which participate in specific functions and, following injury to a part of the brain or spinal cord, there is often impairment of an ability or skill such as vision, motor control, or speech. We also know, however, that functional recovery can occur in some neurological disorders. For example, many individuals with multiple sclerosis experience remissions in which they recover functions that had been lost. In these patients, vision may be regained in an eye that had been blind due to demyelination of the optic nerve, or motor power may be restored in a previously paralyzed limb. Partial functional recovery also frequently occurs in patients who have had strokes and in some cases there can be full recovery, of the ability to walk or use the hand, for example. In each of these cases, if the brain or spinal cord were examined with a microscope, the injury would be seen to persist—the damage becomes, however, clinically "silent" as functional recovery occurs. The two following papers deal with these remarkable phenomena.

In the Hume and Waxman (1988) study we searched for evidence of self-repair of the brain and spinal cord in patients referred to our hospital because of suspected multiple sclerosis. We studied these patients by measuring evoked potentials, which are small electrical changes, recorded using electrodes placed on the scalp, that are elicited in response to various stimuli. Visual evoked potentials can be triggered in response to visual stimuli, for example, the flashing of a checkerboard on a screen in front of the patient. Somatosensory evoked potentials are elicited by small electrical stimuli which are delivered to a nerve such as the median nerve at the wrist. And auditory evoked potentials are elicited by sound (usually in the form of a click) delivered to the ear. The evoked potential appears as an electrical wave which can be recorded through the scalp, and the shape and size of the evoked potential provide information about activity in the nerve cells within the brain underlying the electrode. By measuring the latency of the evoked potential (the time that it takes to occur following stimulation) it is possible to measure the conduction time that is needed for information to travel from the site of stimulation, through the appropriate nerves and fiber tracts within the nervous system, to the part of the brain under the electrode.

The speed of impulse conduction is decreased in nerve fibers whose myelin has been damaged. Earlier investigators, including Ian McDonald and his colleagues at the Institute of Neurology in Queen Square, London, had demonstrated that evoked potentials provide a convenient, noninvasive method for inferring the presence of demyelination along specific nerve fiber tracts within the human brain and spinal cord. They also showed that following remissions in multiple sclerosis, the latencies of evoked potentials can remain prolonged, providing a "footprint" of the now-silent lesion (Halliday, McDonald, and Mushin 1973). This was a remarkable finding because the increase in latency, which corresponds to the extra time needed for the message to reach its destination, was often tens of milliseconds, which is a large amount of time in the context of neural coding. Computation in the brain has usually been considered to be a process in which synaptic signals—which can be excitatory or inhibitory—are integrated by a process somewhat like algebraic summation, a process that requires that they impinge on postsynaptic target neurons at about the same time. It was not clear how, in the face of conduction times that can be prolonged by tens of milliseconds, function of the nervous system can be reestablished. But the early studies on evoked potentials showed clearly that this can occur—testimony to the nervous system's robust capability to extract the information that is inherent in a message.

Inspired by the work of McDonald and his colleagues, in the Hume and Waxman (1988) study we explored the degree to which evoked potentials can demonstrate silent damage of the central nervous system of people with multiple sclerosis. One of our questions concerned the degree to which evoked potentials could provide a diagnostic clue in individuals suspected of having multiple sclerosis. In this study we found that, as predicted by McDonald and his coworkers, evoked potentials can have significant predictive value in this group of patients: an evoked potential demonstrating a clinically silent lesion in a patient with suspected multiple sclerosis was associated with a 71 percent chance of clinical worsening, and a 48 percent chance of developing clinically definite multiple sclerosis. We also, however, were interested in learning about the frequency of subclinical lesions, and our results in this respect were especially exciting. Fifty percent of the abnormal evoked potentials were not accompanied by clinical abnormalities. Thus at least one-half of the demyelinated lesions were subclinical. Our data suggested that demyelinated lesions in certain tracts were more likely to be clinically silent than those in other tracts, implying differences in the mode of neural coding, in redundancy, or in the physiology of the nerve fibers themselves; but we could not make this point with certitude, and we did not mention it in the paper. Irrespective of this latter point, this study taught us that "clinically silent" lesions in multiple sclerosis are not a curiosity—indeed, clinically inapparent damage is quite common in this disease. My own bias is that these silent lesions may provide "model systems" which can teach us about reparative mechanisms within the brain and spinal cord. This paper thus provides a link, to humans, for the laboratory experiments described in part VIII.

The Waxman and Toole (1983) paper discussed recovery of function in another disorder, stroke, which is the third most frequent cause of death in industrialized societies. Stroke results from loss of crucial blood supply to a part of the brain. Stroke produces clinical deficits because it causes infarction, or loss of nerve cells within this portion of the brain. Ischemia, on the other hand, is the impairment of the blood supply to an organ such as the brain; ischemia can temporarily exhaust nerve cells so they cannot generate impulses—and thus are silent—without killing them. It was known, when this article was written in 1983, that ischemia could produce "warning strokes," which were also called transient ischemic attacks (TIAs). The concept of the TIA had been developed, in part, to accommodate patients in whom there was ischemia, but not infarction, of brain tissue; and the definition of TIA had been refined over the years to the generally accepted clinical definition of focal neurologic dysfunction, which resolves completely within twenty-four hours.

Occasionally, however, patients could sustain brain infarctions and nevertheless recover within twenty-four hours, so that clinical deficits could not be detected after this time. The older literature had demonstrated this on the basis of postmortem examinations, and we now could observe this phenomenon in living patients by comparing their clinical courses with their CT scans. The existence of patients who recovered from neurological deficits as in a TIA, but in whom we knew there was brain infarction, raised a number of issues. These included clinical questions (concerning, for example, decisions about medical or surgical management). And there were also experimental issues (for example, whether a patient with transient—less than twenty-four hours' duration—neurologic dysfunction, but with a cerebral infarct visible on CT scan, should be categorized as having sustained a TIA, or a cerebral infarct, in a clinical trial?). I was on the faculty at the school of medicine of Stanford University at the time, and, during a visit by Jim Toole, an authority on stroke from Wake Forest University, I mentioned this problem to him. Having spent most of his career thinking about stroke, Toole had also begun to worry about this problem. We decided to combine our thoughts, and thus published this paper in which we described three examples of patients who met the criteria for TIA from a clinical point of view, but who had, from an anatomical point of view, sustained brain infarction.

The presence of silent damage, in patients with stroke as described in this paper, provides a dramatic example of the adaptive capability of the human brain. Following loss of neurons—even in the dominant hemisphere in some patients—the human brain can reorganize to take over the functions of some compromised circuits, so that there are no persistent sequelae. We included only a few cases, which we thought were illustrative, in this paper. Our ideas were initially received with incredulity by some of our colleagues and we had to send the manuscript to several journals before it was accepted. Now, fifteen years later, there have been many elegant demonstrations of silent brain infarctions (e.g. Brott et al. 1995).

The methods used in these two studies—evoked potentials and early techniques for CT scanning—have been supplanted, in part, by other methods of non-invasively studying the human brain and spinal cord, such as high-resolution CT and MR scanning. I thus doubt whether these papers will continue to be cited in the future. Nevertheless, I consider these early studies important because they permitted us to see subclinical injury or "silent damage" in the human central nervous system, and illustrated that although our brains and spinal cords are complex and fragile, they possess immense flexibility and can utilize it to recover after injury. We want, as physicians, to preserve or restore function. Neuroprotection will one day limit damage to the nervous system, thus preserving function. Neurorehabilitation, on the other hand, has the goal of restoring function in people with damaged brains and spinal cords. Silent damage shows us that the human nervous system possesses its own mechanisms for self-repair, reminding us that this latter goal is a very realistic one.

References

Brott, T., Tomsick, T., Feinberg, W., Johnson, C., et al. for the ACAS Investigators. Baseline silent cerebral infarction in ACAS. *Stroke* 25: 1122–1129, 1995.

Halliday, A. M., McDonald, W. I., and Mushin, J. Visual evoked response in diagnosis of multiple sclerosis. *Br. Med. J.* 4: 661–664, 1973.

Hume, A. L., and Waxman, S. G. Evoked potentials in suspected multiple sclerosis: diagnostic value and prediction of clinical course. *J. Neurol. Sci.* 83: 191–210, 1988.

Waxman, S. G., and Toole, J. F. Temporal profile resembling TIA in the setting of cerebral infarction. *Stroke* 14: 433–437, 1983.

11 Evoked Potentials in Suspected Multiple Sclerosis: Diagnostic Value and Prediction of Clinical Course

Ann L. Hume and Stephen G. Waxman

Summary Pattern visual, somatosensory and brainstem auditory evoked potentials (EPs) of 14 patients with definite multiple sclerosis, 222 patients suspected of having multiple sclerosis, 26 patients with isolated optic neuritis and 40 patients with a chronic not diagnosed neurologic disorder, were compared with their clinical diagnoses on $2\frac{1}{2}$-year follow-up. In the MS suspects, an EP abnormality demonstrating a clinically silent lesion in any modality (65 patients) was associated with a 71% chance of clinical deterioration (48% chance of definite MS within the follow-up period). Normal EPs (121 patients) were associated with a 16% chance of deterioration (4% chance of definite MS). EPs in patients in whom the only abnormalities confirmed known lesions (36 patients) did not predict follow-up status. Visual EPs demonstrated clinically silent lesions more frequently than somatosensory and auditory EPs (22%, 12% and 5% of patients). Only one of the patients with optic neuritis and 3 of the chronic not diagnosed group had EPs demonstrating clinically silent lesions. CSF and NMR studies also correlated with follow-up in subseries of the patients.

Introduction

Evoked potentials (EPs) are used widely in the assessment of patients suspected of having multiple sclerosis (MS) because of their ability to demonstrate clinically silent lesions within the central nervous system (Halliday et al. 1973; Chiappa 1983; Matthews et al. 1985). Rigorous validation of the accuracy and utility of EPs in this context is lacking, however, and to date only 2 studies have attempted to determine by long-term follow-up whether diagnoses of MS indicated by EPs are correct (Matthews et al. 1982; Deltenre et al. 1984). Moreover, the utility of EPs in assessing prognosis in patients with MS has not been, to date, evaluated.

Reprinted with permission from *Journal of the Neurological Sciences* 83: 191–210, 1988.

The current study examines the clinical presentation, the pattern visual, somatosensory and brainstem auditory EPs, and the subsequent clinical course in a series of patients suspected of having MS. The principal aim of this retrospective analysis was to determine how many patients with normal EPs, and how many with abnormal EPs (either confirming known dysfunction (termed confirmatory) or suggesting a clinically silent lesion (termed positive), would deteriorate or develop clinically definite disease within 2–4 years. Results of cerebrospinal fluid (CSF) and nuclear magnetic resonance (NMR) imaging studies were available for comparison in some of the patients.

Methods

Patients

This study is based on data derived from a population of 347 patients referred to Yale–New Haven Hospital by neurological specialists for EP studies because of suspected MS. The series is consecutive except that patients under 15 years of age or over 60, and patients whose symptoms began after the age of 50, are excluded. Thirty-three patients from a single clinic whose records were not available for review are also not included. Approval for review was granted institutionally and by the referring physicians. Of the 347 patients reviewed, 45 were lost to follow-up and their results are excluded from further consideration. Thus, follow-ups were obtained for 302 patients who are analyzed in this paper (table 11.1).

The patients' histories at referral were reviewed and 153 (51 male, 102 female; mean age, 37 years) were classified according to the criteria of McAlpine (1972): 14 had clinically definite MS, 29 had probable MS, and 110 had

Table 11.1

Initial clinical diagnoses and evoked potentials in 236 patients with or suspected of multiple sclerosis, 26 patients with definite or possible optic neuritis (ON) and 40 patients with a chronic not diagnosed neurological disorder (CND)

Initial diagnosis	n	Abnormal EP No. abnormal/No. tested (No. diagnostic)			EPs overall		
		PVEP	SEP	BAEP	Normal	Confirm only	Diagnostic[a]
Definite MS	14	14/14 (2)	11/14 (1)	6/12 (1)	0	10	4
Suspected MS							
Probable	29	26/29 (9)	17/29 (8)	5/29 (0)	2	13	14
Possible	56	19/51 (11)	18/54 (10)	4/52 (2)	31	9	16
Spinal cord	32	12/30 (12)	19/32 (0)	5/32 (5)	11	7	14
Poss. Sp.C.	22	3/21 (3)	2/22 (2)	0/21 (0)	18	0	4
AND	83	14/79 (11)	13/80 (7)	5/80 (3)	59	7	17
Total	222	74/210[b] (46)	69/217 (27)	19/214 (10)	121[c]	36	65
Other							
ON	15	13/15 (0)	0/12 (0)	0/12 (0)	2	13	0
Poss. ON	11	4/11 (4)	0/6 (0)	1/6 (1)	7[d]	0	4
CND	40	1/40 (0)	2/40 (2)	2/39 (2)	36	1	3

[a] Patients with diagnostic EP in one modality may have confirmatory abnormality in another.
[b] Excludes 5 patients with abnormal PVEPs and history of amblyopia (4 others with amblyopia had normal PVEPs), one with blindness 2° to granulomatous disease and one with nystagmus.
[c] 110 normal in all 3 modalities; 3 patients had non-diagnostic PVEPs in one eye (amblyopia), 5 were tested in only 2 modalities and 3 in only 1 modality.
[d] Includes 5 patients with PVEPs tested only.

possible MS by these criteria. Within the possible group, 32 had a history and signs only of spinal cord disease, and 22 had an equivocal history or symptoms suggestive of spinal cord disease.

Three additional diagnostic categories were adopted to include the range of patients referred and because the McAlpine classification excludes patients with isolated optic neuritis (ON) and patients with an initial episode of neurological symptoms. Twenty-six patients (8 male; mean age, 33 years) had ON, in 11 of whom the history was equivocal; none had signs or symptoms to suggest a lesion elsewhere in the central nervous system. Eighty-three patients (28 male; mean age, 31 years) were classified as "acute not diagnosed": this category was defined by Small

et al. (1978) and includes patients with a single episode of symptoms, of a nature compatible with MS of less than 3 months duration at the time of examination. A further 40 patients (7 male; mean age, 36 years) with a history of neurological symptoms or signs lasting more than 3 months without remission or relapse, for which no cause had been found, were classified as "chronic not diagnosed." (Within this series the 22 patients who either met the McAlpine criteria for possible or probable MS or were AND are classified as MS suspects; the patients who had ON or were CND are considered separately.)

The optic nerve, spinal cord and brainstem function of each patient was rated from the medical record as indicating a definite history of dysfunction, equivocal signs or symptoms only, or as being normal. For the optic nerve a clear history of decreased corrected visual acuity with or without recovery, scotoma, unilateral color deficit or afferent pupil defect were considered definitive evidence of dysfunction; transient or episodic visual disturbance or symptoms without documented signs, questionable disc pallor or questionable afferent pupil defect were considered equivocal. Corrected visual acuity was recorded, and a history of ocular or retinal abnormalities, or of amblyopia, was noted. For the spinal cord, objective sensory or motor changes at any level of the neuraxis below the foramen magnum and excluding the peripheral nerves, or spasticity, were considered definitive; sensory or motor symptoms alone or isolated reflex asymmetry were defined as equivocal. For the brainstem, documented diplopia, nystagmus, abnormalities of ocular motility, internuclear ophthalmoplegia, cerebellar signs, or central cranial nerve dysfunction (V, VI, VII) were considered definitive; symptoms or questionable evidence of diplopia, nystagmus, dizziness, unsteadiness or cranial nerve dysfunction were considered equivocal.

Evoked Potentials

EPs in all 3 modalities were recorded in 277 of the patients; 12 had only two and 13 only one modality studied. Standard methods and norms used for recording and interpreting the pattern visual and somatosensory EPs are those of Allison et al. (1983), whose equipment was replicated in this laboratory. The methods and norms for the brainstem auditory EPs are those published by Stockard et al. (1978), the norms being similar to those recorded from 20 normal volunteers in this laboratory.

The visual stimulus, presented monocularly, was a reversing checker-pattern, generated by a galvanometer-mirror system (2 reversals/sec; luminance of white squares 1750 ± 50 cd/m^2, dark squares 45 cd/m^2). Each check subtended

50$'$ and the total field subtended 16° at the eye. Patients fixated a small central spot and their cooperation and alertness were monitored continuously. Averages of 128 samples from each of 4 derivations were recorded simultaneously in order to observe the occipital distribution of the EPs and to ensure correct identification of the major occipital positive potential, P100 (O_z-F_{P_z}, O_1-F_{P_z}, O_2-F_{P_z}, F_{P_z}-linked earlobes); the bandpass was 1–300 Hz (sampling interval, 1 msec). Peak latencies of P100 which were 3 SD or more above normal mean values after correction for age and sex and including right–left differences, W-shaped P100s, or the failure to record P100 given adequate fixation were considered abnormal.

Somatosensory stimuli were 0.5-msec square-wave pulses delivered to the median nerve at the wrist (4/sec) at an intensity just producing a thumb twitch. Averages of 512 samples were recorded from 4 derivations (contralateral parietal scalp, P_4 or P_3, C2 and C7 spinous processes and midclavicle ipsilateral to stimulation, with common electrode at F_{P_z}); the bandpass was 30–3000 Hz (sampling interval, 80 μsec). Interpeak latencies, N20–N10, N20–N13 or N13–N10, which were 3 SD or more above the normal means were defined as abnormal; instances in which the initial cerebral complex from the scalp, N20–P30, or the major negative complex from the neck, N13, were markedly attenuated or could not be recorded were also considered abnormal, provided N10 was normal.

Auditory stimuli were 0.1-msec clicks delivered monaurally through TDH-49P headphones (11/sec) at 65 dB SL; rarefaction clicks were used below 85 dB HL, and alternate polarity clicks at higher intensities. The contralateral ear was masked with white noise at 40 dB HL. Averages of 2000 samples were recorded from 2 derivations (A_2-C_z, A_1-C_z; ear electrodes on medial surface of lobe); the bandpass was 25–3000 Hz (sampling interval, 20 μsec). Interpeak latencies I–V, I–III or III–V, which were 3 SD or more above the normal means were defined as abnormal; instances in which component sequences were severely attenuated or could not be recorded or the V:I amplitude ratio was less than 0.5 on replication were also considered abnormal.

EPs in each modality were defined as *positive* if they were abnormal in the absence of clinical evidence of dysfunction in that system, irrespective of symptoms, *confirmatory* if they were abnormal in the presence of clinical evidence of involvement, or *normal*. Lateralization of either clinical signs or EP abnormalities was not taken into account.

Follow-Up

Clinical follow-ups were obtained in 3 ways: (i) by chart review of patients who continued to see their referring specialist (141 patients), (ii) by writing to a patient's general practitioner if the patient was no longer seeing the specialist (36), or (iii) by directly writing or telephoning the patient if he or she had not recently seen either the specialist or general practitioner (111). Most of the patients contacted directly were either clinically stable or, more frequently, had had no further symptoms or problems relating to their initial referral; in no instance was the possibility of MS suggested to them. Classifications at follow-up were based solely on clinical criteria. Patients were thus recategorized according to the McAlpine criteria as having developed clinically definite MS, as having deteriorated but not having clinically definite disease or as having had no clinical progression or relapse; patients who had recovered and had had no further symptoms were considered separately.

Patients with clinically definite MS at follow-up were followed for an average of 27 months (range, 3–56 months). Excluding those in whom a diagnosis other than MS was established, the other MS-suspect patients were followed for an average of 32 months (12–55 months), the patients with ON, excluding those who became definite, for 33 months (12–56 months), and those in the CND category also for 33 months (11–55 months).

NMR and CSF Studies

Results of NMR brain imaging, undertaken up to 44 months after the EPs (from 1984 on), were available in 41 patients. These studies were done in a private radiological practice, using a 0.15 T imaging device (Technicare) based on a resistive magnet and utilizing standard 2-D FT multislice spin echo imaging sequences. Typical studies involved both T_1- and T_2-weighted images (TR 100–1700, TE 30–100 msec) of the entire brain in the axial plane, supplemented with sagittal or coronal images or with other sequences (i.e., inversion recovery) in selected cases. Studies were interpreted as consistent with MS only in the presence of multiple white matter lesions.

Results of CSF studies undertaken within 3 months of the EPs were available for 117 patients. The presence of multiple oligoclonal bands, or elevations of the IgG/albumin ratio (>0.17), the IgG index (>0.7) or myelin basic protein (MBP; >6.1 ng/ml) were considered abnormal. Not all patients had all 3 CSF parameters studied.

Results

In the following sections, the patients' EPs are compared with their initial clinical presentation and with their clinical evolution. In subsets of patients, the EPs are also compared with the results of NMR and CSF studies.

Clinical Presentation

Results of the EP studies are summarized according to clinical presentation in table 11.1. Ten of the 14 patients with definite MS had EPs which confirmed clinically known lesions, and 4 had EPs which were positive in indicating a clinically silent lesion.

Overall, 93% (27/29) of the patients with probable MS had abnormal EPs, 45% (50/110) of the patients with possible MS including the 54 with spinal cord disease did, and 29% (24/83) of the patients classified as "acute not diagnosed" (AND) did. The EPs were positive and hence of diagnostic value in indicating clinically silent CNS dysfunction in one half of the probable patients (14/29), one third of the possible group (34/110) and one fifth of the AND patients (17/83).

Both overall and within the groups, the visual EP was more frequently abnormal and positive than the somatosensory EP, which, in turn, was more frequently abnormal and positive than the brainstem auditory EP. Thus, 22% (46/210) of all suspect patients had positive visual EPs, 12% (27/217) had positive somatosensory EPs, and 5% (10/214) had positive brainstem auditory EPs. The visual EP was the only positive EP in 15% of the patients, the somatosensory in 7% and the auditory in 1%.

It is striking that 14 of the 32 patients presenting with clinical evidence of isolated spinal cord disease had positive visual or brainstem auditory EPs. Another 3 of the 22 patients with symptoms only of spinal cord dysfunction (table 11.1, Poss Sp C) and 5 of the 18 patients who were AND with a clinically isolated myelopathy had similarly positive visual or auditory EPs (3 others with symptoms only had abnormal somatosensory EPs).

In the patients with ON, 13 of the 15 with clinically definite optic nerve dysfunction had had abnormal visual EPs and all of the 12 tested had had normal somatosensory and brainstem auditory EPs. Four of the 11 with clinically equivocal optic nerve dysfunction had had abnormal visual EPs and one also had an abnormal brainstem auditory EP. Only 4 of the 40 patients with a chronic not diagnosed disorder (CND) had abnormal EPs; their results are discussed below.

Follow-Up and Prognosis

Table 11.2 shows the initial and follow-up clinical diagnoses and the EPs of 204 of the 222 patients initially suspected of MS (data for the 18 receiving a diagnosis other than MS are shown in table 11.3). Table 11.3A shows the corresponding data for the patients with optic neuritis and CND disorders, and table 11.3B for the 28 patients in whom a diagnosis other than MS was established (18 were initially MS-suspects, 2 had ON and 8 were CND).

Forty-eight of the 222 patients initially suspected of MS developed clinically definite MS within the average $2\frac{1}{2}$ year period to follow-up (table 11.2). Thirty-one of these 48 patients who developed clinically definite MS, or 65%, had had positive EPs, 25% had had confirmatory EPs only, and 10% had had totally normal EPs. Within this group developing definite MS, the visual EPs had been positive in 53% (25/47), the somatosensory in 26%, and the auditory in 13%. The visual EP was uniquely positive in 14 patients (30% of patients who developed definite MS), the somatosensory in 5 (11%) and the auditory in none.

Thirty-eight patients had deteriorated on follow-up but did not have clinically definite MS: 16 or 42% had had positive EPs, 21% confirmatory EPs and 37% normal EPs. Increasingly more of the patients who were unchanged or without further symptoms on follow-up had had normal EPs in all modalities.

Greater proportions of patients with definite MS on follow-up had had EP abnormalities in two or more modalities compared with the proportions in the other groups. However, given an EP abnormality, abnormalities in two or more modalities, whether positive or confirmatory, did not significantly increase diagnostic accuracy. For example, 12 of the 48 patients who became definite had had positive EPs in two or more modalities compared with 5 of the 98 who deteriorated or were unchanged ($\chi^2 = 10.4$, $P < 0.001$). However, this 12 as a proportion of the 31 who had had a positive EP and became definite is not significantly different from the 5 as a proportion of the other 32 patients with positive EPs who did not develop definite MS ($\chi^2 = 3.2$, NS).

The 4 EP abnormalities in the AND group with no further symptoms on follow-up were all in the somatosensory modality (table 11.2,

Table 11.2
Initial and follow-up clinical diagnoses, average period to follow-up and EPs of 204 MS-suspects followed for an average of 30 months

| Diagnosis | | n | Follow-up (mth) | Abnormal EP No. abnormal/No. tested (No. diagnostic) | | | EPs overall | | |
Initial	Follow-up			PVEP	SEP	BAEP	Normal	Confirm only	Diagnostic
Became definite									
Probable	—Definite	19	23	18/19 (6)	10/19 (4)	3/19 (0)	1	9	9
Possible	—Definite	15	32	10/14 (9)	12/14 (8)	4/14 (2)	2	1	12
SpC	—Definite	4	25	4/4 (4)	4/4 (0)	2/4 (2)	0	0	4
AND	—Definite	10	28	7/10 (6)	3/9 (0)	3/10 (2)	2	2	6
Total		48		39/47 (25)	29/46 (12)	12/47 (6)	5	12	31
Deterioration									
Possible	—Probable	8	30	2/8 (1)	4/8 (1)	0/7 (0)	3	3	2
SpC	—Progr[a]	11	28	4/9 (4)	8/11 (0)	3/11 (3)	3	2	6
Poss SpC	—SpC	4	40	2/4 (2)	1/4 (1)	0/4 (0)	2	0	2
AND	—Possible	15	35	5/14 (4)	5/15 (3)	2/15 (1)	6	3	6
Total		38		13/35 (11)	18/38 (5)	5/37 (4)	14	8	16
No change									
Probable	—Probable	10	29	8/10 (3)	7/10 (4)	2/10 (0)	1	4	5
Possible	—Possible	29	30	7/26 (1)	2/28 (1)	0/28 (0)	22	5	2
SpC	—SpC	11	32	4/11 (4)	5/11 (0)	0/11 (0)	4	3	4
Poss SpC	—Poss SpC	10	35	1/9 (1)	1/10 (1)	0/9 (0)	8	0	2
Total		60		20/56 (9)	15/59 (6)	2/58 (0)	35	12	13
No further symptoms									
SpC		3	34	0/3 (0)	0/3 (0)	0/3 (0)	3	0	0
Poss SpC		7	31	0/7 (0)	0/7 (0)	0/7 (0)	7	0	0
AND		48	32	0/46 (0)	4/46 (3)	0/45 (0)	44	1	3
Total		58		0/56 (0)	4/56 (3)	0/55 (0)	54	1	3

[a] Progressive spinal cord disease, no other lesions.

Table 11.3
Initial and follow-up clinical diagnoses, average period to follow-up and EPs of (A) patients initially with or suspected of optic neuritis, or with a chronic not diagnosed neurological disorder and (B) patients in whom a diagnosis other than MS was made

Diagnosis		n	Follow-up (mth)	Abnormal EP No. abnormal/No. tested (No. diagnostic)			EPs overall		
Initial	Follow-up			PVEP	SEP	BAEP	Normal	Confirm only	Diagnostic
(A)									
ON-Def(3)/Pr/Poss MS		5	39	4/5 (0)	0/5 (0)	0/5 (0)	1	4	0
	—Residual	5	37	4/5 (0)	0/3 (0)	0/3 (0)	1	4	0
	—Recovery	3	35	3/3 (0)	0/3 (0)	0/3 (0)	0	3	0
Poss ON	—Residual	3	18	2/3 (2)	0/2 (0)	0/2 (0)	1	0	2
	—Recovery	8	32	2/8 (2)	0/4 (0)	1/4 (1)	6	0	2
CND	—Definite MS	1	36	0/1 (0)	0/1 (0)	0/1 (0)	1	0	0
	—No change	19	32	0/19 (0)	0/19 (0)	1/19 (1)	18	0	1
	—Recovery	12	34	0/12 (0)	1/12 (1)	0/12 (0)	11	0	1
(B)									
—OTHER Dx									
Possible—		4[a]	20	0/3 (0)	0/4 (0)	0/3 (0)	4	0	0
SpC (1 Poss SpC)—		4[b]	4	0/4 (0)	2/4 (0)	0/4 (0)	2	2	0
AND—		10[c]	26	2/9 (1)	1/10 (1)	0/10 (0)	7	1	2
ON—		2[d]	2	2/2 (0)	0/1 (0)	0/1 (0)	0	2	0
CND—		8[e]	16	1/8 (0)	1/8 (1)	1/7 (1)	6	1	1

[a] Cerebrovascular disease (2); Arnold Chiari; functional.
[b] Cervical disc disease (2); cervical cord tumor; foramen magnum meningioma.
[c] Vascular disease (4); cervical spondylosis with recovery after surgery (2); myasthenia gravis; ALS; cervical disc; barbiturate abuse.
[d] Chiasmal meningioma; craniopharyngioma.
[e] Vascular disease (3); functional (2); Epstein-Barr; myasthenia gravis; olivopontocerebellar degeneration.

lowest panel). One patient had had abnormal N20–N13 intervals and 2 had had attenuated and variable cervical EPs; all 3 had had associated symptoms or signs, and CSF abnormalities (2 had elevated IgG and multiple oligoclonal bands, and the other, an IgG index of 0.18 with a total protein of 29 mg/dl). The fourth patient had had an asymmetric N20–N13 interval (6.6 vs 5.6 msec) which, as he was also epileptic, was not considered of certain significance.

Spinal Cord Dysfunction

Of the patients who had presented with signs or symptoms of spinal cord dysfunction, 31 had deteriorated on follow-up (9 developed clinically definite MS), 37 were unchanged or had had no further symptoms, and 4 had a diagnosis other than MS. Seventeen of the 31 who deteriorated had had positive EPs compared with 5 of the 37 who did not deteriorate ($\chi^2 = 11.3$, $P < 0.001$).

Optic Neuritis

Three of the patients who presented with clinically certain ON developed definite MS, one became probable and one possible MS; 4 of these had had abnormal visual EPs but none had had other EP abnormalities (table 11.3). The only patient of the entire ON group whose EPs had indicated dysfunction outside the optic nerves, namely in the brainstem auditory pathways, had no further symptoms during the ensuing 3 years to follow-up.

Chronic Not Diagnosed

One of the patients initially categorized as CND had developed clinically definite MS after 3 years; she had had normal EPs. Nineteen others had not changed on follow-up and 12 had had no further symptoms. Two had had abnormal EPs. Both had presented with symptoms of brainstem dysfunction. One of these patients,

with an abnormal auditory EP (I–III interval) was unchanged clinically after 3 years, as were her EPs, and the other who had had asymmetric N20–N13 intervals reported no symptoms after 4 years.

Other Final Diagnoses

Eighteen of the MS suspects received an alternative diagnosis at some stage after the EP study. Two of these patients, both of whom were initially AND, had had EPs which met the criteria for "positive": one with clinical evidence of brainstem disease had an abnormal N20–N13 interval and normal auditory EPs; angiography subsequently demonstrated basilar artery thrombosis. The other with an abnormal occipital distribution of his visual EPs was finally considered to have vasospastic disease and had recovered on follow-up. Three others had had confirmatory EPs: one of 2 with a cervical myelopathy had no recordable cervical somatosensory EPs and was found to have a C1–2 cord tumor, and the other with bilaterally absent cerebral somatosensory EPs had a foramen magnum meningioma. The third patient with cerebellar signs and a visual field defect had a corroborative visual EP; angiography subsequently demonstrated inflammatory vasculitis of the CNS and retina.

Of the 2 CND patients with abnormal EPs and other eventual diagnoses, one, with a family history of MS, had had W-shaped pattern visual EPs which were consistent with her bitemporal disc pallor; CT later showed a middle cerebral artery aneurysm. The other patient had symptoms suggesting right hemisphere dysfunction: he had a prolonged N20–N13 interval to his left hemisphere and bilaterally prolonged I–V intervals; his diagnosis was ophthalmic migraine.

CSF and EPs

Considering all patients in whom the CSF was examined, both the IgG (IgG/albumin ratio or

Table 11.4
Clinical course, CSF (IgG, OB, MBP) and evoked potentials in MS-suspects

Course	IgG result/EP result				OB[a] result/EP result				MBP result/EP result			
	+/+	−/−	+/−	−/+	+/+	−/−	+/−	−/+	+/+	−/−	+/−	−/+
Became definite	16		3	4	11	1	2	6	3	1	1	5
Deteriorated	11	2	4	3	4	3	1	5	1	2	1	9
No change	5	8	4	4	4	8	3	5	2	5	1	1
No > symptoms	3	20		1	2	15	1	1		13	2	1
Total	35	30	11	12	21	27	7	17	6	21	5	16

[a] OB, oligoclonal bands.

IgG index) and the oligoclonal bands tended to be correlated with the patients' status on follow-up (table 11.4). Seventy-nine percent of the patients who developed clinically definite MS or deteriorated (34/43) had had elevated IgG while 73% who were unchanged or had no further symptoms (33/45) had had normal CSF IgG ($\chi^2 = 22.2$, $P < 0.001$). Similarly, 55% of the patients who deteriorated (18/33) had had multiple oligoclonal bands while 74% of those who did not deteriorate (29/39) had had no bands ($\chi^2 = 5.1$, $P < 0.025$). The CSF MBP did not correlate with the patients' follow-ups.

If the patients presenting with spinal cord disease are considered separately, the CSF IgG but not the oligoclonal bands predicted follow-up. Thus 15 of the 19 who deteriorated had had elevated IgG and 8 of the 11 who did not deteriorate had had normal IgG (Fisher exact $P = 0.007$). However, although 8 of the 10 patients who did not deteriorate had had no oligoclonal bands, 8 of the 15 who did deteriorate also had had no bands ($P = 0.17$).

Consistent with the prediction of the patients' follow-ups by the EPs and by the CSF IgG and oligoclonal bands, there is a good concordance between these parameters themselves. Concordance between the CSF IgG and EPs was observed in 65 patients or 74% of the 88 patients studied ($\chi^2 = 18.1$, $P < 0.001$), and between the oligoclonal bands and EPs, in 67% of the 72

patients studied ($\chi^2 = 7.7$, $P < 0.01$). The CSF MBP was unrelated to the EPs in the 48 patients studied.

Patients with spinal cord disease are disproportionately represented in the groups with negative CSF findings and abnormal EPs. They accounted for one-third of the patients who had CSF studies but for one-half with such results (6 of the 12 with normal IgG and abnormal EPs, 8 of the 17 without oligoclonal bands and with abnormal EPs, and 8 of the 16 with normal MBP and abnormal EPs). There were no other factors in the clinical history or EP studies which might account for the discrepancies between the CSF and EP studies.

The CSF studies of the patients with optic neuritis were striking for their lack of abnormality. Although 5 of the 7 patients studied had had abnormal visual EPs, only one had had positive CSF findings; this patient had elevated IgG but normal MBP and no oligoclonal bands within a month of her EP study, and at about the time she developed clinical evidence of spinal cord disease. One of the other 6 with normal CSF studies also developed clinically definite MS; one had residual visual loss with optic atrophy and four recovered with no recurrences.

Of the 10 MS-suspects with CSF studies and diagnoses other than MS on follow-up, 3 had had CSF abnormalities, namely IgG elevation in association with cervical myelopathy. Two of the

Table 11.5

Clinical course, NMR imaging and evoked potentials in 31 MS-suspects

Course	NMR result/EP result			
	+/+	−/−	+/−	−/+
Became definite	11		2	
Deteriorated		2	1	4
No change	2	4	1	2
No > symptoms		2		
Total	13	8	4	6

8 CND patients tested also had IgG elevation but none had multiple oligoclonal bands.

NMR and EPs

Results of the NMR studies were consistent with the patients' follow-up diagnoses and with their EPs (table 11.5). Thus 14 of the 20 patients who deteriorated had had NMR scans which were consistent with a diagnosis of MS (15 had had abnormal EPs, 11 positive EPs) compared with 3 of the 11 who were unchanged or had had no further symptoms (4 had had abnormal EPs, 2 positive EPs). Overall concordance between the NMR and EP studies was 68% (21/31 patients). These comparisons are limited, however, since there were intervals between the EP and NMR studies of up to 44 months (median, 16 months). Such delays, for example, may account for discrepancies between the studies in 3 of the 4 patients who had normal EPs and abnormal NMR studies: delays were 30–44 months and all 3 had deteriorated on follow-up.

Five of the 6 patients with normal NMR and abnormal EP studies had myelopathy at both presentation and follow-up: 2 had had positive visual or auditory EPs and had progressive disease, and 3 had had abnormal somatosensory EPs only (2 had progressive disease, one was unchanged).

Two patients with optic neuritis and corroborative EP changes had normal NMR studies; neither had developed other signs or symptoms on follow-up. Three MS-suspects who received a diagnosis other than MS had NMR studies: one whose NMR demonstrated an Arnold-Chiari malformation had had normal EPs, one whose NMR showed cerebral atrophy had inflammatory vasculitis and an abnormal visual EP, and the other who was diagnosed as having ALS had normal NMR and EP studies. Five CND patients had NMR studies. The one who developed definite MS had had a positive NMR scan 3 years after her normal EPs. The other 4 had each presented with brainstem dysfunction and were unchanged or partially improved on follow-up; all had had normal NMR and EP studies.

Discussion

This study provides indices of both the utility and the limitations of EPs in the diagnosis and prognosis of patients suspected of having MS. It also provides some estimate of the relative diagnostic and prognostic value of CSF studies in subsets of the patients and some limited comparisons of the EPs with NMR studies.

In admitting patients to the study, care was taken to apply the McAlpine criteria rigorously, albeit retrospectively. A significant limitation of our study, like that of Matthews et al. (1982), is that it was based, for ethical as well as logistic reasons, on our retrospective analysis of patient follow-up that did not involve a neurologist in all cases. Nevertheless, comparisons of the clinical profiles, the relapse rates and the incidence of EP abnormalities in the present series with those described in the literature indicate that these patients may indeed be considered representative of patients with early or suspected MS and at least comparable to those in other reports. First, considering the clinical profiles, 79% of the 139 patients carrying the diagnosis of possible or probable MS at referral had no optic signs, 64% had no evidence of spinal cord disease and 80% had no brainstem signs. Comparable reported ranges for each system are 64–92%, 51–62% and 41–77% (Purves et al. 1981; Bauer 1978; Chiappa 1980), and vary with criteria for abnormality. Second, approximately one quarter of the patients developed clinically definite MS within the average $2\frac{1}{2}$-year follow-up. Similar or slightly higher rates of relapse have been reported by McAlpine (1972), and in the EP and follow-up studies of Matthews et al. (1982) and Deltenre et al. (1984). Third, incidences of abnormal and positive EPs in the series (table 11.1) are within or slightly below the recently reported ranges for MS suspects: 41–55% for the pattern visual EP (31–46% positive), 24–58% for the somatosensory (6–33%), and 14–40% for the brainstem auditory (9–29%) (Chiappa 1980; Khoshbin and Hallett 1981; Purves et al. 1981; Matthews et al. 1982; Bartel et al. 1983; Deltenre et al. 1984).

Differences between these studies may be attributable to differences in patient populations, diagnostic schema, and EP techniques and criteria for abnormality. It would be useful, in the future, to carry out a prospective study on EPs in a large population of MS suspects, and in fact such a study is planned. Differences in the criteria for defining clinically silent lesions may also be critical. In the present study, for example, the somatosensory EPs were considered positive only if there was no objective evidence of spinal cord dysfunction at any level; Matthews et al.

(1982) adopted similar standards but other groups have used different criteria.

Having established that this patient series is comparable to others reported, the questions posed in the Introduction concerning the significance of the EPs may be considered. Comparison of the patients' follow-up diagnoses with their EPs in table 11.6 provides an estimate of the predictive significance of each type of EP observation. Overall, 65 patients had had a positive EP: 71% of these patients had deteriorated on follow-up (48% of patients with a positive EP developed clinically definite MS), 20% were unchanged, 5% had had no further symptoms and 3% had a diagnosis other than MS. In contrast, 121 patients had had normal EPs in all modalities: only 16% of these patients deteriorated (4% of patients with normal EPs in all modalities developed definite MS), 75% were unchanged or had had no further symptoms and 11% were given another diagnosis. Thirty-six patients had had only confirmatory EPs: 56% had deteriorated (33% became definite) and 36% were unchanged or had had no further symptoms on follow-up. Overall, there was a 71% chance of deterioration given a positive EP and a 16% chance of deterioration given normal EPs ($\chi^2 = 56.7$, $P < 0.001$). Confirmatory EPs did not predict whether a patient would deteriorate.

Comparing modalities, the pattern visual EPs provided the best prediction of follow-up status, the somatosensory an intermediate level, and the brainstem auditory little or no prediction. Visual EPs were more frequently positive than the somatosensory and auditory EPs (22%, 12% and 5% of patients), and they were more frequently the only positive EP (15%, 7% and 1% of patients). In addition, proportionally more patients with positive visual EPs than with positive somatosensory EPs had deteriorated on follow-up (78%, 63%). Although all 10, or 100%, of the patients with positive auditory EPs later deteriorated, the very low positive rate of these EPs limits their usefulness. The observation that

Table 11.6

Patients (%) with different clinical courses on follow-up given initial EPs defined as diagnostic, confirmatory only or normal

EPs	n	Clinical course				
		Became definite (48)	Deteriorated not definite (38)	No change (60)	No > symptoms (58)	Other diagnosis (18)
Overall (222)						
Diagnostic	65	47.7 (31)	24.6 (16)	20.0 (13)	4.6 (3)	3.1 (2)
Confirmatory	36	33.3 (12)	22.2 (8)	33.3 (12)	2.8 (1)	8.3 (3)
Normal	121	4.1 (5)	11.6 (14)	28.9 (35)	44.6 (54)	10.7 (13)
PVEP (210)						
Diagnostic	46	54.5 (25)	23.9 (11)	19.6 (9)	0.0 (0)	2.2 (1)
Confirmatory	28	50.0 (14)	7.1 (2)	39.3 (11)	0.0 (0)	3.6 (1)
Normal	136	5.9 (8)	16.2 (22)	26.5 (36)	41.2 (56)	10.3 (14)
SEP (217)						
Diagnostic	27	44.4 (12)	18.5 (5)	22.2 (6)	11.1 (3)	3.7 (1)
Confirmatory	42	40.5 (17)	31.0 (13)	21.4 (9)	2.4 (1)	4.8 (2)
Normal	148	11.5 (17)	13.5 (20)	29.7 (44)	35.1 (52)	10.1 (15)
BAEP (214)						
Diagnostic	10	60.0 (6)	40.0 (4)	0.0 (0)	0.0 (0)	0.0 (0)
Confirmatory	9	66.7 (6)	11.1 (1)	22.2 (2)	0.0 (0)	0.0 (0)
Normal	195	18.0 (35)	16.4 (32)	28.7 (56)	28.2 (55)	8.7 (17)

Results overall and in each modality are shown separately. Number of patients in each category is shown in parentheses.

78% of the 86 patients who deteriorated had had normal auditory EPs compared with the 35% who had had normal visual EPs and the 43% who had had normal somatosensory EPs is also consistent with this conclusion.

Considering the different groups of patients, two points may be made. First, within the subgroups who had deteriorated on follow-up, the higher incidences of positive EPs were not, surprisingly, observed in the patients whose diagnoses were least certain initially (table 11.2). Thus, while only 47% (9/17) of the patients who progressed from probable to definite MS had had positive EPs, 80% of the initially possible group, all four of the spinal cord group and 60% of the AND group who became definite did.

Second, there were striking differences in the incidence and type of EP abnormality between the two groups of patients presenting with signs or symptoms of a single lesion, namely those with spinal cord and those with optic nerve dysfunction. One third of the 68 patients with spinal cord dysfunction had EPs which indicated lesions in the optic nerves or brainstem while only one of the 24 patients with optic nerve dysfunction had EPs which indicated another lesion, namely in the brainstem. These clinical and electro-physiological differences suggest that the pathogenesis and the pattern of lesion dissemination in the subsets of patients with isolated optic neuritis and with spinal cord disease who go on to develop clinical evidence of multiple lesions may in fact differ. Differences in the bilateral distribution of the EP abnormalities are consistent with this suggestion and will be described in a separate report.

In their EP-follow-up study, Matthews et al. (1982) reported a positive EP rate of 58% for the 24 patients of their series who were initially possible or probable and became definite, and of 50% if the results of 4 who were "acute not diagnosed" and became definite are included. Comparable rates in the current study (table 11.2) are 66% for the possible and probable patients (25/38) and 65% overall (31/48). In the study by Matthews et al. the chance of deterioration, given a positive EP, was 70% (14 of 20 patients) and similar to that in the present study (71%); however, given a normal EP (44 patients), it was 36% (16% in this study). Deltenre et al. (1984), in their follow-up study, reported that 48, or 86%, of their 56 patients who developed clinically definite MS had had EPs which demonstrated subclinical lesions. They do not, however, indicate how "subclinical lesions" in each modality were defined. Bottcher and Trojaborg (1982) in a follow-up of 21 MS suspects found that almost all with abnormalities of both CSF IgG and visual or somatosensory EPs had deteriorated after 2–4 years; their study did not, however, include any patients with normal IgG and normal EPs.

The true false positive rate of any test for MS which is not specific to the disease cannot be determined and any estimate is necessarily dependent upon exactly which patients are considered and the duration of follow-up. A conservative estimate of the rate for the EPs of this study may be obtained by considering the 60 MS-suspects whose diagnostic categories had not changed on $2\frac{1}{2}$-year follow-up, the 58 who had had no further symptoms and the 18 with an alternate diagnosis: 18 of these 136 patients had had positive EPs, giving a false positive rate of 13%. The comparable rate for the study of Matthews et al. (1982) is 14%. Notably, the incidence of positive EPs in the 40 patients classified as CND and not

defined as MS-suspects in this study was lower, three or 7.5% having positive EPs.

We would emphasize that, in the present study, individual signs and symptoms were not analyzed, so that it is not possible to comment on whether EPs are useful in predicting the development of particular signs and symptoms. Moreover, while the present study demonstrates a clear relationship between EPs and clinical course in a population of MS suspects, our study does not permit a definitive diagnosis to be established in any given patient on the basis of EPs alone. EPs must obviously be interpreted in the context of the overall clinical picture. Nevertheless, the important point is that, considering the population of MS suspects, there is a significant trend between EPs and clinical course.

Both the incidence of CSF abnormalities and their correlation with the patients' diagnoses at follow-up (table 11.4) are similar to those previously described (Trojaborg et al. 1981; Hutchinson et al. 1983, 1984; Moulin et al. 1983; Ebers 1984; Thompson et al. 1985b). The IgG correlated with the follow-up status in 76% of the patients, and the oligoclonal bands in 65%. In the patients with spinal cord disease alone, the IgG but not the oligoclonal bands predicted follow-up status. Both Moulin et al. (1983) and Thompson et al. (1985b) reported that oligoclonal bands predict whether MS-suspects presenting with unifocal disease will deteriorate within 2–3 years. Neither study, however, considered patients with spinal cord disease separately. Also, Thompson's group did find that the IgG index did not correlate with the follow-up status of their patients.

Levels of concordance between the CSF IgG and oligoclonal bands and the EPs were similar to each other (67–74%) and to those published. Moulin et al. (1983) and Thompson et al. (1985b) have found concordances of 58–68% between the oligoclonal bands and the visual and brainstem auditory EPs in patients with suspected MS. The absence of association between the CSF MBP and the EPs is consistent with demonstrations that levels of MBP are related to disease activity, as indexed by relapses and remissions (Cohen et al. 1980; Thompson et al. 1985a), while EPs in general are not (Matthews and Small 1979; Davis et al. 1985).

Results of the NMR brain imaging studies are included principally to demonstrate their 68% concordance with the earlier recorded EPs (table 11.5). Several other groups have recently reported similar concordance between NMR and EP studies, of 67–78%, in comparable groups of patients (Cutler et al. 1986; Farlow et al. 1986; Giesser et al. 1987). The prognostic value of NMR imaging is not assessed in the present study, however, since several of the patients did not have the imaging studies until 3–4 years after their presentation for EPs and when some had, by clinical criteria, developed definite MS.

A considerable discrepancy between the EP and NMR studies was seen in patients with spinal cord disease. Only 2 of the 10 patients imaged in this group had scans demonstrating multiple cerebral lesions; both had positive visual EPs. Three of the 8 with normal scans had normal EPs. The others accounted for 5 of the 6 patients with normal NMR studies and abnormal EPs: positive in 2 and confirmatory in 3; on follow-up, 4 had deteriorated with progressive spinal cord disease and one was unchanged. These results, although the numbers are small, when compared with observations that one-third to one-half of patients with undiagnosed spinal cord disease have abnormal visual or auditory EPs (table 11.1; Halliday et al. 1974; Paty et al. 1979; Blumhardt et al. 1982) suggest that NMR brain imaging may be less likely, and certainly no more likely, than EPs to demonstrate disseminated disease in patients with spinal MS.

Summary of Conclusions

(1) Incidences of EP abnormality, according to diagnostic classification at presentation, were: probable MS (29 patients)—93% EP abnormality (48% positive EPs); possible MS (111 patients)—45% (31%); AND (83 patients)—29%

(20%); isolated optic neuritis (26 patients)—65% (4%); CND (40 patients)—10% (8%).

(2) In the MS suspects (probable and possible MS, AND), a positive EP (i.e., an EP demonstrating a clinically silent lesion) in any modality (65 patients) was associated with a 71% chance of clinical deterioration (including a 48% chance of developing clinically definite MS), and normal EPs (121 patients) with a 16% chance of deterioration (4% definite MS). Confirmatory EPs (36 patients), i.e., EPs that were abnormal in the presence of clinical evidence of dysfunction of that tract, did not predict whether a patient would deteriorate.

(3) Pattern visual EPs were more frequently positive than the somatosensory and auditory EPs (22%, 12% and 5% of patients), and proportionally more patients with positive visual EPs (78%) than with positive somatosensory EPs (63%) had deteriorated on follow-up.

(4) The "false positive rate" for EPs was 13%.

(5) The EPs differed markedly between patients presenting with spinal cord dysfunction and patients with optic nerve dysfunction: 32% of the 68 patients in the former group had positive visual or auditory EPs while only one of the 24 in the latter group had EPs indicating a lesion outside the visual system.

(6) The CSF IgG predicted outcome in 76% of the patients studied (abnormal in 79% who deteriorated, normal in 73% who did not deteriorate) and the oligoclonal bands predicted outcome in 65% (present in 55% who deteriorated, absent in 74% who did not). The CSF MBP did not correlate with the patients' outcomes or with the EPs.

(7) NMR brain imaging was consistent with the EPs in 68% of the 31 MS-suspects who had both studies although there were some delays between the studies.

Acknowledgments

Supported in part by the Medical Research Service, Veterans Administration, and by a grant from the Folger Foundation. We thank the Paralyzed Veterans of America for support. The authors thank physicians of the Yale–New Haven Hospital and southern Connecticut area who agreed to review of their patients, Kathleen McPadden for technical assistance, and Drs. Truett Allison and John Booss for helpful discussion.

References

Allison, T., C. C. Wood and W. R. Goff (1983) Brain stem auditory, pattern-reversal visual, and short-latency somatosensory evoked potentials: latencies in relation to age, sex, and brain and body size. *Electroenceph. Clin. Neurophysiol.*, 55: 619–636.

Bartel, D. R., O. N. Markand and O. J. Oldrich (1983) The diagnosis and classification of multiple sclerosis: evoked responses and spinal fluid electrophoresis. *Neurology*, 33: 611–617.

Bauer, H. J. (1978) Problems of symptomatic therapy in multiple sclerosis. *Neurology*, 28: 8–20.

Blumhardt, L. D., G. Barrett and A. M. Halliday (1982) The pattern visual evoked potential in the clinical assessment of undiagnosed spinal cord disease. In: J. Courjon, F. Mauguière and M. Revol (Eds.), *Clinical Applications of Evoked Potentials in Neurology*, Raven Press, New York, pp. 463–471.

Chiappa, K. H. (1980) Pattern shift visual, brainstem auditory, and short-latency somatosensory evoked potentials in multiple sclerosis. *Neurology*, 30: 110–123.

Chiappa, K. H. (1983) *Evoked Potentials in Clinical Medicine*, Raven Press, New York.

Cohen, S. R., B. R. Brooks, R. M. Herndon and G. M. McKhann (1980) A diagnostic index of active demyelination: myelin basic protein in cerebrospinal fluid. *Ann. Neurol.*, 8: 25–31.

Cutler, J. R., M. J. Aminoff and M. Brant-Zawadzki (1986) Evaluation of patients with multiple sclerosis by evoked potentials and magnetic resonance imaging: a comparative study. *Ann. Neurol.*, 20: 645–648.

Davis, S. L., M. J. Aminoff and H. S. Panitch (1985) Clinical correlations of serial somatosensory evoked potentials in multiple sclerosis. *Neurology*, 35: 359–365.

Deltenre, P., C. Van Nechel, S. Strul and P. Ketelaer (1984) A five-year prospective study on the value of multimodal evoked potentials and blink reflex, as an aid to the diagnosis of suspected multiple sclerosis. In: R. H. Nodar and C. Barber (Eds.), *Evoked Potentials II: The Second International Evoked Potentials Symposium*, Butterworth, Boston, pp. 603–608.

Ebers, G. C. (1984) Oligoclonal banding in MS. *Ann. N. Y. Acad. Sci.*, 436: 206–212.

Farlow, M. R., O. N. Markand, M. K. Edwards, J. C. Stevens and O. J. Kolar (1986) Multiple sclerosis: magnetic resonance imaging, evoked responses, and spinal fluid electrophoresis. *Neurology*, 36: 828–831.

Giesser, B. S., D. Kurtzberg, H. G. Vaughan, J. C. Arezzo, M. L. Aisen, C. R. Smith, N. G. LaRocca and L. C. Scheinberg (1987) Trimodal evoked potentials compared with magnetic resonance imaging in the diagnosis of multiple sclerosis. *Arch. Neurol.*, 44: 281–284.

Halliday, A. M., W. I. McDonald and J. Mushin (1973) Visual evoked response in diagnosis of multiple sclerosis. *Brit. Med. J.*, 4: 661–664.

Halliday, A. M., W. I. McDonald and J. Mushin (1974) Delayed visual evoked responses in progressive spastic paraparesis. *Electroenceph. Clin. Neurophysiol.*, 37: 328.

Hutchinson, M., S. Blandford, D. Glynn and E. A. Martin (1984) Clinical correlates of abnormal brainstem auditory evoked responses in multiple sclerosis. *Acta Neurol. Scand.*, 69: 90–95.

Hutchinson, M., E. A. Martin, P. Maguire, D. Glynn, M. Mansfield and C. Feighery (1983) Visual evoked responses and immunoglobulin abnormalities in the diagnosis of multiple sclerosis. *Acta Neurol. Scand.*, 68: 90–95.

Khoshbin, S. and M. Hallett (1981) Multimodality evoked potentials and blink reflex in multiple sclerosis. *Neurology*, 31: 138–144.

Matthews, W. B. (1985) Clinical aspects. In: W. B. Matthews, E. D. Acheson, J. R. Batchelor and R. O. Weller (Eds.), *McAlpine's Multiple Sclerosis*, Churchill Livingstone, Edinburgh, pp. 49–232.

Matthews, W. B. and D. G. Small (1979) Serial recording of visual and somatosensory evoked potentials in multiple sclerosis. *J. Neurol. Sci.*, 40: 11–21.

Matthews, W. B., J. R. B. Wattam-Bell and E. Pountney (1982) Evoked potentials in the diagnosis of multiple sclerosis: a follow up study. *J. Neurol. Neurosurg. Psychiat.*, 45: 303–307.

McAlpine, D. (1972) Course and prognosis. In: D. McAlpine, C. E. Lumsden and E. D. Acheson (Eds.), *Multiple Sclerosis: A Reappraisal*, Williams Wilkins, Baltimore, pp. 197–223.

Moulin, D., D. W. Paty and G. C. Ebers (1983) The predictive value of cerebrospinal fluid electrophoresis in 'possible' multiple sclerosis. *Brain*, 106: 809–816.

Paty, D. W., W. T. Blume, W. F. Brown, N. Jaatoul, A. Kertesz and W. McInnis (1979) Chronic progressive myelopathy: investigation with CSF electrophoresis, evoked potentials, and CT scan. *Ann. Neurol.*, 6: 419–424.

Purves, S. J., M. D. Low, J. Galloway and B. Reeves (1981) A comparison of visual, brainstem auditory, and somatosensory evoked potentials in multiple sclerosis. *Can. J. Neurol. Sci.*, 8: 15–19.

Small, D. G., W. B. Matthews and M. Small (1978) The cervical somatosensory evoked potential in the diagnosis of multiple sclerosis. *J. Neurol. Sci.*, 35: 211–224.

Stockard, J. J., J. E. Stockard and F. W. Sharbrough (1978) Non-pathologic factors influencing brainstem auditory evoked potentials. *Am. J. EEG Technol.*, 18: 177–209.

Thompson, A. J., J. Brazil, C. Feighery, A. Whelan, J. Kellet, E. A. Martin and M. Hutchinson (1985) CSF myelin basic protein in multiple sclerosis. *Acta Neurol. Scand.*, 72: 577–583.

Thompson, A. J., M. Hutchinson, E. A. Martin, M. Mansfield, A. Whelan and C. Feighery (1985) Suspected and clinically definite multiple sclerosis: the relationship between CSF immunoglobulins and clinical course. *J. Neurol. Neurosurg. Psychiat.*, 48: 989–994.

Trojaborg, W., J. Bottcher and O. Saxtrup (1981) Evoked potentials and immunoglobulin abnormalities in multiple sclerosis. *Neurology*, 31: 866–871.

12 Temporal Profile Resembling TIA in the Setting of Cerebral Infarction

Stephen G. Waxman and James F. Toole

The development of the concept of transient ischemic attack (TIA) was an extremely important advance in the understanding and management of cerebrovascular disease, which has been refined over the years to the generally accepted clinical definition of a focal neurological dysfunction which resolves completely within 24 hours. While there is almost certainly a spectrum of pathophysiologies underlying TIA, it is clear than in many cases TIAs are caused by emboli or microemboli from atherosclerotic plaques and are the harbinger of cerebral infarction.[1-3] The entity, however, is a clinical concept rather than an anatomical one and includes at least several pathological entities, often with different diagnostic, therapeutic and prognostic implications. In particular, the term TIA is currently used to describe a variety of symptomatically transient neurological disturbances of focal nature due to local ischemia caused by a variety of pathophysiologic mechanisms such as hypotension, "hemodynamic crisis," microembolism, or abnormality of blood constituents. They range from potentially reversible ischemia, on the one hand, to infarction on the other.

It is the purpose of this article to demonstrate that, in some cases, the clinician cannot accurately differentiate between a TIA without infarction and an infarction with minor residua, and to suggest the hypothesis that this distinction may have clinical significance. In this article, we call attention to episodes with the temporal profile of TIA, and a demonstrable pathological substrate, *transient neurologic dysfunction in the setting of cerebral infarction*.

TIAs are defined as episodes of focal neurological deficit of sudden onset, referable to a specific arterial territory, lasting no longer than 24 hours. As early as 1914, Hunt referred to

Reprinted with permission from *Stroke* 14: 433–437, 1983.

"cerebral intermittent claudication" due to disease of the carotid artery.[4] Nearly forty years later Denny-Brown[5] described hemodynamic crises or "episodic insufficiency in the circle of Willis of a temporary nature." Millikan, Siekert, and their colleagues,[6] Fisher,[7] and Marshall[8] among others have more recently elaborated and refined the concept. They have agreed that only transient neurological dysfunction, resolving within 24 hours, can be considered. "Fundamentals of Stroke Care,"[9] published under the sponsorship of the National Institute of Neurological and Communicative Disorders and Stroke, states that the diagnosis of TIAs is made by the history and occasional observation of an episode by the physician, and that furthermore, during the intervals between episodes, examination reveals no evidence of neurological disorder. This description specifically states that radionuclide and computed cranial tomography (CCT) are normal in patients with TIA unless there is residual undetected infarction. Biller et al[10] noted that CCT is normal in the majority of patients with TIAs. Allen and Preziosi[11] reported abnormal CCT in 12% of patients with a clinical diagnosis of TIA. Buonanno and Toole[12] emphasized that the diagnosis of TIA can only be made retrospectively after the episode has cleared within the arbitrarily set time limit and that it must be made with qualifying terms pending the outcome of special laboratory procedures such as CCT. They believe that the diagnosis of TIA and reversible ischemic neurological deficit (RIND) signify ischemia with preserved viability of neural tissue and that infarction represents ischemia prolonged beyond the length of time that involved tissue can survive. Hossmann and collaborators[13,14] have experimentally confirmed the reversibility of neuronal dysfunction after transient ischemia, underscoring the importance of the distinction between ischemia and infarction.

This article will focus on the occasional patient who, from a clinical point of view, presents with a neurological syndrome with a temporal profile similar to that seen in TIA, but in whom laboratory investigations show clear evidence of infarction. Representative examples of two such patients, illustrating different aspects of this situation, follow.

Case Reports

Case 1

A 59-year-old hypertensive righthanded man developed a 3-hour episode of slurred speech, weakness and "numbness" of the left arm and leg. The crural weakness was so severe that the patient could not stand. When examined by a neurologist 3 days later, the sole residuum was intermittent left-sided extinction on double simultaneous stimulation. A right carotid bruit was heard by some examiners. The hematocrit was 54, with normal white blood cell and platelet counts. RPR and erythrocyte sedimentation rate were normal. Electrocardiogram was suggestive of ischemia but did not show infarction. CCT revealed a low density area consistent with evolving infarction in the right parietal lobe (figure 12.1). Angiography (figure 12.2) revealed occlusion of the right internal carotid artery with perfusion of the right hemisphere via ophthalmic retrograde flow from the external carotid artery.

Case 2

A 50-year-old professor, while conversing with a friend on 7-7-80, suddenly developed inability to express himself and weakness of the right hand. He walked to his bedroom and lay down. His wife and friend, who had been with him at the initiation of the event, observed that his mental processes seemed slow. For example, when the emergency squad arrived 15 minutes later, the patient was of the impression that only one or two minutes had elapsed. When examined by a

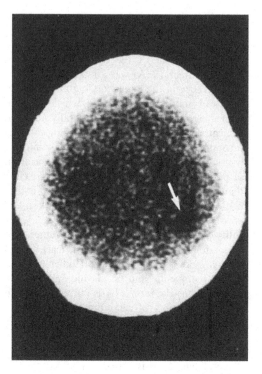

Figure 12.1
CT scan showing right parietal infarction (arrow) in patient no. 1.

neurologist within the hour of onset of the episode, he was noted to have a Broca's aphasia and a right hemiparesis, with a right central facial paresis. It was felt that he had a mild sensory deficit to light touch in the right hand and fingers. Neurovascular examination was normal and he had no bruits in the neck. Blood pressure was 130/80 mm Hg and the pulse regular.

All of these defects resolved completely within 20 hours. CCT performed within 24 hours was compatible with evolving infarction of the left posterior frontal region. Cervical cranial arteriography showed normal extracranial arteries without atheromatosis. In the left posterior frontal region there was a focal area of luxury perfusion involving the short gyri of the insula.

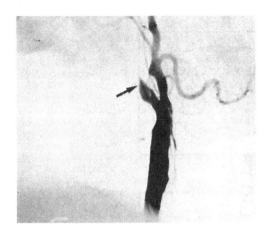

Figure 12.2
Recent carotid arteriogram showing recent occlusion (arrow) from Patient No. 1.

Electroencephalogram, electrocardiogram, echocardiogram, RPR, complete blood count, platelet count and erythrocyte sedimentation rate were all normal. Radioisotopic brain scan on 7-9-80 was normal. Repeated on 7-30-80, it showed increased uptake in the left frontal parietal temporal region, compatible with a small area of infarction. CCT on 8-1-80 demonstrated a hypodense lesion in the anterior part of the left insula, and a dilated frontal horn, suggesting focal infarction which had evolved from the time of the previous scan on 7-8-80. Speech testing on 7-30-80, with a Porch index of communicative abilities and the Boston Diagnostic Aphasia Examination was entirely normal.

Xeon inhalation regional cerebral blood flow studies were performed seriatum (figure 12.3). Baseline Flow Gray pattern and distribution were normal bilaterally on 7-8-80. CO_2 stress test was abnormal with paradoxically reduced flow response in Broca's area and hyperperfusion responses in adjacent areas. The rest of the left hemisphere was non-reactive. On 7-15-80 the left hemisphere baseline pattern was normal, but the CO_2 response remained decreased in Broca's

area, although improved from the previous test of 7-8-80. On 7-31-80 the left hemisphere was still decreased in response to 5% CO_2, with paradoxical CO_2 response in parietal and occipital lobes. Right hemisphere was normal. In review of all three cerebral blood flow studies, the pattern of baseline flow remained low normal quite consistently over the three studies. Vasomotor reactivity to CO_2 improved dramatically over time.

Of incidental interest is the fact that the patient now remembered that he had had several episodes of tingling as well as numbness and unsteadiness of his right hand which had occurred in the month preceding the acute event.

Discussion

From a *clinical* point of view, these patients had transient focal neurologic dysfunction with a time course corresponding to that of TIA. The deficit was focal, the time course appropriate and resolution was nearly complete in Case 1 and complete in Case 2. On the other hand, from an *anatomical* point of view, CCT showed evolving infarction and in one case the regional cerebral blood flow studies were disturbed for six weeks. Should these patients be classified clinically as having sustained a TIA or pathologically as having suffered cerebral infarction, or both? It is unlikely that the pathogenesis of the cerebral insult in these two patients was identical. Nevertheless, from the point of view of clinical phenomenology, the diagnosis of TIA would be correct, whereas with respect to the structural findings, a more proper diagnosis would be completed infarction. An old "silent" infarct with a new episode of borderzone ischemia resulting in a TIA is another possibility. In the case of cerebral infarction, should the patient with clinical resolution within 24 hours despite infarction in a "silent" region be classified and possibly treated differently from the patient with functional recovery after infarction in a less

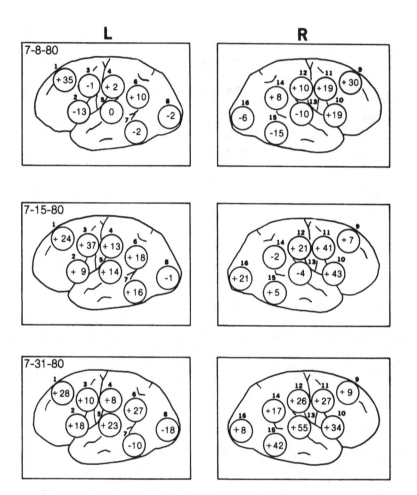

Figure 12.3

Serial determinations of regional cerebral blood flow showing the evolution of described hemodynamics in Patient No. 2. Figures within circles represent the percent change to CO_2 activation from baseline at each probe location.

silent area? In cases such as this, the term "transient ischemic attack" is only partially correct—neurologic dysfunction is indeed transient, but the pathology may be that of a cerebral infarction.

These questions are not purely semantic or academic. Decisions for medical and surgical intervention, as well as prognosis, may differ significantly. The patients described above may be viewed as representing a good surgical risk because of absence of clinical deficits. Yet, from a pathological point of view, the disease process is one of infarction and the risk of surgical conversion of anemic to hemorrhagic infarction must be considered.

Patients such as these are not rare and their classification hinges upon one's decision about CCT findings in TIAs. The interpretation of CCT findings is, of course, also evolving, and with the development of refined imaging methods, it is likely that the accuracy of diagnosis of structural pathology will improve. Few currently available series of patients with TIA take into account the possible differences between those patients with ischemic lesions, and those with infarctions without residual clinical findings. Yet the distinction between pathologically verified TIA, in which the neurological dysfunction is both transient and due to ischemia—a potentially reversible parenchymatous lesion, and cerebral infarction—in which there is irreversible loss of brain tissue—is a crucial, if poorly understood, one. It would not be surprising to find different vascular lesions, prognoses, or response to medical or surgical intervention.

We believe that one root of the problem resides in some cases in inexactitudes of the clinical history and the neurological examination. Regarding history we must, for example, consider the difficulty that patients have in expressing their symptoms, particularly if the event affects the nondominant hemisphere, or if the attack begins during sleep. The moment of beginning of the attack may not be precise and of course, its complete resolution may also be a matter of interpretation. This is illustrated by visual observations described as blurring of vision. Is this partial amaurosis fugax? Another example is provided by the patient with intermittent vertigo. Because of difficulty in its evaluation, clinicians customarily eliminate this symptom from consideration as a TIA unless it is accompanied by other phenomena. Frequently patients will describe visual observations which may include evanescent diplopia. Opinions are divided about whether to classify such patients as TIA. This difficulty with classification is demonstrated by the findings of the cooperative group for study of TIA chaired by Dyken[15] who found that fully 1/3 of patients admitted to the hospital with a diagnosis of TIA were misclassified.

Furthermore, whether the patient has residua of the attack is again judgmental. We have repeatedly encountered patients who by their own account are completely without sequellae, but whose close associates describe as having altered judgment or a personality change. Cognitive changes as a residuum have not been adequately considered in classification of cerebrovascular events as TIA or cerebral infarction. Nevertheless, this consideration is an important one in decisions regarding classification. The objective modalities used for assessing whether a patient has recovered fully within the 24-hour-time constraints are subjective and perhaps arbitrary.

Regarding patient examination for "complete" recovery, this at times is exceedingly difficult. Patients' baseline neurological status, particularly regarding higher cortical function, is often not known so that comparisons cannot be made. What one is left with following examination is a series of observations which, if normal, suggest intact neural function. But if the neurological examination remains abnormal, one must speculate as to whether the ictus or a more remote event(s) caused the abnormality.

This difficulty in classification occurs commonly, with physicians all interested in cerebral circulatory disease disagreeing on the basis of history as to whether an event was a TIA, Ménière's disease, presyncope or even a functional event. This difficulty is magnified when patients consult a physician some weeks after the event. By then the patient's memory has faded and residual deficits may be resolved. Most studies have accepted patients who have had TIA within one to two months of entry. Therefore clinical description and findings may be inexact.

Obviously, there is a need for further careful work in this area. Until further data are available, it seems prudent to us to reserve the term TIA to describe episodes of focal deficit which resolve completely within 24 hours, in which the purported brain lesion is one of an ischemic nature, and which on CCT leaves no visible evidence of its presence. A separate and specific category, cerebral infarction with transient signs (CITS), might appropriately be used to describe patients who (i) fit the temporal profile of TIA but (ii) in whom there is evidence for infarction on CCT. It should be emphasized that this category is an operational one, since the accuracy of diagnosis of structural cerebral lesions is improving with the development of new generation CCT scanners, positron emission tomography, and nuclear magnetic resonance, and may vary from center to center. CCT is only one of a number of laboratory tests that can demonstrate structural pathology, and it is likely that other tests will in the future be widely available. Nevertheless, this distinction may prove useful for the diagnosis and study of patients with cerebrovascular disease, because it may permit the explicit differentiation of one type of transient neurological dysfunction with a well-defined basis in terms of parenchymal pathology. While it is unlikely that transient episodes of neurological dysfunction due to cerebral infarctions represent a single pathophysiological entity, it may be important to place patients with such episodes in a different diagnostic category from those with TIA, since this categorization may have important implications for prognosis and therapy.

Acknowledgments

We wish to thank Larry A. Pearce, M.D. for Case 2 and David Stump, Ph.D. for the cerebral blood flow determinations and interpretations.

References

1. Whisnant JP, Matsumoto N, Elveback LR: Cerebral ischemia attacks in a community. Mayo Clin Proc 48: 194–198, 1973

2. Toole JF, Yuson CP, Janeway R, Johnston F, Davis C, Cordell AR, Howard G: Transient ischemic attacks: A prospective study of 225 patients. Neurology 28: 746–753, 1978

3. Barnett HJM: Progress towards stroke prevention. Neurology 30: 1212–1225, 1980

4. Hunt JR: The role of the carotid arteries in the causation of vascular lesions of the brain with remarks on certain special features of the symptomatology. Amer J Med Sci 147: 704–713, 1914

5. Denny-Brown D: The treatment of recurrent cerebrovascular symptoms and the question of 'vasospasm.' Med Clin N Amer 35: 1457–1474, 1951

6. Millikan CH, Siekert RG, Shick RM: Studies in cerebrovascular disease. V. The use of anticoagulant drugs in the treatment of intermittent insufficiency of the internal carotid arterial system. Proc Mayo Clin 30: 578–586, 1955

7. Fisher CM: Transient monocular blindness associated with hemiplegia. Arch Ophthal 47: 167–203, 1952

8. Marshall J: The natural history of transient ischaemic cerebrovascular attacks. Quart J Med 33: 309–324, 1964

9. Sahs AL, Hartman EC: Fundamentals of Stroke Care. DHEW Publication no. (HRA) 76-14016, 1976

10. Biller J, Laster DW, Howard G, Toole JF, McHenry LC Jr: Cranial computerized tomography in carotid artery transient ischemic attacks. Eur Neurol. In press

11. Allen GS, Preziosi TJ: Carotid endarterectomy: a prospective study of its efficacy and safety. Medicine 60: 298–309, 1981

12. Buonanno F, Toole JF: Management of patients with established ("completed") cerebral infarction. Stroke 12: 7–16, 1981

13. Hossmann KA, Kleihues P: Reversibility of ischaemic brain damage. Arch Neurol 29: 375–384, 1973

14. Hossmann KA, Sato K: Recovery of neuronal function after prolonged cerebral ischaemia. Science 168: 375–378, 1970

15. Dyken ML, Conneally PM, Haerer EF, et al: Cooperative study of hospital frequency and character of transient ischemic attacks. I. Background, organization, and clinical survey. J Am Med Assoc 237: 882–886, 1977

IX HIDE AND SEEK ALONG THE BRAIN'S HIGHWAYS

Nearly 50,000 genes—more than in any other organ—are expressed within the brain. Each of these genes encodes a different protein. Thus, the brain is unique in containing an unusually large number of protein molecules, each with a different structure and each subserving a different function. What is also unique about the brain, however, is the precise placement of its molecules. Rather than being strewn uniformly or randomly throughout the nervous system, molecules within it are highly localized and, in some cases, are anchored in place so that they are present only in well-circumscribed domains. The papers that follow (Kocsis and Waxman 1980; Eng et al. 1988) are part of a series, from our laboratory and others, that mapped the locations and examined the functions of a family of molecules called potassium channels within myelinated nerve fibers. Potassium channels act as conduits for the flow of potassium ions. When these channels open, the flow of potassium ions tends to stabilize the nerve cell, maintaining it in or returning it to a resting state, or inhibiting impulse generation. Thus potassium channels, in a broad-brush sense, can be considered to be molecular brakes.

A nerve fiber runs, like a tiny cable, from one site in the nervous system to another. Where, along this cable, are potassium channels located? The early research on this question, carried out before antibodies were available as markers for these channels, was largely carried out by three research groups spread around the world: Hugh Bostock and Tom Sears at the Institute of Neurology, London; S-Y Chiu and J. Murdoch Ritchie at Yale; and Jeffery Kocsis, me, and our students, then working at Stanford. In an important early experiment Bostock and Sears (1978) used a technique for measuring externally recorded currents in chronically demyelinated nerve fibers close to their entrance into the spinal cord, and made observations that suggested that potassium channels were present in parts of the axons that had lost their myelin. Chiu and Ritchie (1980) built upon these findings and used voltage-clamp to study myelinated axons dissected from a peripheral nerve, the sciatic nerve. When they placed normal myelinated nerve fibers in the voltage-clamp, they did not see evidence for activity of potassium channels, even at the small gaps called nodes of Ranvier where the myelin is absent; but when they acutely removed the myelin, they were able to record activity in potassium channels. They concluded from these experiments that potassium channels were present in the internodal axon membrane, where they are usually covered by the myelin sheath. Ritchie was deservedly excited about these recordings and generously sent copies to Tom Sears and me shortly after he obtained them and before they were published.

My coworkers and I were, however, interested in multiple sclerosis. This disorder affects myelinated nerve fibers within the brain and spinal cord, and we made a strategic decision to focus on these small fibers even though they were too fragile and intertwined to be studied by voltage clamp or longitudinal current analysis. The problem of how to study these delicate nerve fibers was solved by Kocsis' technical ingenuity. He provided us with methodology that utilized very fine microelectrodes, small enough to place inside of axons within the spinal cord so that we could eavesdrop on them. Using these tiny probes we demonstrated that potassium channels were either not expressed at significant levels along intact myelinated nerve fibers in the spinal cord, or were hidden, invisible to the neurophysiologist's microelectrode and inaccessible to drugs that are introduced into the fluid bathing the nerve (Kocsis and Waxman 1980). In other experiments we showed that potassium channels were present so that they could help to shape the nerve impulse prior to the formation of myelin in the optic nerve of newborn rats, but did not contribute to the shaping of the nerve impulse in the mature optic nerve, after myelin has been formed; these experiments provided another line of evidence indicating that these potassium channels were located in the internodal axon membrane where they were covered by the myelin (Waxman and Foster 1980). A few years later we observed a similar developmental sequence which suggested that potassium channels were localized within the internodal axon membrane of regenerating nerve fibers (Kocsis et al. 1982).

Experiments on peripheral nerve and the central nervous system, carried out in three laboratories separated from each other by thousands of miles, thus converged, and taught us that potassium channels are present in myelinated nerve fibers, but are not strewn randomly along them. Indeed, the potassium channels that we could discern at that time were only detectable when the myelin was absent, and were otherwise hidden because of their placement in internodal parts of the axon, under the myelin. Electrophysiological recording methods had allowed us to find them.

We now know that the story is more complicated than this. It has become clear that there are several types of potassium channels with different localizations in myelinated nerve fibers. By 1987 it was known that one type of potassium channel acts to shape the nerve impulse by terminating it to insure that it is brief, while another type modulates the pattern of impulses within a train, preventing echoing or inappropriate after-bursting (Baker et al. 1987; Kocsis et al. 1987). In Eng et al. (1988) we extended this analysis and demonstrated that prior to the formation of myelin, the potassium channels which terminate the nerve impulse are accessible to the extracellular milieu. As myelin forms around the nerve fiber and covers these channels, their activity is masked. And following damage to the myelin that covers them, they are unmasked and again become accessible to the extracellular space. These are the "hidden" internodal channels. Potassium channels that prevent inappropriate repetitive bursting, on the other hand, continue to be accessible to the extracellular milieu even after myelination is complete, placing them at the nodes of Ranvier (Eng et al. 1988). Thus the two types of potassium channels are located in different places, a structural feature of nerve fibers which presumably reflects their different functions.

Early parts of this work resulted in the publication of the diagram (figure 10.4 in Waxman 1982) shown on page 112 of this book. This blueprint of the nerve fiber illustrates, once again, that the nervous system is precisely designed, this time in terms of the locations of the molecules that make it up. Might it be possible to exploit this design plan, to develop new treatments for diseases of the brain and spinal cord? When potassium channels in nerve fibers are uncovered due to damage to the overlying myelin, their function is unmasked and it is as if the molecular brakes are locked. This interferes with the propagation of nerve impulses. Drugs that block the unmasked potassium channels, such as 4-aminopyridine (4-AP), prolong the nerve impulse in demyelinated nerve fibers so that it generates more electrical current (Sherratt, Bostock, and Sears 1980). Thus it was not surprising when it became clear that these drugs can improve conduction in demyelinated fibers *in vitro*, i.e. studied in dishes (Targ and Kocsis 1985; Bowe et al. 1987) and in animal models of multiple sclerosis and spinal cord injury (Blight 1989). Careful clinical studies are needed—and are underway—to determine whether these drugs can be used as symptomatic therapies that improve function in patients with demyelinating disorders such as multiple sclerosis and spinal cord injury.

It is not enough to show that a particular type of molecule is *present* in the brain or spinal cord—the placement of a molecule may be as important as its presence. In some cases it has been necessary to infer the location of critical molecules since they cannot be seen but, like children playing hide-and-seek, neuroscientists have been able to do this, using clues that are present along the way. Ultimately it will be possible to find, with subcellular precision, the hiding places of many of the molecules within the nervous system.

References

Baker, M., Bostock, H., Grafe, P., and Martius, P. Function and distribution of three types of rectifying channel in rat spinal root myelinated axons. *J. Physiol. (Lond.)* 383: 46–67, 1987.

Blight, A. R. Effect of 4-AP on axonal conduction block in chronic spinal cord injury. *Brain Res. Bull.* 22: 47–52, 1989.

Bostock, H., and Sears, T. A. The internodal axon membrane: electrical excitability and continuous conduction in segmental demyelination. *J. Physiol. (Lond.)* 280: 273–301, 1978.

Bostock, H., Sears, T. A., and Sherratt, R. M. The effects of 4-aminopyridine and tetraethylammonium ions on normal and demyelinated mammalian nerve fibers. *J. Physiol. (Lond.)* 313: 301–315, 1981.

Bowe, C. M., Kocsis, J. D., Targ, E. F., and Waxman, S. G. Physiological effects of 4-aminopyridine on demyelinated mammalian motor and sensory fibers. *Ann. Neurol.* 22: 264–268, 1987.

Chiu, S. Y., and Ritchie, J. M. Potassium channels in nodal and internodal axonal membrane of mammalian myelinated fibres. *Nature* 284: 170–171, 1980.

Eng, D. L., Gordon, T. R., Kocsis, J. D., and Waxman, S. G. Development of 4-AP and TEA sensitivities in mammalian myelinated nerve fibers. *J. Neurophysiol.* 60: 2168–2179, 1988.

Kocsis, J. D., Eng, D. L., Gordon, T. R., and Waxman, S. G. Functional differences between 4-aminopyridine and tetraethylammonium-sensitive potassium channels in myelinated axons. *Neurosci. Lett.* 75: 193–198, 1987.

Kocsis, J. D., and Waxman, S. G. Absence of potassium conductance in central myelinated axons. *Nature* 287: 348–349, 1980.

Kocsis, J. D., Waxman, S. G., Hildebrand, C., and Ruiz, J. A. Regenerating mammalian nerve fibres: changes in action potential waveform and firing characteristics following blockage of potassium conductance. *Proc. Roy. Soc. (Lond.) B.* 217: 277–287, 1982.

Sherratt, R. M., Bostock, H., and Sears, T. A. Effects of 4-aminopyridine on normal and demyelinated mammalian nerve fibres. *Nature* 283: 570–572, 1980.

Targ, E. F., and Kocsis, J. D. 4-Aminopyridine leads to restoration of conduction in demyelinated rat sciatic nerve. *Brain Res.* 328: 358–361, 1985.

Waxman, S. G. Current concepts in neurology: membranes, myelin and the pathophysiology of multiple sclerosis. *N. Engl. J. Med.* 306: 1529–1533, 1982.

Waxman, S. G., and Foster, R. E. Ionic channel distribution and heterogeneity of the axon membrane in myelinated fibers. *Brain Res. Rev.* 2: 205–234, 1980.

Waxman, S. G., and Ritchie, J. M. Organization of ion channels in the myelinated nerve fiber. *Science* 228: 1502–1507, 1985.

13 Absence of Potassium Conductance in Central Myelinated Axons

Jeffery D. Kocsis and Stephen G. Waxman

Abstract Two voltage-dependent changes in ionic permeability are responsible for the action potential in squid giant axon.[1] The depolarization phase of the action potential is due to an initial increase in sodium ion permeability, and repolarization is primarily the result of a later increase in potassium permeability. However, voltage-clamp experiments on mammalian peripheral nodes of Ranvier indicate that potassium conductances (g_k) may be minimal or lacking for intact mammalian peripheral myelinated axons.[2-4] Repolarization for these fibres has been explained in terms of a rapid sodium inactivation and large leakage current.[3] When the myelin around these fibres is acutely disrupted, an immediate and prominent g_k appears.[4] Following demyelination, g_k blocking agents have been shown to reduce late outward currents that are not present in normal myelinated fibres.[5] This suggests that K^+ channels are present in the axonal membrane under the myelin but are "masked" in normal peripheral myelinated axons. Previous studies have not investigated the presence or role of K^+ channels in central myelinated axons. We here establish that g_k is not detectable in mammalian dorsal column axons.

The effects of superfusion of myelinated axons in the rat dorsal columns (DCs) with the voltage-dependent g_k blocking agents tetraethylammonium hydrochloride (TEA) and 4-aminopyridine (4-AP) were studied. We also recorded intra-axonally from the axons with glass microelectrodes filled with TEA. This allowed us to reach internodal as well as nodal axon membrane in the intact myelinated central axon. Although TEA injection into spinal motoneurones elicited a rapid and powerful prolongation of the motoneurone (soma-dendritic) action potential, the axonal action potential recorded from DC axons remained virtually unchanged even after prolonged TEA injection. In addition, superfusion of the spinal cord with 4-AP or TEA neither changed the action potential waveform nor altered the fibre refractory period.

Reprinted with permission from *Nature* 287: 348–349, 1980. © *Macmillan Journals Ltd., 1980.*

Extra- and intra-axonal potentials were recorded from the DCs of the rat spinal cord following local DC or sciatic nerve stimulation. The animals were deeply anaesthetized with urethane (1.5 g kg^{-1}) and prepared for acute experimentation. An agar pool was built around the exposed lumbar spinal cord to allow for superfusion of the DC surface with oxygenated and warmed (38 °C) normal Ringer solution (NS) into which 4-AP or TEA could be added.[6] Recordings were confined to within 50 μm of the surface of the spinal cord for the superfusion experiments.

Glass microelectrodes were filled with 3.0 M NaCl for field potential recordings and 2.0 M TEA for intracellular or intra-axonal recordings. Figure 13.1a shows the DC fibre field potential elicited from local surface stimulation of the DC superfused with normal Ringer. The early positive-negative component of the field corresponds to the collective action potential activity of fast conducting myelinated DC axons. The field remains virtually unchanged after introduction of 4-AP (figure 13.1b) or TEA (figure 13.1c) into the superfusion pool. When the potassium concentration of the NS was increased from 3.0–30 mM, a reversible conduction block occurred promptly, thus indicating the efficacy of the superfusion (figure 13.1d). In addition to not affecting the field potential waveform elicited from a single stimulus, external 4-AP or TEA application also did not alter the refractory period of the fibres as determined from paired stimulation experiments (data not shown). In contrast to the absence of response of the myelinated DC fibres to superfusion with TEA and 4-AP, the compound action potential of nonmyelinated cerebellar parallel fibres is markedly altered by both of these agents.[7] Although 4-AP,[8-10] and in some instances TEA,[11] have been shown to block voltage-dependent g_k by external application, the accessibility of either 4-AP or TEA to K^+ channel sites following external application

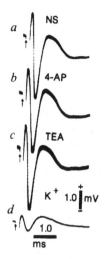

Figure 13.1

Field potentials elicited from surface stimulation of the lumbar DC and recorded 3 mm anterior to the stimulation site within 20 μm of the surface. (*a*) Responses recorded when the spinal cord was continuously superfused with normal Ringer solution NS. The early positive-negative components of the field correspond to action potential activity of the fast conducting myelinated fibres of the DC. The responses in (*b*) and (*c*) were obtained after 30 min of superfusion in 4-AP (3.0 mM) and TEA (10 mM) solutions, respectively. Virtually no change occurs in the waveform of the early positive-negative field component, thus indicating the ineffectiveness of these voltage-dependent g_k blocking agents on these fibres. (*d*) A response recorded within 2 min after the K⁺ concentration was increased from 3 to 30 mM. A significant reduction in the field occurs at high K⁺ concentrations. This effect is reversible within minutes after superfusion with NS. The K⁺ blocking action indicates the efficacy of the superfusion system, and shows that the superfusate gains access to the nodal extracellular space. The calibration in (*e*) pertains to all records.

is open to question. This is particularly important in view of the recent studies of Chiu and Ritchie[4] showing that K⁺ channel distribution may be inhomogeneous, with K⁺ channels present at internodal or paranodal membrane regions but not at nodal membrane.

Prolongation of the somatic action potential has been reported[12-14] following intracellular recordings from neuronal cell bodies with TEA electrodes. This effect appears rapidly after diffusion of TEA from the microelectrode or is facilitated by depolarizing currents. Figure 13.2*a* shows an action potential recorded from a motoneurone immediately after impalement with a TEA microelectrode. The responses shown in figure 13.2*b* and *c* were recorded 4.0 and 12.0 min later, respectively. The action potentials are much prolonged (compare figure 13.2*b* and *c* to *a*), indicating a block of g_k (ref. 12). The same microelectrode was used for recording the intra-axonal responses from DC axons shown in figure 13.2*d–f*. All electrode probes for DC axons were confined to the dorsal 200 μm of the spinal cord, within 300 μm of the spinal cord midline. Intra-axonal impalements were identified by: (1) the presence of negative resting potential; (2) the all-or-none character of the action potential with no underlying synaptic potential; and (3) when possible, collision of directly induced action potentials with those induced from sciatic nerve stimulation. Conduction velocities for these fibres were greater than 15 m s⁻¹, indicating their myelinated nature. After 25 min of impalement with a TEA microelectrode, virtually no change in the axonal action potential duration can be seen (figure 13.2*f*). We also passed depolarization pulses through the microelectrode to facilitate TEA entry, but still no change in action potential waveform occurred. For five axons, intra-axonal penetrations were held for over 45 min each. No significant change in spike waveform or refractory period was seen in these axons or in 26 other axons held for periods greater than 5 min but less than 45 min. During the passage of depo-

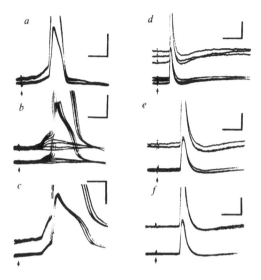

Figure 13.2

(a–c) Intracellular recordings obtained from spinal motoneurones with TEA microelectrodes following stimulation of the ipsilateral sciatic nerve. Orthodromic action potentials can be seen arising from an excitatory postsynaptic potential (EPSP). The upper traces correspond to high gain recordings and the lower traces to low gain recordings. (a) Records obtained immediately after impalement of the motoneurone. (b) Records obtained at about 4 min after impalement. Stimulation intensity was varied to demonstrate the graded nature of the EPSP and all-or-none properties of the action potential. Note the broadening of the action potential as the TEA diffuses into the cell. (c) Records from same cell at about 12 min post-impalement. A marked prolongation of the action potential is evident. (d–f) Intra-axonal action potentials recorded with same TEA microelectrode as used for (a–c) from a DC axon near the midline surface of the lumbar cord. (d) and (e) show the axonal action potential at different oscilloscope sweeps, near the time of axonal impalement. (f) Responses recorded about 25 min after impalement. Depolarizing currents were passed at the time between the records of (e) and (f). No appreciable prolongation of the axon action potential can be seen after TEA injection. Vertical calibrations indicate 20 mV for lower traces and 10 mV for upper traces for (a–f). Horizontal calibrations indicate 4 ms in (a–d) and 2 ms in (e) and (f). Positive voltage deflection is upward.

larization currents, the action potential amplitude was decreased, and hyperpolarization increased the action potential amplitude, thus indicating that the site of impalement was electrotonically close to the site of impulse origin.

The observation here, that external application of either TEA or 4-AP does not prolong the action potential of DC myelinated axons, extends observations made in peripheral nerves to DC axons in the mammalian central nervous system. Also, the lack of action potential prolongation or changes in refractory period after direct intra-axonal injections of TEA into these central myelinated axons suggests that K^+ channels contribute little to action potential waveform and recovery for these axons. One might question whether TEA effectively passed from our microelectrode into the axons, and once inside if it diffused sufficiently to present itself to nearby internodal as well as nodal axon surfaces. However, other observations[12-14] and this study show that TEA readily diffuses from electrode to cytoplasm of neurone somata. Although geometrical differences are present between somadendritic and axonal regions that could vary diffusion properties, the rapidity of the TEA action on large volume motoneurones, the facilitation of TEA ejection by depolarization pulses, and the relatively long duration impalements of the axons (several over 45 min), suggest that TEA may have passed over a significant axonal length.

Voltage-clamp experiments in mammalian peripheral nerve[4] reveal an immediate appearance of g_k after acute myelin disruption, suggesting that K^+ channels are present under the myelin in normal myelinated axons. The absence of demonstrable g_k at intact mammalian peripheral nodes of Ranvier[3] and the lack of effect on the action potential of direct intra-axonal injections of TEA into DC fibres suggest that g_k does not contribute significantly to spike electrogenesis in at least several types of intact mammalian myelinated fibres. Chiu and Ritchie (personal communication) have suggested that potassium channels in the internodal axon membrane may have a normal role in preventing repetitive firing at the node. Although we did not observe repetitive firing after TEA or 4-AP application, our experiments cannot rule this out.

Acknowledgments

This work was supported in part by the Medical Research Service, Veterans Administration, National Institutes of Health grants RR-5353 and NS-15320, and National Multiple Sclerosis Society grant RG-1231. We thank Professor J. M. Ritchie for helpful discussions.

References

1. Hodgkin, A. L. & Huxley, A. F. *J. Physiol., Lond.* 117: 500–544 (1952).

2. Horakova, M., Nonner, W. & Stämpfli, R. *Proc. int. Un. physiol. Sci.* 7: 198 (1968).

3. Chiu, S. Y., Ritchie, J. M., Rogart, R. B. & Stagg, D. *J. Physiol., Lond.* 292: 149–166 (1979)

4. Chiu, S. Y. & Ritchie, J. M. *Nature* 284: 170–171 (1980).

5. Sherratt, R. M., Bostock, H. & Sears, T. A. *Nature* 283: 570–572 (1980).

6. Kocsis, J. D., Malenka, R. C. & Waxman, S. G. *Brain Res.* 195: 511–516, 1980.

7. Kocsis, J. D., Malenka, R. C. & Waxman, S. G. Brain Res. 207: 321–331 (1981).

8. Pelhate, M. & Pichon, *J. Physiol., Lond.* 242: 90–91P (1974).

9. Nicholson, C. G., ten Bruggencate, G. & Senekowitsch, R. *Brain Res.* 113: 606–610 (1976).

10. Llinás, R., Walton, K. & Bohr, V. *Biophys. J.* 16: 83–86 (1976).

11. Hille, B. *J. gen. Physiol.* 50: 1287–1302 (1967).

12. Shapovalov, A. I. & Kurchavyi, C. G. *Brain Res.* 82: 49–67 (1974).

13. Sugimori, M., Preston, R. J. & Kitai, S. T. *J. Neurophysiol.* 41: 1662–1675 (1978).

14. Schwartzkroin, P. A. & Prince, D. A. *Brain Res.* 85: 169–181 (1980).

14 Development of 4-AP and TEA Sensitivities in Mammalian Myelinated Nerve Fibers

Douglas L. Eng, Thomas R. Gordon, Jeffery D. Kocsis, and Stephen G. Waxman

Summary and Conclusions

1. The sensitivities of mammalian myelinated axons to potassium channel blockers were studied over the course of development using in vitro sucrose gap and intra-axonal recording techniques.

2. Application of 4-aminopyridine (4-AP; 1.0 mM) to young nerves led to a delay in return to base line of the sciatic nerve compound action potential and to a post-spike positivity (indicative of hyperpolarization) lasting for tens of milliseconds. These effects were very much attenuated during the course of maturation.

3. Tetraethylammonium chloride (TEA; 10 mM) application alone had little effect on the waveform of the compound action potential at any age. However, the 4-AP-induced postspike positivity was blocked by TEA, Ba^{2+}, and Cs^+. This block was observed in Ca^{2+}-free electrolyte solutions containing EGTA (1.0 mM).

4. Immature sciatic nerves (~3 wk postnatal) were incubated in a potassium-free electrolyte solution containing 120 mM CsCl for up to 1 h in an attempt to replace internal potassium with cesium. When the nerves were tested in the sucrose gap chamber using solutions containing 3.0 mM CsCl substituted for KCl, the compound action potential was broadened and a prolonged depolarization appeared, but there was no postspike positivity; the CsCl effect was similar to the combined effects of 4-AP and TEA.

5. Intra-axonal recordings were obtained to study the effects of 4-AP and TEA on individual axons. In the presence of 4-AP a single stimulus led to a burst of action potentials followed by a pronounced after-hyperpolarization (AHP) in sensory fibers. The AHP was blocked by TEA. In motor fibers 4-AP application resulted in action potential broadening with no AHP.

6. Repetitive stimulation (200–500 Hz; 100 ms) was followed by a pronounced AHP in both sensory and motor fibers at all ages studied. This activity-elicited AHP was sensitive to TEA at all ages.

7. The results indicate that 4-AP and TEA sensitivity change over the course of development in rat sciatic nerve. The effects of 4-AP are much more pronounced in immature nerves than in mature nerves, suggesting that 4-AP-sensitive channels become masked as they are covered by myelin during maturation. However, the TEA-sensitive channels, demonstrable after repetitive firing, remain accessible to TEA after myelination. These channels therefore may have a nodal representation.

Reprinted with permission from *Journal of Neurophysiology* 60: 2168–2179, 1988.

Introduction

Recent studies indicate that two pharmacologically distinct types of potassium channels are present on mammalian myelinated axons in both the peripheral (1, 2, 21) and central nervous system (15, 22); one is sensitive to 4-aminopyridine (4-AP) and the other to tetraethylammonium chloride (TEA). It has been suggested that these potassium channels have different functional roles because the 4-AP-sensitive channel contributes to action potential repolarization whereas the TEA-sensitive channel results in a prolonged afterhyperpolarization (AHP) following repetitive activity (21).

These two pharmacologically defined types of potassium channels on mammalian axons have not as yet been distinguished in voltage-clamp analysis. In fact, voltage clamp studies indicate a relative paucity of voltage-sensitive potassium conductance at the mammalian node as compared to the amphibian node (8–11), where a variety of potassium channel types have been identified (12, 17). This discrepancy may be indicative of the nonuniform spatial distribution of ionic channels along nodal and internodal axon regions (27), the greater difficulty of voltage-clamping mammalian axons, or inherent differences between mammalian and amphibian myelinated axons. Studies utilizing electrotonus measurements (1, 2, 5) and analysis of action potential waveform and firing characteristics (6, 16, 23, 26) following blockade with relatively specific potassium channel-blocking agents provide compelling evidence for the presence of diverse potassium conductances on mammalian myelinated axons.

It is well established that the sensitivity of myelinated axons to 4-AP is very pronounced in immature myelinated axons but attenuates during the course of maturation (14, 23, 26, 31). Moreover, following demyelination of mature myelinated axons the previously insensitive fibers become sensitive to 4-AP (5, 6, 10, 27, 30). The implication of these results is that 4-AP-sensitive potassium channels are localized at the internodal axon membrane which becomes exposed after demyelination (6, 8, 10, 30, 33). The purpose of the present study is to determine the developmental sequence of TEA sensitivity of myelinated axons of rat sciatic nerve and compare it to that of 4-AP. The results indicate that 4-AP and TEA sensitivity develop with different time-courses during the course of sciatic nerve maturation, and have implications for localization of the two types of potassium channels.

Materials and Methods

Wistar rats (6 day–14 mo) were deeply anesthetized with pentobarbital sodium (60 mg/kg) and exsanguinated by carotid section. The sciatic nerves were exposed and a 1.0- to 3.0-cm segment of nerve was excised distal to the sciatic notch. Nerves were carefully desheathed in a modified Krebs' solution (in mM: 124, NaCl; 3.0, KCl; 1.3, NaH_2PO_4; 2.0, $MgCl_2$; 2.0, $CaCl_2$; 26.0, $NaHCO_3$; and 10.0, dextrose), saturated with 95% O_2 and 5% CO_2. Only nerves that could be removed and desheathed with no apparent disruption were used for this study.

4-AP, TEA, CsCl, $BaCl_2$, and EGTA solutions were made by adding appropriate concentrations to the Krebs solution. Isotonic KCl solutions contained (in mM): 120, KCl; 7.0, NaCl; 1.3, NaH_2PO_4; 2.0, $MgCl_2$; 26.0, $NaHCO_3$; and 10, dextrose. Isotonic sucrose solution contained 320 mM sucrose.

Modified Sucrose Gap

Sucrose gap recordings were used to study action potentials and indirectly monitor changes in membrane potential (13, 24). The nerve was placed in a test chamber divided into three compartments by petroleum jelly seals. The end of the nerve which was to be activated was positioned into a compartment which contained oxygenated Krebs solution or a test solution. The opposite end was positioned into a compartment containing isotonic KCl. The central region was continuously washed with isotonic sucrose. Solutions flowed continuously at a rate of 1–2 ml/min. The nerve was stimulated with a bipolar Teflon-coated stainless steel stimulation electrode cut flush and placed directly on the nerve segment in the test compartment. Whole nerve stimulation pulses were delivered by constant current stimulus isolation units which were controlled by a digital timing device. Whole nerve responses and DC potentials were recorded between the outer compartments using a high input impedance differential electrometer which was connected by calomel electrodes to the outer compartments of the sucrose gap chamber.

Intra-Axonal Recordings

Nerves were placed in a brain slice chamber which had provisions for whole nerve stimulation and recording. The whole nerve recording apparatus consisted of two pairs of Ag-AgCl electrodes with 2-mm separation of the two electrodes in each pair. One electrode pair was used for stimulating and the other pair was used for recording the whole nerve response. The electrode pairs were separated by a distance of 1 cm. Aluminosilicate glass microelectrodes for intracellular recording were pulled on a Brown-Flaming P-80 puller, bevelled on a diamond wheel and filled with 2.0 M KCl or 4.0 M K-acetate. DC resistances ranged from 180 to 250 MΩ.

Intra-axonal recordings with resting potentials >55 mV and action potential amplitudes exceeding resting potential were chosen for analysis. Identification of intra-axonal recordings utilized criteria that have been discussed previously (25). An impalement was considered to be intracellular if the passage of a constant hyperpolarizing current led to an increase in action potential amplitude compared to that elicited in the resting state, and passage of a depolarizing current led to a decrease in action potential amplitude. We encountered many axons that had spike amplitudes >60 mV but showed virtually no resting potential. The amplitude of these action potentials was minimally influenced by current passage through the microelectrode, and these spikes were considered to be recorded extra-axonally.

Intracellular studies have established that sensory and motor fibers respond differently to potassium channel blockade with 4-AP (2, 7, 20); sensory fibers give rise to a delayed depolarization with subsequent repetitive firing, whereas motor fibers exhibit broadening of action potentials. These criteria were used to distinguish sensory and motor fibers in the present study.

Results

The potassium channel blocker 4-AP substantially alters the compound action potential of young sciatic nerves (figure 14.1*A1*; 3 wk), but only modestly affects mature nerves (figure 14.1*B1*; 17 wk). The effect of 4-AP is to delay the return to base line of the compound action potential. In addition, the response recorded in immature nerves in the presence of 4-AP demonstrates an overshoot of the base line following the compound action potential (figure 14.1*A2*). This 4-AP-elicited overshoot, which we refer to as the "postspike positivity," is several millivolts in amplitude and >100 ms in duration. With our recording convention, the postspike positivity represents membrane hyperpolarization. It is virtually absent in recordings from mature nerves as shown in figure 14.1*B2*.

Another potassium channel blocker, tetraethylammonium ion (TEA), has little effect on the compound action potential waveform in both young (figure 14.1*A3*) and mature (figure 14.1*B3*) rat sciatic nerves. In contrast to 4-AP, 10 mM TEA did not delay the return to base line of the action potential. TEA did on occasion lead to a slight depolarization and amplitude reduction.

The amplitude of the postspike positivity following a single stimulus in the presence of 4-AP was age-dependent (figure 14.2*A*). The postspike positivity amplitude was initially relatively small (<3 wk postnatal), but reached a maximum absolute amplitude at ∼3 wk of age. From this point on, the amplitude progressively attenuated with age. In figure 14.2*B*, note that the amplitude of the compound action potential is small for nerves <3 wk of age when myelin has not yet formed, but rapidly increases during the third week when myelin is being formed (4, 34). From 3 wk on there is a progressive increase in compound action potential amplitude with maturation. However, although compound action potential amplitude approaches its adult value at 3–4 wk when myelination is well underway, the postspike positivity progressively attenuates after 3 wk. Indeed, when the postspike positivity is scaled for action potential amplitude at a given age by establishing a ratio of the amplitude of the 4-AP-elicited postspike positivity to compound action potential amplitude, the ratio progressively diminishes with age (figure 14.3). These data suggest that the postspike positivity, elicited by a single stimulus in the presence of 4-AP, progressively attenuates during maturation.

Although TEA alone had little effect on the compound action potential waveform of mature nor immature nerves (see figures 14.1*A3* and 14.1*B3*), a striking effect of TEA became manifest when TEA was applied to 4-AP-treated immature nerves. Namely, the 4-AP-induced postspike positivity was eliminated by TEA

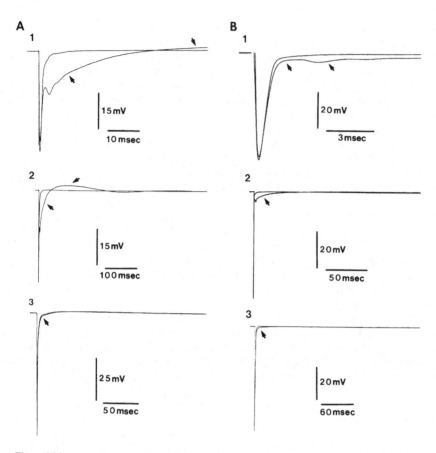

Figure 14.1
Sucrose gap recordings obtained from sciatic nerves of an immature (3-wk-old) and mature (>17-wk-old) rat, shown in columns (*A*) and (*B*), respectively. The superimposed traces in (*A1*) and (*A2*) (immature) and (*B1*) and (*B2*) (mature) are before and after (arrows) application of 4-AP (1.0 mM). 4-AP has a very large effect on the immature nerve (*A1*), but only a modest effect on the mature nerve (*B1*). Note the different time scales in (*A1*) and (*B1*). A prominent postspike positivity (top arrow) is present following a single stimulus to an immature nerve in the presence of 4-AP (*A2*), that is not present in mature nerves (*B2*). TEA (arrows) has little effect on the action potential waveform of immature (*A3*) or mature (*B3*).

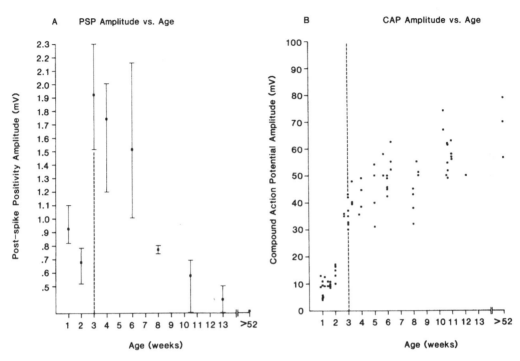

Figure 14.2
Graphs showing the amplitude of the postspike positivity (*A*) and compound action potential amplitude (*B*) vs. age. The vertical dashed line at 3 wk indicates the approximate time when all fibers that are to be myelinated display signs of early myelination (Webster, 34). Note that prior to 3 wk the postspike positivity and the compound action potential are both relatively small. However, after 3 wk the postspike positivity progressively attenuates, whereas the compound action potential amplitude steadily increases in amplitude.

(10 mM). In figure 14.4*A*, three responses are shown superimposed: a normal compound action potential (unlabeled); the compound action potential following 1.0 mM 4-AP application which displays the postspike positivity (labeled 1); and one in the presence of 1.0 mM 4-AP and 10 mM TEA in which the postspike positivity is eliminated (labeled 2). Note that the delay in the return to base line of the compound action potential is increased by 4-AP and is further increased with the addition of TEA. The 4-AP-induced postspike positivity was also blocked by other K-channel blockers such as

Ba$^+$ (2.0 mM; figure 14.4*B*) and Cs$^+$ (10 mM; figure 14.4*C*).

The next set of experiments examined the effects of 4-AP and TEA in the absence of calcium ion. In a calcium-free Krebs' solution containing 6.0 mM MgCl$_2$, both 4-AP and 4-AP in combination with TEA have qualitatively the same effects as in calcium-containing Krebs' solution. Figure 14.4*D* shows the 4-AP-induced postspike positivity and its elimination with the addition of 10 mM TEA in the absence of Ca^{2+}. Another experiment was carried out using Ca^{2+}-free Krebs' containing 1 mM EGTA (incubated

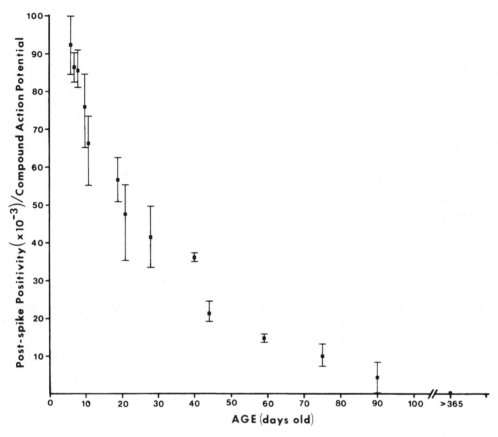

Figure 14.3

A graph showing the ratio established by dividing the postspike positivity amplitude by the compound action potential amplitude, plotted vs. age. Note that when the postspike positivity is scaled for compound action potential amplitude in this manner, it progressively attenuates with maturation.

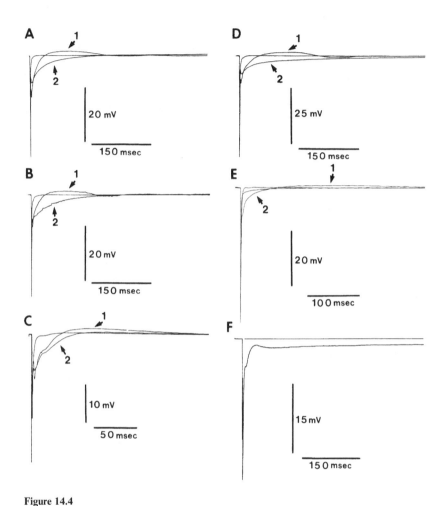

Figure 14.4

Pharmacological properties of the postspike positivity. (*A–C*) Superimposed traces of compound action potentials in normal Krebs (unlabeled) and Krebs containing 4-AP (labeled 1). The responses labeled 2 are in solutions containing TEA (*A*; 10 mM), Ba^{2+} (*B*; 2 mM), Cs (*C*; 10 mM). Note that TEA, Ba^{2+}, and Cs all eliminate the postspike positivity. The induction of the postspike positivity does not require the presence of calcium in the bathing solution. This is evident in (*D*), where 4-AP (labeled 1) can elicit a postspike positivity in a calcium-free solution containing 6.0 mM $MgCl_2$. The response is blocked by TEA (labeled 2). When the nerves are incubated in a calcium-free solution containing the chelating agent EGTA (*E*), a postspike positivity can still be elicited (labeled 1), by 4-AP further suggesting the postspike positivity is independent of calcium. The trace labeled 2 is after TEA application: the postspike positivity is blocked. (*F*) In an attempt to remove all intracellular and extracellular potassium, nerves were incubated in an osmotically balanced potassium-free solution that contained 120 mM CsCl. The nerves were then returned to a potassium-free Krebs solution containing 3.0 mM CsCl. The response in *F* was recorded from such a nerve and shows a response with a pronounced delay in return to base line following the action potential and an absence of the postspike positivity.

0.5–1.0 h) in order to chelate any residual Ca^{2+} (figure 14.4*E*). Although the 4-AP-elicited postspike positivity is slightly reduced in amplitude and increased in duration, the postspike positivity is present in this solution (figure 14.4*E*, 1).

In another set of experiments, nerves were incubated in osmotically balanced potassium-free solution containing 120 mM CsCl in an attempt to replace intracellular potassium with cesium. The sucrose gap recording in figure 14.4*F* is from a 3-wk-old rat sciatic nerve recorded in a potassium-free solution containing 3.0 mM CsCl after a 30-min preincubation in an isotonic CsCl, potassium-free solution. This treatment led to a pronounced broadening of the compound action potential and to prolonged depolarization. A postspike positivity was not present, further supporting the role of potassium conductance in generating the postspike positivity.

A positivity was also elicited by repetitive electrical stimulation of the nerve in normal Krebs' solution. This positivity is referred to as the "posttrain positivity" to distinguish it from the postspike positivity elicited by a single stimulus in 4-AP. In figure 14.5*A* a 200-Hz stimulus train of 100-ms duration elicited a posttrain positivity of several millivolts amplitude, lasting >100 ms in an immature sciatic nerve (3 wk). This posttrain positivity was abolished by 10 mM TEA (figure 14.5*D*). Figure 14.5*B* illustrates a posttrain positivity elicited by a similar stimulus train in a mature (>14 wk) sciatic nerve; the posttrain positivity is similar to that seen in immature nerves. This response was also blocked by TEA (figure 14.5*E*). Increased stimulus frequency applied to young (not illustrated) or mature nerve (figure 14.5*C*) produced a posttrain positivity of greater amplitude (500-Hz train of 100 ms duration). This positivity was also abolished by 10 mM TEA (figure 14.5*F*).

The posttrain positivity and the 4-AP-induced postspike positivity are very similar since they both occur following a prolonged depolarization, have similar amplitudes and durations, and are both abolished by TEA application. However, the posttrain positivity was clearly present at all ages and was present in the absence of 4-AP. Moreover, the posttrain positivity was sensitive to TEA at all ages. Amplitude of the posttrain positivity vs. age is shown graphically in figure 14.5*G*.

An intra-axonal recording obtained in the presence of 4-AP (1.0 mM) from a sensory fiber of a 5-wk-old rat is shown in figure 14.6*A*. A single stimulus elicited a burst of action potentials followed by a prominent afterhyperpolarization (AHP). The AHP was sensitive to TEA (figure 14. 6*B*, arrow). Although an AHP is not seen in motor fibers in 4-AP following a single stimulus, an AHP can be elicited from motor fibers following repetitive stimulation (figure 14.6*C*). The AHP from both sensory and motor axons is TEA-sensitive: simultaneous application of 4-AP and TEA abolishes the AHP seen in sensory axons treated with 4-AP (figure 14.6*B*) and the activity-dependent AHP in motor fibers (figure 14.6*D*). In addition to blocking the AHP, TEA also leads to increased spontaneous action potential activity for both sensory (figure 14.6*B*) and motor (figure 14.6*D*) fibers.

Furthermore, the TEA-sensitive activity-dependent AHP can be activated in virtually all fibers, without 4-AP application, in adult as well as immature sciatic nerve. For example, by stimulating at 200 Hz for 100 ms an AHP can be elicited in normal Krebs' solution (figure 14.7*A1*). Higher frequency stimulation (500 Hz) can augment the AHP (figure 14.7*A2*). AHPs are abolished (except for a brief, <10-ms TEA-insensitive hyperpolarization; see below) following application 10 mM TEA (figure 14.7*A3*). The TEA-sensitive AHP elicited by high-frequency stimulation is not calcium-dependent; repetitive stimulation (200 Hz, 100 ms) can elicit an AHP in Ca^{2+}-free Krebs' solution containing 6 mM $MgCl_2$ (figure 14.7*B1*). Higher frequency (500 Hz, 100 ms) stimulation again augments the AHP (figure 14.7*B2*), and 10 mM TEA abolishes the AHP in the absence of Ca^{2+} (figure

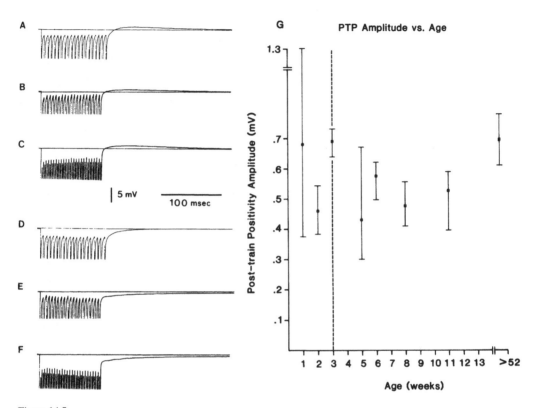

Figure 14.5
Repetitive stimulation elicits a posttrain positivity in the absence of 4-AP. The posttrain positivity and the 4-AP-induced postspike positivity are very similar for they both occur following a prolonged depolarization. The posttrain positivity was clearly present and was attenuated by TEA at all ages studied. (*A–C*) Sucrose gap recordings of trains of action potentials followed by a delayed hyperpolarization are displayed. (*A*) A posttrain positivity obtained from an immature sciatic nerve (3-wk-old). (*B*) Displays a posttrain positivity from a mature sciatic nerve (>14-wk-old) following 200-Hz 100-ms train, which is similar to the immature posttrain positivity. (*C*) Higher frequency stimulation (500-Hz 100-ms) elicits a larger posttrain positivity in this recording from a mature nerve. (*D–F*) 10 mM TEA abolishes the corresponding posttrain positivity in both mature and immature nerves. (*D–F*) Corresponds to *A–C*. Amplitude of the posttrain positivity, shown graphically in *G*, remains relatively constant through development, yet sensitivity of the posttrain positivity to TEA is maintained even in adult sciatic nerves.

A

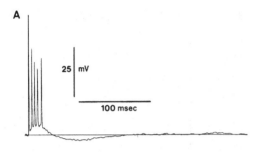

B

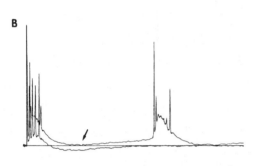

C

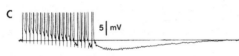

D

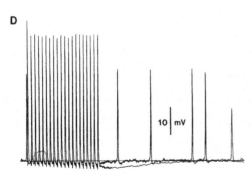

14.7*B3*). In addition to the long duration TEA-sensitive AHP, a brief TEA-insensitive AHP was noted (figure 14.7*A1 arrow*). This AHP is sensitive to 4-AP and has been demonstrated by previous investigators (2).

Discussion

It is well established that the broadening of the action potential and the development of delayed depolarizations elicited by 4-AP attenuate during the course of maturation (14, 23, 26, 31). In the present study it was found that in addition to the attenuation of these effects of 4-AP, the 4-AP-induced postspike positivity also attenuates in amplitude after an age of 3 wk. However, the amplitude of the activity-elicited posttrain positivity and its sensitivity to TEA remain relatively stable over the course of development. These findings can be explained, in part, by physiological changes secondary to myelination and fiber diameter growth.

The 4-AP-elicited postspike positivity increases in amplitude over the first few postnatal weeks to reach a maximum at 3 wk and subsequently shows a reduction in amplitude. Several factors may contribute to this sequence of development. First is the change during development of the compound action potential amplitude. As shown in figure 14.3*B*, the compound action potential initially is of small amplitude (<20 mV) and

Figure 14.6
Intra-axonal recordings of rat sciatic nerve fibers are shown. (*A*) Action potentials of a sensory fiber in the presence of 1 mM 4-AP. Notice the burst of action potentials resulting from a single stimulus and the following afterhyperpolarization (AHP) which lasts almost 100 ms. (*B*) Recorded from the same sensory axon: action potential burst with AHP in the presence of 1 mM 4-AP, superimposed on an action potential burst in the presence of 1 mM 4-AP plus 10 mM TEA. Notice that TEA abolishes the AHP and results in spontaneous activity. (*C*) Intra-axonal recording of AHP in motor fiber induced by repetitive stimulation (200 Hz 100 ms). A motor axon will not spontaneously fire bursts of action potentials. (*D*) Superimposed are train of action potentials (200 Hz 100 ms) and the AHP from a motor axon in 1 mM 4-AP, and the response with the addition of 10 mM TEA. Notice that TEA can abolish the AHP.

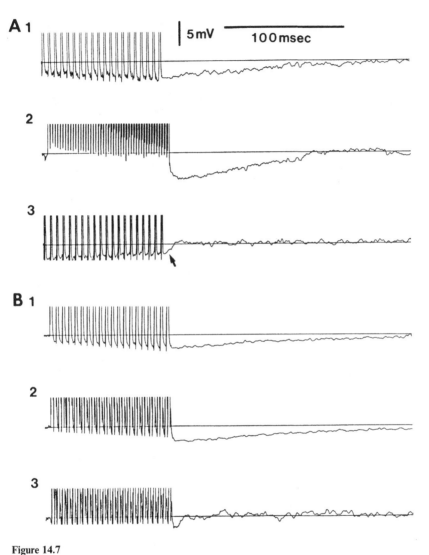

Figure 14.7

Intra-axonal recordings of repetitive stimulation. (*A*) Normal Krebs solution. (*A1*) Repetitive stimulation of 200 Hz for 100 ms followed by an AHP of several millivolts and of 100-ms duration. (*A2*) Repetitive stimulation of 500 Hz for 100 ms elicits a larger AHP than in *A1*. (*A3*) Repetitive stimulation of 200 Hz for 100 ms in the presence of 10 mM TEA. Notice that the AHP is abolished or absent except for a small 4-AP sensitive notch. (*B*) Krebs solution without Ca^{2+} but with the addition of 6 mM $MgCl_2$. (*B1*) Repetitive stimulation of 200 Hz for 100 ms elicits characteristic AHP. (*B2*) Higher frequency stimulation (500 Hz for 100 ms) increases AHP. (*B3*) In the presence of 10 mM TEA, repetitive stimulation (200 Hz for 100 ms) fails to elicit AHP.

approaches its adult value at 3 wk postnatal. The low amplitude of the postspike positivity in nerves younger than 3 wk may parallel the reduced amplitude of the compound action potential in these nerves. Another factor may be the accessibility of the 4-AP-sensitive potassium channels to extracellularly applied pharmacological agents over the course of development. Several lines of evidence suggest that, in mature myelinated fibers, the 4-AP-sensitive potassium channels are located within the internodal membrane where they are "masked" by the overlying myelin sheath (6, 9, 10, 23). Assuming such a localization for 4-AP-sensitive channels, one would expect the effects of 4-AP to be attenuated as these channels are masked by the myelin sheath, with a time-course paralleling that of maturation of the paranodal axon-Schwann cell junctions which isolate the internodal axon from the extracellular space (19, 29). Berthold (3) has shown, in developing sciatic nerve, that there is a transient period of myelin remodeling which is completed ∼12 wk postnatal. During this period of remodeling the paranodal junctions are loosened (3, 4, 18). Thus the morphological and physiological results are in agreement in terms of explaining the alterations in 4-AP sensitivity that occur during development.

In contrast to the postspike positivity observed in the presence of 4-AP following a single stimulus, the posttrain positivity, induced in the absence of 4-AP by repetitive stimulation, showed relatively stable amplitude at all ages studied. Thus the posttrain positivity is relatively larger than the postspike positivity in young premyelinated axons. We are uncertain as to why this may be. One possibility is that factors such as electrogenic pump activity may contribute to the posttrain positivity in immature nerves. Since the surface:volume ratio is greater in small fibers prior to myelination, it might be expected that transmembrane ion fluxes would lead to greater pump activation prior to myelination.

Only the sensory fibers gave rise to a distinct TEA-sensitive AHP in the presence of 4-AP fol-

lowing a single stimulus. This intracellularly recorded AHP corresponds in time-course and relative amplitude to the postspike positivity in the compound action potential that was blocked by TEA. However, in motor fibers studied after 4-AP application, an AHP was not present following a single stimulus, but it could be induced in both motor and sensory fibers during and following repetitive stimulation. This type of activity-evoked hyperpolarization was blocked by TEA in both sensory and motor fibers. These findings demonstrate that the TEA-sensitive AHP requires prolonged depolarization for its appearance; this depolarization can be elicited in motor fibers by a stimulus train and in sensory fibers by 4-AP-induced depolarization and consequent burst firing (7, 20) or by repetitive stimulation. All fibers tested with repetitive stimulation in normal solution developed an AHP.

The changes in 4-AP and TEA sensitivity seen during maturation provide some insight into the possible localization of the two classes of potassium channels identified by selective sensitivity to these agents. The 4-AP sensitivity of young rat sciatic nerves to 4-AP, its progressive decline with maturation (23), and the enhancement of this sensitivity in demyelinated (6, 28, 30) and regenerated (24, 26) mammalian nerve suggest that the 4-AP-sensitive channels have a greater representation at the internode on mature myelinated fibers. The available data do not demonstrate whether or not there are 4-AP-sensitive potassium channels in premyelinated fibers at regions destined to develop into nodes, but the data show that 4-AP is not significantly active in mature nodes.

In contrast, TEA-sensitivity of the posttrain positivity and of the activity-elicited AHP is present in both young and mature nerves. The persistence of TEA-sensitivity, after myelin and axon-Schwann cell junctions are formed, is consistent with the idea that TEA-sensitive channels have a significant nodal representation. Baker et al. (2) suggested a similar localization of TEA-sensitive channels from electrotonus measurements. The present analysis cannot predict whether or not TEA-sensitive channels are present in the internodal axon membrane as has been posited by others (2). However, the results do indicate that mammalian myelinated axons display different ontological sequences with respect to development of sensitivities to various potassium channel-blocking agents.

Acknowledgments

This work was supported in part by grants from the National Institute of Neurological and Communicative Disorders and Stroke and National Multiple Sclerosis Society, and by the Medical Research Service, Veterans Administration.

References

1. Baker, M., Bostock, H., and Grafe, P. Accommodation in rat myelinated axons depend on two pharmacologically distinct types of potassium channels. *J. Physiol. Lond.* 369: 102P, 1985.

2. Baker, M., Bostock, H., Grafe, P., and Martius, P. Function and distribution of three types of rectifying channel in rat spinal root myelinated axons. *J. Physiol. Lond.* 383: 45–67, 1987.

3. Berthold, C. H. Morphology of normal peripheral axons. In: *Physiology and Pathobiology of Axons*, edited by S. G. Waxman. New York: Raven, 1978, pp. 3–63.

4. Berthold, C. H. and Skoglund, S. Postnatal development of feline paranodal myelin sheath segments. *Acta Soc. Med. Ups.* 73: 127–144, 1968.

5. Bostock, H. and Grafe, P. Activity-dependent excitability changes in normal and demyelinated rat spinal root axons. *J. Physiol. Lond.* 365: 239–257, 1985.

6. Bostock, H., Sears, T. A., and Sherratt, R. M. The effect of 4-aminopyridine and tetraethylammonium ions on normal and demyelinated mammalian nerve fibers. *J. Physiol. Lond.* 313: 301–315, 1981.

7. Bowe, C. M., Kocsis, J. D., and Waxman, S. G. Differences between ventral and dorsal spinal roots in response to blockade of potassium channels during maturation. *Proc. R. Soc. Lond. B Biol. Sci.* 224: 355–366, 1985.

8. Brismar, T. Potential clamp experiments on myelinated nerve fibers from alloxan diabetic rats. *Acta Physiol. Scand.* 105: 384–386, 1979.

9. Chiu, S. Y. and Ritchie, J. M. Potassium channels in nodal and internodal axonal membrane of mammalian myelinated fibers. *Nature Lond.* 284: 170–171, 1980.

10. Chiu, S. Y. and Ritchie, J. M. Evidence for the presence of potassium channels in the paranodal region of acutely demyelinated mammalian nerve fibers. *J. Physiol. Lond.* 313: 415–437, 1981.

11. Chiu, S. Y., Ritchie, J. M., Rogart, R. B., and Stagg, D. A quantitative description of membrane currents in rabbit myelinated nerve. *J. Physiol. Lond.* 292: 149–166, 1979.

12. Dubois, J. M. Evidence for the existence of three types of potassium channels in frog Ranvier node membrane. *J. Physiol. Lond.* 318: 297–316, 1981.

13. Eng, D. L. and Kocsis, J. D. Activity-dependent changes in extracellular potassium and excitability in turtle olfactory nerve. *J. Neurophysiol.* 57: 740–754, 1987.

14. Foster, R. E., Connors, B., and Waxman, S. G. Rat optic nerve: electrophysiological, pharmacological and anatomical studies during development. *Dev. Brain Res.* 3: 371–386, 1982.

15. Gordon, T. R., Kocsis, J. D., and Waxman, S. G. Evidence for the presence of two types of potassium channels in the rat optic nerve. *Brain Res.* 447: 1–9, 1988.

16. Grafe, P., Martius, P., and Bostock, H. Three types of potassium channels in rat spinal axons. *Pfluegers Arch.* 405: R53, 1985.

17. Grissmer, S. Properties of potassium and sodium channels in frog internode. *J. Physiol. Lond.* 381: 119–134, 1986.

18. Hildebrand, C., Kocsis, J. D., Berglund, S., and Waxman, S. G. Myelin sheath remodelling in regenerated rat sciatic nerve. *Brain Res.* 358: 163–170, 1985.

19. Hirano, A. and Dembitzer, H. M. The transverse bands as a means of access to the periaxonal space of the central myelinated nerve fiber. *J. Ultrastruct. Res.* 28: 141–149, 1969.

20. Kocsis, J. D., Bowe, C. M., and Waxman, S. G. Different effects of 4-aminopyridine on sensory and motor fibers: pathogenesis of paresthesias. *Neurology* 36: 117–120, 1986.

21. Kocsis, J. D., Eng, D. L. Gordon, T. R., and Waxman, S. G. Functional differences between 4-aminopyridine and tetraethylammonium-sensitive potassium channels in myelinated axons. *Neurosci. Lett.* 75: 193–198, 1987.

22. Kocsis, J. D., Gordon, T. R., and Waxman, S. G. Mammalian optic nerve fibers display two pharmacologically distinct potassium channels. *Brain Res.* 383: 357–361, 1986.

23. Kocsis, J. D., Ruiz, J. A., and Waxman, S. G. Maturation of mammalian myelinated fibers: changes in action potential characteristics following 4-aminopyridine application. *J. Neurophysiol.* 50: 449–463, 1983.

24. Kocsis, J. D. and Waxman, S. G. Long-term regenerated nerve fibres retain sensitivity to potassium channel blocking agents. *Nature Lond.* 304: 640–642, 1982.

25. Kocsis, J. D. and Waxman, S. G. Intra-axonal recordings in rat dorsal column axons: membrane hyperpolarization and decreased excitability precede the primary afferent depolarization. *Brain Res.* 238: 222–227, 1982.

26. Ritchie, J. M. Sodium and potassium channels in regenerating and developing mammalian myelinated nerves. *Proc. R. Soc. Lond. B. Biol. Sci.* 215: 273–287, 1982.

27. Ritchie, J. M. and Chiu, S. Y. Distribution of sodium and potassium channels in mammalian myelinated nerve. In: *Demyelinating Disease: Basic and Clinical Electrophysiology,* edited by S. G. Waxman and J. M. Ritchie. New York: Raven, 1981, pp. 329–342.

28. Ritchie, J. M., Rang, H. P., and Pellegrino, R. Sodium and potassium channels in demyelinated and remyelinated mammalian nerve. *Nature Lond.* 294: 257–259, 1981.

29. Schnapp, B. and Mugnaini, E. Membrane architecture of myelinated fibers as seen by freeze-fracture. In: *Physiology and Pathobiology of Axons,* edited by S. G. Waxman. New York: Raven, 1978, pp. 83–123.

30. Targ, E. G. and Kocsis, J. D. 4-Aminopyridine leads to restoration of conduction in demyelinated rat sciatic nerve. *Brain Res.* 328: 358–361, 1984.

31. Waxman, S. G. and Foster, R. E. Ionic channel distribution and heterogeneity of the axon membrane in myelinated fibers. *Brain Res. Rev.* 2: 205–234, 1980.

32. Waxman, S. G., Kocsis, J. D., and Eng, D. L. Ligature-induced injury in peripheral nerve: changes in action potential characteristics following blockade of potassium conductance. *Muscle & Nerve* 8: 85–92, 1985.

33. Waxman, S. G. and Ritchie, J. M. Organization of ion channels in the myelinated nerve fiber. *Science Wash. DC* 228: 1502–1507, 1985.

34. Webster, H. DeF. The geometry of peripheral myelin sheaths during their formation and growth in rat sciatic nerves. *J. Cell Biol.* 48: 348–367, 1971.

X THE GLUE WITHIN THE BRAIN

The brain is notable for its abilities to process and interpret information, to control a variety of complex behaviors, to engage in deductive and inductive logic, to make complex decisions, and to generalize. In carrying out these processes the brain depends, in large part, on the ability of nerve cells to communicate with each other via the generation of all-or-none electrical impulses. Nerve cells, or neurons, are unique in being able to generate these signals. Their ability to generate electrical impulses is called electrical "excitability," and because of this excitability, neurons have classically been viewed as the "thinking" cells within the brain and the spinal cord. However, neurons are not the only cells within the nervous system. They are surrounded by other cells that, unlike neurons, do not give rise to nerve fibers, and are not usually considered to be excitable. Classically, these non-neuronal cells were considered to be the putty or glue that holds the brain together, and they were thus named "glia." Glial cells are not rare within the brain and spinal cord—they outnumber neurons ten to one. What do these enigmatic cells really do?

One type of glial cell, the oligodendrocyte, forms myelin sheaths that act as insulation around axons in its vicinity. Each oligodendrocyte extends 2–50 tentaclelike processes, each contacting an axon and wrapping around it so as to produce a myelin sheath. As discussed in part I, there is an "optimal" value for myelin sheath thickness for an axon with any given diameter, and, if an axon's myelin has this thickness, the axon will conduct action potentials with the fastest speed possible. For most axons, the myelin has this optimal thickness, an arrangement that makes functional sense. But how is myelin sheath thickness matched to axon diameter to achieve this optimal value? How does the myelin-forming oligodendrocyte "know" how thick its myelin should be? One possibility is that a single oligodendrocyte is programmed to produce myelin sheaths of one particular thickness at the ends of all of its processes, and that the oligodendrocyte seeks out axons of an appropriate diameter and myelinates them. Alternatively, it is possible that each axon specifies the diameter of its myelin sheath, signaling the oligodendrocyte process that encircles it to make the correct number of wraps around it.

In 1983, our laboratory was joined by Terry Sims, a new postdoc interested in the spinal cord and the glial cells within it. One of his projects, we decided, would be to study the development of oligodendrocytes to help us to tell which of these hypotheses is correct. Waxman and Sims (1984) present the results of this study. It shows that a single oligodendrocyte can myelinate axons of many different diameters within its neighborhood. Remarkably, the oligodendrocyte adjusts the thickness of each myelin sheath as desired for its axon. This indicates that the axon tells the oligodendrocyte how thick to make its myelin. Consistent with this hypothesis of *axonal specification* of myelin sheath thickness, parts of the protein-synthesizing apparatus (ribosome-studded endoplasmic reticulum and polyribosomes) can be found in distal parts of each of the oligodendrocyte's tentacles, very close to the forming myelin sheaths. The machinery for production of myelin sheaths by oligodendrocytes thus appears to be decentralized, deployed to the oligodendrocyte's many processes where it is close to, and subject to local control by, the axon.

We still do not know the details of the code which the axon uses to tell the oligodendrocyte how thick to make its myelin. We do know, however, that the conversation between the axon and the oligodendrocyte is not a monologue. When the axon is covered by insulating myelin, there are changes in the molecular structure of the axon membrane; these changes in the axon are not intrinsic to it, though, and only occur after it is ensheathed by myelin (Black et al. 1986). We also know that the changes in structure of the axon membrane are confined to areas of face-to-face contact where the oligodendrocyte touches the axon (Black et al. 1985). Thus, the axon and the oligodendrocyte both participate in a highly precise conversation in which they give each other detailed instructions, sculpting each other into just the right configuration as the myelinated nerve fiber matures. Specialized "signal molecules," produced by the axon and the oligodendrocyte, and possibly located on their surfaces, appear to carry the information necessary for this transcellular dialogue (Waxman 1987). When we, or others, are able to characterize these molecular signals we will be closer to understanding how nerve fibers build themselves so that they can function in an "optimal" or "smart" manner.

A second type of glial cell, the astrocyte, also contributes to the formation of myelinated fibers. The original observation of this phenomenon had been made by Claes Hildebrand at the Karolinska Institute (see Hildebrand 1971), and he convinced us of its importance during a year he spent on sabbatical in our laboratories. The paper by Waxman and Black (1984) used freeze-fracture, a method that is especially useful for visualizing cell membranes and their relationships, to examine the finger-like processes that extend from astrocytes to cover the axon membrane at nodes of Ranvier, the tiny (approximately 1/1000 of a millimeter) gaps that punctuate myelin sheaths. We learned that the relationship between the astrocyte and the axon is not a grazing blow or a casual touch; it is, on the contrary, an intimate embrace. Sims subsequently showed that this glial-axonal relationship appears very early during development, immediately after astrocytes differentiate and before the myelin matures (Sims et al. 1985), and we subsequently showed that astrocyte processes will travel far, up to a millimeter or more (a long distance for an extension of a cell to travel) in order to contact their axonal partners (Sims, Gilmore, and Waxman 1991).

The functional implications of the close relationship between astrocytes and the myelinated axons they contact at the nodes of Ranvier are not yet fully understood. One possibility is that astrocytes serve a homeostatic or housekeeping role, mopping up excess potassium that is released by axons during repetitive activity so as to maintain a concentration in the extracellular fluid that permits electrical activity to continue. Another, more speculative hypothesis is that astrocytes may function as sites for the synthesis of sodium channels, which are then transferred to nearby axons where they are inserted within the axonal membrane at the node of Ranvier. This hypothesis was first suggested by Ritchie and his colleagues (Chiu, Shrager, and Ritchie 1984; Bevan et al. 1985; Shrager, et al. 1985). The presence of astrocyte processes, contacting the axons at nodes of Ranvier, is consistent with this suggestion. But do astrocytes, in fact, have the capability to produce sodium channels?

To answer this question, my colleagues and I used a variety of techniques. By studying the mRNA within astrocytes, we were able to demonstrate that these cells do, in fact, activate the genes for sodium channels (Black et al. 1994b; Oh and Waxman 1994). Using antibodies that recognize sodium channels, we were further able to demonstrate that, as a result of expression of these sodium channel genes, astrocytes produce sodium channel protein (Black et al. 1994a, 1995). We were fortunate at this time to be joined by Harry Sontheimer, who had just completed his Ph.D. in biophysics and molecular biology as part of a small vanguard of "glial" biologists in Heidelberg. Using a method called patch-clamp recording, which permits the recording of the electrical currents produced by sodium channels in single cells, he was able to characterize, in great detail, the sodium channels that astrocytes insert within their membranes. Interestingly, astrocytes from different parts of the brain and spinal cord produced sodium channels with different properties, and they produced them in different numbers. This was a novel finding at the time, but because nerve cells from different regions of the brain and spinal cord have markedly different properties, it was not entirely unexpected.

In 1992 we observed that spinal cord astrocytes produce more sodium channels than other types of astrocytes (Sontheimer and Waxman 1992). Using spinal cord astrocytes as a model, Sontheimer and I carried out a detailed biophysical analysis of astrocytic sodium channels and showed that some of these channels, like those in neurons, have actions that can be fit by the Hodgkin-Huxley equations. We also made the surprising observation that, because of the presence of these channels in their membranes, astrocytes are capable of generating impulses (Sontheimer and Waxman 1992); under resting conditions the channels, however, are inactivated, and do not function in this way.

In a subsequent paper (Thio, Waxman, and Sontheimer 1993) we demonstrated that the synthesis of sodium channels by astrocytes is subject to control by neurons. We showed this by placing astrocytes in tissue culture, where we could use patch-clamp methods to measure their sodium currents, which provide an estimate of the number of sodium channels in their membranes. In order to determine whether neurons effect the number of sodium channels produced by astrocytes, we first studied astrocytes cultured alone, and then compared the results to those obtained from astrocytes that had been co-cultured, together with neurons. These experiments showed us that neurons have a strong modulatory effect on sodium channel expression in astrocytes. Although we do not yet understand the details of the dialogue between neurons and glial cells that is responsible for this signaling, the results in Thio, Waxman, and Sontheimer (1993) provide a clue: contact with neurons is not necessary in order to alter the expression of sodium channels in astrocytes. If the culture medium bathing neurons is collected, and if astrocytes are exposed to it in isolation from neurons, then there is still a significant effect on the expression of sodium channels within the astrocytes. A soluble factor, secreted by neurons, seems to be involved. Future studies will almost certainly elucidate the nature of this factor.

Most of the electrophysiological studies that had been carried out on sodium channels in glial cells, including our own, had focused on astrocytes in culture where they can be studied in a highly controlled environment. But this raised the question of whether sodium channels might be an artifact of tissue culture. To address this question, Sontheimer and I used patch clamp to study astrocytes in their native environment, within the slices taken from the brain. This study (Sontheimer and Waxman 1993) provided clear evidence for the presence of functional sodium channels within astrocytes within their normal environment, in the brain.

Although our studies had clearly demonstrated that astrocytes have the capability to produce sodium channels, the transfer of these channels to neurons, as suggested by Ritchie and his colleagues, had not been demonstrated. It was important, therefore, to consider other roles for sodium channels within astrocytes. Na^+/K^+-ATPase is a molecule, present in the membranes of glial cells as well as other cells, that acts as a pump, taking up excess potassium from the extracellular space and exchanging it for sodium. Noting that Na^+/K^+-ATPase requires a supply of sodium ions within the cell in order to operate, Sontheimer suggested that sodium channels within glial cells might function as a pathway for sodium entry that is necessary for the maintenance Na^+/K^+-ATPase activity. We did patch clamp studies, together with imaging studies which permitted the measurement of intracellular sodium, and the results supported this hypothesis (Sontheimer et al. 1994). Other studies, however, have given conflicting results (Rose, Ransom, and Waxman 1997). The role of sodium channels in glial cells remains enigmatic.

Neuroscientists have paid more attention to neurons and, as a consequence, know less about glia. But we do know that glial cells possess a rich architecture, interact intimately with nerve cells, and are highly dynamic. There now is a scientific journal, *Glia,* devoted to glial cells, and several recent monographs (e.g. Kettenmann and Ransom, 1995; Laming et al. 1998) highlight them. We will soon learn more about how glial cells work and we may ultimately find out how they contribute to the ability of the brain and spinal cord to carry out its complex activities. Although these fascinating cells have only begun to reveal their secrets, they are clearly much more than glue.

References

Bevan, S., Chiu, S. Y., Gray, P. T. A., and Ritchie, J. M. The presence of voltage-gated sodium, potassium and chloride channels in rat cultured astrocytes. *Proc. R. Soc. Lond. B* 225: 299–313, 1985.

Black, J. A., Waxman, S. G., and Hildebrand, C. Axo-glial relations in the retina-optic nerve junction of the adult rat: freeze-fracture observations. *J. Neurocytol.* 14: 887–907, 1985.

Black, J. A., Waxman, S. G., Sims, T. J., and Gilmore, S. A. Effects of delayed myelination by oligodendrocytes and Schwann cells on the macromolecular structure of axonal membrane in rat spinal cord. *J. Neurocytol.* 15: 745–762, 1986.

Black, J. A., Westenbroek, R., Minturn, J. E., Ransom, B. R., Catterall, W. A., and Waxman, S. G. Isoform-specific expression of sodium channels in astrocytes in vitro: immunocytochemical observations. *Glia* 14: 133–144, 1995.

Black, J. A., Westenbroek, R., Ransom, B. R., Catterall, W. A., and Waxman, S. G. Type II sodium channels in spinal cord astrocytes in situ: immunocytochemical observations. *Glia* 12: 219–227, 1994a.

Black, J. A., Yokoyama, S., Waxman, S. G., Oh, Y., Zur, K. B., Sontheimer, H., Higashida, H., and Ransom, B. R. Sodium channel mRNAs in cultured spinal cord astrocytes: in situ hybridization in identified cell types. *Molec. Brain Res.* 23: 235–245, 1994b.

Chiu, S. Y., Shrager, P., and Ritchie, J. M. Neuronal-type Na^+ and K^+ channels in rabbit cultured Schwann cells. *Nature* 311: 156–157, 1984.

Hildebrand, C. Ultrastructural and light microscopic studies of the nodal region in large myelinated fibres of the feline spinal cord white matter. *Acta Physiol. Scand.* Suppl. 364: 43–71, 1971.

Kettenmann, H., and Ransom, B. R. *Neuroglia.* New York: Oxford University Press, 1995.

Laming, P. R., Sykova E., Reichenbach, A., Hatton, G. I., and Bauer, H. *Glial Cells: Their Role in Behavior.* New York: Cambridge University Press, 1998.

Oh, Y., and Waxman, S. G. The $\beta 1$ subunit mRNA of the rat brain Na^+ channel is expressed in glial cells. *Proc. Natl Acad. Sci. U.S.A.* 91: 9985–9989, 1994.

Rose, C. R., Ransom, B. R., and Waxman, S. G. Pharmacological characterization of Na^+ influx via voltage-gated Na^+ channels in spinal cord astrocytes. *J. Neurophysiol.* 78: 3249–3259, 1997.

Shrager, P., Chiu, S. Y., and Ritchie, J. M. Voltage-dependent sodium and potassium channels in mammalian cultured Schwann cells. *Proc. Natl. Acad. Sci. U.S.A.* 82: 948–952, 1985.

Sims, T. J., Gilmore, S. A., and Waxman, S. G. Radial glia give rise to perinodal processes. *Brain Res.* 549: 25–36, 1991.

Sims, T. J., Waxman, S. G., Black, J. A., and Gilmore, S. A. Perinodal astrocytic processes at nodes of Ranvier in developing glial cell deficient rat spinal cord. *Brain Res.* 337: 321–333, 1985.

Sontheimer, H., Black, J. A., Ransom, B. R., and Waxman, S. G. Ion channels in spinal cord astrocytes in vitro: I. Transient expression of high levels of Na^+ and K^+ channels. *J. Neurophysiol.* 68: 985–999, 1992.

Sontheimer, H., Fernandez-Marques, E., Ullrich, N., Pappas, C., and Waxman, S. G. Astrocyte Na^+ channels are required for maintenance of Na^+/K^+-ATPase activity. *J. Neurosci.* 14: 464–2475, 1994.

Sontheimer, H., and Waxman, S. G. Ion channels in spinal cord astrocytes in vitro: II. Biophysical and pharmacological analysis of two Na^+ current types. *J. Neurophysiol.* 68: 1000–1011, 1992.

Sontheimer, H., and Waxman, S. G. Expression of voltage-activated ion channels by astrocytes and oligodendrocytes in the hippocampal slice. *J. Neurophysiol.* 70: 1863–1873, 1993.

Thio, C. L., Waxman, S. G., and Sontheimer, H. Ion channels in spinal cord astrocytes in vitro: III. Modulation of channel expression by co-culture with neurons and neuron-conditioned medium. *J. Neurophysiol.* 69: 819–831, 1993.

Waxman, S. G. Molecular neurobiology of the myelinated nerve fiber: ion-channel distributions and their implications for demyelinating diseases. In: *Molecular Neurobiology in Neurology and Psychiatry*, Kandel, E. R. (ed.). New York: Raven Press, pp. 7–37, 1987.

Waxman, S. G., and Black, J. A. Freeze-fracture ultrastructure of the perinodal astrocyte and associated glial junctions. *Brain Res.* 308: 77–87, 1984.

Waxman, S. G., and Sims, T. J. Specificity in central myelination: evidence for local regulation of myelin thickness. *Brain Res.* 292: 179–185, 1984.

15 Specificity in Central Myelination: Evidence for Local Regulation of Myelin Thickness

Stephen G. Waxman and Terry J. Sims

Abstract The ventral funiculi of normal and X-irradiated 13-day-old rats were studied by electron microscopy. In both tissues, oligodendrocytes form myelin sheaths around multiple axons, with a single oligodendrocyte associated with several axons of different sizes. Despite their origin from the same glial cell, the myelin sheaths are thicker for larger axons. Polyribosomes and rough endoplasmic reticulum are observed in distal oligodendrocyte processes, in proximity to the forming myelin sheaths. These results indicate that myelin sheath thickness is matched to axon size via local mechanisms, and suggest a role of polyribosomes and/or rough endoplasmic reticulum in myelin formation.

It is well established that myelin sheaths in the central nervous system are produced by oligodendrocytes,[2,7,10,11] although the details of the mechanisms which initiate, and control, myelination remain incompletely understood. Myelination probably involves highly specific interactions between axons and glial cells.[14,16] Myelin sheath thickness, for example, is related to fiber size.[1,3,17,19] However, the nature of the mechanism(s) which determine myelin thickness remain unexplained. One hypothesis would hold that myelin sheath thickness is adjusted to the caliber (possibly by a cell surface-mediated or related signal[14,18,21]) of each axon myelinated by a given oligodendrocyte. Alternatively, a second hypothesis argues that a given oligodendrocyte myelinates axons of only one specified size, and produces myelin sheaths of predetermined thickness around these axons. Data available to date do not distinguish between these hypotheses. In addition, myelination involves a significant increase in membrane area of the myelin-forming cell; the mechanisms underlying this membrane elaboration are not completely understood. In the present communication, we

Reprinted with permission from *Brain Research* 292: 179–185, 1984.

describe several previously unreported aspects of the relationship between central axons and their myelinating oligodendrocytes in normal developing and X-irradiated developing spinal cord; the latter tissue is especially suitable for examination of these interrelationships due to the lower density of glial cells.[5] These findings indicate that a single oligodendrocyte can myelinate axons of varying caliber within its vicinity, and provide data supporting the hypothesis that myelin thickness is specified independently for each axon. It is likely that this specification is mediated by local mechanisms; in this context, the present results suggest that glial polyribosomes and/or intracellular membrane-bound organelles such as endoplasmic reticulum, located in oligodendrocytic processes in proximity to the forming myelin but at a distance from the glial cell body, may play a role in membrane biosynthesis during myelination.

Two normal Charles Rivers CD rats and two litter-mates, X-irradiated on the 3rd postnatal day with 4000 R over the lumbar spinal cord,[5] were anesthetized at 13 days of age by intraperitoneal injection (0.2 ml/100 g) of a 35% solution of chloral hydrate. The rats were then perfused via the left ventricle with 2% paraformaldehyde, 2% glutaraldehyde, 0.5% acrolein and 0.5% dimethylsulfoxide in 0.12 M Sorensen's phosphate buffer at pH 7.2. Two hours following perfusion, the lumbar spinal cords were removed, cut into 2 mm segments and stored in fixative overnight at 4 °C. The tissues were post-fixed in 2% OsO_4 (in buffer) for 2 h at 4 °C, rinsed in buffer and stained en bloc with 2% uranyl acetate for 1.5 h. The spinal cord segments were then dehydrated in a graded series of ethanol washes, rinsed in acetone and infiltrated and embedded in Spurr plastic. Transverse sections, 1 μm thick, were stained with toluidine blue and examined by light microscopy to locate areas of the ventral funiculus for subsequent thin

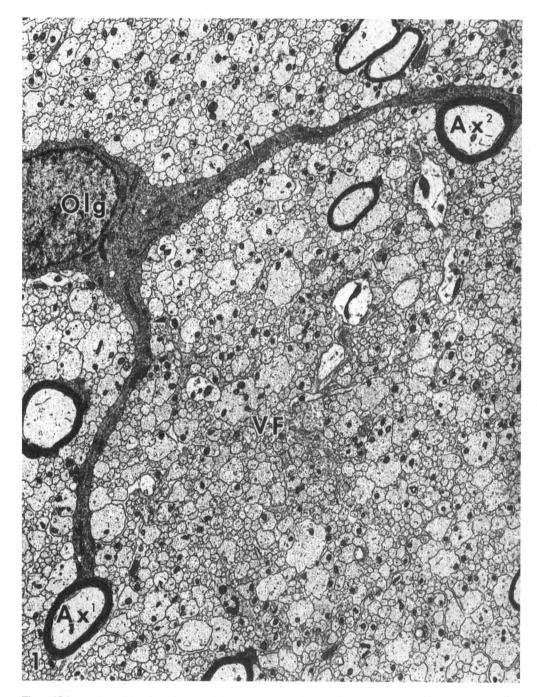

Figure 15.1
The ventral funiculus (VF) of a 13-day-old normal rat in which the majority of axons have not been myelinated. In this fortuitous plane of section an oligodendrocyte (Olg) is shown myelinating two axons (Ax^1 and Ax^2). The oligodendrocyte processes contain Golgi apparatus (arrow-heads) and other organelles which are shown at higher magnification in figures 15.2 and 15.3. Magnification ×6750.

sectioning. Thin sections were post-stained in uranyl acetate and lead citrate and examined with a JEOL 100C electron microscope. Equivalent axon diameters were measured by averaging major and minor cross sectional axon diameters.

In contrast to white matter in the adult, the ventral funiculus of the normal developing rat at several weeks after birth contains relatively few oligodendrocytes, and only a minority of axons are myelinated; however, myelination has proceeded to the formation of compact sheaths around some axons. Thus, this tissue is especially suitable for studying early interactions between glial cells and axons. Irradiation of the spinal cord at 3 days of age has been shown to decrease the number of oligodendroglia while leaving the neuronal elements relatively uneffected; fewer axons are myelinated at early postnatal ages after irradiation.[6,13] As a result of the much lower density of oligodendroglia, myelin sheaths clustered around a given oligodendrocyte can be associated with that cell with a high degree of certainty.

Several important features of oligodendroglial organization, and of the relation between the oligodendrocyte and myelin sheaths, can be seen in figure 15.1. Two myelinated axons, the oligodendroglial cell of origin of their myelin sheaths, and the thin cytoplasmic processes connecting the oligodendroglial cell to the myelin sheaths, are shown. The connections between the myelin sheaths and the plasma membrane of the oligodendrocyte can be seen at higher magnification in figures 15.2 and 15.3. The myelinated fibers are both located along thin processes extending approximately 12 μm from the oligodendroglial cell body from which the myelin sheaths are derived. The two myelin sheaths exhibit different rotational polarities, one extending clockwise and the other counterclockwise from their glial processes of origin. The myelinating glial processes contain a number of membrane-bound organelles. In figure 15.1, a Golgi complex is present in the oligodendroglial process connect-

ing the glial cell with its myelin sheath. This oligodendroglial process also contains microtubules, tubular reticulum, and occasional mitochondria, oriented roughly parallel to the axis of the glial process. More distally within these processes, polyribosomes are present in the oligodendroglial cytoplasm (figure 15.3). The second glial myelin-forming process (figure 15.2) contains polyribosomes in addition to cisternae of rough endoplasmic reticulum. These cisternae, which are studded with ribosomes, are located within 2 μm of the forming myelin sheath.

In other cases oligodendrocytes form myelin sheaths around multiple axons of differing diameter. Figure 15.4 shows part of a myelinating oligodendrocyte from 13-day postnatal ventral funiculus of normal rat. The oligodendrocyte is characterized by relatively dense cytoplasm and the high nucleo-cytoplasmic ratio characteristic for this cell type. Cisternae of rough endoplasmic reticulum are scattered through the cytoplasm, which also is characterized by a high density of polyribosomes. Two axons (Ax^1, Ax^2) are seen, in this section, to be directly contiguous to this oligodendroglial cell; it is highly likely that this glial cell is the cell of origin of these myelin sheaths. Axon Ax^2, which is connected to the oligodendroglial cell body by a tapering cytoplasmic process, is 2.4 μm in diameter. Polyribosomes and rough endoplasmic reticulum are located distally in the myelinating glial cell process in proximity to axon Ax^2. Axon Ax^1 is 1.4 μm in diameter. It is located adjacent to the cell body of the oligodendrocyte. Myelin thickness is correlated with diameter. The myelin sheath of axon Ax^2 (0.4 μm thick) is thicker than that of axon Ax^1 (0.16 μm).

An oligodendrocyte from the ventral funiculus of a 10-day post-irradiation rat (13 days old) is shown in figure 15.5. Few other oligodendrocytes were present in the vicinity of this oligodendrocyte. Two axons (Ax^1, Ax^2) can be observed to be directly contiguous to (and very probably myelinated by) this oligodendrocyte. These axons are of different size (axon diameter

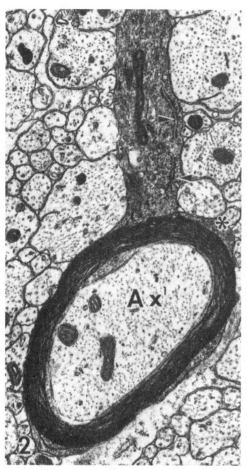 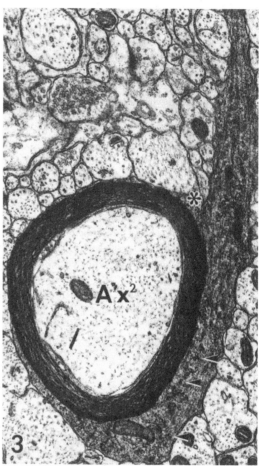

Figure 15.2
Axon (Ax^1) from figure 15.1 with rough endoplasmic reticulum (arrow-head) in the distal oligodendrocyte process. The myelin spirals about this axon in a counterclockwise direction with a cytoplasm-filled portion of the outer layer (*) to the right of the primary oligodendroglial process. Magnification ×20,250.

Figure 15.3
Axon (Ax^2) from figure 15.1 with polyribosomes (arrowheads) in the outer cytoplasmic-glial layer and distal portion of oligodendroglial process, with which it is continuous. The myelin sheath spirals in a clockwise direction with a cytoplasm-filled portion of the outer layer (*) abutting the main glial process from left. Microtubules can be observed oriented longitudinally within the oligodendroglial process. Magnification ×20,250.

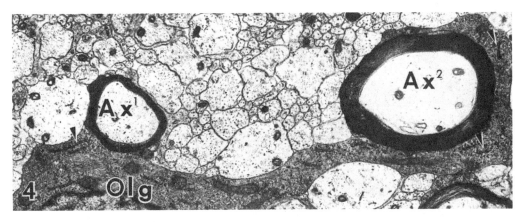

Figure 15.4

An oligodendrocyte (Olg) in the ventral funiculus of a 13-day-old normal rat. Two myelinated axons (Ax[1] and Ax[2]) of different calibers are directly adjacent to this oligodendrocyte, which very likely is the cell of origin of these myelin sheaths. The smaller myelinated axon (Ax[1]) has a thinner myelin sheath than the larger axon (Ax[2]). Cisternae of rough endoplasmic reticulum (arrow-heads) are located in proximity to the myelin sheaths. Magnification ×11,200.

of $Ax^1 = 2.5$ μm; $Ax^2 = 1.6$ μm). Myelin thickness ($Ax^1 = 0.32$ μm; $Ax^2 = 0.24$ μm) is, as in figure 15.4, greater for the larger axon. Rough endoplasmic reticulum is present in the glial cytoplasm in proximity to the myelin sheath.

In the examples shown in figures 15.4 and 15.5, a single oligodendrocyte forms myelin sheaths around two nearby axons of different diameter; thicker myelin sheaths have been formed around the larger axons. While it is possible that diameters of these axons are less strikingly different in other sections,[8] we have observed a number of oligodendrocytes which myelinate several axons of different caliber. These observations lead to the conclusion that formation of myelin by an oligodendroglial cell is not limited to axons of a single diameter. On the contrary, a single oligodendrocyte can myelinate axons of varying diameter within its vicinity. Moreover, myelin thickness is regulated such that it is not invariant for all the sheaths produced by a given oligodendrocyte, but on the contrary is matched to axonal size. This

finding extends the observation by Friedrich and Mugnaini[4] of two myelin sheaths of different thicknesses formed by one glial process (around axons of roughly the same diameter). The latter authors interpreted this finding as suggesting that myelin thickness is regulated independently by each axon, at a site close to the axon. In this context, the high degree of specificity in myelination has previously been interpreted as suggesting that myelin sheath geometry is signalled, at least in part, by the axon.[14,16] In addition, the available evidence indicates that factors in addition to axon size play a role in initiating myelin formation.[9,19] The conclusion that myelination by a single oligodendrocyte is not limited to one size, or class, of axons, is also suggested by immunocytochemical observations which demonstrate myelination of fibers from intersecting tracts (tectospinal and pontocerebellar) by a single oligodendroglial cell.[15]

As noted by Peters et al.,[11] it is extremely difficult to demonstrate continuity between the oligodendrocyte membrane and the outer myelin

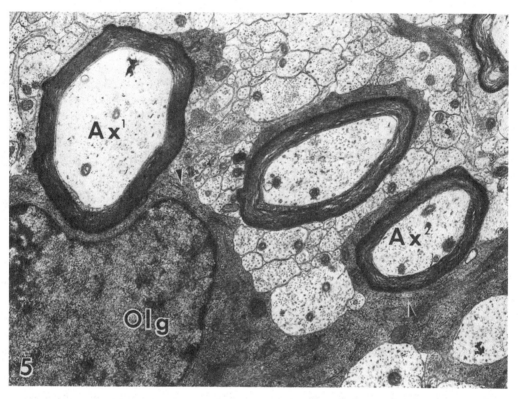

Figure 15.5

Oligodendrocyte (Olg) from ventral funiculus of 13-day-old X-irradiated rat. Few other oligodendrocytes were present in the vicinity of this cell. Two axons (Ax^1, and Ax^2) are in close proximity to, and probably myelinated by this oligodendrocyte. The calibers of these axons are different, and there are corresponding differences in myelin thickness. The arrow-heads point to cisternae of ribosome-studded endoplasmic reticulum, located close to the myelin sheaths. Magnification ×14,700.

layer (figures 15.1–15.3 above represent an unusually fortuitous plane of section in this respect). It was for this reason that X-irradiated tissue was examined. The density of oligodendrocytes is decreased (compared to normal), thus increasing the probability that myelinated axons, clustered about a given oligodendrocyte, derive their myelin sheath from that cell. There were few other oligodendrocytes in the vicinity of the myelinated fibers shown in figure 15.5. Thus axons Ax^1 and Ax^2, and possibly other axons,

derive their myelin from the oligodendrocyte shown in this figure.

The present findings suggest local specification of myelin thickness, such that each sheath acquires dimensions which meet specific functional requirements (cf. ref. 17). It is interesting, in this context, that polyribosomes and cisternae of rough endoplasmic reticulum are present in distal glial processes in proximity to the forming myelin sheaths (figures 15.2 and 15.4). As noted by a number of workers,[11,12,20] myelination involves a marked increase in membrane area of the myelin-forming cell. Robertson[12] commented on the proliferation of ribosome-studded endoplasmic reticulum in Schwann cells during myelination; he also noted the presence of spirals of rough endoplasmic reticulum during myelination, and suggested that these membrane specializations might play a role in membrane synthesis during peripheral myelin formation. The present observations suggest a similar conclusion for central myelinated fibers, i.e. that polyribosomes and/or rough endoplasmic reticulum, located in proximity to the developing sheath, may be involved in membrane synthesis or assembly during myelination. These results further suggest that myelin formation is, at least in part, under local control by the axon.

Acknowledgments

This work was supported in part by Grants NS-15320 and NS-04761 from the National Institutes of Health and by the Medical Research Service, Veterans Administration. We thank Dr. Shirley A. Gilmore for the X-irradiated rats and M. E. Smith and C. Choy for excellent technical assistance. T.J.S. is supported in part by the Neural Plasticity Program.

References

1. Bishop, G. H., Clare M. H. and Landau, W. M., The relation of axon sheath thickness to fiber size in the central nervous system of vertebrates, *Int. J. Neurosci.*, 2 (1971) 69–78.

2. Bunge, M. B., Bunge, R. P. and Pappas, G. D., Electron microscopic demonstration of connections between glia and myelin sheaths in the developing mammalian central nervous system, *J. Cell Biol.*, 12 (1962) 448–453.

3. Friede, R. L. and Samorajski, T., Relation between the number of myelin lamellae and axon circumference in fibers of vagus and sciatic nerves of mice, *J. comp. Neurol.*, 130 (1967) 223–232.

4. Friedrich, V. L. and Mugnaini, E., Myelin sheath thickness in the CNS is regulated near the axon. *Brain Research*, 274 (1983) 329–331.

5. Gilmore, S. A., The effects of X-irradiation on the spinal cords of neonatal rats. I. Neurological observations, *J. Neuropath. exp. Neurol.*, 22 (1963) 285–293.

6. Gilmore, S. A., The effects of X-irradiation on the spinal cords of neonatal rats. II. Histological observations, *J. Neuropath. exp. Neurol.*, 22 (1963) 294–301.

7. Hirano, A., A confirmation of the oligodendroglial origin of myelin in the adult rat, *J. Cell Biol.*, 38 (1968) 637–640.

8. Knobler, R. L., Stempak, J. G. and Laurencin, M., Oligodendroglial ensheathment of axons during myelination in the developing rat central nervous system: a serial section electron microscopical study, *J. Ultrastruct. Res.*, 49 (1974) 34–49.

9. Matthews, M. A. and Duncan, D., A quantitative study of morphological changes accompanying the initiation and progress of myelin production in the dorsal funiculus of the rat spinal cord, *J. comp. Neurol.*, 142 (1971) 1–22.

10. Peters, A., Observations on the connexions between myelin sheaths and glial cells in the optic nerves of young rats, *J. Anat. (Lond.)*, 98 (1964) 125–134.

11. Peters, A., Palay, S. L. and Webster, H. deF., *The Fine Structure of the Nervous System*, W. B. Saunders Co., Philadelphia, 1976.

12. Robertson, J. D., New unit membrane organelle of Schwann cells. In *Biophysics of Physiological and Pharmacological Actions*, American Association for the Advancement of Science, Washington, DC 1961, pp. 63–96.

13. Sims, T. J. and Gilmore, S. A., Interactions between intraspinal Schwann cells and cellular constituents normally occurring in the irradiated rat, *Brain Research*, 276 (1983) 17–30.

14. Spencer, P. S. and Weinberg, H. J., Axonal specification of Schwann cell expression and myelination. In S. G. Waxman (Ed.), *Physiology and Pathobiology of Axons*, Raven Press, New York, NY, 1978, pp. 389–405.

15. Sternberger, N. H., Itoyama, Y., Kies, M. W. and Webster, H. deF., Immunocytochemical method to identify basic protein in myelin-forming oligodendrocytes of newborn rat C.N.S., *J. Neurocytol.*, 7 (1978) 251–263.

16. Waxman, S. G., Regional differentiation of the axon: a review with special reference to the concept of the multiplex neuron, *Brain Research*, 47 (1972) 269–288.

17. Waxman, S. G. and Bennett, M. V. L., Relative conduction velocities of small myelinated and non-myelinated fibres in the central nervous system, *Nature New Biol.*, 238 (1972) 217–219.

18. Waxman, S. G. and Foster, R. E., Development of the axon membrane during differentiation of myelinated fibres in spinal nerve roots, *Proc. roy. Soc. B*, 209 (1980) 441–446.

19. Waxman, S. G. and Swadlow, H. A., Ultrastructure of visual callosal axons in the rabbit, *Exp. Neurol.*, 53 (1976) 115–127.

20. Webster, H. deF., The geometry of peripheral myelin sheaths during their formation and growth in rat sciatic nerves, *J. Cell Biol.*, 48 (1971) 348–367.

21. Wiley-Livingston, C. A. and Ellisman, M. H., Development of axonal membrane specializations defines nodes of Ranvier and precedes Schwann cell myelin elaboration, *Develop. Biol.*, 79 (1980) 334–355.

16 Freeze-Fracture Ultrastructure of the Perinodal Astrocyte and Associated Glial Junctions

Stephen G. Waxman and Joel A. Black

Abstract Freeze-fracture examination of nodes of Ranvier from adult rat optic nerve demonstrates the presence of astrocytic processes at the majority of nodes of Ranvier. Astrocytic processes often run along the entire length of the nodal gap, although they do not necessarily encircle the entire nodal circumference. The E- and P-fracture faces and the cross-fractured cytoplasm of these astrocytes (termed 'perinodal astrocytes') were examined. The cytoplasm of perinodal astrocytes contains 10-nm filaments. The P-faces of perinodal astrocytic membranes are characterized by orthogonal arrays of intramembranous particles ('assemblies'), with a center-to-center periodicity of ≈ 6 nm. Complementary orthogonally arranged pits are observed on the E-faces of the astrocytic membranes. The density of these arrays in perinodal astrocytic membranes is similar to that in parenchymal astrocytic membranes, but is substantially lower than that at pericapillary astrocytic membranes. In addition, gap junctions are present between astrocytes, and between astrocytes and paranodal oligodendroglial layers. These findings indicate that astrocytic processes comprise an important structural component of central nodes of Ranvier, and provide a morphological basis for a possible astrocytic role in nodal function.

Introduction

The node of Ranvier in the central nervous system exhibits a complex morphology, characterized by structural differentiation of both the oligodendroglial cell and myelin, and of the axon membrane.[38,40,45] In the peripheral nervous system, finger-like processes extend from the Schwann cell to form a network surrounding the axon at the node of Ranvier.[30,35,41] In contrast, such processes do not extend from the oligodendroglial cell into the nodal gap in the central nervous system. However, an association between astrocytic processes and the node

Reprinted with permission from *Brain Research* 308: 77–87, 1984.

of Ranvier within spinal cord has been described.[8,17,18,36] Astrocytic processes in association with the node of Ranvier have also been described in the optic nerve.[20] Previous studies on this astrocytic component of central nodes of Ranvier, which we have termed the 'perinodal astrocyte', have been confined to transmission electron microscopic examination of sectioned tissue. As part of a program to further explore axo-glial relationships at the node of Ranvier, we have examined perinodal astrocytes and associated glial membrane specializations using freeze-fracture methods, which permit an analysis of intercellular relationships at the node and also provide information about the ultrastructure of neuronal and glial membranes.

Materials and Methods

Long-Evans rats (Simonsen Labs., Gilroy, CA) weighing 250–350 g were anesthetized with sodium pentobarbital (10 mg/100 g body weight) and artificially respirated. Tissue was fixed by transcardiac perfusion with a room temperature, physiological saline solution followed by 5% glutaraldehyde in 0.2 M sodium cacodylate buffer (pH 7.4, buffer osmolarity = 420 mOsm; fixative osmolarity = 920 mOsm), containing 0.03% $CaCl_2$. Following perfusion, the optic nerves were carefully dissected free and placed into fresh fixative within 30 s. Tissue samples for freeze-fracture analysis were placed in fresh fixative (room temperature) for 1 h following in situ fixation. Tissue was then washed in 0.2 M sodium cacodylate buffer for 30 min (several changes). Cryoprotection was provided by infiltration with 10% glycerol in 0.2 M cacodylate buffer (1 h) followed by 30% glycerol in buffer (2–3 h). Tissue was mounted on gold–brass specimen holders, rapidly frozen in a slush of Freon 22, and stored in liquid nitrogen. Freeze-

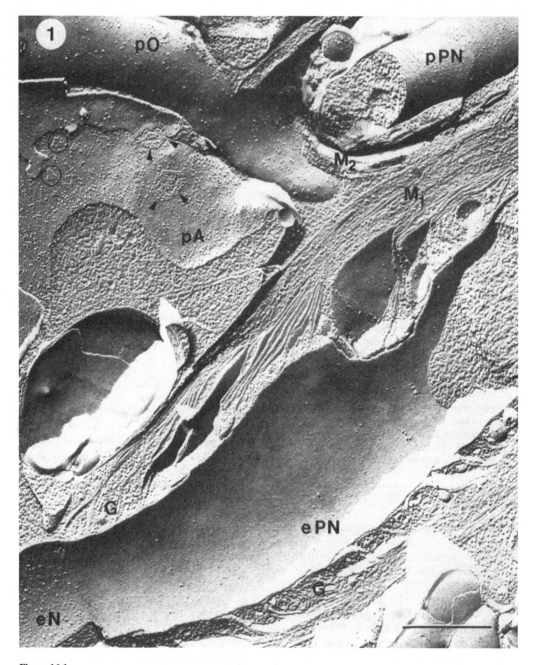

Figure 16.1

Freeze-fracture electron micrograph of adult Long–Evans rat optic nerve. The nodal regions of two adjacent axons are present. The E-face of a node (eN) and paranode (ePN) of one axon, and the P-face of the paranode (pPN) of an adjacent axon, are exposed. Paranodal terminal glial loops (G) and compact myelin (M_1) are cross-fractured. The P-face of an oligodendroglial process (pO) is seen to be continuous with myelin sheath M_2. Note the gap junctions (arrowheads) and assemblies (circled) present on the P-face (pA) of an astrocytic membrane. Bar = 0.5 μm. ×49,200.

fracturing was performed in a Balzers BAF 301 freeze-etch device, with the stage temperature maintained at $-110\,°C$ and vacuum below 2×10^{-6} Torr. Platinum (≈ 2 nm) was deposited ($45°$ angle) on freshly fractured surfaces and stabilized with a layer of carbon. Replicas were cleaned in Clorox, rinsed several times in double-distilled water, and mounted on copper grids. The grids were examined in a JEOL 100CX electron microscope operating at 100 kV. The nomenclature of freeze-fracture membrane faces is that of Branton et al.[7]

Results

Nodes of Ranvier are commonly encountered in the optic nerve, and appear to be clustered,[33] so that they often appear in groups within freeze-fracture replicas. Axolemmal E- and P-faces at the nodes and paranodes are readily exposed by freeze-fracture, which also exposes the membrane structure of surrounding glial elements (figure 16.1). The quantitative freeze-fracture structure of the nodal axon membrane in rat optic nerve has been described in detail previously[6] and will not be described here. Oligodendroglial and astrocytic processes are easily distinguished in freeze-fracture replicas on the basis of their differing membrane ultrastructure[1,12,27,31] and cytoplasmic characteristics. Examples of the membrane ultrastructure of oligodendroglia and astrocytes are shown in figure 16.2. Astrocytes are unequivocably identified by the presence of 'assemblies'[27] on P-fracture faces, and by complementary orthogonal arrays of pits on E-faces. Oligodendrocytes are distinguished on the basis of the population of intramembranous particles present on the respective fracture faces.[31] The plasmalemmal P-face contains ≈ -1000 particles/μm^2 in an heterogeneous mixture, consisting of large and tall particles, small and short particles, small ellipsoidal particles, and polymers of 2–5 small subunits. The E-face of oligodendrocytes contains approximately half as many particles as the P-face, and the particles are largely of moderate size and height.

In many cases, as previously described in thin-sectioned tissue,[3,39,44] an enlarged extracellular space (asterisk, figure 16.3) surrounds part of the nodal axon. However, this enlargement of the extra-cellular space does not extend around the entire circumference of the nodal axon, since astrocytic processes often approach, and appear to cover, part of the axon at the node. Perinodal astrocytic profiles in some cases appear to be oriented parallel to (eA_1, figure 16.6) or slightly obliquely to (figure 16.3) the axon. In other cases, small projections extend from larger astrocytic processes and approach the node (eA_2, figure 16.6). Figure 16.3 shows some characteristic features of cellular relationships and membrane ultrastructure in a freeze-fracture replica of a node of Ranvier from adult rat optic nerve. The P-face of the nodal axolemma, and the E-face of the terminating oligodendrocytic lamella at one side of the node, are shown. An enlarged extracellular space is present adjacent to the node but this space does not surround the entire nodal axon. Several astrocytic processes can be seen approaching the node of Ranvier. The cross-fractured astrocytic cytoplasm contains 10 nm filaments (arrowheads, figure 16.3). The E-faces of astrocytic membrane (eA_1, eA_2, figure 16.3) contain orthogonal arrays of pits. These arrays of pits, which have ≈ 6 nm center-to-center periodicity, are most likely the imprints of P-face assemblies. There are ≈ 15–35 pits per array. The astrocytic membrane (eA_1) in figure 16.3 includes at least 11 orthogonal arrays in a membrane area of 0.83 μm^2 (≈ 13 arrays/μm^2).

The density of arrays observed on perinodal astrocytes is similar to that reported previously for intraparenchymal astrocytic processes.[1,29] It has been reported that the number of orthogonal arrays decreases in anoxic tissue.[28] We therefore also examined astrocytic surfaces abutting

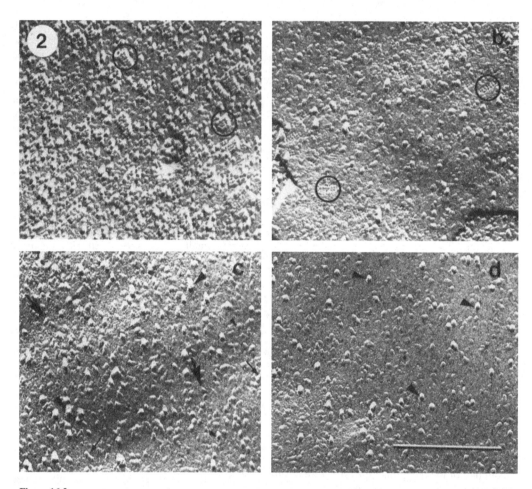

Figure 16.2

(a) P-fracture face of astrocyte. Assemblies of intramembranous particles (circled) are prevalent on the membrane. There is a moderately high density of background particles. (b) E-fracture face of astrocyte. Orthogonal arrays of pits (circled), the "imprints" of P-face assemblies, are apparent on the membrane. (c) P-fracture face of oligodendrocyte. The heterogeneous population of particles is composed of large and tall particles (large arrowheads), small and short particles (small arrowheads), small ellipsoid particles (large arrows), and linear polymers of 2–5 subunits (small arrows). (d) E-fracture face of oligodendrocyte. The moderate density of particles is composed primarily of particles of medium height and width. Bar = 0.25 μm. ×116,000.

capillaries, where the density of orthogonal arrays is known to be high.[12,27] Figure 16.4 illustrates this specialized juxtavascular astrocytic membrane from the same optic nerve as shown in figures 16.3 and 16.5. The density of orthogonal arrays is high, and is similar to that previously reported.[12,27,29] Thus, the densities of arrays observed within the perinodal astrocytic membranes examined in this study do not appear to have been reduced as a result of tissue anoxia.

The freeze-fracture faces converse to those shown in figure 16.3, i.e. the E-face of the nodal axolemma, and the P-face of an associated astrocytic process, are shown in figure 16.5. In this figure, the high density of intramembranous particles in the nodal E-face[6,25,40] can be appreciated. In contrast to the E-face of nodal axolemma, the E-face of paranodal axolemma contains a low density of intramembranous particles. Periodic indentations of the paranodal membrane run around the paranodal axon, and can be seen to coincide with the edges of cross-fractured terminating oligodendroglial loops. The fracture plane shown in figure 16.5 passes from the axolemma through the perinodal extracellular space to expose the P-face of an associated astrocytic process. The fracture plane thus exposes a 'window' in the nodal axolemma, and permits visualization of the elements lying immediately adjacent to (outside of) the axon membrane at the node. Note that the nodal membrane (eN) and perinodal astrocytic membrane (pA) appear to run parallel to each other. The astrocyte membrane P-face exhibits an intramembranous particle density (excluding assembly particles) of approximately $1000/\mu m^2$. The number of assemblies on the astrocytic P-face membrane is quite low, and is in stark contrast to perivascular astrocytic membrane (cf. figure 16.4).

Gap junctions are often present in astrocytic membranes close to nodes of Ranvier (figures 16.6 and 16.7). As seen en face, these junctions are usually round to ellipsoid in shape, and measure approximately 0.25 μm in diameter. In

some cases, it is possible to identify both of the cells participating in this junctional membrane specialization. As described previously,[31] gap junctions between astrocytes and oligodendroglial cell bodies, processes, and outer turns of myelin are present. Inter-astrocytic gap junctions are also observed. In figure 16.6, the fracture plane exposes (from left to right): the P-face of the outermost layer of oligodendroglial membrane at the paranodal termination, the P-face of the nodal axolemma, and several oligodendroglial layers of the second paranode (to right of micrograph). Tight junctions between apposing oligodendroglial loops are present. Several astrocytic profiles are associated with the node. One of these (eA_2) is a projection of a larger astrocytic process, which extends toward the node. A thin astrocytic profile (eA_1) extends parallel to the axon, adjacent to the node, which it appears to partially cover. This astrocytic process extends over the entire length of the node of Ranvier, although it is not possible to determine, from this replica, whether this glial profile covers the entire circumference of the node. A gap junction, fractured so as to expose closely spaced connexons on the P-face of the outermost oligodendroglial layer at the paranode and complementary regularly arranged pits on the E-face of the adjoining cell, is present. On the basis of the configuration of the astrocytic process (eA_1), and its proximity to the gap junction, it is likely that the E-face component of this gap junction originates from the perinodal astrocytic process.

Another example of an astrocytic–oligodendrocytic gap junction, at a paranode from rat optic nerve, is shown in figure 16.7. The P-face of a node of Ranvier and the adjacent paranode can be visualized. The fracture plane passes directly from the E-face of an astrocytic membrane (which can be identified on the basis of orthogonally arranged pits) to the P-face of paranodal oligodendroglial membrane; a gap junction connects these two glial membranes. As with the previous examples shown here, the astrocytic

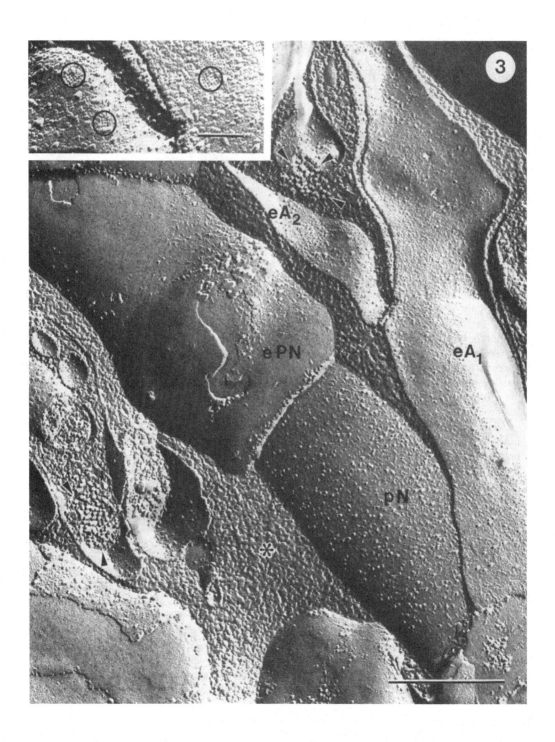

process is located in proximity to the nodal region of the axon.

Discussion

The results shown above demonstrate the presence of astrocytic processes at central nodes of Ranvier. Astrocytic processes and membranes can be identified and distinguished from those of other glial cell types in freeze-fracture replicas on the basis of both 10-nm cytoplasmic filaments and characteristic membrane structure.[31] Earlier observations on thin-sectioned tissue[4,8,17,18,20,36] suggested the presence of astrocytic processes at nodes of Ranvier in the central nervous system. The freeze-fracture method, however, exposes relatively large membrane surfaces not necessarily constrained to a single sectional level, and thus provides a clear demonstration of the close morphological relationship between astrocytes and central nodes. The present results also extend the earlier findings by indicating that the astrocytic component of the node of Ranvier is characterized by several membrane specializations. These include orthogonal arrays[1,12,27,31] and gap junctions,[15,31] which have previously been described as occurring on mammalian parenchymal astrocytic membranes.

In the case of the perinodal astrocyte, the density of orthogonal arrays is considerably lower than reported for the specialized astrocytic membrane in subpial regions and on the glial face surrounding capillaries.[1,12,27,31] The number of assemblies on perinodal astrocytic membrane is similar to that reported for parenchymal astrocytes,[1,29] and within the sarcolemma at nonsynaptic regions of fast-twitch muscle fibers[14] and the lateral plasmalemma of several epithelial cell types.[22,43] While several physiological roles for these orthogonal arrays of intramembranous particles have been suggested, including active transport,[21,27] coordination of cellular activities,[22] and intramembranous enzyme activity,[37] the function or functions of these arrays remain unclear.

The presence of inter-astrocytic gap junctions on perinodal astrocytes suggests that, as for astrocytes in general,[16] there is coupling between astrocytes in the nodal region. It is also interesting that there appears to be coupling between perinodal astrocytes and the outermost layer of terminating oligodendroglial cytoplasm at the paranode. The occurrence of gap junctions between astrocytes and oligodendrocytes has been previously noted.[13,31] Our results indicate that these junctions occur close to nodes of Ranvier. It has been suggested that astrocytes may act as a spatial buffer in terms of extracellular ionic concentrations.[2,26] In this regard, although voltage-sensitive potassium conductance at central nodes of Ranvier is highly attenuated,[23] an increase in extracellular potassium concentration due to passage of ions via the leak conductance[9] might be expected following impulse conduction. If astrocytic processes buffer the extracellular ionic milieu by uptake of potassium ions,[10] it might be expected that changes in electrolyte and/or water flux would also occur in astrocyte-coupled paranodal oligodendrocytic loops; this could account, at least in part, for the loosening

Figure 16.3
Freeze-fracture electron micrograph of nodal region from adult rat optic nerve. The nodal P-face (pN) and the E-face (ePN) of the terminal oligodendroglial loop are shown. An enlarged extracellular space (asterisk) is associated with the node. Several astrocytic processes are present in proximity to the node. The E-fracture faces of two astrocytic processes (eA$_1$ and eA$_2$) are exposed; 10-nm filaments (arrowheads) are observed in cross-fractured astrocytic cytoplasm. Bar = 0.5 μm. ×70,000. Inset: the E-face of part of the astrocytic membrane is shown at increased magnification. Several orthogonal arrays of pits are circled. Bar = 0.1 μm. ×122,850.

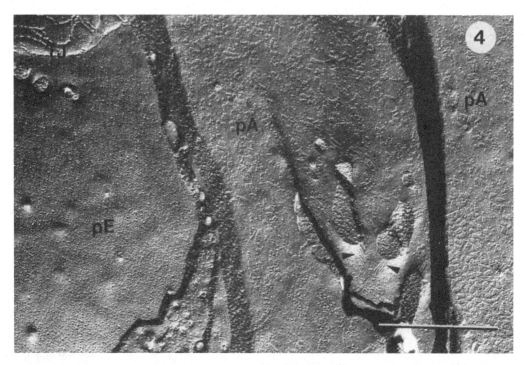

Figure 16.4
Freeze-fracture electron micrograph of pericapillary astrocytic membrane from adult rat optic nerve. The P-face of the pericapillary astrocytic membrane (pA) contains numerous orthogonal arrays of intramembranous particles. Several rows of particles are present at sites of membrane invagination (arrowheads). The P-face of an endothelial cell (pE), and a tight junction (TJ) between adjacent endothelial cells, are exposed. Bar = 0.5 μm. ×32,500.

of paranodal myelin following repetitive action potential activity which has been reported by Moran and Mateu.[32]

As shown in the present study, astrocytic processes comprise a relatively constant component of the extra-axonal region at central nodes of Ranvier. Astrocytic processes have also been described surrounding the axon initial segment;[11,19] the initial segment membrane is known to exhibit morphological[45] and physiological[24] properties similar to those of nodal membrane. Similarly, radially oriented processes of Müller astrocytes are specifically associated

with the specialized foci of node-like membrane which are found along non-myelinated ganglion cell axons in the rat retinal nerve fiber layer.[19] These observations suggest a specific relationship of astrocytic elements to regions of nodal-type membrane. The functional implications of this relationship are not yet understood. As noted above, the perinodal astrocyte may function so as to buffer ionic concentrations in the perinodal extracellular compartment, or to elaborate and/or maintain the nodal gap substance.[17,30] Alternatively, perinodal astrocytes may play a role in metabolic maintenance of the axon and/or oli-

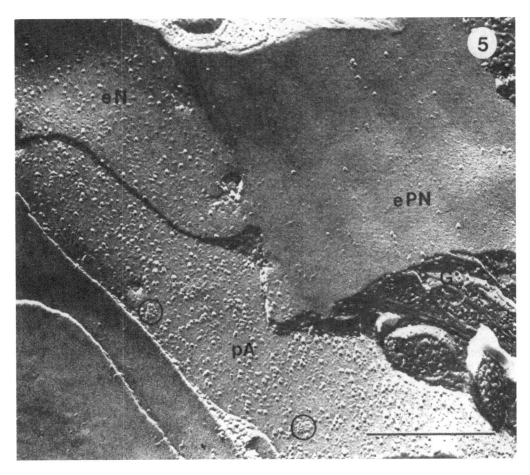

Figure 16.5

Freeze-fracture electron micrograph of nodal region from adult rat optic nerve. The E-faces of nodal (eN) and adjacent paranodal (ePN) membrane are exposed. Note the scalloped contour of the paranodal axon membrane and the large E-face particles in grooves between terminating myelin loops (G) which are cross-fractured. The P-face of an astrocytic process (pA) is observed in close association to the node; several orthogonal arrays (circled) are present on the astrocytic membrane. Bar = 0.5 μm. ×72,750.

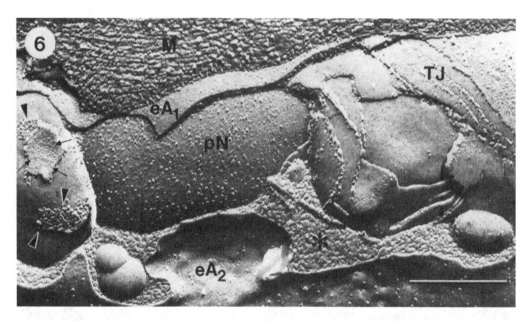

Figure 16.6

Freeze-fracture electron micrograph of nodal region from adult rat optic nerve. Several astrocytic profiles are observed in proximity to the node. The E-face of an astrocytic process (eA₁) is located adjacent to the P-face of the node (pN). A small projection (eA₂) also extends from a larger astrocytic process, and approaches the node. Compact myelin (M) encompassing another fiber is seen above the astrocytic process. An enlarged extracellular space (asterisk) is present adjacent to the node. A tight junction (TJ) is observed between outer layers of the myelin sheath to the right of the node. To the left of the node, the P-face of the outer terminal oligodendroglial loop is exposed, and two gap junctions are present. The gap junction is formed between the P-face (arrowheads) of the oligodendrocyte and the E-face (arrows) of an adjacent cell. Bar = 0.5 μm. ×53,000.

godendroglial cell. It is also notable that some oligodendrocyte-specific markers increase substantially following co-culturing of oligodendroglial cells with astrocytes.[5] In this context, it is interesting that, concomitant with the differentiation of the nodal axon membrane, astrocytic processes appear in proximity to central nodes of Ranvier in developing optic nerve.[20] These latter observations suggest that astrocytes may play a role in the development and/or maturation of central myelinated fibers. While details of the functional role of perinodal astrocytes remain to be elaborated, it seems clear from the morphological findings that at least three cell types (axon, oligodendrocyte, astrocyte) are involved in the formation of nodes of Ranvier in the central nervous system.

Acknowledgments

This work was supported in part by Grant NS-15320 from the National Institutes of Health, and by the Medical Research Service, Veterans Administration. Dr. Black is a fellow of the Neural Plasticity Program.

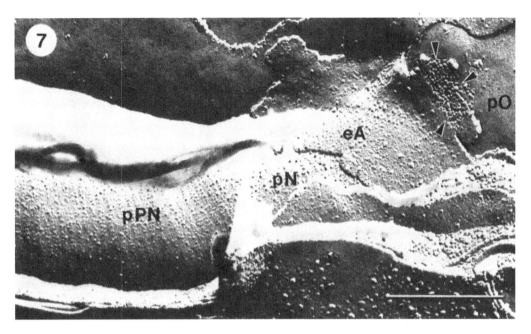

Figure 16.7
Freeze-fracture electron micrograph of nodal and paranodal region from adult rat optic nerve. The P-faces of the paranodal axolemma (pPN) to the left of the node, as well as the P-face nodal axolemma (pN), are exposed. To the right of the node, the P-face of the outer terminal oligodendroglial loop (pO) is seen. Overlying the node and forming a gap junction (arrowheads) with the outermost glial loop, is the E-face of an astrocytic process (eA). At higher magnification (not shown), orthogonal arrays of pits are present on this astrocytic membrane. Bar = 0.5 μm. ×65,000.

References

1. Anders, J. J. and Brightman, M. W., Assemblies of particles in the cell membranes of developing, mature and reactive astrocytes, *J. Neurocytol.*, 8 (1979) 777–795.

2. Baylor, D. A. and Nicholls, J. G., Changes in extracellular potassium concentration produced by neuronal activity in the central nervous system of the leech, *J. Physiol. (Lond.)*, 203 (1969) 555–569.

3. Bennett, M. V. L., Pappas, G. D., Gimenez, M. and Nakajima, Y., Physiology and ultrastructure of electrotonic junctions. IV. Medullary electromotor nuclei in gymnotid fish, *J. Neurophysiol.*, 30 (1967) 238–300.

4. Berthold, C.-H. and Carlstedt, T., Observations on the morphology at the transition between the peripheral and the central nervous system in the cat. III. Myelinated fibres in S₁ dorsal rootlets, *Acta physiol. scand.*, Suppl. 446 (1977) 43–60.

5. Bhat, S., Barbarese, E. and Pfeiffer, S. E., Requirement for non-oligodendrocyte cell signals for enhanced myelinogenic gene expression in long term cultures of purified rat oligodendrocytes, *Proc. nat. Acad. Sci. U.S.A.*, 78 (1981) 1283–1287.

6. Black, J. A., Foster, R. E. and Waxman, S. G., Rat optic nerve: freeze-fracture studies during development of myelinated axons, *Brain Research*, 250 (1982) 1–20.

7. Branton, D., Bullivant, S., Gilula, N. B., Karnovsky, M. J., Moor, H., Muhlethaler, K., Northcote,

D. H., Packer, L., Satir, B., Satir, P., Speth, V., Staehelin, L. A., Steere, R. L. and Weinstein, R. S., Freeze-etching nomenclature, *Science*, 190 (1975) 54–56.

8. Carlstedt, T., Observations on the morphology at the transition between the peripheral and the central nervous system in the cat. IV. Unmyelinated fibres in S_1 dorsal rootlets, *Acta physiol. scand.*, Suppl. 446 (1977) 61–71.

9. Chiu, S. Y., Ritchie, J. M., Rogart, R. B. and Stagg, D., A quantitative description of membrane currents in rabbit myelinated nerve, *J. Physiol. (Lond.)*, 292 (1979) 149–166.

10. Connors, B. W., Ransom, B. R., Kunis, D. M. and Gutnick, M. J., Activity-dependent K^+ accumulation in developing rat optic nerve, *Science*, 216 (1982) 1341–1343.

11. Conradi, S., Observations on the ultrastructure of the axon hillock and initial axon segment of lumbosacral motoneurons in the cat, *Acta physiol. scand.*, Suppl. 332 (1969) 65–84.

12. Dermietzel, R., Junctions in the central nervous system of the cat. III. Gap junctions and membrane-associated orthogonal particle complexes (MOPC) in astrocytic membranes, *Cell Tiss. Res.*, 149 (1974) 121–135.

13. Dermietzel, R., Schunke, D. and Leibstein, A., The oligodendrocytic junctional complex, *Cell Tiss. Res.*, 193 (1978) 61–72.

14. Ellisman, M. H., Rash, J. E., Staehelin, L. A. and Porter, K. R., Studies of excitable membranes. II. A comparison of specializations at neuromuscular junctions and nonjunctional sarcolemmas of mammalian fast and slow twitch muscle fibers, *J. Cell Biol.*, 68 (1976) 752–774.

15. Griffiths, I. R., Duncan, I. D. and McCulloch, M., Shaking pups: a disorder of central myelination in the spanial dog. II. Ultrastructural observations on the white matter of the cervical spinal cord, *J. Neurocytol.*, 10 (1981) 847–858.

16. Gutnick, M. J., Connors, B. W. and Ransom, B. R., Dye-coupling between glial cells in the guinea pig neocortical slice, *Brain Research*, 213 (1981) 486–492.

17. Hildebrand, C., Ultrastructural and light microscopic studies of the nodal region in large myelinated fibres of the feline spinal cord white matter, *Acta physiol. scand.*, Suppl. 364 (1971) 43–71.

18. Hildebrand, C., Ultrastructural and light-microscopic studies of the developing feline spinal cord white matter. I. The nodes of Ranvier, *Acta physiol. scand.*, Suppl. 364 (1971) 81–101.

19. Hildebrand, C. and Waxman, S. G., Regional node-like membrane specializations in non-myelinated axons of rat retinal nerve fiber layer, *Brain Research*, 258 (1983) 23–32.

20. Hildebrand, C. and Waxman, S. G., Postnatal differentiation of rat optic nerve fibres: electron microscopic observations on the development of nodes of Ranvier and axoglial relations, *J. comp. Neurol.*, 224 (1984) 25–37.

21. Humbert, F., Pricam, C., Perrelet, A. and Orci, L., Specific plasma membrane differentiation in the cells of the kidney collecting tubule, *J. Ultrastruct. Res.*, 52 (1975) 13–20.

22. Inoue, S. and Hogg, J. C., Freeze-etch study of the tracheal epithelium of normal guinea pigs with particular reference to intercellular junctions, *J. Ultrastruct. Res.*, 61 (1977) 89–99.

23. Kocsis, J. D. and Waxman, S. G., Absence of potassium conductance in central myelinated axons, *Nature (Lond.)*, 287 (1980) 348–349.

24. Kocsis, J. D. and Waxman, S. G., Action potential electrogenesis in mammalian central axons. In S. G. Waxman and J. M. Ritchie (Eds.), *Demyelinating Disease: Basic and Clinical Electrophysiology*, Raven Press, New York, 1981, pp. 299–312.

25. Kristol, C., Sandri, C. and Akert, K., Intramembranous particles at the nodes of Ranvier of the cat spinal cord: a morphometric study, *Brain Research*, 142 (1978) 391–400.

26. Kuffler, S. W. and Nicholls, J. G., The physiology of neuroglial cells, *Ergebn. Physiol.*, 57 (1966) 1–90.

27. Landis, D. M. D. and Reese, T. S., Arrays of particles in freeze-fractured astrocytic membranes, *J. Cell Biol.*, 60 (1974) 316–320.

28. Landis, D. M. D. and Reese, T. S., Astrocyte membrane structure: changes after circulatory arrest, *J. Cell Biol.*, 88 (1981) 660–663.

29. Landis, D. M. D. and Reese, T. S., Regional organization of astrocytic membranes in cerebellar cortex, *Neuroscience*, 7 (1982) 937–950.

30. Landon, D. N., Structure of normal peripheral myelinated nerve fibers. In S. G. Waxman and J. M.

Ritchie (Eds.), *Demyelinating Disease: Basic and Clinical Electrophysiology*, Raven Press, New York, 1981, pp. 25–50.

31. Massa, P. T. and Mugnaini, E., Cell junctions and intramembrane particles of astrocytes and oligodendrocytes: a freeze-fracture study, *Neuroscience*, 7 (1982) 523–538.

32. Moran, O. and Mateu, L., Loosening of paranodal myelin by repetitive propagation of action potentials, *Nature (Lond.)*, 304 (1983) 344–345.

33. Peters, A., The node of Ranvier in the central nervous system, *Quart. J. exp. Physiol.*, 51 (1966) 229–236.

34. Quick, D. C. and Waxman, S. G., Specific staining of the axon membrane at nodes of Ranvier with ferric ion and ferrocyanide, *J. Neurol. Sci.*, 31 (1977) 1–11.

35. Raine, C. S., Differences between the nodes of Ranvier of large and small diameter fibres in the P.N.S., *J. Neurocytol.*, 11 (1982) 935–947.

36. Raine, C. S., On the association between perinodal astrocytic processes and the node of Ranvier in the CNS, *J. Neurocytol.*, 13 (1984) 21–27.

37. Rash, J. E. and Ellisman, M. H., Studies of excitable membranes. I. Macromolecular specializations of the neuromuscular junction and nonjunctional sarcolemma, *J. Cell Biol.*, 63 (1974) 567–586.

38. Ritchie, J. M. and Rogart, R. B., Density of sodium channels in mammalian myelinated nerve fibers and nature of the axonal membrane under the myelin sheath, *Proc. nat. Acad. Sci. U.S.A.*, 74 (1977) 211–215.

39. Robertson, J. D., Bodenheimer, T. S. and Stage, D. E., The ultrastructure of Mauthner cell synapses and nodes in goldfish brains, *J. Cell Biol.*, 19 (1963) 159–199.

40. Rosenbluth, J., Intramembranous particle distribution at the node of Ranvier and adjacent axolemma in myelinated axons of the frog brain, *J. Neurocytol.*, 5 (1976) 731–745.

41. Rydmark, M. and Berthold, C.-H., Electron microscopic serial section analysis of nodes of Ranvier in lumbar spinal roots of the cat: a morphometric study of nodal compartments in fibres of different sizes, *J. Neurocytol.*, 12 (1983) 537–565.

42. Schnapp, B. and Mugnaini, E., Membrane architecture of myelinated fibers as seen by freeze-fracture.

In S. G. Waxman (Ed.), *Physiology and Pathobiology of Axons*, Raven Press, New York, 1978, pp. 83–123.

43. Staehelin, L. A., Three types of gap junctions interconnecting intestinal epithelial cells visualized by freeze-fracture, *Proc. nat. Acad. Sci. U.S.A.*, 69 (1972) 1318–1321.

44. Waxman, S. G., Regional differentiation of the axon: a review with special reference to the concept of the multiplex neuron, *Brain Research*, 47 (1972) 269–288.

45. Waxman, S. G. and Quick, D. C., Intra-axonal ferric ion-ferrocyanide staining of nodes of Ranvier and initial segments in central myelinated fibers, *Brain Research*, 144 (1978) 1–10.

17 Ion Channels in Spinal Cord Astrocytes In Vitro. II. Biophysical and Pharmacological Analysis of Two Na⁺ Current Types

Harald Sontheimer and Stephen G. Waxman

Summary and Conclusions

1. Na⁺ currents expressed in astrocytes cultured from spinal cord were studied by whole cell patch-clamp recording. Two subtypes of astrocytes, pancake and stellate cells, were morphologically differentiated and showed expression of Na⁺ channels at densities that are unusually high for glial cells (2–8 channels/μm^2) and comparable to cultured neurons.

2. Na⁺ currents in stellate and pancake astrocytes were comparable to neuronal Na⁺ currents with regard to Na⁺-current activation (τ_m) and inactivation (τ_h) time constants, which were equally fast in both astrocyte types. However, they differed with respect to voltage dependence of activation, and current-voltage ($I–V$) curves were ~10 mV more positive in stellate cells (-11.1 ± 5.6 mV, mean $\pm$ SD) than in pancake cells (19.7 ± 4.5 mV). Steady-state activation (m_∞ curves) was 16 mV more negative in pancake (mean $V_{1/2} = -48.8$ mV) than in stellate cells (mean $V_{1/2} = -32.7$ mV).

3. Steady-state inactivation (h_∞ curves) of Na⁺ currents was distinctly different in the two astrocyte types. In stellate astrocytes h_∞ curves had midpoints close to -65 mV (-64.6 ± 6.5 mV), similar to most cultured neurons. In pancake astrocytes h_∞-curves were ~25 mV more negative, with midpoints close to -85 mV (84.5 ± 9.5 mV).

4. The two forms of Na⁺ currents were additionally distinguishable by their sensitivity to tetrodotoxin (TTX). Na⁺ currents in stellate astrocytes were highly TTX sensitive [half-maximal inhibition (K_d) = 5.7 nM] whereas Na⁺ currents in pancake astrocytes were relatively TTX resistant, requiring 100- to 1,000-fold higher concentrations for blockage ($K_d = 1,007$ nM).

5. Na⁺ currents were fit by the Hodgkin-Huxley (HH) model. In pancake astrocytes, as in squid gigant axons, Na⁺-current kinetics could be well described with an m^3h model, whereas in stellate astrocytes Na⁺ currents were better described with higher-order power terms for activation (m). On average, best fits were obtained using an m^4h model.

Reprinted with permission from *Journal of Neurophysiology* 68: 1001–1011, 1992.

6. Pancake astrocytes were capable of generating action-potential (AP)-like responses under current clamp whereas stellate astrocytes were not. The h_∞ curve for APs shows that membrane potentials more negative than -70 mV are required to allow these responses to occur. Because the cells' resting potential was much more depolarized (-40 mV), this mismatch between the steady-state inactivation (h_∞ curve) and resting potential, which results in Na⁺ current inactivation, does not allow these responses to occur spontaneously and makes it unlikely that AP-like responses occur in spinal cord pancake astrocytes in vivo.

7. Although Na⁺ currents expressed in stellate astrocytes resembled, in all their features, Na⁺ currents observed in cultured neurons, the combination of negative h_∞ curve and TTX insensitivity characterizing Na⁺ currents in pancake astrocytes has not been observed in excitable cells, suggesting the existence of an astrocyte-specific Na⁺ channel in these cells.

Introduction

Na⁺ conductances in astrocytes are typically about two to three orders of magnitude smaller than in neurons, with astrocytes usually expressing a Na⁺ channel density of $<1/\mu m^2$ (Barres et al. 1988, 1990; Sontheimer et al. 1991*a, b*), compared with a density of 10–100 channels/μm^2 in cultured neurons (see table 1 in Sontheimer et al. 1992). This suggested that astrocytes typically lack the channel complement necessary for electrogenesis and prompted the speculation that astrocytes may synthesize Na⁺ channels destined to be inserted into the axolemma of neighboring axons (Bevan et al. 1985). If this were the case, one would expect that astrocytic Na⁺ currents should be similar to Na⁺ currents in axons. Accumulating evidence suggests, however, that astrocytes may express multiple forms of Na⁺ channels (Barres et al. 1989, 1990; Minturn et al. 1992; Sontheimer 1992; Sontheimer et al. 1991*a, b*) and may synthesize Na⁺ channels that have properties different from Na⁺ channels in excitable cells. On the basis of recent advances in molecular biology, the observation of multiple types of Na^+ channels within one cell preparation is not surprising. Thus far, six isoforms of Na^+ channels have been cloned and characterized, most of which differ with respect to features of their macroscopic current. The existence of multiple forms of Na^+ channels in neurons has long been suspected on the basis of observations that currents in different cell preparations and species can be differentially modulated (Strichartz et al. 1987). Tetrodotoxin (TTX), in particular, has been used to distinguish two classes of Na^+ currents in neurons (Ikeda and Schofield 1987; Kostyuk et al. 1981; Roy and Narahashi 1991, 1992). Studies on cultured dorsal root ganglion (DRG) neurons demonstrated that multiple types of Na^+ currents can be expressed within the same cell or cell type (Caffrey et al. 1991, 1992; McLean et al. 1988; Roy and Narahashi 1991; Schwartz et al. 1990). Recent observations on expression of the rat brain II Na^+ channel after point mutations in *Xenopus* oocytes (Noda et al. 1989), and on the expression of Na^+ channels in mammalian cells after transfection with cDNA encoding the IIA Na^+ channel α-subunit (Yang et al. 1992), suggest that the TTX-binding site of the rat brain II and IIA Na^+ channels is conferred by their primary amino acid sequence. Thus the appearance of TTX-sensitive and TTX-resistant Na^+ channels in a cell population may indicate the expression of two distinct Na^+ channel proteins.

In this paper, we provide evidence that indicates that certain subtypes of spinal cord astrocytes in vitro express Na^+ channels that differ pharmacologically and kinetically from axonal and neuronal Na^+ channels, whereas other subtypes of spinal cord astrocytes express Na^+ channels indistinguishable from their neuronal counterparts. In making these observations, we took advantage of the discovery that spinal cord astrocytes in vitro express unusually high levels of Na^+ channels, up to 1,000-fold higher than astrocytes from other areas of the brain (Sontheimer et al. 1992). This spinal cord preparation

contains subtypes of astrocyte that are easily distinguishable morphologically. Two clearly distinct forms of Na^+ currents are selectively expressed and confined to morphologically different types of cells in these cultures, stellate and pancake astrocytes, respectively.

Methods

Cultured spinal cord astrocytes, derived from neonatal Sprague-Dawley rats, were investigated in this study. Cells were cultured at 37°C on polyornithine-laminin–coated glass cover slips in complete medium [Earle's minimum essential medium containing 10% fetal calf serum (Hyclone), penicillin/streptomycin (500 U/ml each), and 20 mM glucose containing trypsin inhibitor and bovine serum albumin (each 1.5 mg/ml)] in a 5% CO_2-95% air atmosphere. Methods used for cell culture and identification are described more fully in the companion paper (Sontheimer et al. 1992).

Whole cell patch-clamp recordings were obtained using thin-walled borosilicate electrodes (WPI, TW150F-40; OD 1.5 mm, ID 1.2 mm) coated with silicone elastomer (Sylgard; Dow Corning) and filled with a solution containing (in mM) 145 KCl, 1 $MgCl_2$, 0.2 $CaCl_2$, 10 EGTA, 10 N-2-hydroxyethylpiperazine-N'-2-ethane-sulfonic acid (HEPES; sodium salt), pH adjusted to 7.4 using tris(hydroxymethyl)aminomethane (Tris); these electrodes had resistances of 2–3 MΩ. Some recordings were obtained with a pipette solution in which KCl was replaced by N-methyl-D-glucamine (NmDg) 125 mM and tetraethylammonium chloride (TEA-Cl) 20 mM to inhibit outward currents, and these had resistances of 3–5 MΩ. Cells were continuously superfused at room temperature with a solution containing (in mM) 125 NaCl, 5.0 KCl, 1.2 $MgSO_4$, 1.0 $CaCl_2$, 1.6 Na_2HPO_4, 0.4 NaH_2PO_4, 10.5 glucose, 32.5 HEPES (acid), pH 7.4 adjusted with NaOH. Special care was taken to ensure sufficient voltage-clamp conditions; for details see Sontheimer et al. (1992). Only recordings that met the following criteria were included in our analysis. *1*) Series resistance before compensation of errors was <10 MΩ. *2*) Na$^+$ currents reached their peak within <800 μs. *3*) Na$^+$ currents reversed within 5–10 mV of the mean current reversal potential, which was close to the theoretical equilibrium potential for Na$^+$.

Data Analysis and Curve Fitting

Data analysis was performed on leak-subtracted current traces, after P/4 leak subtraction had been obtained (Bezanilla and Armstrong 1977). Analysis of digitized data traces and curve fitting to those traces as well as fitting to cumulative data were done using the script interpreter of a scientific plotting program (Origin, MicroCal). All these fits were obtained using a Marquard-Levenberg non-linear-squares algorithm. The models and equations to which sets of data were fit are given below. Cumulative data analysis was performed by exporting measures obtained with Clampan (Axon Instruments) to a spreadsheet (Excel) and computing statistical values (mean, SD, and SE) for spreadsheet data. These values were exported for graphing and curve fitting to the same plotting program (Origin) used for analysis of digitized data.

Hodgkin and Huxley Parameters

Time constants for current activation and inactivation were obtained by fitting data to the empirically derived Hodgkin-Huxley (HH) model (Hodgkin and Huxley 1952). Current kinetics were described by an $m^p h$ model. Na$^+$ currents were converted to conductances by dividing digitized traces point-by-point by $(V_m - E_{Na^+})$. Current reversal potential was considered to be E_{Na^+}. The derived Na$^+$ conductances were fit by the following equation

$$f(t) = A0 + A1 \cdot \{1 - \exp[-(t - t0)/\tau_m]\}^P$$
$$\cdot \{\exp[-(t - t0)/\tau_h]\}$$

where $A0$ and $A1$ were amplitude factors, $t0$ was a time-offset factor, and $\tau_m \tau_h$ were the time constants for activation and inactivation, respectively. p was the power factor for the activation (m) term.

Na$^+$ currents were initially fit to an $m^3 h$ model, thus p was set to 3. However, in stellate astrocytes better fits could be obtained with p values >3. If p was included as a fitting parameter, and thus determined through the fitting algorithm, best fits were typically obtained with $4 < p < 6$ for stellate astrocytes. However, because fits did not improve considerably at $p > 4$ as judged by comparing ω^2 values, we chose to use $m^4 h$ as the model to fit activation and inactivation in these cells. All pancake cells were fit with an $m^3 h$ model.

In some instances we compared τ_h values obtained from the HH model to values obtained from fitting the decay phase of Na$^+$ currents. In these instances, the data were fit to single exponentials of the form

$$f(t) = A0 + A1 \cdot \exp\{-[(x - x0)/\tau]\}$$

Normalized P_{Na} relationships (figures 17.1 and 17.6) were calculated by dividing conductances, derived from peak currents divided by $V_m - E_{Na^+}$, by the largest conductances measured. Steady-state inactivation curves (h_∞) and activation curves were fit to a modified Boltzmann equation of the form

$$h(V) \text{ or } m(V) = 1/\{1 + \exp[(V - V_{1/2})/a]\}$$

with $V_{1/2}$ representing the midpoint of the sigmoidal curve.

Other Parameters

TTX used in these studies was obtained from Sigma. TTX inhibition curves were fit to a Langmuir binding isotherm of the form

$$I(X) = A \cdot X/(B + X)$$

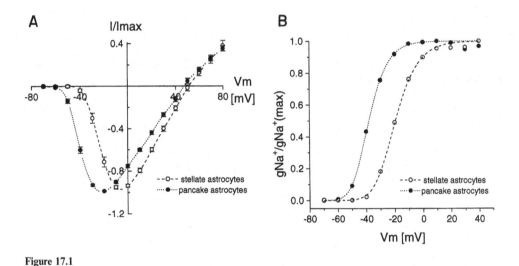

Figure 17.1

Na⁺ current activation. Cells were voltage-clamped at −80 mV, and 10-ms voltage steps were applied to potentials ranging from −70 to 80 mV. To remove channel inactivation, we preceded test voltage steps by 200-ms conditioning voltage steps to −110 mV. (A) Recordings obtained from 23 pancake and 24 stellate astrocytes were averaged and their mean peak currents in response to these voltage steps were plotted as a function of step potential. Error bars indicate SE. In pancake astrocytes (··· in A), voltage steps more positive than −60 mV activated transient inward currents that inactivated rapidly. Currents were largest at test potentials close to −20 mV and decreased at more positive test potentials. Similar recordings were obtained in stellate astrocytes (––– in A). In stellate cells, thresholds for both activation (−40 mV) and peak (−10 mV) were ~10 mV more positive than in pancake cells. In both cell types currents reversed close to 50 mV. (B) From same data plotted in (A), normalized activation curves were constructed as follows. Peak currents were converted to conductances by dividing peak currents by driving force $V_m − E_{Na^+}$. These values were normalized to the largest conductance value [$gNa^+(max)$]. Normalized conductance values for every potential step were averaged for the 23 and 24 cells studied, respectively, and plotted as a function of step potential. Dashed and dotted curves were obtained by fitting the data to Boltzmann-like equations (see Methods). These activation curves indicate that Na⁺ current in the two cell types differs substantially with regard to voltage dependence of activation. Activation curves were ~16 mV more negative in pancake cells than in stellate cells. For clarity, SE bars were omitted, but were identical to those of (A).

Results

Na⁺ currents were recorded in pancake and stellate astrocytes at up to 37 days in vitro (DIV; 32 DIV for stellate astrocytes). As noted previously (Sontheimer et al. 1992), Na⁺ currents could be observed only after >3 DIV in pancake astrocytes, and current densities were largest at 6–10 DIV in these cells. We have therefore confined our analysis and comparison of Na⁺ current characteristics to astrocytes between 6 and 10 DIV. We did not include recordings obtained at later times in culture, because cells were often too large to assure sufficient voltage clamp.

Voltage Dependence of Na⁺-Current Activation

Na⁺-current activation was studied by voltage-clamping cells at −80 mV and applying voltage steps to potentials ranging from −70 to 80 mV. To ensure that Na⁺-channel inactivation was completely removed, voltage steps were preceded by a prepulse potential of -110 mV (200-ms duration). Recordings on stellate astrocytes were obtained in the presence of 2–5 mM 4-aminopyridine (4-AP) to reduce outward currents. Pancake astrocytes typically did not require blockage, because outward currents were very small.

Current-voltage (I–V) curves were obtained for 23 pancake and 24 stellate astrocytes, respectively. Normalized mean I–V curves for both cell types are illustrated in figure 17.1A. Voltage steps more positive than -60 mV in pancake cells and -40 mV in stellate astrocytes activated transient inward currents. Currents were largest at potentials close to -20 mV in pancake astrocytes and -10 mV in stellate astrocytes (figure 17.1A). At more positive potentials, currents decreased in size and reversed at close to 50 mV. Both peak of activation and the threshold for activation were consistently more positive in stellate astrocytes (figure 17.1A). Comparing 36 pancake and 50 stellate cells, the mean I–V curves were significantly different ($P < 0.0001$) with mean peak values of -19.7 ± 4.5 (SD) mV for pancake and -11.1 ± 5.6 (SD) mV for stellate astrocytes. The current reversal potential was close to 55 mV [pancake astrocytes: 50.7 ± 6.34 (SD) mV$_0$ stellate astrocytes: 57.4 ± 8.9 (SD) 8.9] and reasonably close to the calculated Na$^+$ equilibrium potential ($E_{Na} = 63.8$ mV). We used the close fit of current reversal potentials to E_{Na^+} as criteria to establish that voltage-clamp conditions were adequate to control currents (for further detail on voltage control see Methods and Sontheimer et al. 1992). From the same data, we derived the steady-state activation (m_∞) curves displayed in figure 17.1B by dividing peak currents by ($V_m - E_{Na^+}$), thus deriving conductances (gNa$^+$) from peak currents, and normalizing the conductances to the largest conductance [gNa$^+$(max)] observed. The data were fit by sigmoidal, Boltzmann-like functions (continuous lines; see Methods). The values derived from the fits show a shift by 16 mV to more negative

potentials in pancake cells (mean $V_{1/2} = -48.8$) compared with stellate cells (mean $V_{1/2} = -32.7$ mV), whereas the slopes were similar in both cell types.

To determine the time constants of Na$^+$-current activation and inactivation, kinetic analysis of activation and inactivation was carried out by determining the HH parameters τ_m and τ_h, respectively. Values for τ_m and τ_h were obtained by fitting the data traces to an HH model of the form $m^p h$. In their study of Na$^+$ currents in the squid giant axon, Hodgkin and Huxley (1952) used a model in which m was raised to the third power ($m^3 h$). Although this model gave acceptable fits to Na$^+$ currents in pancake cells (figure 17.2A), in stellate astrocytes better fits were obtained for $p > 3$ (figure 17.2B). We therefore decided to include the power term p as a variable and approximate its value from least-squared fits. In pancake astrocytes, as in the squid giant axon, the fitted value for p was always close to 3 (3.22 ± 0.08 (SD), $n = 11$). In contrast, values of p were consistently higher in stellate astrocytes ($4.18 \pm$ (SD), $n = 10$). This difference between pancake and stellate cells was highly significant ($P < 0.00001$).

Examples of conductances and superimposed fitted curves are displayed for representative stellate and pancake cells in figure 17.2. Conductances (gNa) were plotted for three voltage steps for both cell types, respectively. The p values yielding best fits in the $m^p h$ model (dotted lines) were approximated as 3.21, 3.0, and 2.89 in the pancake cell and 4.21, 5.4, and 4.4 in the stellate cell. Comparing the quality of fits for various p values indicated that at $p > 4$ the fits did not improve significantly for stellate cells. We therefore used $m^3 h$ as the model to fit Na$^+$ currents in pancake cells and $m^4 h$ for Na$^+$ currents in stellate cells, and all time constants were derived using these two models.

To illustrate the voltage dependence of τ_m and τ_h, we determined these parameters for representative examples of the two astrocyte types [original traces displayed in figure 8 of compan-

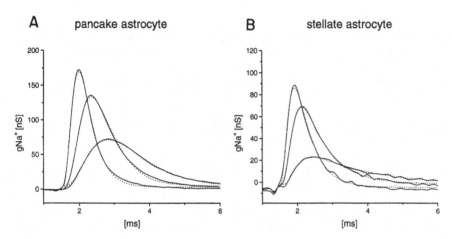

Figure 17.2

Hodgkin and Huxley (HH) parameters for Na^+ currents. Time constants for Na^+-current activation and inactivation were determined by fitting the data to the Hodgkin and Huxley model (Hodgkin and Huxley 1952). Current traces were converted to conductances as described in Methods, and conductance traces were fit to the HH model using the following equation

$$(t) = A0 + A1 \cdot \{1 - \exp[-(t - t0)/\tau_m]\}^P \cdot \{\exp[-(t - t0)/\tau_h]\},$$

as described in Methods. Best fits were obtained in pancake cells if the activation term m was raised to the 3rd power (e.g., $P = 3$), whereas in stellate cells $P = 4$ (or greater) gave better fits. Families of conductance traces displayed for a pancake astrocyte (*A*) and a stellate astrocyte (*B*) were obtained from the same cells as displayed in fig. 8 of the companion paper (Sontheimer et al. 1992). Fitted traces were superimposed ($\cdots$) on data (——). *P* values yielding best fits were 3.21 (−30 mV), 3.0 (−10 mV), and 2.89 (0 mV) for the pancake cell (*A*) and 4.21 (−20 mV), 5.4 (−10 mV), and 4.4 (0 mV) for the stellate cell (*B*).

ion paper (Sontheimer et al. 1992)] and plotted τ_h and τ_m as a function of voltage in figure 17.3. For comparative purposes we also determined the time-to-peak values (figure 17.3, *A* and *B*) as a function of membrane potential. The latter values did not differ significantly between the two cell types ($P < 0.01$). This was also true for inactivation time constants τ_h, which were between 1.5 and 0.25 ms (depending on voltage) in both cell types, and which changed e-fold for a potential change of 10.7 and 14.5 mV, respectively (figure 17.3, *E* and *F*). As expected from the similarity of time-to-peak values in both cell types, with currents following different activation models (m^3h vs m^4h), values for activation τ_m were faster in stellate cells than in pancake cells

(figure 17.3, *C* and *D*). In both cell types τ_m plots could be fit by exponentials that indicate an e-fold change of τ_m for about a 10-mV voltage change.

Because Na^+-current inactivation is often determined by fitting an exponential decay to the falling phase of the current (e.g., Chiu et al. 1979), rather than fitting the HH model to Na^+ conductances, to account for both activation and inactivation, we obtained τ_h using this approach for comparison with the values derived via the HH model (figure 17.4). As indicated for Na^+ currents at two potentials (−30 and −10 mV) these values (τ) were up to 40% larger than τ_h determined from the HH model, suggesting an apparently slower current inactivation. Varying

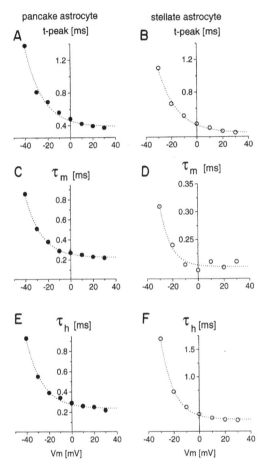

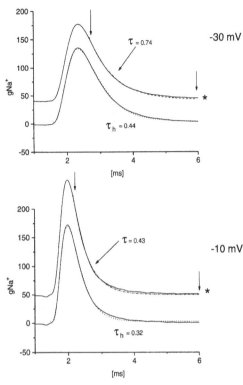

Figure 17.3

Na$^+$-current kinetics. Using the HH model, we analyzed Na$^+$ currents kinetically. Displayed examples were obtained from same cells shown in fig. 8 of the companion paper (Sontheimer et al. 1992). For each cell, time-to-peak (*A* and *B*), activation τ_m (*C* and *D*), and inactivation time constant τ_h (*E* and *F*) were determined for potentials between −40 and 30 mV. Values were plotted as a function of step potentials. These values could be fit by exponential decay functions (····· in *A–F*). For examples displayed, time-to-peak did not differ, τ_m was somewhat faster in the stellate astrocyte, and τ_h was slower in the stellate than in the pancake cell. Analysis of 11 pancake and 10 stellate astrocytes, however, did not show significant differences in these parameters between pancake and stellate astrocytes.

Figure 17.4

Determination of Na$^+$-current inactivation. Inactivation time constant τ_h of Na$^+$ currents was determined by 2 methods and compared. *1*) τ_h was derived from fitting the data to the HH model as described in figure 17.2. Examples of data (——) and superimposed fits (·····) are shown (*bottom* traces in *top* and *bottom* panels, 0 intercept) for 2 potentials (−30 and −10 mV). *2*) τ_h was derived from fitting a single exponential to the decay phase, namely, the range at which conductances were between 80 and 0% of maximal. For display purposes, these traces were offset upward by ∼50 nS (*). Arrows indicate the fitting region used: dashed lines are superimposed fits. Values obtained differed substantially and were ∼30% larger if only the decay phase were fit.

the fit-region for the current decay reduced this discrepancy only if the very tail of the decay (the portion between 0 and 10% of peak conductance) were used for the fit. These experiments suggest that τ_h of macroscopic currents can be determined more accurately from HH model fits and are otherwise overestimated.

The results demonstrated in figures 17.2–17.4 were representative for all other recordings analyzed. A comparison of τ_h and τ_m for 11 pancake and 10 stellate astrocytes, analyzed by fitting HH models to the data, indicates that these values did not differ significantly between pancake and stellate astrocytes when compared at the same potential: τ_m (at −10 mV), pancake cells: 0.222 ± 0.017 (SD); stellate cells: 0.227 ± 0.019 (SD); $P = 0.93$; τ_h (at −10 mV), pancake cells: 0.425 ± 0.04 (SD); stellate cells: 0.483 ± 0.06 (SD); $P = 0.55$. Note, however, that, because of the shift in steady-state activation, τ values, as a function of membrane potential, differed at potentials between −40 and −20 mV.

Steady-State Na$^+$-Current Inactivation (h_∞)

To study the steady-state inactivation of Na$^+$ currents, we obtained recordings after a conditional prepulse protocol. Cells were voltage-clamped at −80 mV. Na$^+$ currents were activated by stepping the membrane to −20 mV, the potential resulting in the largest inward currents (figure 17.1). This voltage step was preceded by a series of increasingly more positive prepulse potentials ranging from −130 to −30 mV (10-mV increments; indicated in figure 17.5, *inset*). Currents recorded were largest at very negative prepulse potentials (−130 to −100 mV) and decreased at more positive potentials (figure 17.5, *A* and *B*). In pancake astrocytes, currents were completely inactivated at prepulse potentials of −60 mV. In contrast, more than one-half of the current was still activatable at this potential in stellate astrocytes, where currents did not become completely inactivated until the prepulse potential was more positive than −40 mV.

To illustrate these differences more clearly, we constructed h_∞ curves for both cell types (figure 17.5C). Peak currents were normalized to the largest current (typically at −130 mV) and plotted as a function of prepulse potential. The data were fit to Boltzmann equations (———, as described in Methods) to yield the h_∞ curves. These curves differed for the two types of astrocytes by 20 mV, being more negative in pancake than in stellate cells. The h_∞ curve midpoint for the stellate astrocyte shown was close to −65 mV, whereas the midpoint for the pancake astrocyte shown was about −85 mV (dashed lines in figure 17.5C). Mean values for 28 pancake and 34 stellate astrocytes yielded h_∞ midpoints of −84.5 ± 9.5 (SD) mV and −64.6 ± 6.5 (SD) mV, respectively. This difference was highly significant ($P < 0.0001$).

Because we have observed previously that h_∞ curves can shift with time in vitro for hippocampal astrocytes (Sontheimer et al. 1991b), we studied h_∞ curves in astrocytes of both types at 1–37 DIV (figure 17.5D). h_∞ curves were constructed for all cells in which Na$^+$ currents were large enough to allow construction of complete h_∞ curves, and their midpoints were determined as described above. Mean values were computed for both cell types at every timepoint studied, and these were plotted as a function of time in vitro (figure 17.5D). The h_∞ midpoints for the two populations of astrocytes did not overlap and were significantly different (0.0004 < P < 0.012) at each timepoint except at 9 DIV ($P = 0.34$). Moreover, h_∞ midpoints for the two populations did not change significantly with time in vitro. Values were always around −85 mV for pancake astrocytes and −65 mV in stellate astrocytes (figure 17.5D).

Overlap of h_∞ and m_∞ Curves ("Window Currents")

To evaluate the overlap of steady-state activation and inactivation, we constructed m_∞ and h_∞ curves for both cell types from 11 pancake

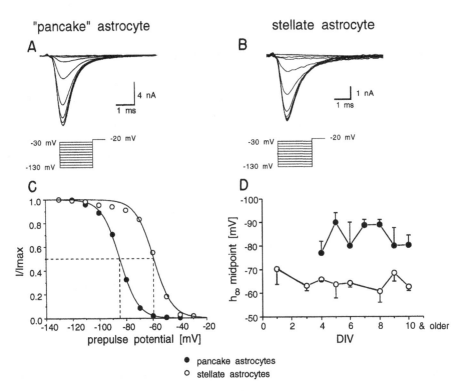

Figure 17.5
Steady-state Na$^+$-current inactivation. Steady-state inactivation (h_∞) curves were obtained by altering the prepulse potential from which currents were activated between −130 and −30 mV (A and B) as described in METHODS. Currents were largest at very negative prepulse potentials (e.g., −130 mV), and these were used to normalize peak currents (I/I_{max}). Normalized peak currents were plotted as a function of prepulse potential and yielded h_∞ curves (C). These were fit by the Boltzmann equation (C, ——). h_∞ curves of pancake and stellate astrocytes differed significantly and were ~25 mV more positive in stellate than in pancake astrocytes. Midpoints of these curves (− − −) were −84 mV for the pancake astrocyte (C, ●) and −59 mV for the stellate astrocyte (C, ○). Midpoints of h_∞ curves were compared in pancake and stellate astrocytes during in vitro development at 1–37 days in vitro (DIV; D). Midpoints were close to −85 mV in pancake astrocytes (D, ●) and close to −65 mV in stellate astrocytes (○) and did not change with time in vitro.

cells and 10 stellate cells, respectively (figure 17.6). h_∞ curves were constructed as described above. m_∞ curves were constructed by plotting normalized $gNa[gNa/gNa(max)]$ values as a function of membrane potential. Values for gNa were calculated as described in METHODS.

Both h_∞ and m_∞ curves differed by ∼20 mV in the two cell types in that both curves were more positive in stellate cells (figure 17.6B) than in pancake cells (figure 17.6A). Overlapping areas of m and h ("windows") were similar in size in both cell types, but again the membrane potential range of such overlaps differed by ∼20 mV and was −75 to −50 mV in pancake astrocytes and −60 to −30 mV in stellate astrocytes. The largest values for m and h within the window of overlap were <0.5 and <0.4, respectively. The maximal conductance at those potentials $[g = g \cdot (m^3h)$ for pancake cells or $g = g \cdot (m^4h)$ for stellate cells] would therefore be small.

TTX Sensitivity of Astrocyte Na⁺ Currents

Na⁺ currents in pancake and stellate astrocytes were investigated with respect to sensitivity to TTX, a highly specific toxin known to block voltage-activated Na⁺ currents. Figure 17.7 shows effects of TTX on representative examples of a stellate and a pancake astrocyte. In stellate astrocytes Na⁺ currents were reduced ∼60% by 10 nM TTX and were completely blocked in the presence of 100 nM TTX (figure 17.7A). In contrast, 1 μM TTX did not abolish Na⁺ currents in pancake astrocytes and typically reduced inward currents by only 50% (figure 17.7B), and even at 10 μM TTX, Na⁺ currents were still observable. Although TTX reduced the peak Na⁺ currents in both types of cells, it did not alter the voltage dependence of activation (figure 17.7, C and D), current kinetics or the current reversal potential (figure 17.7, C and D). To better compare effects of TTX on the two subtypes of astrocytes, we obtained recordings in the presence of various concentrations of TTX and mean TTX inhibi-

tion curves were established. Currents in the presence of TTX were normalized to the control current before TTX application, and mean values of current inhibition were plotted as a function of TTX concentration for 19 stellate and 20 pancake cells (figure 17.8). The data were fit to Langmuir binding isotherms (———, weighted fit). The values for half-maximal TTX inhibition (K_d) were derived from the fitted curves and had values of 5.7 nM for stellate astrocytes and 1,007 nM for pancake astrocytes. Thus the Na⁺ currents in the two subtypes of astrocytes differed by more than two orders of magnitude with respect to their TTX sensitivity.

AP-like Responses Require Negative Resting Potentials

In the companion paper (Sontheimer et al. 1992) we demonstrated that, because of their high Na⁺-current densities, pancake astrocytes, but not stellate astrocytes, were capable of generating AP-like responses under current-clamp recording, which resembled APs in excitable cells. Because we observed (see above) unusually negative h_∞ curves in pancake astrocytes, we expected that AP-like responses would be initiated only from very negative membrane potentials in these cells. To examine the voltage dependence of AP-like responses, we current clamped pancake astrocytes at various potentials ranging from −50 to −130 mV, and constant-current steps of 1 nA were applied. A representative recording obtained in this way is displayed in figure 17.9. At −61 mV, the 1-nA current step depolarized the membrane but did not elicit an AP-like response; at −71 mV, a small response could be elicited with an amplitude of ∼55 mV. At −77 mV, the AP-like nature of the response became apparent, with an amplitude of 105 mV and an overshooting peak close to 30 mV. The largest responses were observed at potentials more negative than −90 mV where the peak of the response was close to E_{Na}. The amplitudes of AP-like responses recorded in this way were

pancake astrocytes

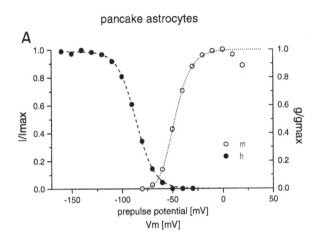

stellate astrocytes

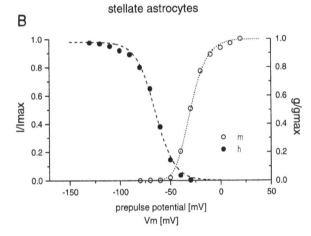

Figure 17.6

h_∞ and m_∞ curves show Na$^+$ "window" currents. To test whether an overlapping region ("window") exists in which nonzero values for Na$^+$ current activation (m) and inactivation (h) overlap, we analyzed these parameters in cultured astrocytes as follows: h_∞ curves were obtained as described in the legend to figure 17.5, for 11 pancake (A, ●) and 10 stellate astrocytes (B, ●). Steady-state activation (m_∞) curves were obtained by determining the peak Na$^+$ current in response to depolarizing voltage steps (○, A and B) as described in legend to Fig. 8 of the companion paper (Sontheimer et al. 1992). For every voltage step, conductance (g) was calculated from peak current by dividing by $V_m - E_{Na^+}$. This value was divided by the largest conductance (g_{max}) typically observed at step-potentials more positive than -20 mV. The normalized values (g/g_{max}) for 11 pancake (A, ○) and 10 stellate astrocytes (B, ○) were plotted as a function of step potential. Both h_∞ and m_∞ data were fit to the Boltzmann equation. In pancake cells both curves are $\sim$20 mV more negative than in stellate astrocytes. For both cell types "windows" are present, at which both m and h are >0, thus where Na$^+$ currents flow at steady-state. These windows were between -75 and -45 mV in pancake astrocytes and between -60 and -30 mV in stellate astrocytes.

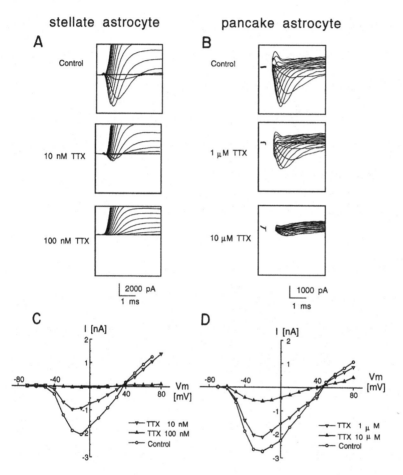

Figure 17.7

Na$^+$ currents in stellate and pancake cells show different tetrodotoxin (TTX) sensitivity. Na$^+$ currents were recorded in pancake and stellate astrocytes in the presence of 10 nM–100 μM TTX and compared with control currents in the absence of TTX. Examples are displayed for a stellate astrocyte (*A*) and a pancake astrocyte (*B*). Na$^+$ currents in stellate astrocytes were more sensitive to TTX than Na$^+$ currents in pancake cells, and 10 nM TTX reduced Na$^+$ currents by >60% (*A, middle*). At 100 nM, Na$^+$ currents were completely blocked in stellate astrocytes (*A, bottom*). In pancake astrocytes a much higher concentration of TTX had to be used to diminish Na$^+$ currents; in the example demonstrated, 1 μM TTX reduced Na$^+$ currents by only 25% (*B, middle*), and even at 10 μM, 15% of the current persisted (*B, bottom*). TTX did not alter the threshold of activation or current reversal potential in stellate (*C*) or pancake astrocytes (*D*).

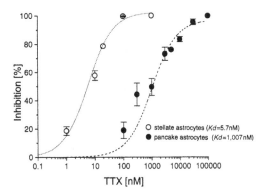

Figure 17.8
TTX inhibition curves for spinal cord astrocytes. To better compare effects of TTX on the 2 subtypes of astrocytes, we obtained recordings in the presence of various concentrations of TTX and established mean TTX inhibition curves. Currents in the presence of TTX were normalized to the control current before TTX application, and mean values of current inhibition were plotted as a function of TTX concentration for 19 stellate and 20 pancake cells on a semilogarithmic scale. Data were fit to Langmuir binding isotherms (---, weighted fit, see Methods). Values for half-maximal TTX inhibition (K_d) were derived from fitted curves and had values of 5.7 nM for stellate astrocytes and 1,007 nM for pancake astrocytes. TTX sensitivity of Na^+ currents in the 2 subtypes of astrocytes differed by >2 orders of magnitude.

normalized to the largest response (at -90 mV) and plotted as a function of membrane potential. The data were fit to the Boltzmann equation (——, figure 17.9, *left*) and yielded a midpoint at -77.1 mV. This value is remarkably close to the midpoint obtained for Na^+-current inactivation curves in voltage-clamp recordings (about -85 mV; figure 17.5C). Thus membrane potentials more negative than -70 mV are required to allow AP-like responses to occur in these cells. It is important to note, however, that in those pancake astrocytes in which AP-like responses could be recorded, membrane potentials (measured as the potential recorded on rupturing the

patch and establishing whole-cell recording) were between -10 and -40 mV. Even when intracellular contents were dialyzed during whole cell patch-clamp recordings, these cells always assumed potentials close to -40 mV, much more depolarized than required for the initiation of AP-like responses.

Discussion

Stellate and Pancake Astrocytes Express Different Na^+ Current Types

Na^+ currents were expressed in almost all stellate astrocytes regardless of time in vitro, and in pancake astrocytes after >3 DIV and up to 37 DIV, the latest timepoint examined. Because pancake astrocytes expressed the largest densities of currents in a time window of 6–10 DIV (Sontheimer et al. 1992), and because during this period cells were small enough to obtain sufficient voltage control, we obtained most of our data characterizing Na^+ currents during this time period. Stellate astrocytes showed Na^+ currents that were similar to Na^+ currents most typically recorded in cultured neurons (Carbone and Lux 1986; MacDermott and Westbrook 1986; Sontheimer et al. 1991b). Currents were transient and showed fast activation and inactivation, threshold for activation was around -40 mV, and largest currents were evoked close to -10 mV. Furthermore, the Na^+-current steady-state inactivation (h_∞) curves had midpoints close to -65 mV. In contrast, in pancake astrocytes the activation curve was ~ 10 mV more negative, with activation threshold at -50 mV, and a peak at -20 mV. Additionally, the midpoints of h_∞ curves were centered close to -85 mV, ~ 20 mV more negative than in stellate astrocytes.

Similar differences in Na^+ current properties have been reported for the two types of rat optic nerve (RON) astrocytes cultured from RON

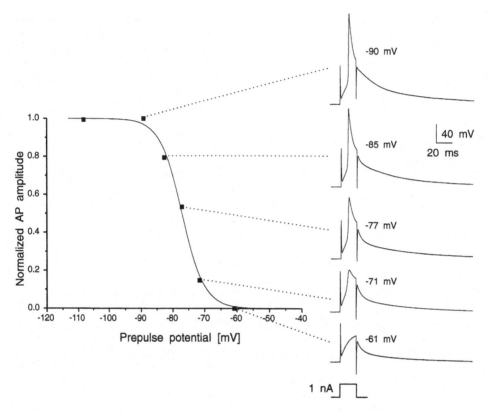

Figure 17.9

Voltage dependence of action-potential (AP)-like responses. To study the voltage dependence of AP-like responses in pancake astrocytes, we obtained current-clamp recordings as described in the legend to Fig. 10 of the companion paper (Sontheimer et al. 1992), and recordings from the same cell are displayed. Constant-current injections of 1 nA were applied at various prepulse potentials ranging from −61 to −110 mV. At −61 mV the current step depolarized the membrane but did not elicit an AP-like response; at −71 mV, a small response could be elicited with an amplitude of ∼55 mV. At −77 mV the AP-like nature of the response became apparent, with an amplitude of 105 mV and an overshooting peak close to 30 mV. Largest responses were observed at potentials more negative than −90 mV, where the peak of the response was close to E_{Na}. Amplitudes of AP-like responses recorded in this way were normalized to the largest response (at −90 mV) and plotted as a function of membrane potential. Data were fit to the Boltzmann equation (——) and yielded a midpoint at −77.1 mV. Although membrane potentials more negative than −70 mV were required to allow AP-like responses to occur in this cell, the membrane potential was only −25 mV, much more depolarized than required for the initiation of AP-like responses.

(Barres et al. 1989; Sontheimer et al. 1991a). In comparing activation and h_∞ curves of RON astrocytes to retinal ganglion cells, Barres et al. (1989) concluded that type 1 RON astrocyte Na^+ channels have different properties not only from type 2 astrocytes, but also from neurons, and thus termed the Na^+ channels in type 1 RON astrocytes a "glial type" of Na^+ channel. RON type 2 astrocytes showed currents that were very similar to those expressed by ganglion cells and these were therefore termed "neuronal type" Na^+ channels. Characteristics of Na^+ currents were also described for rat cerebral astrocytes (Bevan et al. 1985, 1987), and Na^+ currents in these astrocytes had h_∞ midpoints close to -80 mV, similar to spinal cord pancake astrocytes or RON type 1 astrocytes. From all these studies it appears that most flat, non-process-bearing astrocytes express similar Na^+ current types, which are different from typical neuronal Na^+ currents. However, in hippocampal cultures flat, non-process-bearing astrocytes sequentially expressed both types of Na^+ currents. At 1–5 DIV, hippocampal astrocytes expressed "neuronal type" Na^+ currents, whereas at 6–20 DIV Na^+ currents were of the "glial" type (Sontheimer et al. 1991b).

Changes in activation (I–V) and h_∞ curves, similar to the differences described here between stellate and pancake astrocytes, can be observed in response to changes in temperature and $[pH]_0$ (Carbone and Lux 1986). However, because the two current types observed in the present study could always be recorded on the same cover slip and in adjacent cells, they cannot be accounted for by these factors. Several types of Na^+ currents with similar properties and h_∞ midpoints close to -80 and -55 mV have been observed in DRG neurons, either within different size classes of DRG neurons or within the same cell (Caffrey et al. 1991, 1992; Kostyuk et al. 1981; McLean et al. 1988; Roy and Narahashi 1991, 1992; Schwartz et al. 1990). In contrast to pancake astrocytes, the Na^+ channels in DRG neurons mediating currents with an h_∞ curve midpoint at

-80 mV were considerably slower than Na^+ channels mediating currents with a midpoint at -65 mV. Our recordings indicate that both types of Na^+ currents were almost equally fast in terms of activation and inactivation in spinal cord astrocytes. These observations suggest that various subtypes of Na^+ channels, with different voltage dependence of inactivation, exist in neurons and glia. Because Na^+ channels with the hyperpolarized h_∞ curve have been observed in both neurons and glial cells, it is not clear whether it is appropriate to use nomenclature that divides Na^+ channels into "glial" and "neuronal" types on the basis of h_∞ curves. Nevertheless, the combination of low TTX sensitivity (see below) and negative h_∞ curve, which characterizes Na^+ currents in pancake cells, has not been described for excitable cells to date, and thus suggests that it may represent an isoform of Na^+ channel unique to astrocytes.

HH Parameters and Na^+-Channel Densities

In determining the HH parameters for Na^+ currents (τ_h, τ_m, h_∞, and m_∞), we were surprised that the two astrocyte types require different models to fit the observed Na^+ conductances. Pancake astrocyte Na^+ conductances could be fit well to an m^3h model, as proposed for Na^+ currents in the squid giant axon (Hodgkin and Huxley 1952). In contrast, Na^+ conductances in stellate cells were better fit by a m^4h model. These differences could not be explained by insufficient voltage clamp for two reasons: 1) Na^+ currents showed a clear reversal potential that was close to E_{Na}, and 2) time-to-peak was fast (<800 μs at V_m more positive than -30 mV) and similar in both cell types.

Na^+ currents that follow different HH kinetics have been reported previously. In rabbit nodes of Ranvier, Na^+ currents were best fit to m^2h kinetics, whereas frog nodal Na^+ currents followed m^3h kinetics (Chiu et al. 1979). The physiological implications of differences in the power term are twofold. 1) Na^+ currents are faster in cells with m^3h than with m^4h characteristics, because the rise of the activation term m^p is steeper. This is illustrated in figure 17.10 (*inset*), where the rise of Na^+ conductance is plotted for various powers of m in the absence of inactivation. With higher values for m the rise is slower. 2) Peak Na^+ conductances increase with decreasing powers of m. This is indicated in figure 17.10 where the Na^+ conductance from a pancake cell was superimposed by a series of calculated conductances in which the power term p of the HH model (m^ph) was varied for constant values of τ_m and τ_h. The data could be fit best to a kinetic model with p values close to 3 (3.2). The model predicts differences in peak Na^+ conductances at constant channel density (the amplitude factor was constant) for different values of p. In fact, increasing p from 3 to 4 decreases peak conductance by $\sim$30% at constant channel density. Because the largest conductances recorded in both astrocyte types were about equal, we have to assume that channel densities were actually greater in stellate cells (m^4h) than in pancake cells (m^3h).

Na^+ Channels of Stellate and Pancake Astrocytes Have Different TTX Sensitivity

Interestingly, we found that the forms of Na^+ channels expressed in the two astrocyte morphologies also differed markedly in their TTX sensitivity. Although Na^+ channels in both types of cell could be blocked by high concentrations of TTX, Na^+ currents in stellate astrocytes, which were characterized by an h_∞ midpoint of -60 mV, were highly sensitive to TTX (average $K_d = 5.7$ nM). In contrast, pancake astrocytes, which showed h_∞ midpoints close to -85 mV, were up to 1,000-fold more resistant to TTX (average $K_d = 1,007$ nM). Na^+ channels with comparatively low TTX sensitivities have also been described in rat (Bevan et al. 1985, $K_d = 520$ nM) and mouse (Nowak et al. 1987, $K_d = 400$ nM) cerebral astrocytes. A difference in TTX sensitivity characterizes two Na^+ channel types in DRG neurons (Caffrey et al. 1991, 1992;

Kostyuk et al. 1981; Roy and Narahashi 1991). In contrast to spinal cord astrocytes, the relationship between TTX sensitivity and h_∞ characteristics is reversed in DRG neurons. In DRG neurons the TTX-sensitive Na^+ current is characterized by h_∞ curves with midpoints close to -85 mV (Caffrey et al. 1991; Kostyuk et al. 1981) compared with -65 mV in stellate spinal cord astrocytes, and the TTX-resistant Na^+ current in DRGs had h_∞ midpoints close to -50 mV compared with -85 mV in pancake spinal cord astrocytes. Furthermore, the two forms of DRG Na^+ channels differ dramatically with regard to current inactivation, which is about one order of magnitude slower for the TTX-resistant Na^+ current. The TTX-resistant Na^+ current in pancake astrocytes was indistinguishable with regards to its kinetics from TTX-sensitive currents in stellate cells. It will be interesting to determine whether differences in TTX sensitivity are also observable in hippocampal and RON astrocytes, both of which have been shown to express two types of Na^+ currents with different h_∞ curves (Barres et al. 1989; Sontheimer et al. 1991*a*, *b*). Schwann cells, the principal glial cells of the peripheral nervous system, show only one form of Na^+ current with h_∞ midpoints close to -70 mV (Chiu 1991; Howe and Ritchie 1990), which, like Na^+ currents in stellate astrocytes, are highly TTX sensitive [$K_d \sim 2$ nm for saxitoxin (Howe and Ritchie 1990); $K_d = 7.1$ nM for TTX (Shrager et al. 1985)].

Na^+ Channels in Stellate and Pancake Astrocytes May Have Different Amino Acid Sequences

The different biophysical and pharmacological characteristics of Na^+ channels in DRGs and spinal cord astrocytes suggest that the Na^+ channels in these neural cells may also differ in other respects, possibly including primary amino acid sequence. Studying the type II Na^+ channel, Noda et al. (1989) observed that a single site

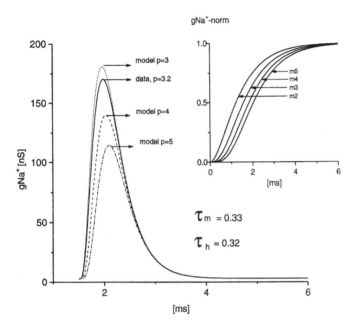

Figure 17.10
Model of Hodgkin-Huxley (HH) parameters for Na$^+$ currents. Pancake astrocyte Na$^+$ conductances could be well fit to an m^3h model as proposed for Na$^+$ currents in the squid giant axon (Hodgkin and Huxley 1952). In contrast, Na$^+$ conductances in stellate cells were better fit by an m^4h model. To illustrate implications of differences in the power term of Na$^+$ current activation (m^p; $2 < p < 5$), we plotted normalized Na$^+$ conductance as a function of time for the HH activation term m raised to the 2nd to 5th power (*inset*). Na$^+$-current activation is faster for smaller powers of m and becomes increasingly slower with increasing powers. Peak Na$^+$ conductances increase with decreasing powers of m. Na$^+$ conductance from a pancake cell (———) was superimposed by a series of calculated conductances in which the power term P of the HH model (m^Ph) was varied for constant values of τ_m and τ_h. Data could best be fit to a kinetic model with P values close to 3 (3.2). Model predicts differences in peak Na$^+$ conductances at constant channel density (the amplitude factor was constant) for different values of P. Increasing P from 3 to 4 decreases peak conductance by $\sim$30%, whereas increasing P from 3 to 5 decreased peak conductance by $>$60%.

(position 387) conferred TTX resistance on the channel. Moreover, the rat heart I (RH-1) and skeletal muscle II (SKM2) Na$^+$ channels, the RNA of which expresses TTX-resistant Na$^+$ channels in oocytes (Cribbs et al. 1990; Krafte et al. 1991), have a glutamine at the same site, i.e., position 387 (Kallen et al. 1990; Rogart et al. 1989). Recently, Yang et al. (1992) expressed the brain IIA Na$^+$ channel a-subunit in Chinese hamster ovary (CHO) cells and rat ventricular myocytes in vitro. Gating properties of the IIA Na$^+$ currents, especially inactivation, were different in CHO cells and cardiac myocytes, suggesting that these properties are modulated by cell-specific post-translational processing of the Na$^+$ channel a-subunit. In contrast, IIA Na$^+$ channels were blocked to 90% by 90 nM TTX in both CHO cells and cardiac myocytes, although the latter cells continued to express endogenous TTX-resistant Na$^+$ channels. These results support the hypothesis that TTX sensitivity, at least in type II Na$^+$ channels, depends on the channels' primary amino acid sequence. If this reasoning applies to Na$^+$ channels in glial cells, it would suggest that pancake and stellate astrocytes express Na$^+$ channels that differ in terms of their primary amino acid sequence. It might also be speculated that differences in the amino acid sequence could confer different fixed-charge properties in the voltage-sensor region of the channel, thus accounting for the differences in HH kinetics (m^3h vs. m^4h) that we observed. Definitive demonstration of differences between channels on the structural level will, however, require molecular cloning approaches.

Mismatch of Resting Potential and h_∞ Curve Prevents Astrocyte Electrogenesis

Pancake astrocytes, which expressed Na$^+$ currents at high densities (>100 pA/pF), were capable of generating AP-like responses under current-clamp recordings in the absence of channel blockers. However, spontaneous AP-like responses were never observed and current

injections were required to depolarize cells by $\sim$20 mV (Sontheimer et al. 1992). The voltage dependence of Na$^+$-channel inactivation required that cells were current clamped to potentials more negative than -70 mV, and peak responses required voltages more negative than -90 mV. The resting potential of these cells was much more depolarized (more positive than -40 mV), explaining why AP-like responses never occurred spontaneously, because Na$^+$ currents were completely inactive at potentials more positive than -50 mV (figure 17.6A) where $h_\infty = 0$. This brings into question the relevance of AP-like responses for astrocytes in vivo. Resting potential measurements were obtained with low-resistance patch-clamp recordings, which may not allow accurate determination of the resting potentials of cells, particularly because ionic gradients are imposed. Two arguments suggest, however, that such errors cannot account for the depolarized membrane potentials observed. *1*) Even 10–15 min after rupturing the patch, when a new equilibrium should have been achieved, membrane potentials usually did not exceed -40 mV, a potential >40 mV more positive than E_K ($E_K = -84$ mV) under the imposed ionic gradients. Assuming that the seal resistance, which always exceeded 5 GΩ, did not change while rupturing the patch, potentials should have been closer to E_{K^+}. *2*) A more likely explanation suggests that the depolarized membrane potentials result from the unusually high pNa$^+$-to-pK$^+$ ratios in these cells, which have a much larger pNa$^+$ than pK$^+$ (Sontheimer et al. 1992). We can only speculate about conditions that could alter the resting potential to more permissive levels. Because a high pNa$^+$ is required to carry the upstroke of the AP, a larger pK$^+$ would be required for a more negative resting potentials. We are currently examining factors that modulate Na$^+$ and K$^+$ channel expression in spinal cord astrocytes.

Regardless of whether AP-like responses occur in astrocytes in vivo, the data presented here suggest that spinal cord astrocytes are, in principle, capable of expressing Na^+ channels at high levels, comparable to cultured neurons. In our previous studies of hippocampal (Sontheimer et al. 1991b), optic nerve (Minturn et al. 1992; Sontheimer et al. 1991a), and cortical astrocytes (unpublished), we never encountered comparable Na^+-channel densities. We are thus encouraged to assume that Na^+-channel expression in astrocytes is heterogeneous and dependent on cell origin. Alternatively, differences in the modulation of channel expression by extrinsic factors could account for the differences observed. Experiments studying the influence of neurons, substrate, and activation of second-messenger pathways on astrocyte Na^+ channel expression are presently underway. Preliminary data suggest that the presence of DRG neurons down-regulates Na^+ channel expression in spinal cord astrocytes (C. L. Thio, H. Sontheimer, and S. G. Waxman, in preparation), suggesting that channel expression is tightly modulated and dependent on environmental factors.

Acknowledgments

The authors thank Dr. Chloe Thio, who recorded some of the TTX data presented, and K. Zur, who assisted with the spinal cord cultures.

This work was supported in part by grants from the National Multiple Sclerosis Society, and the National Institutes of Health and by the Medical Research Service, Department of Veterans Affairs. H. Sontheimer was supported in part by a Spinal Cord Research fellowship from the Eastern Paralyzed Veterans Administration.

References

Barres, B. A., Chun, L. L. Y., and Corey, D. P. Ion channel expression by white matter glia. I. Type 2 astrocytes and oligodendrocytes. *Glia* 1: 10–30, 1988.

Barres, B. A., Chun, L. L. Y., and Corey, D. P. Glial and neuronal forms of the voltage-dependent sodium channel: characteristics and cell type distribution. *Neuron* 2: 1375–1388, 1989.

Barres, B. A., Chun, L. L. Y., and Corey, D. P. Ion channels in vertebrate glia. *Annu. Rev. Neurosci.* 13: 441–474, 1990.

Bevan, S., Chiu, S. Y., Gray, P. T. A., and Ritchie, J. M. The presence of voltage-gated sodium, potassium and chloride channels in rat cultured astrocytes. *Proc. R. Soc. Lond B Biol. Sci.* 225: 299–313, 1985.

Bevan, S., Lindsay, R. M., Perkins, M. N., and Raff, M. C. Voltage gated ionic channels in rat cultured astrocytes, reactive astrocytes and an astrocyte-oligodendrocyte progenitor cell. *J. Physiol. Paris* 82: 327–335, 1987.

Bezanilla, F. and Armstrong, C. M. Inactivation of the sodium channel. I. Sodium current experiments. *J. Gen. Physiol.* 70: 549–566, 1977.

Caffrey, J. M., Brown, L. D., Emanuel, J. G. R., Eng, D. L., Waxman, S. G., and Kocsis, J. D. Na^+ channel isotypes in rat dorsal root ganglion neurons identified by electrophysiological and molecular biological techniques. *Soc. Neurosci. Abstr.* 17: 381, 1991.

Caffrey, J. M., Eng, D. L., Black, J. A., Waxman, S. G., and Kocsis, J. D. Three types of sodium channels in adult rat dorsal root ganglion neurons. *Brain Res.* 592: 283–297, 1992.

Carbone, E. and Lux, H. D. Sodium channels in cultured chick dorsal root ganglion neurons. *Eur. Biophys. J.* 13: 259–271, 1986.

Chiu, S. Y. Functions and distribution of voltage-gated sodium and potassium channels in mammalian Schwann cells. *Glia* 4: 541–558, 1991.

Chiu, S. Y., Ritchie, J. M., Rogart, R. B., and Stagg, D. A quantitative description of membrane currents in rabbit myelinated nerve. *J. Physiol. Lond.* 292: 149–166, 1979.

Cribbs, L. L., Satin, J., Fozzard, H. A., and Rogart, R. B. Functional expression of the rat heart I Na^+ channel isoform: demonstration of properties characteristic of native cardiac Na^+ channels. *FEBS Lett.* 275: 195–200, 1990.

Hodgkin, A. L. and Huxley, A. F. A quantitative description of membrane current and its application to conduction and excitation in nerve. *J. Physiol. Lond.* 117: 500–544, 1952.

Howe, J. R. and Ritchie, J. M. Sodium currents in Schwann cells from myelinated and non-myelinated nerves of neonatal and adult rabbits. *J. Physiol. Lond.* 425: 169–210, 1990.

Ikeda, S. R. and Schofield, G. G. Tetrodotoxin-resistant sodium current of rat nodose neurones: monovalent cation selectivity and divalent cation block. *J. Physiol. Lond.* 389: 255–270, 1987.

Kallen, R. G., Sheng, Z.-H., Yang, J., Chen, L., Rogart, R. B., and Barchi, R. L. Primary structure and expression of a sodium channel characteristic of denervated and immature skeletal muscle. *Neuron* 4: 233–242, 1990.

Kostyuk, P. G., Veselovsky, N. S., and Tsyndrenko, A. Y. Ionic currents in the somatic membrane of rat dorsal root ganglion neurons. I. Sodium currents. *Neuroscience* 6: 2423–2430, 1981.

Krafte, D. S., Volberg, W. A., Dillon, K., and Ezrin, A. M. Expression of cardiac Na$^+$ channels with appropriate physiological and pharmacological properties in *Xenopus* oocytes. *Proc. Natl. Acad. Sci. USA* 88: 4071–4074, 1991.

MacDermott, A. B. and Westbrook, G. L. Early development of voltage-dependent sodium currents in cultured mouse spinal cord neurons. *Dev. Biol.* 113: 317–326, 1986.

McLean, M. J., Bennett, P. B., and Thomas, R. M. Subtypes of dorsal root ganglion neurons based on different inward currents as measured by whole-cell voltage-clamp. *Mol. Cell Biochem.* 80: 95–107, 1988.

Minturn, J. E., Sontheimer, H., Black, J. A., Ransom, B. R., and Waxman, S. G. Sodium channel expression in optic nerve astrocytes chronically-deprived of axonal contact. *Glia* 6: 19–30, 1992.

Noda, M., Suzuki, H., Numa, S., and Stühmer, W. A single point mutation confers tetrodotoxin and saxotoxin insensitivity on the sodium channel II. *FEBS Lett.* 259: 213–216, 1989.

Nowak, L., Ascher, P., and Berwald-Netter, Y. Ionic channels in mouse astrocytes in culture. *J. Neurosci.* 7: 101–109, 1987.

Rogart, R. B., Cribbs, L. L., Muglia, L. K., Kephart, D. D., and Kaiser, M. W. Molecular cloning of a putative tetrodotoxin-resistant rat heart Na$^+$ channel isoform. *Proc. Natl. Acad. Sci. USA* 86: 8170–8174, 1989.

Roy, M.-L. and Narahashi, T. Effects of scorpion venom, sea anemone toxin and chlorpromazine on tetrodotoxin-sensitive and tetrodotoxin-resistant sodium channels. *Soc. Neurosci. Abstr.* 17: 382, 1991.

Roy, M.-L. and Narahashi, T. Differential properties of tetrodotoxin-sensitive and tetrodotoxin-resistant sodium channels in rat dorsal root ganglion neurons. *J. Neurosci.* 12: 2104–2111, 1992.

Schwartz, A., Palti, Y., and Meivi, H. Structural and developmental difference between three types of Na$^+$ channels in dorsal root ganglion cells of newborn rats. *J. Membr. Biol.* 116: 117–128, 1990.

Shrager, P., Chiu, S. Y., and Ritchie, J. M. Voltage-dependent sodium and potassium channels in mammalian cultured Schwann cells. *Proc. Natl. Acad. Sci. USA* 82: 948–952, 1985.

Sontheimer, H. Astrocytes, as well as neurons, express a diversity of ion channels. *Can. J. Physiol. Pharmacol.* 70: 5223–5238, 1992.

Sontheimer, H., Black, J. A., Ransom, B. R., and Waxman, S. G. Ion channels in spinal cord astrocytes in vitro. I. Transient expression of high levels of Na$^+$ and K$^+$ channels. *J. Neurophysiol.* 68: 985–1000, 1992.

Sontheimer, H., Minturn, J. E., Black, J. A., Ransom, B. R., and Waxman, S. G. Two types of Na$^+$-currents in cultured rat optic nerve astrocytes: changes with time in culture and with age of culture derivation. *J. Neurosci. Res.* 30: 275–287, 1991a.

Sontheimer, H., Ransom, B. R., Cornell-Bell, A. H., Black, J. A., and Waxman, S. G. Na$^+$-current expression in rat hippocampal astrocytes in vitro: alterations during development. *J. Neurophysiol.* 65: 3–19, 1991b.

Strichartz, G., Rando, T., and Wang, G. K. An integrated view of the molecular toxinology of sodium channel gating in excitable cells. *Annu. Rev. Neurosci.* 10: 237–267, 1987.

Yang, X. C., Labarca, C., Nargeot, J., Ho, B. Y., Elroy, S. O., Moss, B., Davidson, N., and Lester, H. A. Cell-specific posttranslational events affect functional expression at the plasma membrane but not tetrodotoxin sensitivity of the rat brain IIA sodium channel alpha-sub-unit expressed in mammalian cells. *J. Neurosci.* 12: 268–277, 1992.

XI SPINAL CORD INJURY AND MULTIPLE SCLEROSIS: NEW PATHOLOGIES, NEW THERAPEUTIC TARGETS

One of the exciting things about research is that we keep learning, keep rethinking, and even keep redefining. When I went to medical school, we were taught that spinal cord injury is a disorder in which descending and ascending axons within the spinal cord are severed as a result of trauma. And we were also taught that multiple sclerosis is a "demyelinating" disease, in which the myelin insulation surrounding axons is lost and never replaced. These teachings about pathology were accompanied by a nihilistic approach to therapy: severed axons and missing myelin, we were told, meant that spinal cord injury and multiple sclerosis could not be treated. The following papers challenge these teachings.

Spinal cord injury comes in several forms: penetrating injuries are most common during military conflicts, and result from missile wounds, stab injuries, and similar forms of trauma. During peacetime, most spinal cord injuries arise from motor vehicle accidents, athletic injuries and falls, and are non-penetrating. There were hints, in the classical medical literature, that in nonpenetrating injuries some axons might survive and maintain their continuity through the area of damage. But these early reports were eclipsed by growing interest in the biology of severed nerve fibers and in strategies that might promote the regrowth of severed spinal cord axons and their reconnection with appropriate targets. If achieved, this would be a major step forward toward the restoration of function in people with spinal cord injuries. In Waxman (1993) I summarized evidence for a second, less severe form of pathology in nonpenetrating spinal cord injury: a population of axons that survives and runs through the level of damage, even in patients who are classified as "clinically complete" (i.e. who have lost all motor and sensory function below the level of the injury and appear, on clinical grounds, to have severed their spinal cords). These residual axons have not been severed. But they are unable to function because they have lost their myelin.

The nervous system possesses significant redundancy, and the spinal cord is no exception. It has been estimated that, if only ten percent of the descending motor axons were to survive and retain function after a spinal cord injury, an afflicted individual would retain the capability to stand and walk, albeit with a somewhat clumsy gait. Especially when viewed in the context of redundancy, the redefinition of the pathology of spinal cord injury suggests that restoration of function may be more realistic than previously thought. The presence of surviving but demyelinated axons within the injured spinal cord presents the challenge: can we coax these axons to conduct impulses successfully from one end to the other, despite the loss of myelin? Part IX describes attempts to develop drugs that restore secure impulse conduction in demyelinated fibers. And as described in part XVIII, research efforts around the world are now examining cell transplantation as a strategy for producing myelin around demyelinated spinal cord axons, in an attempt to promote recovery of impulse conduction in them. Therapeutic nihilism has been replaced by an active search for treatments that will reverse paralysis and sensory loss after injury to the spinal cord.

We are also redefining our understanding of multiple sclerosis. Virtually every textbook of neurology classifies multiple sclerosis as a "demyelinating disease," with the brunt of the injury being borne by the myelin and/or the oligodendrocyte, the cell that forms myelin within the central nervous system. There is now evidence, however, that nerve fibers also degenerate in multiple sclerosis (McDonald, Miller, and Barnes 1992; Trapp et al. 1998). As outlined in Waxman (1998), axonal degeneration may not be bad news. We know a lot about how axons respond to injury and may be able to devise strategies that protect them so that they do not degenerate (Stys, Waxman, and Ransom 1992; Stys, Ransom, and Waxman 1992; Fern et al. 1993, 1994; George, Glass, and Griffin 1995). This approach is discussed in part XV.

Axonal degeneration is not the only maladaptive neuronal change in disorders that have been thought to be "demyelinating." Just prior to writing this book, my colleagues and I demonstrated changes in sodium channel expression in a genetic model of demyelination (Black et al. 1999). Remarkably, in this model, Purkinje neurons in the cerebellum produce the wrong type of sodium channels, Sensory Neuron Specific (SNS) sodium channels. SNS channels are normally not present in Purkinje cells, which are responsible for coordination, and if present should alter their behavior. In the months following delivery of the manuscript to the publisher we demonstrated abnormal expression of sodium channels within neurons in two other "demyelinating" diseases. Using in situ hybridization and immunocytochemistry, we first studied chronic-relapsing experimental allergic encephalomyelitis (EAE), a model of multiple sclerosis in mice prepared by David Baker at the Institute of Neurology, London. These experiments showed us that SNS channels are present within Purkinje cells of mice with EAE. We also studied precious human tissue, obtained post mortem by Jia Newcombe and Louise Cuzner at the Institute of Neurology, and found SNS channels within Purkinje cells in patients with multiple sclerosis (Black et al. 2000). These results suggest that there is an "acquired channelopathy" in multiple sclerosis, a molecular abnormality that is likely to result in distorted impulse trafficking in the affected neurons. This could have important therapeutic implications—drugs that selectively modulate various sodium channel subtypes should soon be available, and may restore relatively normal electrogenic properties in these neurons, thereby reversing some of the symptoms in multiple sclerosis (Waxman 2000).

The idea that molecular changes in neurons contribute to symptoms in multiple sclerosis, and the suggestion that it may be possible to develop new therapeutic strategies that target neurons, rather than myelin, are still speculative. I am not convinced, however, that it is bad to speculate. One of the gifts of my teacher Norman Geschwind was his willingness to put new ideas—right or wrong—on the table where they could stimulate discussion and research; and my friend Hal Weintraub, a remarkably innovative molecular biologist, once told me "I know I'm doing creative science if I feel anxious—I have to be near the edge." Part of the value—and part of the fun of science—comes from suggesting new ideas, trying new things, and taking new risks.[1]

References

Black, J. A., Fjell, J., Dib-Hajj, S., Duncan, I. D., O'Connor, L. T., Fried, K., Gladwell, Z., Tate, S., and Waxman, S. G. Abnormal expression of SNS/PN3 sodium channel in cerebellar Purkinje cells following loss of myelin in the taiep rat. *NeuroReport* 10: 913–918, 1999.

Black, J. A., Dib-Hajj, S., Baker, D., Newcombe, J., Cuzner, M. L., and Waxman, S. G. Sensory Neuron Specific sodium channel (SNS) is abnormally expressed in the brains of mice with experimental allergic encephalomyelitis and humans with multiple sclerosis. *Proc. Natl. Acad. Sci. U.S.A.*, in press.

Fern, R., Ransom, B. R., Stys, P. K., and Waxman, S. G. Pharmacological protection of CNS white matter during anoxia: Actions of phenytoin, carbamazepine and diazepam. *J. Pharmacol. Exper. Ther.* 266: 1549–1555, 1993.

Fern, R., Waxman, S. G., and Ransom, B. R. Modulation of anoxic injury in CNS white matter by adenosine and GABA. *J. Neurophysiol.* 72: 2609–2616, 1994.

George, E. B., Glass, J. D., and Griffin, J. W. Axotomy-induced axonal degeneration is mediated by calcium influx through ion-specific channels. *J. Neurosci.* 15: 6445–6452, 1995.

McDonald, W. I., Miller, D. H., and Barnes, D. The pathological evolution of multiple sclerosis. *Neuropathol. Appl. Neurobiol.* 18: 319–334, 1992.

1. This chapter was revised in the proof stage, in July 2000, to incorporate new research results. It illustrates the rapid pace of progress in neuroscience.

Stys, P. K., Ransom, B. R., and Waxman, S. G. Tertiary and quaternary local anesthetics protect CNS white matter from anoxic injury at concentrations that do not block excitability. *J. Neurophysiol.* 67: 236–240, 1992.

Stys, P. K., Waxman, S. G., and Ransom, B. R. Ionic mechanisms of anoxic injury in mammalian CNS white matter: role of Na^+ channels and Na^+-Ca^{2+} exchanger. *J. Neurosci.* 12: 430–439, 1992.

Trapp, B. D., Peterson, J., Ransohoff, R. M., Rudick, R., Mörk, S., and Bö, L. Axonal transection in the lesions of multiple sclerosis. *N. Engl. J. Med.* 338: 278–285, 1998.

Waxman, S. G. Aminopyridines and the treatment of spinal cord injury. *J. Neurotrauma* 10: 19–24, 1993.

Waxman, S. G. Demyelinating diseases: new pathological insights, new therapeutic targets. *N. Engl. J. Med.* 338: 323–325, 1998.

Waxman, S. G. Multiple sclerosis as a neuronal disease. *Arch. Neurol.* 57: 22–24, 2000.

18 Aminopyridines and the Treatment of Spinal Cord Injury

Stephen G. Waxman

Research on the treatment of spinal cord injury is in an exciting phase. Progressing in close parallel are several approaches that hold promise of providing more effective treatment of acute injuries and restoring function in patients with chronically-injured spinal cords. One rapidly-advancing research area focuses on understanding, and limiting, secondary injury after trauma to the central nervous system (CNS). In this area, there has been exciting progress in terms of understanding the roles of excitatory transmitters (Choi, 1988; Faden and Simon, 1988) and of calcium (Ballentine and Spector, 1977; Young and Koreh, 1986; Waxman et al., 1991) and free radicals (Hall and Braughler, 1993) in producing secondary injury after trauma to the spinal cord. The complexity of the cascade of events, which leads from the initial traumatic insult to eventual irreversible dysfunction of nerve cells and their axonal processes, provides a multiplicity of opportunities for therapeutic intervention.

A second avenue of research focuses on regeneration and plasticity of the CNS. It is becoming increasingly clear that, under the right circumstances, neurites within the brain and spinal cord may have the capability to regrow, at least over short domains, and to establish functional synaptic connections with target neurons (Aguayo et al., 1990; Bray et al., 1991). Our understanding of inhibition and promotion of CNS axon regeneration by Schwann cells (Bunge, 1991), oligodendrocytes (Cadelli and Schwab, 1991), and astrocytes (Liesi and Silver, 1988) is increasing. The role of immediate early (early response) genes in CNS regeneration is also being elucidated (de Felipe et al., 1993; Sagar and Sharp, 1993), and there is evidence suggesting that, during neurite regeneration, intranuclear

Reprinted with permission from *Journal of Neurotrauma* 10: 19–24, 1993.

calcium transients may be involved in the activation of these genes (Birch et al., 1992), which suggests that their activation may be subject to therapeutic modulation.

A third area of research focuses on the possibility that the function of residual neurons, or circuits of neurons, that have survived the injury may be favorably altered. One approach has examined "fictive locomotion," and the neural circuits (central pattern generators) that underlie this phenomenon, as well as the pharmacologic manipulation of these circuits (Grillner and Dubuc, 1988). A second approach, which utilizes pharmacologic manipulation of injured axons to enhance their ability to transmit action potentials, has arisen from the delineation of the molecular architecture of myelinated axons within CNX white matter (Waxman and Ritchie, 1993). This approach is being actively explored by a number of research groups. In this issue Hansebout et al. (1993) report an important advance in this approach: their article provides initial data suggesting that aminopyridine drugs, which block a specific type of K^+ channel, may enhance the conduction of action potentials and thus improve clinical status in humans with spinal cord injury.

Early electrophysiologic studies in the mammalian peripheral nervous system (PNS) demonstrated that repolarization of the action potential in myelinated axons is not prolonged by exposure to 4-aminopyridine (4-AP) (Ritchie, 1982; Kocsis et al., 1982; Eng et al., 1988). Following the early studies in PNS, this approach was extended to the CNS, and it was demonstrated that 4-AP has a much smaller effect on action potential repolarization in mature CNS myelinated axons than in their premyelinated precursors (Kocsis and Waxman, 1980; Foster et al., 1982). These observations suggested that 4-AP–sensitive K^+ channels (termed "fast" K^+ channels by some because of their rapid kinetics) are not present, or are present in only low densities, in the axon membrane at the node of Ranvier. Interestingly, the physiologic studies also provided evidence that 4-AP–sensitive K$^+$ channels are located in paranodal or internodal parts of the axon membrane, under the myelin sheath. These studies demonstrated a larger effect of 4-AP on action potential repolarization prior to myelination, than on mature myelinated fibers where the 4-AP–sensitive K$^+$ channels are "masked" by the overlying myelin sheath (Ritchie, 1982; Kocsis et al., 1982; Foster et al., 1982). Voltage-clamp studies on acutely demyelinated axons, which permitted the examination of the internodal axon membrane as the overlying myelin was being damaged, demonstrated the appearance of a voltage-dependent K$^+$ conductance concomitant with demyelination (Chiu and Ritchie, 1980; Chiu and Ritchie, 1981).

The demonstration that fast K$^+$ channels are present in the internodal axon membrane under the myelin, and the recognition that these channels could become functional following demyelination, led to the hypothesis that fast K$^+$ channels "clamp" the membrane close to the K$^+$ equilibrium potential E$_k$, thus opposing depolarization and interfering with conduction in demyelinated axons. This reasoning further suggested that pharmacologic blockade of fast K$^+$ channels might produce a prolongation of the action potential that would increase the safety factor and thereby enhance conduction in demyelinated axons (Schauf and Davis, 1974; Davis and Schauf, 1981; Sears and Bostock, 1981). The early research demonstrated that K$^+$ channel blockade might enhance action potential conduction not only within demyelinated regions, but also at the transition zones at the boundary between normal demyelinated regions; thus, biophysical studies suggested that 4-AP should facilitate invasion of impulses into focally demyelinated axon regions (Waxman and Wood, 1984).

In experimentally demyelinated peripheral nerve, Bostock and co-workers (Sherratt et al., 1980; Bostock et al., 1981) showed that 4-AP increases the temperature at which conduction block occurs in demyelinated ventral root axons, in some cases reversing conduction block at physiologic temperatures. In experiments at the single-fiber level, Targ and Kocsis (1985) demonstrated the reversal of conduction block, with restoration of secure impulse conduction, following treatment of experimentally-demyelinated sciatic nerve axons with 4-AP. These early basic findings were rapidly followed by clinical studies, which showed that 4-AP can produce transient improvements in clinical status in patients with inflammatory demyelinating diseases at doses that do not produce unacceptable adverse effects. For example, Stefoski et al. (1987) observed transient improvement in visual fields and critical flicker fusion frequency in multiple sclerosis patients following intravenous treatment with 4-AP. More recently, Davis et al. (1990) observed similar improvements following oral administration of 4-AP. Based on a similar rationale (increased duration of the action potential, which is normally terminated by fast K$^+$ channels localized in nonmyelinated preterminal axons close to synaptic terminals), the aminopyridines have been studied as possible symptomatic therapies for the treatment of the Lambert-Eaton syndrome, and clinical improvement has been observed at clinically acceptable doses (Lundh et al., 1984; McEvoy et al., 1989).

These findings are part of the background for an important set of observations on spinal cord injury, published in this and other journals over the past several years, that culminate in this issue's study by Hansebout et al. (1993). These investigations have provided evidence that, in some cases of spinal cord injury and spinal cord compression in both experimental animals (Gledhill et al., 1973; McDonald, 1974; Harrison and McDonald, 1977; Blight, 1983*a*; Griffiths and McCulloch, 1983) and in humans (Byrne and Waxman, 1990; Bunge et al., 1993), there is demyelination of axons that maintain continuity through the lesion. The function of these demyelinated spinal cord axons has been studied in electrophysiologic investigations (Blight, 1983b) in experimental animals. These studies have demonstrated decreased conduction velocity, prolonged refractory period, and decreased safety factor consistent with the presence of demyelination. In some patients in whom spinal cord injury appears to be clinically complete, these observations provided pathologic and physiologic correlates for the presence of residual descending influences on spinal reflex activity that could be elicited by careful examination (Dimitrijevic, 1988).

Molecular reorganization of demyelinated spinal cord axons has been observed in immunocytochemical studies. These studies have demonstrated that these axons can acquire higher than normal densities of Na^+ channels within several weeks after loss of the myelin sheath (Black et al., 1991). A variety of investigations suggest that this type of membrane plasticity can facilitate the recovery of conduction through demyelinated axons (Bostock and Sears, 1978; Waxman and Brill, 1978); microelectrode studies in the spinal cord have, in fact, demonstrated that action potentials will propagate within spinal cord axons, suggesting Na^+ channel reorganization following demyelination (Black et al., 1991). The uniquely high Na^+ channel densities expressed by spinal cord astrocytes under some conditions (Sontheimer et al., 1992) and the plasticity of Na^+ channel expression, which in spinal cord astrocytes is subject to very strong modulation by neuronal factors (Thio et al., 1993), are consistent with the idea that astrocytes play a role in the recovery of conduction in demyelinated axons after injury to the spinal cord. It has been speculated that astrocytes may synthesize Na^+ channels that are subsequently transferred to demyelinated axons (Bevan et al., 1985; Gray and Ritchie, 1985) or may participate in the anchoring of Na^+ channels along demyelinated axons (Waxman, 1993).

Studies by Blight (1989) demonstrated that conduction block in demyelinated axons within the injured spinal cord is labile and can be overcome with 4-AP. Administration of 4-AP in dogs with experimental and nonexperimental spinal cord injuries produced significant improvement in behavioral function (Blight et al., 1991). In the context of these important observations in isolated spinal cords and in subhuman models of spinal cord injury, it is natural to ask whether 4-AP might prove beneficial in human spinal cord injury. Hansebout et al. (1993) hint that ion channel modulation with aminopyridines may provide an approach to the symptomatic therapy of spinal cord injury that merits careful exploration.

In this study, 4-AP was administered, using a randomized, double-blind crossover design, to eight patients with chronic spinal cord injury. 4-AP was given in escalating total doses that ranged from 18 to 33.5 mg IV. Beneficial effects were not detected in the two patients with complete paraplegia who were studied. In five of the six patients with incomplete spinal cord injury, however, the researchers reported significant transient neurologic improvement. This included improvement in sensory scores, as well as reduction in spasticity and in chronic pain and dysesthesias in the lower extremities. There was a tendency toward improvement in motor scores, although this did not reach a statistically significant level in this initial study of a small number of cases. Surprisingly, some of the changes in neurologic status persisted for as long as 48 hours.

As pointed out by its researchers, this study is just a first step; further studies on 4-AP in spinal cord injured patients are clearly needed. Despite this cautionary note, this study is an important one. It emphasizes, as did the earlier studies on multiple sclerosis, that in patients with disorders involving CNS axons, clinical status may be predictably improved on the basis of pharmacologic manipulation of ion channels. For at least some patients with incomplete and dyscomplete spinal cord injury, it may thus be possible to develop symptomatic therapies which will transiently improve neurologic status, thus providing a degree of symptomatic relief.

Much work remains to be done along these lines. These early studies in humans must be repeated. Larger numbers of patients must be studied and the results must be confirmed by other workers. Clearly, it will be important to study pharmacokinetics and dose-response curves for 4-AP in spinal cord injured patients. Other related drugs, such as 3,4-diaminopyridine, may also merit study. Important questions remain concerning the mechanism of action of 4-AP in spinal cord injury: while the early physiologic studies suggest that 4-AP enhances conduction by blocking fast K^+ channels in demyelinated axons, this would not explain (assuming that pharmacokinetics are not altered) the long duration of the changes that were observed in this preliminary study. This raises the question of mechanisms of action that involve synaptic modulation, unmasking of previously silent pathways, or other unanticipated actions of 4-AP. Nootropic effects, and generalized arousal, will have to be differentiated from improved conduction in demyelinated axons. Thus, it will be important to carefully monitor the response to 4-AP in chronically treated patients. Careful electrophysiologic study of spinal cord injury patients, together with biochemical, neuroendocrine, and immunologic studies may provide some clues; K^+ channels are present in many types of cells, and blockade of these channels could have widespread effects. Appropriate studies will have to be performed to rule out mutagenic, carcinogenic, and teratogenic effects.

Selective improvement in sensory function following treatment with 4-AP, and the long-lasting reductions in spasticity and in chronic pain and dysesthesias that were reported, raise some interesting questions about the interaction of 4-AP with various types of axons. The decrease in vibratory sensation seen by Hansebout et al. (1993) may provide some clues about mechanisms of drug action. It is now well-established (Bowe et al., 1985) that there are differences in the ion channel organization of mammalian sensory versus motor axons, and recent studies (Stys et al., 1992c; Kampe et al., 1992; Scholz et al., 1992) suggest that the repertoire of ion channels deployed in mammalian axons may be more complex than currently suspected. If axons in various CNS tracts express different repertoires of ion channels, it may be possible to design pharmacologic interventions that will specifically alter conduction in designated pathways. This would allow selective treatment of symptoms such as spasticity, pain, and sensory loss.

The recent studies on 4-AP in humans should add to the excitement that pervades spinal cord injury research. The leap from bench to bedside will not be an easy one, and we must be cautious as we move ahead. Nevertheless, the study by Hansebout et al. suggests that we may be closer than we think to making that important leap.

References

Aguayo, A. J., Carter, D. A., Zwimpfer, T., Vidal-Sanz, M., and Bray, G. M. (1990). Axonal regeneration and synapse formation in the injured CNS of adult mammals. In: *Brain Symposium Series*. A. J. Björklund, A. J., Aguayo, and D. Ottoson (eds.). Stockton Press: New York, Vol. 56, pp. 252–272.

Ballentine, J. D., and Spector, M. (1977). Calcification of axons in experimental spinal cord trauma. Ann. Neurol. 2: 520–523.

Bevan, S., Chiu, S. Y., Gray, P. T. A., and Ritchie, J. M. (1985). The presence of voltage-gated sodium, potassium and chloride channels in rat cultured astrocytes. Proc. Roy. Soc. Lond. B225: 229–313.

Birch, B., Eng, D. L., and Kocsis, J. D. (1992). Intranuclear Ca^{2+} transients during neurite regeneration in adult mammalian neuron. Proc. Natl. Acad. Sci., USA 89: 7978–7982.

Black, J. A., Felts, P., Smith, K. J., Kocsis, J. D., and Waxman, S. G. (1991). Distribution of sodium channels in chronically demyelinated spinal cord axons: Immuno-ultrastructural localization and electrophysiological observations. Brain Res. 544: 59–70.

Blight, A. R. (1983a). Cellular morphology of chronic spinal cord injury in the cat: Analysis of myelinated axons by line-sampling. Neuroscience 10: 521–543.

Blight, A. R. (1983b). Axonal physiology of chronic spinal cord injury in the cat: Intracellular recording in vitro. Neuroscience 10: 1471–1486.

Blight, A. R. (1989). Effect of 4-AP on axonal conduction block in chronic spinal cord injury. Brain Research Bull. 22: 47–52.

Blight, A. R., Toombs, J. P., Bauer, M. S., and Widmer, W. R. (1991). The effects of 4-aminopyridine on neurological deficits in chronic cases of traumatic spinal cord injury in dogs: A Phase I clinical trial. J. Neurotraum. 8(2): 103–119.

Bostock, H., and Sears, T. A. (1978). The internodal axon membrane: Electrical excitability and continuous conduction in segmental demyelination. J. Physiol. Lond. 280: 273–301.

Bostock, H., Sears, T. A., and Sherratt, R. M. (1981). The effects of 4-aminopyridine and tetraethylammonium ions on normal and demyelinated mammalian nerve fibers. J. Physiol. (Lond.) 313: 301–315.

Bowe, C. M., Kocsis, J. D., and Waxman, S. G. (1985). Differences between mammalian ventral and dorsal spinal roots in response to blockade of potassium channels during maturation. Proc. Roy. Soc. Lond. B224: 355–366.

Bray, G. M., Villegas-Pérez, M. P., Vidal-Sanz, M., Carter, D. A., and Aguayo, A. J. (1991). Neuronal and nonneuronal influences on retinal ganglion cell survival, axonal regrowth and connectivity after axotomy. In: Glial–Neuronal Interaction. N. J. Abbott (ed). New York Academy of Sciences: New York, pp. 214–228.

Bunge, R. P. (1991). Schwann cells in central regeneration. In: Glial–Neuronal Interaction. N. J. Abbott (ed.). New York Academy of Sciences: New York, pp. 229–233.

Bunge, R. P., Puckett, W. R., Becerra, J. L., Marcillo, A., and Quencer, R. M. (1993). Observations on the pathology of human spinal cord injury. A review and classification of 22 new cases with details from a case of chronic cord compression with extensive focal demyelination. In: Advances in Neurology, Vol. 59. Neural Injury and Regeneration. F. J. Seil (ed.). Raven Press: New York, pp. 75–89.

Byrne, T. N., and Waxman, S. G. (1990). Spinal Cord Compression. F. A. Davis Co.: Philadelphia.

Cadelli, D. S., and Schwab, M. E. (1991). Myelin-associated inhibitors of neurite outgrowth and their role in CNS regeneration. In: Glial–Neuronal Interaction. N. J. Abbott (ed.). New York Academy of Sciences: New York, pp. 234–240.

Chiu, S. Y., and Ritchie, J. M. (1980). Potassium channels in nodal and internodal axonal membrane in mammalian myelinated fibers. Nature 284: 170–171.

Chiu, S. Y., and Ritchie, J. M. (1981). Evidence for the presence of potassium channels in the paranodal region of acutely demyelinated mammalian nerve fibres. J. Physiol. (Lond.) 313: 415–437.

Choi, D. W. (1988). Glutamate neurotoxicity and diseases of the nervous system. Neuron 1: 623–634.

Davis, F. A., and Schauf, C. L. (1981). Approaches to the development of pharmacological interventions in multiple sclerosis. In: Demyelinating Disease: Basic and Clinical Electrophysiology. S. G. Waxman and J. M. Ritchie (eds.). Raven Press: New York, pp. 505–510.

Davis, F. A., Stefoski, D., and Rush, J. (1990). Orally administered 4-aminopyridine improves clinical signs in multiple sclerosis. Ann. Neurol. 27: 186–192.

de Felipe, C., Jenkins, R., O'Shea, R., Williams, T. S. C., and Hunt, S. P. (1993). The role of immediate early genes in the regeneration of the central nervous system. In: Advances in Neurology, Neural Injury and Regeneration. F. J. Seil (ed.). Raven Press: New York, Vol. 59, pp. 263–271.

Dimitrijevic, M. R. (1988). Residual motor functions in spinal cord injury. In: Functional Recovery in Neurological Disease. S. G. Waxman (ed.). Raven Press: New York, pp. 139–155.

Eng, D. L., Gordon, T. R., Kocsis, J. D., and Waxman, S. G. (1988). Development of 4-AP and TEA sensitivities in mammalian myelinated nerve fibers. J. Neurophysiol. 60: 2168–2179.

Faden, A. I., and Simon, R. P. (1988). A potential role for excitotoxins in the pathophysiology of spinal cord injury. Ann. Neurol. 23: 623–626.

Foster, R. E., Connors, B. W., and Waxman, S. G. (1982). Rat optic nerve: Electrophysiological, pharmacological, and anatomical studies during development. Dev. Brain Res. 3: 361–376.

Gledhill, R. F., Harrison, B. M., and McDonald, W. I. (1973). Demyelination and remyelination after acute spinal cord compression. Exp. Neurol. 38: 472–487.

Gray, P. T., and Ritchie, J. M. (1985). Ion channels in Schwann and glial cells. Trends Neurosci. 8: 411–415.

Griffiths, I. R., and McCulloch, M. C. (1983). Nerve fibers in spinal cord impact injuries. 1. Changes in the myelin sheath during the initial five weeks. J. Neurol. Sci. 58: 335–345.

Grillner, S., and Dubuc, R. (1988). Control of locomotion in vertebrates: Spinal and supraspinal mechanisms. In: *Advances in Neurology, Functional Recovery in Neurological Disease*. S. G. Waxman (ed.). Raven Press: New York, Vol. 47, pp. 425–454.

Hall, E. D., and Braughler, J. M. (1993). Free radicals in CNS injury. In: *Molecular and Cellular Approaches to the Treatment of Neurological Disease*. S. G. Waxman (ed.) Raven Press: New York, pp. 81–105.

Hansebout, R. R., Blight, A. R., Fawcett, S., and Reddy, K. (1993). 4-Aminopyridine in chronic spinal cord injury: A controlled, double-blind, crossover study in eight patients. J. Neurotraum. 10: 1–18.

Harrison, B. M., and McDonald, W. I. (1977). Remyelination after transient experimental compression of the spinal cord. Ann. Neurol. 1: 542–551.

Kampe, K., Safronov, B., and Vogel, W. (1992). A Ca-activated and three voltage-dependent K channels identified in mammalian peripheral nerve. Pflügers Arch., Europ. J. Physiol. 420(Suppl. 1), R28.

Kocsis, J. D., and Waxman, S. G. (1980). Absence of potassium conductance in central myelinated axons. Nature 287: 348–349.

Kocsis, J. D., Waxman, S. G., Hildebrand, C., and Ruiz, J. A. (1982). Regenerating mammalian nerve fibres: Changes in action potential waveform and firing characteristics following blockage of potassium conductance. Proc. R. Soc. Lond. B217: 277–287.

Liesi, P., and Silver, J. (1988). Is astrocyte laminin involved in axon guidance in mammalian CNS? Devel. Biol. 130: 774–785.

Lundh, H., Nilsson, O., and Rosen, I. (1984). Treatment of Lambert–Eaton syndrome: 3,4 diaminopyridine and pyridostigmine. Neurol 34: 1324–1330.

McDonald, W. I. (1974). Remyelination in relation to clinical lesions of the central nervous system. Br. Med. Bull. 30: 186–189.

McEvoy, K. M., Windebank, A. J., Daube, J. R., and Low, P. A. (1989). 3,4 Di-aminopyridine in the treatment of Lambert–Eaton myasthenic syndrome. New Engl. J. Med. 321: 1567–1571.

Ritchie, J. M. (1982). Sodium and potassium channels in regenerating and developing mammalian myelinated nerves. Proc. Roy. Soc. B215: 273–287.

Sagar, S. M., and Sharp, F. R. (1993). Early response genes as markers of neuronal activity and growth factor action. In: *Advances in Neurology, Neural Injury and Regeneration*. F. J. Seil (ed.). Raven Press: New York, Vol. 59, pp. 273–284.

Schauf, C. L., and Davis, F. A. (1974). Impulse conduction in multiple sclerosis: A theoretical basis for modification by temperature and pharmacological agents. J. Neurol. Neurosurg. Psychiat. 37: 152–161.

Scholz, A., Reid, G., Bostock, H., and Vogel, W. (1992). Na and K channels in human axons. Pflügers Arch., Europ. J. Physiol. 420(Suppl. 1), R28.

Sears, T. A., and Bostock, H. (1981). Conduction failure in demyelination: Is it inevitable? In: *Demyelinating Diseases: Basic and Clinical Electrophysiology*. S. G. Waxman and J. M. Ritchie (eds.). Raven Press: New York, pp. 357–375.

Sherratt, R. M., Bostock, H., and Sears, T. A. (1980). Effects of 4-aminopyridine on normal and demyelinated mammalian nerve fibers. Nature 283: 570–572.

Sontheimer, H., Black, J. A., Ransom, B. R., and Waxman, S. G. (1992). Ion channels in spinal cord astrocytes in vitro: I. Transient expression of high levels of Na^+ and K^+ channels. J. Neurophysiol. 68: 985–999.

Stefoski, D., Davis, F. A., Faut, M., and Schauf, C. L. (1987). 4-Aminopyridine improves clinical signs in multiple sclerosis. Ann. Neurol. 21: 71–77.

Stys, P. K., Sontheimer, H., Ransom, B. R., and Waxman, S. G. (1992). Non-inactivating, TTX-sensitive Na^+ conductance in rat optic nerve axons: Possible physiological and pathological roles. Abstr. Soc. Neurosci. 18: 1137 (478.25).

Targ, E. F., and Kocsis, J. D. (1985). 4-Aminopyridine leads to restoration of conduction in demyelinated rat sciatic nerve. Brain Res. 328: 358–361.

Thio, C. L., Waxman, S. G., and Sontheimer, H. (1993). Ion channels in spinal cord astrocytes in vitro: III. Modulation of channel expression by co-culture with neurons and neuron-conditioned medium. J. Neurophysiol., 69: 819–831, 1993.

Waxman, S. G. (1993). The perinodal astrocyte: Functional and developmental considerations. In: *Biology and Pathobiology of Astrocyte–Neuron Interactions.* S. Federoff, R. Doucette, and B. H. Juurlink (eds.) Plenum Publishing Corp.: New York, in press.

Waxman, S. G., and Brill, M. H. (1978). Conduction through demyelinated plaques in multiple sclerosis: Computer simulations of facilitation by short internodes. J. Neurol. Neurosurg. Psychiat. 41: 408–417.

Waxman, S. G., Ransom, B. R., and Stys, P. K. (1991). Non-synaptic mechanisms of calcium-mediated injury in CNS white matter. Trends in Neuroscience 14: 461–468.

Waxman, S. G., and Ritchie, J. M. (1993). Molecular dissection of the myelinated axon. Ann. Neurol. 33: 121–136.

Waxman, S. G., and Wood, S. L. (1984). Impulse conduction in inhomogeneous axons: Effects of variation in voltage-sensitive ionic conductances on invasion of demyelinated axon segments and preterminal fibers. Brain Res. 294: 111–122.

Young, W., and Koreh, I. (1986). Potassium and calcium changes in injured spinal cord. Brain Res. 364: 42–53.

19 Demyelinating Diseases—New Pathological Insights, New Therapeutic Targets

Stephen G. Waxman

Virtually every textbook of neurology or general medicine includes chapters on demyelinating diseases, with most of the attention devoted to multiple sclerosis. The concept of multiple sclerosis as a demyelinating disease is deeply ingrained. The early description of multiple sclerosis by Charcot stressed the loss of myelin. The diagnosis of multiple sclerosis rests in part on the demonstration, by measurement of evoked potentials, of slowed action-potential conduction, a physiologic hallmark of demyelination.

The lipid-rich myelin sheath is produced by Schwann cells in peripheral nerves and by oligodendrocytes in the brain and spinal cord, and myelin possesses high electrical resistance and low capacitance and thus acts as an insulator around axons. The myelin is arranged in segments separated by nodes of Ranvier, where sodium channels are clustered in high density in the axon membrane so that they can produce action potentials (figure 19.1A). Myelin covers and masks the internodal parts of the axon, which contain fewer sodium channels and a higher density of potassium channels, which tend to oppose the generation of action potentials. Myelination increases the speed of conduction and improves its metabolic efficiency. Damage to the myelin is accompanied by a decrease in conduction velocity and, when severe, by conduction block (figure 19.1B).[1] In addition, cell-cell interactions between myelin-forming glial cells and their underlying axons actively influence the biochemical properties of the axons; a loss of the myelin is associated with destabilizing changes in the molecular structure of the axonal cytoskeleton.[2]

Multiple sclerosis can take several forms. In the relapsing-remitting type of multiple sclerosis, the patient's course is punctuated by exacerbations or relapses in which there is clinical worsening, but these are followed (within weeks to a few months) by remissions with partial or full recovery from the deficits. The molecular substrate for remissions appears to be provided by a remodeling of the demyelinated (formerly internodal) axonal membrane so that it acquires a higher-than-normal sodium-channel density, which permits conduction of action potentials despite the loss of myelin (figure 19.1C).[3–5] Progressive forms of multiple sclerosis are characterized by a downhill course without remissions, so that the patient acquires more and more clinical deficits, either beginning at presentation (primary progressive form) or after a period of relapsing-remitting disease (secondary progressive form).

Why do the patients with progressive multiple sclerosis not have remissions? An answer to this question might help us to approach the important objective of limiting the development of permanent deficits. In a study reported in this issue of the *Journal*, using confocal microscopy and computer-based, three-dimensional reconstructions, Trapp et al.[6] have provided an elegant demonstration of substantial damage to axons, as well as myelin, in the brains of patients with multiple sclerosis. Using antibodies to nonphosphorylated neurofilaments (a marker of axonal regions that lack myelin), they demonstrate axonal transection throughout active lesions (including acute lesions early in the course of the disease) and within chronic active lesions, particularly at the edges of actively demyelinating lesions, where major-histocompatibility-complex class II–positive inflammatory cells are abundant. They postulate that axonal degeneration (figure 19.1D) is a pathologic correlate of irreversible neurologic impairment in multiple sclerosis.

This demonstration of axonal pathology in multiple sclerosis builds on a history of hints

Reprinted with permission from *The New England Journal of Medicine* 338: 323–325, 1998.

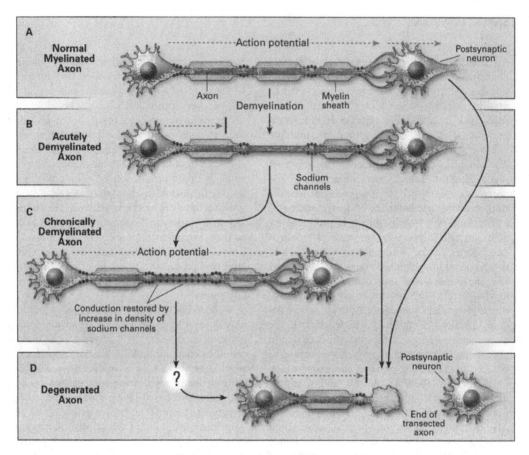

Figure 19.1

Demyelination and axonal degeneration in multiple sclerosis. In a normal myelinated axon (*A*), the action potential (dashed arrow) travels, with high velocity and reliability, to the postsynaptic neuron. In acutely demyelinated axons (*B*), conduction is blocked (black bar). In some chronically demyelinated axons that acquire a higher-than-normal density of sodium channels (*C*), conduction is restored. Axonal degeneration (*D*), by contrast, interrupts action-potential propagation in a permanent manner.

throughout the literature that it is more than just a demyelinating disease. Even Charcot's early description of multiple sclerosis mentioned axonal pathology. In the 1970s, on the basis of more contemporary molecular dissection of myelinated axons, which demonstrated a mutual interdependence of axons and myelin-forming glial cells, some of us speculated that there could be no "pure" demyelinating diseases. McDonald et al.[7] suggested in 1992, on the basis of magnetic resonance imaging and electron microscopy of brain tissue from patients with multiple sclerosis, that as lesions age, there is progressive axonal loss. This group also used magnetic resonance spectroscopy to study cerebellar white matter and found a significant reduction in a neuronal marker (N-acetyl aspartate) that was correlated with the presence of cerebellar deficits; these observations provided evidence that axonal loss is important in the development of persistent neurologic disability in multiple sclerosis.

The studies by Davie et al.[8] and Narayanan et al.[9] also found evidence of axonal degeneration in normal-appearing white matter outside of demyelinating lesions, possibly due to wallerian degeneration of axonal projections that had been disconnected from their origins as a result of transection. Using amyloid precursor protein as a histopathological marker of damaged axons in the brains of patients with multiple sclerosis, Ferguson et al.[10] recently found evidence of axonal injury throughout acute lesions and at the margins of active chronic lesions; like Trapp et al.,[6] they interpret their results as suggesting that axonal damage may be associated with inflammation.

If axonal injury early in the course of disease contributes to the development of irreversible neurologic deficits, the prevention of axonal loss might be expected to prevent persistent disability. Trapp et al.[6] and Ferguson et al.[10] note a relation between axonal injury and inflammation, suggesting that a reduction in the inflammatory response might result in the loss of fewer axons and thus in less clinical deficit. An alternative approach is suggested by studies that have demonstrated that ion channels and exchangers[11-13] together form a "final common pathway," subject to modulation by neurotransmitters,[14] that underlies axonal degeneration after various injuries. Axonal function and integrity can be preserved after acute insults by means of neuroprotective interventions that block or modulate injurious ion fluxes at several stages within this molecular death cascade[12,14,15] or that interfere with "downstream" degenerative events such as activation of calpains and other destructive enzymes.[13] Further studies will be needed to determine whether the reduction in inflammatory responses or the neuroprotection of axons can limit or prevent axonal degeneration in multiple sclerosis and, if so, whether this will reduce or prevent the acquisition of persistent neurologic deficits.

Chapters on "demyelinating" diseases will not necessarily become shorter as a result of the reclassification of multiple sclerosis as an "axonal" disorder. It has recently been recognized that in some patients with traumatic (nonpenetrating) spinal cord injury there are residual axons that maintain continuity through the lesion but fail to conduct impulses as a result of demyelination. These findings have been reported in some patients with "clinically complete" lesions (i.e., those with no function below the level of the lesion), which are classically considered to be due to transection of the spinal cord and its constituent axons within the lesion.[16-18] The demonstration of these preserved, but demyelinated, axons suggests that in spinal cord injury, at least some degree of functional recovery might be achieved by strategies that restore impulse conduction along demyelinated axons.

Recognition that multiple sclerosis is, in part, an axonal disease and that spinal cord injury is, in part, a disorder of myelin should trigger a critical rethinking of these disorders and provides us with new targets for therapy. Ideally, future studies will tell us whether the protection of axons from injury in multiple sclerosis and the repair of demyelinated axons in spinal cord injury are therapeutic strategies that will help preserve neurologic function in patients with these disorders.

References

1. Waxman SG. Pathophysiology of demyelinated and remyelinated axons. In: Cook SD, ed. Handbook of multiple sclerosis. 2nd ed. New York: Marcel Dekker, 1996: 257–94.

2. Kirkpatrick LL, Brady ST. Modulation of the axonal microtubule cytoskeleton by myelinating Schwann cells. J Neurosci 1994; 14: 7440–50.

3. Bostock H, Sears TA. The internodal axon membrane: electrical excitability and continuous conduction in segmental demyelination. J Physiol (Lond) 1978; 280: 273–301.

4. Foster RE, Whalen CC, Waxman SG. Reorganization of the axon membrane in demyelinated peripheral nerve fibers: morphological evidence. Science 1980; 210: 661–3.

5. Felts PA, Baker TA, Smith KJ. Conduction in segmentally demyelinated mammalian central axons. J Neurosci 1997; 17: 7267–77.

6. Trapp BD, Peterson J, Ransohoff RM, Rudick R, Mörk S, Bö L. Axonal transection in the lesions of multiple sclerosis. N Engl J Med 1998; 338: 278–85.

7. McDonald WI, Miller DH, Barnes D. The pathological evolution of multiple sclerosis. Neuropathol Appl Neurobiol 1992; 18: 319–34.

8. Davie CA, Barker GJ, Webb S, et al. Persistent functional deficit in multiple sclerosis and autosomal dominant cerebellar ataxia is associated with axon loss. Brain 1995; 118: 1583–92. [Erratum, Brain 1996; 119: 1415.]

9. Narayanan S, Fu L, Pioro E, et al. Imaging of axonal damage in multiple sclerosis: spatial distribution of magnetic resonance imaging lesions. Ann Neurol 1997; 41: 385–91.

10. Ferguson B, Matyszak MK, Esiri MM, Perry VH. Axonal damage in acute multiple sclerosis lesions. Brain 1997; 120: 393–9.

11. Stys PK, Waxman SG, Ransom BR. Ionic mechanisms of anoxic injury in mammalian CNS white matter: role of Na^+ channels and Na^+–Ca^{2+} exchanger. J Neurosci 1992; 12: 430–9.

12. Stys PK. Anoxic and ischemic injury of myelinated axons in CNS white matter: from mechanistic concepts to therapeutics. J Cereb Blood Flow Metab 1998; 18: 2–25.

13. George EB, Glass JD, Griffin JW. Axotomy-induced axonal degeneration is mediated by calcium influx through ion-specific channels. J Neurosci 1995; 15: 6445–52.

14. Fern R, Ransom BR, Waxman SG. Autoprotective mechanisms in the CNS: some new lessons from white matter. Mol Chem Neuropathol 1996; 27: 107–29.

15. Waxman SG, Ransom BR. Neuroprotection of CNS white matter. In: Bär PR, Beal F, eds. Neuroprotection. New York: Marcel Dekker, 1997: 305–19.

16. Blight AR. Cellular morphology of chronic spinal cord injury in the cat: analysis of myelinated axons by line-sampling. Neuroscience 1983; 10: 521–43.

17. Bunge RP, Puckett WR, Becerra JL, Marcillo A, Quencer RM. Observations on the pathology of human spinal cord injury: a review and classification of 22 new cases with details from a case of chronic cord compression with extensive focal demyelination. Adv Neurol 1993; 59: 75–89.

18. Waxman SG, Kocsis JD. Spinal cord repair: progress towards a daunting goal. Neuroscientist 1997; 3: 263–9.

XII SEEDS OF RECOVERY WITHIN THE SPINAL CORD

It is a remarkable fact that, during development, the entire body and its many billions of constituent cells arise from a single fertilized ovum and that, as part of this process, the more than ten billion nerve cells within the brain and spinal cord develop from primitive, pleuripotent cells called progenitors. One of the more exciting objectives for developmental neuroscience, and a major goal of clinical neuroscience, is to determine whether progenitors, or similar cells, are retained within the adult brain and spinal cord. If so, a more ambitious goal would be to exploit these cells therapeutically so that they differentiate into electrically active nerve cells after injury. If these could be recruited into functional circuits we would be closer to a holy grail of contemporary neuroscience—regeneration of the injured brain and spinal cord.

There are many paths that can lead to this holy grail, and some of them may take advantage of clues from lower species. One of these is the South American knife fish *Sternarchus*, which I learned about while I was a graduate student, working for the summer in Woods Hole. *Sternarchus* lives in the estuaries of the Amazon where it spends its time foraging for food between rocks and plants on the river's floor. *Sternarchus's* tail usually sticks out from among the debris which hide its head, so that it can be seen by predators. A light stripe or band is present on *Sternarchus's* tail (this adornment can be seen in figure 20.1 in Anderson and Waxman 1985), making it, rather than *Sternarchus's* head, an attractive target.

In leaving its tail exposed so that larger fish may devour it, *Sternarchus* is not making an altruistic sacrifice. *Sternarchus* cannot live without its head. But it can survive without a tail, and its tail (which occupies the back one-third of its body) has an extraordinary capability to regenerate or regrow after it has been lost.

Regrowth of the tail of *Sternarchus* is accompanied by regeneration of a new spinal cord. This new spinal cord includes new neurons. Thus, *Sternarchus* presents a unique model of neurogenesis (the generation of new neurons) and regeneration following spinal cord injury in an adult animal. In 1979, encouraged by a request for proposals from the Veterans Administration to examine spinal cord regeneration, I asked Marilyn Anderson, an expert on the growth of nerve fibers and their regrowth after injury, to join our research group so that we could study *Sternarchus* and its capability for spinal cord regeneration. The first step was to establish a colony of *Sternarchus*, some with injured tails, each housed in its own tank in an Amazon-like habitat. Regeneration is not an overnight process; regrowth of the tail occurs at a rate of about one millimeter per week, so we had to wait months before we could study the spinal cords. We were rewarded, however, by results which showed that, following injury to or loss of the spinal cord, *Sternarchus* regenerates a new one which is populated by apparently normal nerve cells with shapes, sizes and axonal branching patterns similar to those in uninjured cells. The new nerve cells, moreover, received synaptic inputs in a normal manner and became functional. We observed that spinal cord regeneration, in contrast to normal growth in *Sternarchus*, is characterized by production of excessive numbers of neurons, but also learned that the cell population is subsequently adjusted by a wave of cell death which kills the supernumerary neurons, leaving a normal number (Anderson, Waxman, and Tadlock 1984; Waxman and Anderson 1985). We also learned that glial scarring does not prevent neuronal regeneration in this species (Anderson et al. 1984).

Having demonstrated that the mature spinal cord, in adult *Sternarchus*, possesses the capability for regeneration, we of course wanted to identify the cells which give rise to the new, regenerated neurons. As a first step we searched for them in tissue culture where, using a molecule called [H^3] thymidine which labels dividing cells, we found that some cells in the spinal cord of adult *Sternarchus* retain the ability to divide and then differentiate into nerve cells, complete with axons (Anderson and Waxman 1985). In fact, 45 percent of the nerve cells that we observed within the cultures had arisen by cell division. Thus it appeared that progenitor cells were present in the adult spinal cord, and that they could survive, divide, and differentiate into nerve cells even after we removed them and placed them in culture. An important next step was to identify these progenitors. By introducing dye molecules that labeled neurons within the *Sternarchus* spinal cord and then culturing them, we were able to show that the neurons themselves were not the progenitors. Which cells, then, were responsible for giving birth to new neurons? Culturing of meticulously dissected fragments of the spinal cord permitted us to localize the progenitor cells to a deep layer of cells, called ependymal cells, which line the fluid-filled central cavity within the spinal cord (Anderson, Waxman, and Fong 1987).

Our studies on neurogenesis in *Sternarchus* were eclipsed a few years later by demonstrations of neurogenesis in adult mammals. It is now well established that progenitor cells, capable of giving rise to neurons, are present within, or just below, the lining of the cavities of the adult mammalian brain, in a location similar to that of ependymal cells (Doetsch et al. 1999). And within a portion of the brain called the hippocampus, there is a population of progenitor cells which can proliferate and give rise to new neurons, even in adulthood. Notably, the rate of neurogenesis in the hippocampus appears to be activity-dependent, and it can be enhanced by learning (Gould et al. 1999) and exposure to an enriched environment (Kempermann, Kuhn, and Gage 1998; Kempermann and Gage 1999). There is also evidence suggesting that transplanted progenitor cells can migrate widely, at least within the young brain, to populate areas that need them (Yandava, Billinghurst, and Snyder 1999). The presence of these progenitor cells within the adult mammalian nervous system has triggered a wave of interest among neuroscientists, since these cells are potentially amenable to being stimulated to divide in vivo by exposure to agents such as growth factors, to clonal expansion in tissue culture, which would provide a supply of cells for transplantation, or to genetic manipulation that would permit them to be "engineered" into designer cells that could be used for specific therapeutic purposes after injury to the brain or spinal cord (see, e.g., Gage, Ray, and Fisher 1995; Morrison et al. 1999).

The mammalian brain and spinal cord, of course, do not rebuild themselves as completely as the spinal cord of *Sternarchus* after injury. But the extraordinary regenerative capability of the *Sternarchus* spinal cord shows us, at a minimum, that rebuilding of the injured brain and spinal cord is not impossible. Progenitor cells—seeds of recovery—are present within the brains and spinal cords of many species, even in adulthood, and the challenge is to utilize them effectively. The nervous systems of lower species may hold some important clues—about facilitatory factors, absent in higher species, that encourage nervous system regeneration; about inhibitory factors in higher species; or about the genes that control cell division by progenitors, for example—that can help us. If we can understand more about the seeds of recovery and the ways they grow within nervous systems that *do* regenerate, perhaps we can come closer to the holy grail of healing injured brains and spinal cords in species that do not regenerate, including our own.

References

Anderson, M. J., Swanson, K. A., Waxman, S. G., and Eng, L. F. Glial fibrillary acidic protein in regenerating teleost spinal cord. *J. Histochem. Cytochem.* 31: 1099–1106, 1984.

Anderson, M. J., and Waxman, S. G. Neurogenesis in tissue cultures of adult teleost spinal cord. *Devel. Brain Res.* 20: 203–212, 1985.

Anderson, M. J., Waxman, S. G., and Fong, H. L. Explant cultures of teleost spinal cord: source of neurite outgrowth. *Devel. Biol.* 119: 601–604, 1987.

Anderson, M. J., Waxman, S. G., and Tadlock, C. H. Cell death of asynaptic neurons in regenerating spinal cord. *Devel. Biol.* 103: 433–455, 1984.

Doetsch, F., Caille, I., Lim, D. A., Garcia-Verduga, J. M., and Alvarez-Buylla, A. Subventricular zone astrocytes are neural stem cells in the adult mammalian brain. *Cell* 97: 703–716, 1999.

Gage, F. H., Ray, J., and Fisher, L. J. Isolation, characterization, and use of stem cells for the CNS. *Annu. Rev. Neurosci.* 18: 159–192, 1995.

Gould, E., Beylin, A., Tanapat, P., Reeves, A., and Shors, T. J. Learning enhances adult neurogenesis in the hippocampal formation. *Nature Neurosci.* 2: 260–265, 1999.

Kempermann, G., and Gage, F. H. New nerve cells for the adult brain. *Sci. Am.* 48–53, 1999.

Kempermann, G., Kuhn, H. G., and Gage, F. H. Experience-induced neurogenesis in the senescent dentate gyrus. *J. Neurosci.* 18: 3206–3212, 1998.

Morrison, S. J., White, P. M., Zock, C., and Anderson, D. J. Prospective identification, isolation by flow cytometry, and in vivo self-renewal of multipotent mammalian neural crest stem cells. *Cell* 96: 737–749, 1999.

Waxman, S. G., and Anderson, M. J. Generation of electromotor neurons in *Sternarchus albifrons*: differences between normal and regenerating spinal cord. *Devel. Biol.* 112: 338–344, 1985.

Yandava, B. D., Billinghurst, L. L., and Snyder, E. Y. "Global" cell replacement is feasible via neural stem cell transplantation: evidence from the dysmyelinated shiverer mouse brain. *Proc. Natl. Acad. Sci. U.S.A.* 96: 7029–7034, 1999.

20 Neurogenesis in Adult Vertebrate Spinal Cord In Situ and In Vitro: A New Model System

Marilyn J. Anderson and Stephen G. Waxman

Introduction

Current clinical management of neurologic disorders, including cerebrovascular disease, degenerative disorders such as amyotrophic lateral sclerosis, and central nervous system trauma, is limited as a result of the fact that, under usual conditions, the number of neurons in the mammalian nervous system is fixed at, or shortly after, birth. Nevertheless, since production of new neurons could, in a manner similar to that of neural transplantation, lead to some degree of functional recovery after damage to the CNS, a number of research groups have recently begun to examine the mechanisms that underlie neurogenesis (production of new neurons) in those sites where it does occur, either as a normal process or in response to CNS injury. To date, the number of demonstrations of postnatal neurogenesis in mammalian CNS has been small; and these have been restricted, moreover, to a limited number of sites, such as rodent olfactory epithelium[1,2] and hippocampus.[3,4] Careful studies of postnatal neurogenesis have also been carried out in other vertebrate systems, such as the telencephalic vocal control nucleus of adult female canaries.[5,6] Nevertheless, the cellular mechanisms controlling postnatal neurogenesis remain poorly understood. In this regard, the development of accessible models of neurogenesis would be of great value.

Phylogenetically lower species in some cases exhibit *compensatory neurogenesis* after injury to the CNS; these species include urodele amphibians and teleosts.[7–10] Furthermore, even though postnatal neurogenesis is absent from most regions of the mammalian CNS, new neurons are produced in adulthood in fish and amphibians.[11] Thus, for example, there is clear evidence

Reprinted with permission from *Annals of the New York Academy of Sciences* 457: 213–233, 1985.

that new neurons are added in the retina[12–14] and its projection zone, the optic tectum,[15–17] in adult fish and amphibia. An increase in the number of neurons in several other areas of postnatal CNS, including spinal cord, has been reported in the guppy,[18] stingray,[19] and gymnotiform teleosts.[29] Since teleosts exhibit compensatory neurogenesis after injury and postnatal neurogenesis during normal growth in the adult, they may provide useful model systems for the study of this process. In the present report, we describe neurogenesis from adult tissue, both in situ and in vitro, in the spinal cord of *Sternarchus albifrons*.

The *Sternarchus* Electromotor System

In the weakly electric gymnotiform teleost *Sternarchus albifrons*, the spinal electromotor system exhibits striking regeneration (figure 20.1) after injury or extirpation in the adult.[9,10,21] In contrast to other vertebrate species in which neurites may regenerate but where neuronal perikarya are not replaced after injury, spinal cord regeneration in *Sternarchus* includes an initial phase of neurogenesis, which is followed by neuronal differentiation and selective neuronal cell death.[22] Synaptic connections, presumably from the appropriate brainstem nuclei, are established with many of these regenerated neurons.[9,22] Moreover, neurogenesis in *Sternarchus* is not limited to the response to injury. In adult *Sternarchus*, ongoing growth of the spinal cord and electric organ, including the production and differentiation of new neurons, occurs concomitant with continued increase in length of the mature adult animal.[20,23] These newly added neurons are contacted by descending axons,[9] and apparently are recruited into functional neural circuits.

The spinal electromotor system in *Sternarchus albifrons*[24–27] contains electromotor neurons (which are specialized spinal motor neurons)

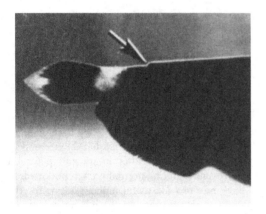

Figure 20.1
Regenerated tail of *Sternarchus albifrons*. Nine months after amputation of the tail. 2.8 cm of tail has regenerated from the amputation site, demarcated by the notch (arrow) at the dorsal surface.

clustered in paired medial columns, located on either side of the central canal and dorsal to the ventral gray matter (figure 20.2*A*). Within the normal spinal cord (except the terminal spinal segment, where neurons are produced; see description below), each transverse section contains profiles of 4–12 electromotor neurons. The cell bodies of electromotor neurons exhibit a characteristic morphologic pattern which permits their identification in normal[28] and regenerated[9,22] spinal cord. In particular, the cells are relatively large and spherical in shape and lack dendrites, and the initial myelin segment extends up to or partially over the cell body so that there is no unmyelinated initial segment. This mode of cell architecture closely reflects the functional role of these cells in terms of firing in response to incoming synaptic information.[28] Cell bodies are contacted by descending bulbospinal axons and are electrically coupled via a presynaptic pathway. While some presumably chemical synapses are present, most axosomatic synapses are characterized by gap junctions.[28,29] Single axons can form gap junctions with several neighboring electromotor neurons.[28] The presynaptic fibers

arise as blunt projections from large myelinated fibers, in some cases forming *en passant* synapses (arising from nodes of Ranvier) with the electromotor neurons. Gap junctions at these synapses are relatively large, often occupying all of the area of apposition between the presynaptic ending and the neuronal cell body. This characteristic morphologic structure facilitates electron microscopic identification of these descending electromotor junctions.

After amputation of the tail in *Sternarchus*, there is a striking degree of spinal cord regeneration.[9,22,30] While individual fish vary significantly with respect to the rate of regeneration, in most fish maintained at 26 °C, 1.0–4.0 cm of tail regenerates in the first year post amputation (figure 20.1). Regeneration of the spinal cord initially occurs at a rate of 0.6–1.5 mm per week; after a period of 3–5 months, the rate slows somewhat. Regenerated cord usually exhibits one or two segmental-type swellings; spinal nerves emerge from the regenerated cord at irregular intervals along the rostral portion. Notably, while ongoing growth of the normal (not operated on) spinal cord occurs in the caudalmost spinal segment (see below), spinal cord regeneration occurs after amputation at levels more than 5 cm rostral to the caudal tip,[30] i.e., from regions of the cord that are no longer actively growing and that are histologically stable. This observation indicates that some cells, even in the mature (rostral) spinal cord, retain the ability to generate new neurons and glia under appropriate conditions.

Compensatory Neurogenesis In Situ

After amputation of the tail, new spinal cord is produced from the regenerated ependymal tube, which is continuous with ependymal tube surrounding the central canal in the spinal cord at the site of injury.[30] Neurogenesis occurs in the caudal region (limited to the caudalmost several millimeters) of the regenerating cord, while rostral to this, cells differentiate into neurons and

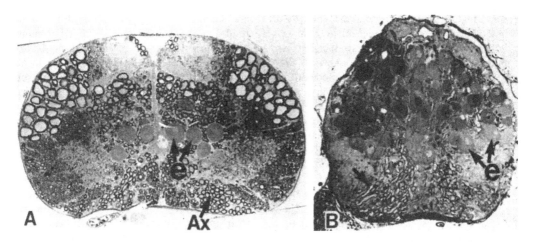

Figure 20.2 (*A* and *B*)

A series of transverse sections through regenerated spinal cords. (*A*) Normal, unregenerated spinal cord. Cell bodies of the electromotor neurons (e) are clustered in a medial column. Axons of the electromotor neurons (Ax) are grouped at the ventral border, prior to exit in the ventral root. Large-diameter myelinated axons are grouped in a dorsolateral column; small-diameter myelinated fibers line the ventrolateral border of the cord. Magnification ×130. (*B*) Two-month regenerated cord. Note the large number of electromotor neurons (e) which virtually fill the dorsal half of the cord. Organized groupings of axons are lacking except for the electrocyte axons (arrow), which run towards the ventral roots (one visible at lower left). Magnification ×160.

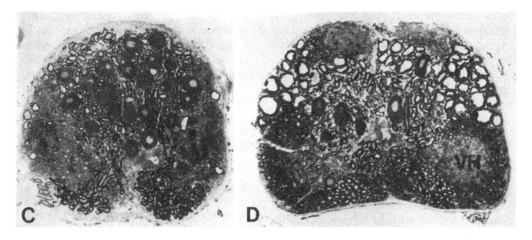

Figure 20.2 (*C* and *D*)

Transverse sections through regenerated spinal cords. (*C*) Section from the mid-regenerated region of a 12-month regenerated cord. The number of electromotor neurons is decreased (compared to the early-regenerated stage in *B*) and small groups of myelinated axons (arrow) are present. Magnification ×120. (*D*) Rostral region of 29-month regenerated cord. Overall morphology is indistinguishable from that of normal cord shown in (*A*). This section contains the normal number of electromotor neurons, dorsolateral tracts of large-diameter myelinated axons, small myelinated axons lining the ventrolateral border, and a distinct ventral horn (VH) region. Magnification ×120.

glia. Thus, there is a rostrocaudal gradient of development along the regenerated cord. As judged along this gradient, rostral regions are more highly differentiated and organized, since they have regenerated for longer periods of time than caudal regions. This report will first briefly describe the morphologic structure of rostral regenerated spinal cord, where the morphologic pattern approaches that of the normal spinal cord. We will then turn attention to caudal zones, where neurogenesis begins.

After long-term regeneration of *Sternarchus* spinal cord, the most mature regenerated tissue (just behind the transition zone between regenerated and nonregenerated cord) exhibits a normal morphology.[22] The rostral, long-term regenerated cord (figure 20.2D) contains the normal number of electromotor neurons, located lateral and dorsal to the central canal (as in normal cord). Axon tracts in rostral long-term regenerated cord are indistinguishable from normal ones (figure 20.2A) in numbers and placement. Moreover, synapses (both chemical and electrical) with a normal morphologic structure are established within the regenerated cord.

In contrast to the rostral long-term regenerated spinal cord, more caudal cord, which has regenerated for shorter periods of time, exhibits a very different morphologic pattern. Cross sections of *Sternarchus* cords which have regenerated for up to 6 months (or sections in the middle of long-term regenerated cords) show an excess number of the electromotor neurons, with neuronal perikarya often filling the dorsal half of the regenerating cord (figure 20.2B and C). Thus, many more electromotor neurons are produced within the regenerating cord than are present in normal cord.[9,22] This overproduction of neurons during spinal cord regeneration in situ can result in a five-fold excess of electromotor neurons. However, continuing morphogenesis of the regenerating cord over time leads to a modulation of the number of electromotor neurons and the establishment of a normal spinal cord organization. Excess electromotor neurons

are eliminated by a process of cell death, which results in the normal number of electromotor neurons in long-term regenerated cord. Cell elimination is selective, in that neurons in abnormal locations are eliminated, while neurons in appropriate locations are retained. This process of selective neuronal death in the regenerating spinal cord is described in detail by Anderson et al.[22] Similar processes of cell death play a role in regulating neuronal numbers in a number of developing systems.[31-34]

The recapitulation of normal morphologic structure in the regenerated spinal cord extends to the structure of the electromotor neurons and their afferent synapses.[9,22] Regenerated electromotor neurons, like normal ones,[28] are spherical in shape, between 25–50 μm in diameter, and lack dendrites. As in the normal cord, myelin extends over the initial segment to contact, or partially cover, the electromotor neuron. Perikarya of the regenerated electromotor neurons receive electrotonic synapses (figure 20.3), as do normal *Sternarchus* electrocytes. These synapses, as in the normal *Sternarchus* spinal cord, arise as blunt endings derived from large myelinated fibers or as *en passant* synapses which originate at nodes of Ranvier. Extensive gap junctions (figure 20.3, inset) are present at these synapses on the electromotor cell bodies, as in normal spinal cord. In addition, after regeneration in situ, the peripheral axons of the electromotor neurons develop a normal ultrastructure; this recapitulation of morphologic structure includes the establishment of several classes of nodes of Ranvier and normal axoglial relationships.[21]

Ependymal Cells as Neuronal Progenitors

Morphologic studies have indicated that cells in the ependymal layer constitute the source of the new neurons (and glia) in the regenerating cord in *Sternarchus*.[9,30] The ependymal layer similarly serves as a source of neurons during embryogenesis in a variety of species, a fact that

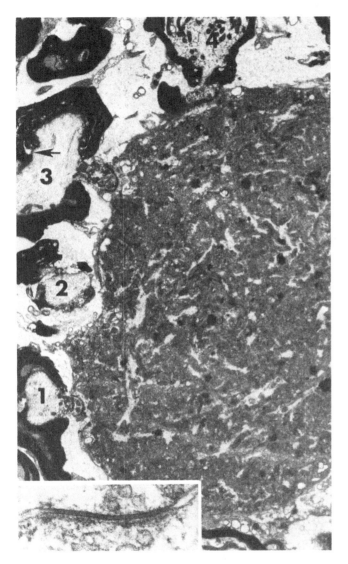

Figure 20.3
Regenerated electromotor neuron receiving four axosomatic synapses. The synapses all arise from large myelinated axons and contain extensive areas of gap junction (inset). One of the synapses (number 3) arises *en passant*, from a node of Ranvier (arrow denotes other side of node). Ultrastructure of the regenerated electromotor neuron is identical to that of normal cells. Magnification ×4575; inset ×69,300.

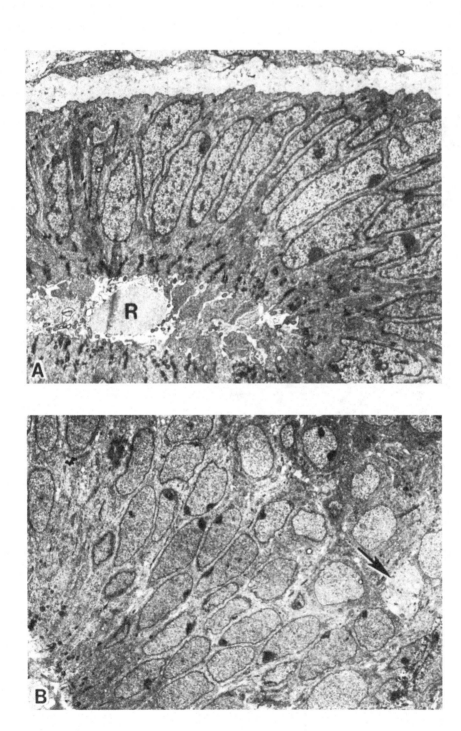

has led some authors to refer to it as the "generative neuroepithelium."[35] Since development proceeds in a rostrocaudal sequence, the caudalmost cord contains the "youngest" (most recently generated) elements. The caudalmost region of regenerated spinal cord, in fact, consists of a single tubular layer of ependymal cells (figure 20.4A). The caudal ependymal cells in regenerating cord are enlarged and are more numerous (80–90 per transverse section) than are those in the unregenerated spinal cord (30–40 per transverse section).[30] The cells in this generative neuroepithelial layer do, however, continue to exhibit the morphologic characteristics of ependymal cells: they give rise to microvillae and cilia which extend into the central canal, they exhibit the cytoplasmic characteristics of ependymal cells, and they are joined via junctional complexes.[30,36]

Rostral to the single-cell ependymal layer, undifferentiated cells radiate away from the ependyma (figure 20.4B) and subsequently differentiate into the neurons and glia of the regenerating spinal cord. Neurites and axons from the rostral part of the regenerated cord and from undamaged cord rostral to the extirpation site grow caudally into and through the regenerating cord, where they establish synapses which exhibit a normal ultrastructure.[9,30] The progression of cell generation from the ependymal layer in Sternarchus is very similar to that observed in regenerating spinal cord of urodele amphibians.[7,37]

These results in both urodele amphibians and teleosts indicate that some of the ependymal cells in adult spinal cord of these species retain the ability to undergo mitosis and produce new neurons as well as glial cells, given the proper stimulus. In this regard, the presence of ependyma has been shown to be a necessary prerequisite for regeneration of spinal axons and non-neuronal structures in the tail of the lizard Lygosoma.[38] In addition, the course of generation of cells from the ependymal layer in regenerating spinal cords of amphibians and teleosts is very similar to the sequence of maturation during normal embryonic development of the spinal cord in some species.[39,40] A comparison with embryonic development in Sternarchus is not presently possible since the fish have not been bred in captivity. However, as described below, ependyma constitutes the stem-cell population from which neurons arise during postnatal growth of the spinal cord in this species.

Postnatal Neurogenesis during Normal Growth In Vivo

Teleosts exhibit growth in size, which continues into adult life; as part of this postnatal growth, neurons are added to many parts of the teleost CNS throughout adult life.[11,18,19] This aspect of teleost growth provides the opportunity to study neurogenesis from adult tissues. In Sternarchus, addition of spinal cord tissue and generation of new neurons during ongoing growth of the adult occurs in the caudalmost segment of spinal cord.[20,23] The source of the new neurons and glia in the caudalmost segment of cord is the ependymal layer,[23] which shows striking morphologic similarity to the ependyma of regenerating cord.[30]

Figure 20.4
Ependymal layer in caudal regenerated cord. (A) Caudalmost regenerated cord, which is constituted solely of a tube of ependymal cells. Ependymal cells are large and nuclei contain patchy or dispersed chromatin. Processes of the ependymal cell cytoplasm extend into the central canal, which also contains numerous ependymal cell cilia and the Reissner's fiber (R). Magnification ×5330. (B) A section of caudal regenerated cord from a specimen with a 3-week regeneration period. Undifferentiated cells radiate away from the cells surrounding the central canal (lower left), creating a multilayered cord. Groups of longitudinally oriented axons (arrow) are present amidst the cells. At this stage there is no clear distinction between the ependymal cells and other cells that have moved away from the ependymal layer. Magnification ×2640.

The caudalmost spinal segment in normal adult *Sternarchus*[23] consists of a single layer of ependymal cells. These cells, as in regenerating cord, are radially enlarged and more numerous than in the more rostral (mature) cord (50–55 cells versus 30–40 cells in rostral cord). Within 1–2 mm rostral from the caudalmost tip, numerous undifferentiated cells are generated from the innermost ependymal layer. Somewhat more rostral, neurons and glia begin to differentiate, while longitudinally oriented axons have grown in from the more rostral cord. Morphologic structure of the cord thus undergoes a gradual transition in the caudalmost two spinal segments from the single-cell layer of ependymal tube to the "mature" morphologic pattern of more rostral, histologically unchanging cord.

Although in most respects the caudalmost (generative) segment of spinal cord in normal adult *Sternarchus* resembles the caudal portion of regenerating spinal cord, it is interesting that the massive overproduction and subsequent cell death of electromotor neurons that are seen in regenerated cord do not occur in the processes of ongoing growth at the tip of normal cord.[20] Apparently, the mechanisms by which neuronal number is modulated are different in normally growing spinal cord compared with regenerating cord. This interesting difference between regeneration and normal growth is currently under study.

The background of demonstrated neurogenesis, which occurs both in situ in normal adult *Sternarchus* cord and during regeneration after injury, suggested that *Sternarchus* spinal cord might also carry on neurogenesis in vitro. Accordingly, an explant culture system was developed in our laboratory and [³H]thymidine incorporation was examined in cultured explants from *Sternarchus* spinal cord.

Neurogenesis from Adult Tissue In Vitro

Previous in vitro studies on CNS neurons have been carried out almost entirely with embryonic tissue, since adult avian or mammalian neuronal tissue has been extremely difficult to grow in culture. Besides, with a few exceptions,[41,42] studies of neuronal tissue in vitro have led to the general conclusion that the growth observed in cultures of even embryonic neuronal tissue represents an outgrowth of neurites from postmitotic neurons, rather than production of neurons in vitro. Thus, in vitro studies have provided an extremely useful model for the study of neuronal differentiation, growth, and interaction with other cells; however, it has not been possible to study neurogenesis in vitro. Recently, however, Kriegstein and Dichter[43] provided autoradiographic evidence for the generation of new neurons in cultures of embryonic brain tissue. This study is important since it demonstrated the possibility of studying in vitro the factors controlling neurogenesis from embryonic CNS tissue.

Whereas in vitro systems for studying CNS tissue (in contrast to embryonic tissue) from adult mammals or birds have not been readily available, CNS tissue from adult teleosts has proved amenable to tissue culture.[44,45] Recently, a culture system has been developed for spinal cord explants from adult *Sternarchus albifrons*.[46] The explants are grown in Leibovitz's L-15 medium on plastic tissue-culture dishes coated with polylysine or polyornithine.[47] These spinal cord cultures have been examined to determine whether neurogenesis occurs in vitro in this system. Examination of the spinal cord explants with [³H]thymidine and antineuronal monoclonal antibodies has demonstrated that thymidine incorporation occurs in cells which, after a further growth period, can unequivocally be identified as neurons.[48] Notably, the neurogenesis occurs in cultures derived from both normal adult spinal cord (i.e., from tissue derived from mature spinal cord regions located rostral to the growing tip) and from regenerated spinal cord.

Neurons in the cultures were identified by a combination of morphologic and behaviorial characteristics and by staining with neuron-specific monoclonal antibodies.[49,50] Neurites could be observed in the cultures after 3–6 days, and typical networks of neurites were formed in the cultures after 6–9 days (figure 20.5A). Despite the formation of neurite networks, individual neurons could clearly be observed at the edges of the outgrowth area or in areas of less dense outgrowth. Cells were identified as neurons (figure 20.5B) on the basis of the following characteristics: rounded cell bodies, the presence of neurites and growth cones, branching and fasciculation of the neurites, and contacts of the cell body or neurites with non-neuronal cells. The morphologic identification of neurons was confirmed, in some cultures, by positive staining with monoclonal antibodies against neurofilaments (figure 20.6A).

Explants derived from regenerating spinal cord start neurite outgrowth sooner (2–4 days versus 5–9 days for normal cord) and show a denser outgrowth than do explants from unregenerated normal adult cord.[46] However, both types of cultures clearly show dense neurite outgrowth after 2–3 weeks. At 3–10 days in culture, groups of closely apposed rounded cells, which are presumably undergoing mitosis, are observed. Cells with short neurites, probably in early stages of outgrowth, are present at the edges of these groups of presumptively postmitotic cells. Mitosis is, in fact, demonstrated by triticated thymidine autoradiography.[48]

For demonstration of neurogenesis, tritiated thymidine (0.5–5 µCi/ml) was added to the culture medium between days 7–14 in culture. After a labeling period of 24–72 hr, the [³H]thymidine was washed out and fresh medium containing $100 \times$ cold unlabeled thymidine was added. The explants were cultured for a period of 2–8 more days, to allow neuronal differentiation, before fixation and autoradiography. Some cultures were fixed in methanol and stained with neuron-specific antineurofilament antibody (RT-97 [Ref. 49] or 02–40 [Ref. 50]) prior to application of the autoradiographic emulsion.

In cultures that were incubated with [³H]thymidine, dense nuclear labeling is ob-

served in cells that can unequivocally be identified as neurons by both morphologic criteria (figure 20.5C and D) and by staining with antineuronal monoclonal antibody (figure 20.6B and C). [³H]-labeled neurons are present in cultures from both unregenerated adult spinal cords and regenerating cords. Many [³H]-labeled neurons can be clearly identified by morphologic criteria alone; however, colabeling with antineurofilament antibody (figure 20.6) makes the case unequivocal. A total of 110 cultures were examined in this study: 98 cultures were [³H]-labeled cultures and 12 cultures were colabeled with tritium plus antibody.[48] Double-labeled neurons were present in each of the 12 antibody-stained cultures that were examined. In counts of 826 normal neurons and 952 regenerated neurons, a mean value of 15% of the neurons are labeled with [³H]thymidine in the cultures derived from normal adult spinal cord. A mean value of 45% of the neurons are [³H]-labeled in cultures derived from regenerating cords.

In order to rule out the possibility that [³H]thymidine could be taken up by already differentiated neurons, autoradiography was carried out on a culture that was exposed to [³H]thymidine for a shorter time period (17 hr) and was fixed immediately; another culture was exposed to [³H]thymidine for 20 hours and then allowed to grow for 4 more days (to allow neuronal differentiation) prior to fixation and autoradiography. In the culture that was fixed immediately after the labeling period, no differentiated neurons exhibited [³H]-labeled nuclei; only rounded cells and non-neuronal cells were labeled with tritium. This finding demonstrates that tritium labeling is not due to uptake of [³H]thymidine into already differentiated neurons. The sister culture, which was allowed to grow for 4 days subsequent to the labeling period, did contain [³H]-labeled neurons. These results indicate that tritiated thymidine incorporation takes place prior to neuronal differentiation.

The results of this study provide strong evidence that neurogenesis occurs in the cultures

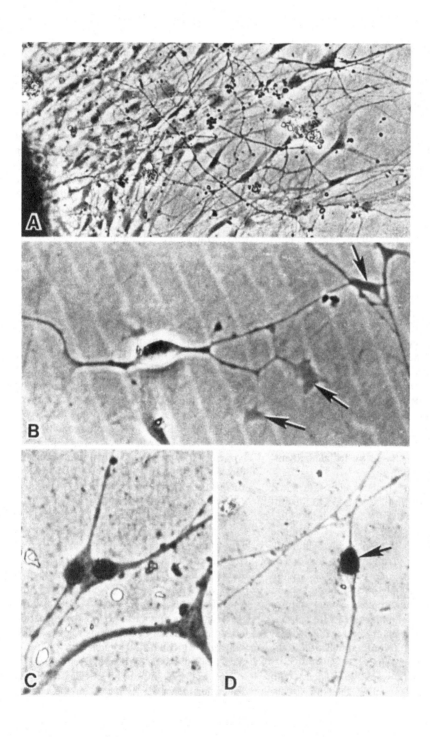

from both normal adult and regenerating *Sternarchus* spinal cord. The possibility of thymidine incorporation into already differentiated neurons is very unlikely for several reasons. First, as noted above, the cultures fixed immediately after the thymidine-labeling period show no tritium-labeled neurons. Instead, the tritium appears only in rounded non-neuronal cells and glia. However, when time is allowed after thymidine uptake, neuronal differentiation occurs in some of the labeled cells. Second, a mitotic origin for the thymidine-labeled neurons is suggested by the appearance of groups of rounded, apparently dividing cells in the cultures at the times when thymidine labeling is obtained. Many of these rounded cells are labeled in cultures fixed immediately after incubation with [³H]thymidine. Third, the in situ evidence for neurogenesis in normal adult and regenerating *Sternarchus* cord strongly implies that some of the ependymal cells within histologically mature cord remain capable of mitosis and the generation of new neurons. The demonstration of thymidine incorporation into cultured *Sternarchus* neurons now suggests that this process can also proceed in vitro.

A prior study by de Boni and coworkers[44] failed to demonstrate thymidine incorporation in cultures of adult goldfish brain. However, species differences or differences in the methods used could account for the disparity between their report and the present results in *Sternarchus* spinal cord cultures. *Sternarchus* spinal cord may have greater capability for regeneration than does

goldfish brain. The study on goldfish brain employed a different medium and different timing of ³H-labeling and autoradiography. And, interestingly, despite their failure to demonstrate [³H]thymidine incorporation, de Boni et al. observed that fragments of goldfish brain that did not contain a portion of the ventricular and subventricular zones resulted in cultures that contained mesenchymal and glial cells, but not neurons.[44]

As in previously reported studies on amphibian[51] and fish[45] retina in culture, neuritic outgrowth was more rapid and more dense from explants of regenerated *Sternarchus* spinal cord as compared to nonregenerated cord. In effect, the explantation procedure to tissue culture may initiate the process of regeneration, which we know occurs in vivo in response to cellular injury. In this sense, the explantation procedure for tissue culture may "prime" the neuronal precursor cells in the explants derived from normal cord to initiate regeneration. Explants from regenerated cord would be expected to grow faster in tissue culture because they are already "primed" and regenerating. The nature of the priming stimulus is not known, although it may be related to tissue injury. With respect to neurogenesis, however, it should be noted that ependymal cells do not give rise to axons, and thus the priming mechanism involved in neurogenesis may not be the same as the mechanism involved in the "priming lesions" which have been shown to stimulate regeneration of axons.[45,51,52]

Figure 20.5

Sternarchus spinal cord in tissue culture. (*A*) Outgrowth of neurites and non-neuronal cells from explant of normal adult spinal cord after 1½ weeks in culture. Explant proper is at left (dark area). Magnification ×245. (*B*) Bipolar neuron from a 4-week culture of regenerated cord. Several prominent growth cone areas (arrows) are present on this neuron. Magnification ×510. (*C*) and (*D*) Autoradiograms of neurons from cultures labeled with [³H]thymidine. (*C*) Two neurons showing dense nuclear labeling with tritium grains. This 18-day culture was from regenerated cord. Magnification ×500. (*D*) Neuron from a 30-day culture from normal adult cord. A dense cap of tritium grains (arrow) is visible over the nuclear area. One neurite from this cell fasciculates with several neurites from other cells near top of figure. Magnification ×420.

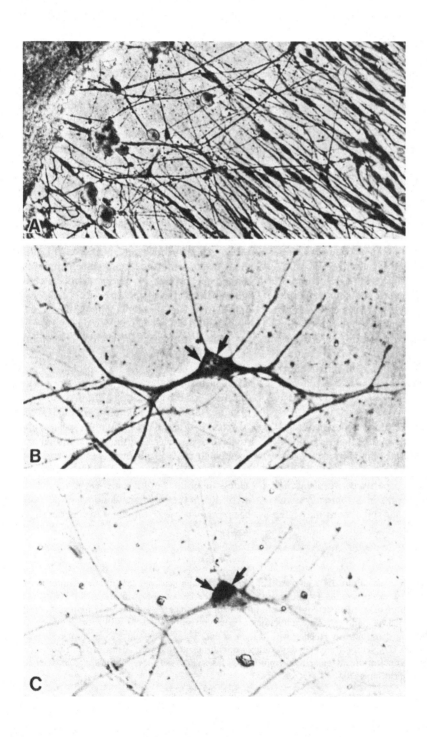

Functional Correlates and Implications for Repair of the Nervous System

As shown above, postnatal neurogenesis continues as an ongoing process in the caudal spinal cord of *Sternarchus*. One obvious question concerns the functional implications of this ongoing production of neurons. Electromotor neurons in *Sternarchus* constitute the effector cells of the electromotor system.[26,27] These cells generate an electric field which is sensed by electroreceptors distributed along the sides of the fish. Given the source-sink arrangement of current flow in the electric organ,[26,27] it is functionally advantageous for the electric organ to increase in size by addition of electromotor neurons concomitant with growth of the fish. Thus, neurogenesis in *Sternarchus* serves to optimize function of the electromotor system.

Compensatory neurogenesis and regeneration after injury have obvious evolutionary advantages. The tail in *Sternarchus* is marked by several white bands (figure 20.1) and these distinguish the tail from the rest of the fish, which is covered with dark skin, and make it a more attractive target for predators. Since the caudal region of the spinal cord is a site of ongoing neurogenesis, it might be speculated that regeneration after injury should occur more rapidly at caudal than at rostral levels of the spinal cord. According to this hypothesis, *Sternarchus* would offer, as a target for predators, caudalmost regions, where the capability for regeneration is greatest. Importantly, however, regeneration after injury is not confined to this caudal region; on the contrary, regenerative capacity is retained even at rostral levels of the spinal cord.

During growth and regeneration of the *Sternarchus* electromotor system, it appears that a basic structural plan is conserved, so that growth yields more neurons of the same type, rather than neurons with an intrinsically different structure or type of connectivity. These new neurons are incorporated into the electromotor circuit in a manner similar to that of preexisting cells, and thus do not appear to qualitatively alter the input-output function of the system in question (in contrast to the example of postnatal neurogenesis in the avian vocal control nuclei[6]). Nevertheless, the important point is that the electromotor system in *Sternarchus* demonstrates the *modifiability of the adult CNS in terms of production of new neurons*. This modifiability may provide an important degree of freedom in terms of functional characteristics, and may have important implications with respect to mechanisms by which the CNS can adapt to injury.

Since the electromotor neurons exhibit a relatively simple and stereotyped morphology, it might be assumed that their production, or regeneration, would require one basic set of genetic instructions, which are expressed iteratively in the production of multiple neurons. Even in this respect, however, neurogenesis must involve a significant degree of regulation in terms of neuronal differentiation. The generation of new electromotor neurons, showing normal relationships with presynaptic fibers (at the cell body)

Figure 20.6
Tritiated thymidine labeling in culture stained with RT-97 antineuronal monoclonal antibody. (*A*) Overview of an explant from regenerated cord fixed and stained with RT-97 after 18 days in culture. The neurite network and neuronal cell bodies stain darkly with the anti-neurofilament antibody. Non-neuronal cells, not clearly visible in this figure, do not stain with the antibody. Magnification ×220. (*B*) and (*C*) Double-labeled neurons from the culture in (*A*). (*B*) Neuron stained with antineurofilament antibody, but before autoradiography. The cell body and neurites are positively stained by the antibody. The nuclear area (arrows) is clear, except for two dark inclusions (nucleoli). Magnification ×435. (*C*) The same cell after autoradiography to visualize [³H]thymidine labeling. Dark tritium grains now cover the nuclear area (arrows). Magnification ×435.

and with myelin-forming oligodendrocytes (at the initial segment) or Schwann cells (in the regenerated electric organ[21]), suggests that the neuronal plasma membrane of newly generated electromotor neurons differentiates in a normal manner with respect to the distribution of "recognition molecules."[53-55] It should also be recalled that the electromotor neurons exhibit a complex and highly specific pattern of synaptic innervation by descending fibers (see below); this implies the need for a more complex set of instructions that can regulate the development of a spectrum of axonal characteristics.

Since electromotor neurons are innervated by medullary control neurons,[26] the occurrence of postnatal neurogenesis in the caudal region of spinal cord leads to a requirement for plasticity at more rostral levels in the medulla. The necessity for reorganization at higher levels is even more acute in the case of regenerating spinal cord, where up to five times the normal number of electromotor neurons can be produced[9] and where synapses are established with at least some of these regenerated neurons. While the functional properties of the regenerated Sternarchus spinal cord and electric organ have not yet been examined, both of these regenerated neural systems do achieve an apparently normal morphologic structure over time. Descending synaptic inputs onto regenerated electromotor neurons are indistinguishable from normal ones in terms of the ultrastructure of the synapses.[22] The relatively sudden introduction of large numbers of new neurons during spinal cord regeneration would, moreover, be expected to place an immediate and increased (relative to normal) demand on higher centers for production and integration of new descending connections.

In normal adult Sternarchus, there is morphologic[28] and physiological[26,56] evidence for synaptic projection of the medullary command nucleus to caudal (more recently generated) electromotor neurons as well as to rostral neurons. Thus, during growth and concomitant addition of neurons to the caudal spinal cord, there

is continuing formation of new axonal projections to, and synaptic connection with, the newly formed neurons in the spinal cord. It is not at present clear whether the new projections reflect production of additional relay neurons in the medulla[56] or collateral formation or branching from preexisting bulbospinal axons that arise from these medullary cells. Irrespective of which of these mechanisms is shown to be correct, reorganization of neural structures in adult Sternarchus must occur at a variety of levels to accommodate newly generated neurons. In this regard, the situation in Sternarchus may be similar to that in telencephalic vocal control nucleus in canaries, where newly generated neurons in the adult brain have been shown to be recruited into functional synaptic circuits.[6] It should be recalled, moreover, that the morphologic pattern (and conduction velocity) of bulbospinal fibers in the Sternarchus electromotor system are matched to functional requirements so that the axons can function as time-delay lines to mediate synchronous firing of electromotor neurons.[57,58] Thus, the ongoing reorganization of the caudal spinal cord and descending projections involves a high degree of specificity at the cellular level.

In summary, spinal cord from the adult teleost Sternarchus albifrons shows a high capacity for neurogenesis, which occurs in situ as an ongoing process and in response to injury, as well as in vitro in explant cultures of spinal cord. Moreover, both regeneration in situ and neurogenesis in vitro can occur from mature spinal cord tissue which is not normally a site of neuron production. This raises the possibility of study of the signals by which neurogenesis is initiated and controlled. In this respect, the Sternarchus culture system should provide a very useful model in which the determinants of neurogenesis and neuronal differentiation can be examined. The occurrence of neurogenesis and regeneration in the Sternarchus electromotor system provides an ideal system in which to address basic questions of neuronal recovery after injury and plasticity in the adult vertebrate central nervous system.

Summary

Phylogenetically "lower" species in some cases use different biological strategies for recovery after injury to the CNS than do "higher" species. One approach that we have taken in our laboratory has been to study the mechanisms of functional recovery of the CNS after injury in those vertebrate species where recovery does occur. The present report reviews recent studies on a model system, the spinal electromotor system of the gymnotiform teleost *Sternarchus albifrons*, which exhibits regeneration and neurogenesis after injury. Regeneration in this system leads to a recapitulation of relatively normal morphologic structure by the damaged or extirpated spinal cord. In *Sternarchus*, new spinal cord is generated from ependymal cells; some ependymal cells in the adult remain pluripotent and retain the capability to generate new neurons. The *Sternarchus* spinal cord thus represents an especially useful model for the study of neurogenesis after injury to the CNS.

Recent studies in our laboratory indicate that neurogenesis in adult *Sternarchus* spinal cord tissue occurs both in vivo and in vitro. Neurogenesis has been demonstrated by incorporation of tritiated thymidine into explant cultures from the spinal cord of adult *Sternarchus*. Autoradiography reveals the presence of thymidine-labeled neurons. Neuronal identity of ^{3}H-labeled cells has been confirmed by positive staining with neuron-specific monoclonal antibodies. Thymidine labeling occurs in cultured neurons derived from both normal (histologically and functionally mature) and regenerating spinal cord of adult *Sternarchus albifrons*. These results provide evidence that some cells in spinal cord of adult *Sternarchus* retain the ability to incorporate thymidine and undergo neuronal differentiation in vitro. This system provides a new model in which neurogenesis from adult tissue can be studied in vivo and in vitro.

Acknowledgments

C. Choy and H. L. Fong provided excellent technical assistance for this research. The RT-97 antibody was the generous gift of Dr. John Wood; 02–40 was the generous gift of Drs. Nancy and Ludwig Sternberger.

This work was supported in part by the Medical Research Service, Veterans Administration, by Grant NS-15320 from the National Institute of Neurological and Communicative Disorders and Stroke, and by the Folger Foundation.

References

1. Graziadei, P. P. C. and G. A. Graziadei. 1979. Neurogenesis and neuron regeneration in the olfactory system of mammals. I. Morphological aspects of differentiation and structural organization of the olfactory sensory neurons. J. Neurocytol. 8: 1–18.

2. Wilson, K. C. P. and G. Raisman. 1980. Age-related changes in the neurosensory epithelium of the mouse vomeronasal organ: Extended period of postnatal growth in size and evidence for rapid cell turnover in the adult. Brain Res. 185: 103–113.

3. Altman, J. and G. D. Das 1965. Postnatal origin of microneurones. Nature 207: 953–956.

4. Kaplan, M. S. and J. W. Hinds. 1977. Neurogenesis in the adult rat: Electron microscopic analysis of light autoradiographs. Science 197: 1092–1094.

5. Goldman, S. A. and F. Nottebohm. 1983. Neuronal production, migration and differentiation in a vocal control nucleus of the adult female canary brain. Proc. Natl. Acad. Sci. USA 80: 2390–2394.

6. Paton, J. A. and F. N. Nottebohm. 1984. Neurons generated in the adult brain are recruited into functional circuits. Science 225: 1046–1048.

7. Nordlander, R. H. and M. Singer. 1978. The role of ependyma in regeneration of the spinal cord in the urodele amphibian tail. J. Comp. Neurol. 180: 349–374.

8. Kirsche, W. 1965. Regenerative Vorgange im Gehirn und Rukkenmark. Ergeb. Anat. Entwicklungsgesch. 38: 143–194.

9. Anderson, M. J. and S. G. Waxman. 1981. Morphology of regenerated spinal cord in *Sternarchus albifrons*. Cell Tissue Res. 219: 1–8.

10. Anderson, M. J. and S. G. Waxman. 1983. Regeneration of spinal neurons in inframammalian vertebrates: morphological and developmental aspects. J. Hirnforsch. 24: 371–398.

11. Easter, S. S., Jr. 1983. Postnatal neurogenesis and changing connections. Trends Neurosci. 6: 53–56.

12. Johns, P. R. 1982. Formation of photoreceptors in larval and adult goldfish. J. Neurosci. 2: 178–198.

13. Johns, P. R. and S. S. Easter. 1977. Growth of the adult goldfish eye. II. Increase in retinal cell number. J. Comp. Neurol. 176: 331–342.

14. Straznicky, K. and R. M. Gaze. 1971. The growth of the retina in *Xenopus laevis*: An autoradiographic study. J. Embryol. Exp. Morphol. 26: 67–79.

15. Raymond, P. A. and S. S. Easter, Jr. 1983. Postembryonic growth of the optic tectum in goldfish. I. Location of germinal cells and numbers of neurons produced. J. Neurosci. 3: 1077–1091.

16. Stevenson, J. and M. G. Yoon. 1980. Kinetics of cell proliferation in the halved tectum of adult goldfish. Brain Res. 184: 11–22.

17. Straznicky, K. and R. M. Gaze. 1972. Development of the optic tectum in *Xenopus laevis*. An autoradiographic study. J. Embryol. Exp. Morphol. 28: 87–115.

18. Birse, S. C., R. B. Leonard and R. E. Coggeshall. 1980. Neuronal increase in various areas of the nervous system of the guppy, *Lebistes*. J. Comp. Neurol. 194: 291–301.

19. Leonard, R. B., R. E. Coggeshall and W. D. Willis. 1978. A documentation of an age related increase in neuronal and axonal numbers in the stingray. J. Comp. Neurol. 179: 13–22.

20. Waxman, S. G. and M. J. Anderson. 1985. Generation of electromotor neurons in *Sternarchus albifrons*: Differences between normally growing and regenerating spinal cord. Dev. Biol. 112: 338–344.

21. Waxman, S. G. and M. J. Anderson. 1980. Regeneration of spinal electrocyte fibers in *Sternarchus albifrons*: Development of axon-Schwann cell relationships and nodes of Ranvier. Cell Tissue Res. 208: 343–352.

22. Anderson, M. J., S. G. Waxman and C. H. Tadlock. 1984. Cell death of asynaptic neurons in regenerating spinal cord. Dev. Biol. 103: 443–455.

23. Anderson, M. J. and S. G. Waxman. 1983. Caudal spinal cord of the teleost *Sternarchus albifrons* resembles regenerating cord. Anat. Rec. 205: 85–92.

24. Oliviera Castro, G. de. 1955. Differentiated nervous fibers that constitute the electric organ of *Sternarchus albifrons*. Linn. Anais Acad. Brasil Cien. 4: 557–562.

25. Bennett, M. V. L. 1970. Comparative physiology: Electric organs. Ann. Rev. Physiol. 32: 471–528.

26. Bennett, M. V. L. 1971. Electric organs. *In* Fish Physiology. W. S. Hoar and D. J. Randall, Eds. Vol. 5: 347–491. Academic Press. New York, NY.

27. Waxman, S. G., G. D. Pappas and M. V. L. Bennett. 1972. Morphological correlates of functional differentiation of nodes of Ranvier along single fibers in the neurogenic electric organ of the knife fish *Sternarchus*. J. Cell Biol. 53: 210–224.

28. Pappas, G. D., S. G. Waxman and M. V. L. Bennett. 1975. Morphology of spinal electromotor neurons and presynaptic coupling in the gymnotid *Sternarchus albifrons*. J. Neurocytol. 4: 469–478.

29. Bennett, M. V. L., C. Sandri and K. Akert. 1978. Neuronal gap junctions and morphologically mixed synapses in the spinal cord of a teleost, *Sternarchus albifrons* (Gymnotoidei). Brain Res. 143: 43–60.

30. Anderson, M. J., S. G. Waxman and M. Laufer. 1983. Fine structure of regenerated ependyma and spinal cord in *Sternarchus albifrons*. Anat Rec. 205: 73–83.

31. Hamburger, V. 1975. Cell death in the development of the lateral motor column of the chick embryo. J. Comp. Neurol. 160: 535–546.

32. Cowan, W. M. 1973. Neuronal death as a regulative mechanism in the control of cell number in the nervous system. *In* Development and Aging in the Nervous System. M. Rockstein, Ed.: 19–41. Academic Press. New York, NY.

33. Oppenheim, R. W. 1981. Neuronal cell death and some related regressive phenomena during neurogenesis: A selective historical review and progress report. *In* Studies in Developmental Neurobiology: Essays in Honor of Viktor Hamburger. W. M. Cowan, Ed.: 74–133. Oxford University Press. London.

34. Cunningham, T. J. 1982. Naturally occurring neuron death and its regulation by developing neural pathways. Int. Rev. Cytol. 74: 163–186.

35. Jacobson, M. 1978. Developmental Neurobiology, 2nd ed.: 1–42. Plenum Press. New York, NY.

36. Sandri, C., K. Akert and M. V. L. Bennett. 1978. Junctional complexes and variations in gap junctions between spinal cord ependymal cells of a teleost, *Sternarchus albifrons* (Gymnotoidei). Brain Res. 143: 27–41.

37. Egar, M. and M. Singer. 1972. The role of ependyma in spinal cord regeneration in the urodele, *Triturus*. Exp. Neurol. 37: 422–430.

38. Simpson, S. B. 1964. Analysis of tail regeneration in the lizard *Lygosoma laterale*. I. Initiation of regeneration and cartilage differentiation: The role of ependyma. J. Morphol. 114: 425–436.

39. Singer, M., R. H. Nordlander and M. Egar. 1979. Axonal guidance during embryogenesis and regeneration in the spinal cord of the newt: The blueprint hypothesis of neuronal patterning. J. Comp. Neurol. 185: 1–22.

40. Nordlander, R. H. and M. Singer. 1982. Spaces precede axons in *Xenopus* embryonic spinal cord. Exp. Neurol. 75: 221–228.

41. Juurlink, B. and S. Federhoff. 1982. The development of mouse spinal cord in tissue culture. II. Development of neuronal precursor cells. In Vitro 18: 179–182.

42. Sensenbrenner, M., E. Wittendorp, I. Barakat and R. Rechenmann. 1980. Autoradiographic study of proliferating brain cells in culture. Dev. Biol. 75: 268–277.

43. Kriegstein, A. and M. A. Dichter. 1984. Neuron generation in dissociated cell cultures from fetal rat cerebral cortex. Brain Res. 295: 184–189.

44. de Boni, U., M. Seger, J. W. Scott and D. R. Crapper. 1976. Neuron cultures from adult goldfish. J. Neurobiol. 7: 495–512.

45. Landreth, G. E. and B. W. Agranoff. 1976. Explant culture of adult goldfish retina: Effect of prior optic nerve crush. Brain Res. 118: 299–303.

46. Anderson, M. J. 1985. Neuronal growth in cultures from adult teleost spinal cord. Submitted for publication.

47. Letourneau, P. C. 1975. Possible roles for cell-to-substrate adhesion in neuronal morphogenesis. Dev. Biol. 44: 77–91.

48. Anderson, M. J. and S. G. Waxman. 1985. Neurogenesis in tissue cultures of adult teleost spinal cord. Dev. Brain Res. 20: 203–212.

49. Wood, J. N. and B. H. Anderton. 1981. Monoclonal antibodies to mammalian neurofilaments. Biosci. Rep. 1: 263–268.

50. Sternberger, L. A., L. W. Harwell and N. H. Sternberger. 1982. Neurotypy: Regional individuality in rat brain detected by immunochemistry with monoclonal antibodies. Proc. Natl. Acad. Sci. USA 79: 1326–1330.

51. Agranoff, B. W., P. Field and R. M. Gaze. 1976. Neurite outgrowth from explanted *Xenopus* retina: an effect of prior optic nerve crush. Brain Res. 113: 225–234.

52. McQuarrie, I. G. and B. Grafstein. 1981. Effect of a conditioning lesion on optic nerve regeneration in goldfish. Brain Res. 216: 253–264.

53. Goodman, C. S., M. J. Bastiani, C. Q. Doe, S. du Lac, S. L. Helford, J. Kuwada, and J. B. Thomas. 1984. Cell recognition during neuronal development. Science 225: 1271–1279.

54. Waxman, S. G. and R. E. Foster. 1980. Development of the axon membrane during differentiation of myelinated fibres in spinal nerve roots. Proc. Roy. Soc. London, Ser. B 209: 441–446.

55. Smith, M. E., J. D. Kocsis and S. G. Waxman. 1983. Myelin protein metabolism in demyelination and remyelination in the sciatic nerve. Brain Res. 270: 37–44.

56. Tokunaga, A., K. Akert, C. Sandri and M. V. L. Bennett. 1980. Cell types and synaptic organization of the medullary electromotor nucleus in a constant frequency weakly electric fish, *Sternarchus albifrons*. J. Comp. Neurol. 192: 407–426.

57. Bennett, M. V. L. 1968. Neural control of electric organs. *In* The Central Nervous System and Fish Behavior. D. Ingle, Ed.: 147–169. The University of Chicago Press. Chicago, IL.

58. Waxman, S. G. 1975. Integrative properties and design principles of axons. Int. Rev. Neurobiol. 18: 1–40.

XIII HOW DOES A BOXER STAND?

One of the remarkable things about living creatures is the ease with which they navigate through and exert actions on the external world. This applies especially to primates who, with their opposing thumbs and facial musculature, can manipulate tools, play the piano or flute, and produce intelligible speech.

How does the brain control motor behavior? This paper (Waxman 1996) builds upon an earlier publication (Trosch et al. 1990) which described a patient with a fascinating clinical syndrome called emotional facial paresis. In this syndrome, half of the face is paralyzed—but only for emotionally generated movements. Only half of the patient's face will smile in response to a humorous remark, and half of the patient's face will show surprise or anger in response to threatening stimuli. The other half is "emotionally paralyzed," in the sense that it does not move in response to these emotional inputs. This syndrome results from damage to particular parts of the brain, and usually from lesions below the cortex, involving the thalamus and surrounding parts of the "deep" brain.

For obvious reasons, the brain regions responsible for these emotionally evoked movements have been called the "emotional motor system" (Holstege, Bandler, and Saper 1996). This set of neural circuits, located below the cerebral cortex, is an old one from the point of view of evolution. It controls the posturing that contributes to mating displays, for example, in birds and reptiles, and the stereotyped movements that various species make, when threatened, to frighten off their enemies. In humans, the emotional motor system can be very clearly seen in infants, where crying occurs frequently because it is not subject to the inhibitions that exist in adults. These inhibitions are provided by the cerebral cortex, which does not mature until after infancy.

The cortex contains a more fine-grained, voluntary motor system, which is superimposed on the emotional motor system like a higher rung on a ladder. The function of the voluntary motor system can be graphically seen in a contrasting form of facial paralysis, termed "voluntary facial paralysis," which is commonly observed in patients who have suffered strokes. In these patients, the face responds fully to emotional stimuli, and both halves laugh, for example, in response to jokes. But voluntary facial movements (in response, for example, to the command "show me your teeth") are impaired, and the half of the face on the side opposite to the injury in the brain cannot respond. The injury in these cases involves the motor control region of the cerebral cortex.

The existence of these two contrasting syndromes, associated with lesions in two parts of the brain, provides an important clue from the clinical domain about how the brain controls motor activity in humans. Motor activity is not controlled by *a* motor control system in the brain. We learn from these patients that there are, in fact, several motor control systems.

Other clinical observations, even of aphasias (disorders of language that result from injury to the brain), also provide hints about the organization of the motor control system in the brain. The existence of multitiered motor systems can be discerned in the description by Geschwind (1965, 1975) of patients with Wernicke's aphasia. In this disorder, patients sustain a severe impairment of the ability to comprehend language and speech, as a result of injury to a language processing center (Wernicke's area, also termed area 22) within the temporal lobe of the left cerebral hemisphere. Medical students are routinely taught that patients with severe Wernicke's aphasia are unable to understand *any* spoken language and, to all intents and purposes, this is nearly true. However, Geschwind pointed out that there is one striking exception: although these patients cannot understand, and therefore do not perform appropriately when asked to carry out actions involving muscles of the hands, feet, and so on ("point at me"; "touch your nose with your finger"; "make a fist"), they retain a striking ability to carry out movements of their trunk, shoulders and hips in response to commands such as "stand up," "bow," or "turn around." These patients can even perform accurately in response to the complex command, "show me how a boxer stands."

What can we learn from these retained movements, which regulate the position of the body-as-a-whole, and tend to "steer" the body in space? What is different about these whole-body movements and the brain's control of them? Our hands, of course, are highly specialized and are capable of carrying out very delicate movements. Evolution of the "opposable thumb" (which allows humans and monkeys to grasp and manipulate tiny objects) was accompanied by the development of a unique degree of dexterity in the hands and, to a lesser degree, in the feet of primates. Paralleling this, there apparently was an enhanced development of a "higher" motor control system within the cortex, called the "pyramidal system," or "corticospinal motor system." This higher-order motor system within the cortex controls the highly individuated, fractionated movements that permit humans to, for instance, play the piano. It is superimposed upon a more primitive motor system, which evolved earlier and is present even in fish, that controls whole-body movement and orientation. The preservation, in patients with Wernicke's aphasia, of the ability to make whole-body movements in response to commands, in contrast to the absence of a similar ability for the muscles involving the hand, provides a clinical demonstration of the existence of multiple motor systems in humans.

We also get hints about these multiple motor systems by watching paralyzed people walk. Stroke victims who sustain severe damage to the motor cortex usually develop hemiplegia, or paralysis of one side of the body. But they almost always walk again, even if the "leg" area in the motor cortex is destroyed. This residual "circumabductive" gait, in which the extensors of the hip and knee remain powerful (or even stuck in a spastic rigidity), allows the weakened leg to act as a strut. It reflects residual activity of the antigravity muscles, which are driven by "lower" motor control centers to keep the body erect and moving forward at all costs. A century ago the pioneering neurophysiologist Sir Charles Sherrington was aware of the robustness of the subcortical systems controlling the antigravity muscles and, allegedly with a pistol at his side, studied a tree sloth after its cortex had been injured. As predicted from its upside-down, arboreal lifestyle, he found residual activity in the flexors of its hips and knees—again illustrating the presence of a primitive motor system that is not responsible for making fine or precise movements but which, rather, opposes gravity, thus helping to keep the sloth in its tree and out of harm's way.

As one watches living organisms act on the world, it is hard not to appreciate the beauty of their movements. This outer beauty, manifested by behavior, is paralleled by an inner beauty reflecting the design of the brain and spinal cord and the motor systems within. Remarkably, we can begin to discern the organization of the nervous system without dissecting it, by careful watching of the movements of normal people, or of people with rare disorders such as emotional facial paresis or common ones like aphasia and hemiplegia. Thus we can begin to see, without even touching a patient, the elegance of design of our brains and spinal cords, and the exquisite coupling between the structure and function of our nervous system.

References

Geschwind, N. Disconnection syndromes in animals and man. *Brain* 88: 237–294, 585–644, 1965.

Geschwind, N. The apraxias: neural mechanisms of disorders of learned movements. *Am Scientist.* 188–195, 1975.

Holstege, G., Bandler, R., and Saper, C. B. The emotional motor system. *Prog. Brain Res.* 107, 1996.

Trosch, R., Sze, G., Brass, L. M., and Waxman, S. G. Emotional facial paresis with striatocapsular infarction. *J. Neurol. Sci.* 98: 195–202, 1990.

Waxman, S. G. Clinical observations on the emotional motor system. In: *The Emotional Motor System,* Holstege, G., Bandler, R., and Saper, C. (eds.), Elsevier, Amsterdam, pp. 595–605, 1996.

21 Clinical Observations on the Emotional Motor System

Stephen G. Waxman

Introduction

Even the most molecularly-oriented neurologist must, sooner or later, come to grips with the questions of how neurons are built so as to confer them with appropriate information-processing capabilities, and how neurons are assembled into circuits that underlie purposeful behavior. In this regard, one of the most important aspects of behavior involves motor activities, i.e., the positioning or movement of body parts in ways that have functional value for the organism. Although motor activity is usually considered, at least at first glance, in terms of its voluntary aspects ("make a fist"; "show me two fingers"; "show me your teeth"), there are other motor activities (e.g., smiling, crying, laughing) which occur spontaneously and are not easily or accurately mimicked on a voluntary basis or in response to verbal instruction. These motor activities are mediated, in large part, by an emotional or non-verbal motor system.

This chapter describes clinical observations, made by the author over the past two decades, on non-verbal aspects of motor control relevant to the emotional motor system. Many of these observations were motivated by Norman Geschwind, an extraordinary neurologist who served, for over fifteen years, as the James Jackson Putnam Professor at the Harvard Neurological Unit at the Boston City Hospital and later, at the Beth Israel Hospital. Geschwind was widely regarded as a remarkably perceptive clinical observer and an outstanding clinical teacher (Waxman, 1985). His most well-known contributions helped to elucidate the neuroanatomical substrates for language, but he was also interested in the verbal and non-verbal control of motor activity (see,

Reprinted with permission from *Progress in Brain Research* 107: 595–604, 1996. © 1996 Elsevier Science B.V. All rights reserved.

e.g., Geschwind, 1965*a, b*, 1975). At his bedside rounds, Geschwind frequently illustrated the relatively independent operation of several anatomically distinct motor systems in man, the first controlling distal appendicular musculature which can be activated volitionally in a highly fractionated manner, the second involving more proximal axial musculature involved in whole body activities such as maintenance of posture, body steering, and orientation. Still a third motor system innervates the facial and bulbar musculature involved in emotional expression and other affective displays. These three systems for motor control utilize relatively independent, descending pathways. Although neuroanatomic studies (see e.g. Chapters 2 and 32, this volume) have provided much of the basis for our understanding of multiple motor systems in primates, the existence of these parallel systems can also be inferred from clinical observation. This chapter discusses some clinical observations which illustrate the presence, in man, of these three motor systems.

Two Motor Systems Controlling the Limbs and Trunk

Figure 21.1 shows, in simplified diagrammatic form, two motor systems: (i) an axial motor system which controls posture, orientation, and body steering; and (ii) an appendicular motor system which controls fine, highly differentiated movements involving distal musculature (e.g. of the digits), in man. The first is controlled via bilateral (crossed and uncrossed) pathways which descend in the anterior and lateral funiculi of the spinal cord, whereas the second is carried predominantly by the crossed fibers which make up most of the lateral corticospinal tract. These two systems are affected differentially in patients with strokes involving the frequently affected

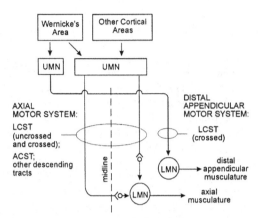

Figure 21.1
Multiple pathways of descending motor control. The axial system for whole-body, steering, and postural muscle activation utilizes both crossed and uncrossed projections (largely polysynaptic) from upper motor neurons (UMN) to lower motor neurons (LMN) in the lateral corticospinal tract (LCST) and anterior corticospinal tract (ACST). Individuated, precise distal appendicular motor control utilizes crossed (largely monosynaptic) pathways that project from upper motor neurons within the lateral corticospinal tract.

portions of the cerebral hemispheres (e.g., strokes in the territory of the middle cerebral artery). In these patients there is usually a stereotyped pattern of motor deficit which does not affect all muscles to an equal degree. The differentiated (rather than uniform) pattern of weakness reflects the pattern of motor control of various muscle groups involved in different functions. For example, in patients with middle cerebral territory infarctions, there is often loss of manual dexterity that can result in loss of function of the hand out of proportion to its weakness, in the context of preservation of gross movements at the shoulder.

The pattern of clinical deficit (or alternatively of recovery of function) reflects the fact that "pyramidal weakness" affects distal limb musculature more than proximal, and extensors more than flexors in the upper extremity and flexors more than extensors in the lower (Kuypers, 1968). Characteristically, recovery of strength in flexors of the fingers and hand precedes recovery of strength of the finger and wrist extensors in patients with pyramidal weakness, e.g., after cerebral infarcts. In fact, if motor function is (incorrectly) assessed by asking the patient to "squeeze my fingers," a hemiparesis may be missed; assessment of extension of the fingers provides a more sensitive measure of pyramidal tract dysfunction. The eventual degree of functional recovery can be predicted, to at least a rough degree, from serial examinations of the various muscle groups that are differentially affected after a cerebral infarct; if flaccidity of hand grip persists for more than seven days following a stroke, it is unlikely that there will be significant functional recovery (Twitchell, 1951). This differentiated pattern of motor dysfunction can be understood in neuroanatomical terms; for example, descending pyramidal innervation is most dense for motor neurons innervating the forearm and hand (Porter, 1968). Neuroanatomic studies suggest that monosynaptic projections from the primary motor cortex to motor neurons in the contralateral ventral horn provide part of the neural substrate for high-precision, fractionated movements of the fingers. (Bortoff and Strick, 1993). Whereas motor neurons innervating distal arm musculature are innervated by descending pathways originating in the contralateral cerebral hemisphere, motor neurons innervating proximal musculature (i.e. musculature controlling the shoulder) are innervated by descending pathways, very possibly polysynaptic, that originate on both sides of the midline (Brinkman and Kuypers, 1973).

Even after severe unilateral damage to the motor cortex or the lateral corticospinal tract, many patients show recovery of the ability to stand, and develop a stiff-legged and circumductive gait in association with abnormally increased extensor tone in the lower extremities. In this abnormal motor state, there is relatively increased tone in antigravity muscle groups (Waxman, 1988). Despite the absence of control from the contralateral motor cortex via the classical decussating pyramidal tract, the residual hemiplegic posture and gait confer the ability to remain upright and, to at least some degree, to propel the body in a forward direction. Interestingly, the hemiplegic posture is not a simple result of spasticity; lesions of the dorsal roots do not abolish the hemiplegic posture (Burke, 1988), and positioning a hemiplegic primate in an upside-down posture may result in extension of the upper limb together with flexion of the lower limb, presumably as a result of vestibulospinal influences (Denny-Brown, 1966).

Patients can recover the capability to walk in this circumductive manner even after large cerebral infarcts involving the territories of the middle and anterior cerebral arteries. The residual gait appears to be triggered, at least in part, by descending influences from the undamaged hemisphere ipsilateral to the paretic leg. In a study on patients who had undergone spinal cordotomy for intractable pain, Nathan and Smith (1969) observed that there was partial recovery of gait, with regression of paresis beginning within hours, in some patients following unilateral damage to the lateral corticospinal tract. Pathological studies showed that this recovery was mediated, in these patients, via descending projections located in the opposite lateral corticospinal tract. Interestingly, in patients in whom the lateral corticospinal tract on the opposite side of the cord was damaged by a subsequent lesion, the recovery was immediately reversed. These observations indicate that the lateral corticospinal tract on each side has bilateral influences on some lower motor neurons, providing a basis for partial recovery of gait after damage to the pyramidal (decussating) component of the corticospinal projections. Together with the phylogenetically older descending tracts in the anterior funiculus of the spinal cord, the uncrossed lateral corticospinal tract provides a substrate for maintenance of posture

and the ability to walk and stand after unilateral damage to the crossed lateral corticospinal tract. Similarly, this axial control system can provide residual motor function at the shoulder, even in patients with profound loss of dexterity in the hand. Following damage to the discriminative, high resolution pyramidal pathway which controls fine motor activities such as fractionated movements of the digits, the more primitive nonpyramidal motor system preserves the capability to activate more proximal musculature that is involved in the maintenance of posture, body steering, and orientation.

Autonomic and Emotional Automatisms in Temporal Lobe Epilepsy

Automatisms involving simple midline actions, often related to the alimentary system, are commonly seen as part of temporal lobe seizures. These can include chewing, swallowing, lip-smacking, and related activities. These autonomically-related motor activities presumably are triggered by abnormal limbic discharges.

It is well appreciated that temporal lobe seizures frequently include an affective component. For example, patients may experience sensations of pleasure, fear, grief, or sexual excitement during seizures (Penfield, 1955; Waxman and Geschwind, 1975; Engel, 1989). Autonomic and emotional automatisms can also occur as part of temporal lobe seizures. The autonomic components can include abnormal bowel activity or penile erection. Stereotyped masturbatory activity may also be seen. The repeated opening and closing of buttons, zippers, or other parts of the clothing seen in other patients presumably represents a fragment of grooming behavior, possibly an outgrowth of phylogenetically older courting or mating displays (see MacLean, 1986). The stereotyped nature of this ictal behavior hints at the existence of a relatively segregated set of motor pathways involved in limbic activity.

In other patients, laughter may occur as an epileptic phenomenon (Wilson, 1935; LeGros Clark et al., 1938; Gibbs and Gibbs, 1952); this has been termed "gelastic epilepsy" (Daly and Mulder, 1957), and is often associated with abnormal temporal lobe discharges (Roger et al., 1967). Kissing can also occur during temporal lobe seizures: smiling and crying are also seen. The pathways mediating these complex ictal facial movements are not known, but may involve the non-verbal input pathway (pathway 3) depicted in figure 21.4 later in this chapter.

Several Motor Systems Control Facial Muscle Activation

The existence of several motor systems controlling facial muscle activation can be inferred from behavioral observations on normal individuals, and from clinical observations on patients with focal brain lesions. As pointed out by Geschwind, and as appreciated by most of us, most normal individuals have difficulty mimicking facial expressions (such as smiling or frowning) when they do not feel the appropriate emotion (Ekman, 1993). Duchenne de Bologne (1862) noted that the orbicularis oculi muscle is activated during spontaneous smiling, but is not contracted during voluntary smiling; in fact, most normal individuals are unable to contract the orbicularis oculi on a voluntary basis (Ekman et al., 1990). The inability to voluntarily activate, in the appropriate sequence, the muscles involved in spontaneous smiling is of course well known to photographers, who are well aware that voluntary (posed) smiles often do not capture the full range of facial muscle activations seen in spontaneous smiling.

The differentiation between voluntary control of facial musculature, and emotionally evoked activation, can be readily appreciated by examination of patients exhibiting the pseudobulbar state. In these patients, as a result of bilateral damage to corticobulbar pathways, voluntary

activation of facial musculature is impaired. Thus, the patient cannot show his teeth, open his mouth, extend his tongue, or smile voluntarily or in response to command. Nevertheless, in the pseudobulbar state, the appropriate facial musculature is activated (often without the usual social inhibitions) in response to emotional stimuli (Poeck, 1969). In some patients, this pattern of activation occurs to an exaggerated degree, so that the patient exhibits "pathological laughing or crying" (Wilson, 1924). This pathologic response, which appears to be due to an impairment of normal inhibitory mechanisms that control facial expression, is frequently seen in patients with multiple sclerosis, and may respond to treatment with amitriptyline (Schiffer, 1985).

The pseudobulbar state demonstrates the presence of multiple systems for the control of facial musculature: a voluntary motor pathway, and an involuntary (emotional) motor pathway. The emotional motor pathway develops earlier during normal ontogenesis, where it seems to play a crucial role in preverbal maternal-infant interactions, and it is likely that it is older in phylogenetic terms since it is involved in primitive social, dominance, and courting behavior (MacLean, 1987). In fact, some lesions can impair emotionally evoked or spontaneous facial movements, while sparing voluntary movements of the face; this syndrome, termed "emotional facial paresis," is described below.

Emotional Facial Paresis

In unilateral upper motor neuron facial paresis, there is damage to upper motor neurons in one cerebral hemisphere associated with contralateral weakness of the face. These patients have difficulty activating the contralateral facial musculature voluntarily or in response to command; thus, some authors have used the term "voluntary facial paresis" to describe the syndrome. Most commonly only the lower half of the face is weak. The sparing of upper facial strength in voluntary facial paresis has classically been explained on the basis of bilateral cortical projections to motor neurons for the upper face, together with a purely contralateral projection to the remainder of the facial motor neurons which control musculature of the lower face (van Gehuchten 1898; Parhon and Minea, 1907). Recent neuroanatomic studies suggest an alternative explanation, that upper facial strength is preserved, like that of proximal limb musculature, because motor neurons for the upper face do not receive (or depend on) strong direct cortical input but are, on the contrary, activated by polysynaptic inputs that pass through the nearby pontine reticular formation (Jenny and Saper, 1987).

The converse of voluntary facial paresis, termed emotional facial paresis, refers to hemifacial paresis of emotionally evoked or spontaneous smiling or weeping in the context of preserved volitional movements of the face. This syndrome, which is much less common than voluntary facial paresis, has been termed amimia, and was first characterized by Stromeyer (cited in Wilson, 1924). Kinear Wilson (1924) described three cases of emotional facial paresis, two with pathologic findings; in one case there was a tumor involving the right internal capsule and subthalamic region, and in the second there was a tumor located in the midbrain tegmentum and rostral pons. Emotional facial paresis has been described in a patient with thalamic infarction limited to the anterolateral thalamus in the distribution of the tuberothalamic artery (Graff-Radford et al., 1984, 1985; Bogousslavsky et al., 1988), a branch of the posterior communicating artery supplying the anterior, ventral anterior, and ventral lateral nuclei (Archer et al., 1981). Adams and Victor (1989) have suggested that "anterior frontothalamopontomedullary connections," descending rostral to the genu of the internal capsule, are involved in the control of emotional expression.

Figure 21.2 shows a patient with emotional facial paresis, described by the author (Trosch

et al., 1990), in whom CT scan and MRI demonstrated infarction limited to the head of the caudate nucleus, putamen and anterior limb of the internal capsule on the contralateral side. The patient, a 15 year old right-handed boy, exhibited intact volitional facial movements, including platysma contraction in response to verbal commands. When asked to smile, he was able to contract the appropriate facial muscles fully and symmetrically. In contrast, in response to humorous or embarrassing comments, or with spontaneous smiling, there was marked facial asymmetry with a right lower facial droop associated with flattening of the nasolabial fold and an increased right palpebral fissure. Dysarthria, mild word-finding difficulties, and a mild right hemiparesis were also present acutely, but resolved in contrast to the emotional facial paresis which persisted as an isolated neurologic deficit.

The lesion in this patient (figure 21.3) was an infarction involving the left caudate, globus pallidus, putamen, and anterior limb of the internal capsule. Notably, the caudal portion of the posterior limb of the internal capsule was spared. Significant thalamic involvement was not evident on follow-up MRI, nor were other lesions observed. Arteriography revealed segmental beading of the anterior cerebral artery, a pattern of involvement that is usually seen in striatocapsular infarction (Bladin and Berkovic, 1984; Caplan et al., 1989) in the distribution of either the lateral lenticulostriate arteries arising from the middle cerebral artery (Damasio, 1983), or the recurrent artery of Heubner or anterior perforators branching from the proximal anterior cerebral (Caplan et al., 1989).

The absence of a voluntary facial paresis, which is usually present in this clinical setting, may have been due in this patient to sparing of the caudal 1/3 of the posterior limb of the internal capsule, which appears to contain the corticobulbar fibers controlling facial musculature in some patients (Englander et al., 1975). Stimulation of the posterior part of the internal capsule

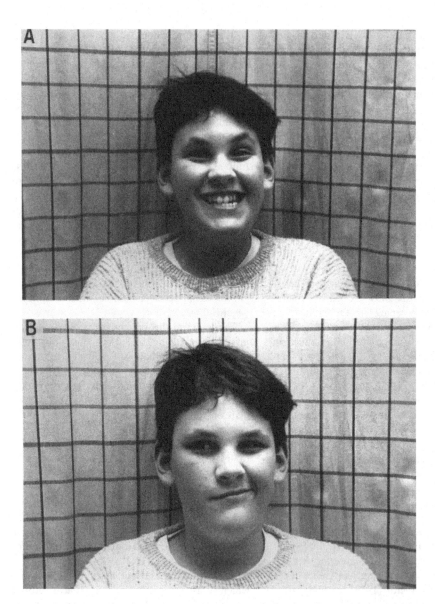

Figure 21.2
Emotional facial paresis. (*A*) Symmetric volitional smile performed in response to verbal command. (*B*) In response to humorous comment, only half of the face smiles. Note the increased right palpebral fissure as well as the flattened nasolabial fold. A similar asymmetry was present in spontaneous smiling. From Trosch et al. (1990).

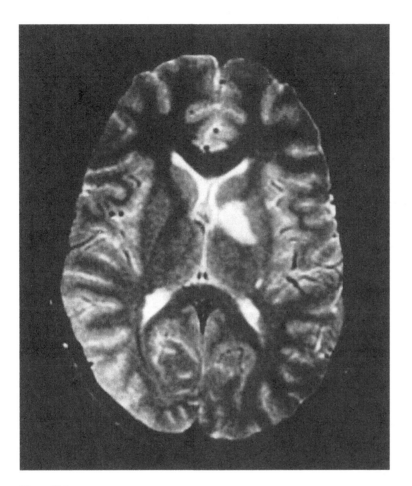

Figure 21.3
T2-weighted MR scan of the patient shown in figure 21.2. The lesion is centered in the globus pallidus and putamen but also involves the caudate and anterior limb of the internal capsule. From Trosch et al. (1990).

during stereotaxic surgery can, in fact, evoke contraction of the contralateral facial muscles (Bertrand, 1966).

The extrathalamic lesion in this patient with emotional facial paresis is consistent with the early cases described by Wilson in which there were lesions involving the internal capsule and subthalamic region, and the midbrain tegmentum and rostral pons, respectively. On the basis of stimulation experiments in subhuman primates, he postulated the presence of two descending pathways for emotional control of "faciorespiratory" motor activity, the first arising from the basal frontal lobe and the second from the somatosensory cortex, converging in the thalamus. The MRI demonstration of a striatocapsular lesion associated with emotional facial paresis (Trosch et al., 1990), however, shows that thalamic involvement is not required for the production of this disorder. In this case, damage to the striatum may have produced emotional facial paresis. The facial masking that occurs in Parkinson's disease, in which there is dopaminergic loss that is most severe within the striatum (Kish et al., 1988), also supports the conclusion that striatal lesions can produce emotional facial paresis.

An alternative localization for a pathway controlling emotionally-driven facial muscle activity, which is supported by the MRI findings in this case, involves the anterior limb of the internal capsule. Such a localization would be consistent with the suggestion of Adams and Victor (1989) of anterior frontothalamopontomedullary connections which descend rostral to the genu of the internal capsule. Since pyramidal tract fibers controlling facial and bulbar musculature are located in the posterior limb (Englander et al., 1975), preservation of the caudal posterior limb of the internal capsule in this case could provide an anatomic basis for retained voluntary facial movements in this patient.

Together with the pseudobulbar syndrome, emotional facial paresis provides evidence for the existence of several distinct descending path-

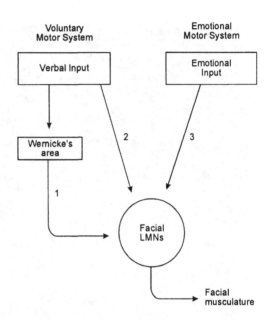

Figure 21.4
Speculative schema showing multiple pathways for facial motor control in man. Pathway 1 can be activated voluntarily in response to verbal command and involves Wernicke's area. Pathway 2 controls simple undifferentiated facial muscle activation (eye opening/closure, mouth opening/closure) in response to verbal command but bypasses Wernicke's area. Pathway 3 is dependent on striatocapsular structures, and activates facial musculature in response to emotional (and not necessarily verbal) stimuli.

ways controlling facial expression (figure 21.4): a voluntarily activated pathway which can be accessed in response to verbal command if function of Wernicke's area is intact (pathway 1); and another, dependent on striatocapsular structures, that activates facial musculature in response to emotional (and not necessarily verbal) state (pathway 3). There is also evidence, based on observations of patients with Wernicke's aphasia, for another pathway (pathway 2) bypassing Wernicke's area, that controls simple facial movements such as closing and opening the eyes, opening the mouth, etc.

Residual Motor Control Pathways in Patients with Wernicke's Aphasia

Patients with Wernicke's aphasia provide an interesting illustration of the operation of multiple motor control systems in humans (Geschwind, 1965b, 1975). Careful examination reveals that many of these patients exhibit a dissociated loss of the ability to perform motor tasks in response to verbal command. As expected from their severely impaired comprehension, these patients usually cannot perform appropriately when asked to carry out actions involving distal appendicular musculature ("point at me"; "touch your nose"; "make a fist"). Despite this, these patients often retain the ability to carry out whole-body movements involving midline or proximal musculature in response to verbal commands, and thus perform correctly when asked to "stand up," "bow," "turn around," "dance," "show me a boxer's stance," or "sit down." As in the case of hemiparetic motor activity, these patients display a dissociated impairment of fine, fractionated motor performance involving distal musculature of the limbs (e.g., the fingers) in response to verbal commands, in the context of preserved proximal, postural and steering functions that utilize axial musculature.

A similar dissociation can be seen in facial motor activity. Simple commands involving midline or bilateral facial musculature, such as "close your eyes," "open your mouth," and "open your eyes" often elicit correct responses in patients with Wernicke's aphasia. On the other hand, complex or lateralizing commands, such as "stick your tongue out and to the right" or "push against your cheek with your tongue" are typically not followed; similarly, these patients are often unable to voluntarily smile, frown, or laugh in response to verbal command. Yet spontaneous facial expression is preserved.

The preservation of responses to midline, whole-body commands in these patients, in contrast to the loss of ability to respond to complex appendicular commands, can be explained on the basis of differential control of axial muscle groups, mediated by different pathways than responses involving distal (pyramidally-innervated) musculature. As described above, neuroanatomic studies (Kuypers, 1968; Lawrence and Kuypers, 1968; Brinkman and Kuypers, 1973) have, in fact, provided evidence indicating that postural movements are controlled by different pathways than those that control distal finger movement. Geschwind (1965b, 1975) has suggested that control of axial of whole-body movements involves non-pyramidal pathways running in association with the bundle of Turck, which arise from multiple sites in the cortex including the superior temporal gyrus. It is possible that this motor control system receives input from regions in the non-dominant hemisphere that retain the capability to respond to fragments of language. Although the detailed organization of the non-pyramidal motor pathways is not understood, the observations from hemiparetic patients, and from non-paretic patients with Wernicke's aphasia, are consistent in indicating the existence of discrete descending motor systems, one controlling fractional or complex movements and requiring the crossed lateral corticospinal tract with strong input from Wernicke's area for verbal activation; and the other controlling midline, whole body movements and utilizing bilateral descending pathways that do not depend on input from Wernicke's area (figure 21.1).

In terms of facial motor control, the clinical observations indicate the existence of at least three independent pathways (figure 21.4). The first (pathway 1) involves Wernicke's area and controls complex voluntary facial muscle activation including the response to complex verbal commands. Pathway 2 activates simple, symmetric or bilateral facial activities such as eye-opening/closure and mouth opening/closure and, while bypassing Wernicke's area, can be accessed by verbal inputs. Pathway 3, the emotional motor pathway, mediates spontaneous and emotionally evoked facial expression. As shown by the preservation of spontaneous and emotionally evoked facial expression in patients with Wernicke's aphasia who can not smile or frown in response to verbal command, pathway 3 is separate from pathways 1 and 2.

As shown in this paper, clinical observations demonstrate the presence in humans of multiple motor systems whose existence has also been demonstrated by neuroanatomic studies in primates. While the traditional neurological examination tends to focus on the precise, highly fractionated outputs of the voluntary, verbally-controlled motor system, careful behavioral observation, including observation of spontaneous and non-verbally-evoked behavior, can provide important information about the function of the emotional motor system. Coupled with modern techniques of neuro-imaging such as fMRI (functional magnetic resonance imaging), it is likely that careful behavioral observations will shed considerable light on the anatomic organization of the emotional motor system in humans.

Acknowledgments

This work was supported in part by the Medical Research Service, Department of Veterans Affairs. This paper is dedicated to D.W., one of my most important teachers.

References

Adams, R. D. and Victor, M. (1989) *Principles of Neurology*, McGraw-Hill, New York.

Archer, C. R., Ilinsky, I. A., Goldfader, P. R. and Smith, K. R. (1981) Aphasia in thalamic stroke: CT stereotactic localization. *J. Comput. Assist. Tomogr., 5:* 427–432.

Bertrand, G. (1966) Stimulation during stereotaxic operations for dyskinesias. *J. Neurosurg., 24:* 419–423.

Bladin, P. F. and Berkovic, S. F. (1984) Striatocapsular infarction: large infarcts in the lenticulostriate arterial territory. *Neurology,* 38: 1423–1430.

Bogousslavsky, J., Regli, F. and Uske, A. (1988) Thalamic infarcts: clinical syndromes, etiology, and prognosis. *Neurology,* 38: 837–848.

Bortoff, G. A. and Strick, P. L. (1993) Corticospinal terminations in two new-world primates: further evidence that corticomotoneuronal connections provide part of the neural substrate for manual dexterity. *J. Neurosci.,* 13: 5105–5118.

Brinkman, J. and Kuypers, H. (1973) Cerebral control of contralateral and ipsilateral arm, hand and finger movements in the split-brain Rhesus monkey. *Brain,* 96: 653–674.

Burke, D. (1988) Spasticity as an adaptation to pyramidal tract injury. In: S. G. Waxman (Ed.), *Functional Recovery in Neurological Disease,* Raven Press, New York, pp. 401–424.

Caplan, L. R., Schahmann, J. D., Kase, C. S., Feldmann, E., Baquir, G., Greenberg, J. P., Gorelick, P. B., Helgasm, C. and Hien, D. B. (1989) Caudate infarcts. *Arch. Neurol.,* 47: 133–143.

Daly, D. D. and Mulder, D. W. (1957) Gelastic epilepsy. *Neurology (Minneapolis),* 7: 189–192.

Damasio, H. (1983) A computed tomographic guide to the identification of cerebral vascular territories. *Arch. Neurol,* 40: 138–142.

Denny-Brown, D. (1966) *The Cerebral Control of Movement,* Liverpool University Press, Liverpool.

Duchenne de Bologne, B. (1862; translated, 1990) *The Mechanism of Human Facial Expression or an Electro-Physiological Analysis of the Expression of the Emotions,* Cambridge University Press, New York.

Ekman, P. (1993) Facial expression and emotion. *Am. Psychol,* 48: 384–392.

Ekman, P., Davidson, R. J. and Friesen, W. V. (1990) The Duchenne smile: emotional expression and brain physiology II. *J. Pers. Soc. Psychol.,* 58: 342–353.

Engel, J. J. (1989) *Seizures and Epilepsy,* F. A. Davis, Philadelphia, PA.

Englander, R. N., Netsky, M. D. and Adelman, L. S. (1975) Location of human pyramidal tract in the internal capsule: anatomic evidence. *Neurology,* 25: 823–826.

Geschwind, N. (1965a) Disconnection syndromes in animals and man, II. *Brain,* 88: 585–644.

Geschwind, N. (1965b) Disconnection syndromes in animals and man, I. *Brain,* 88: 237–294.

Geschwind, N. (1975) The apraxias: neural mechanisms of disorders of learned movements. *Am. Sci.,* 188–195.

Gibbs, F. A. and Gibbs, E. L. (1952) *Atlas of Electroencephalography,* Addison-Wesley, Cambridge.

Graff-Radford, N. R., Eslinger, P. J., Damasio, A. R. and Yamada, T. (1984) Nonhemorrhagic infarction of the thalamus. *Neurology,* 34: 14–23.

Graff-Radford, N. R., Damasio, H., Yamada, T., Eslinger, P. J. and Damasio, A. R. (1985) Nonhemorrhagic thalamic infarction. *Brain,* 108: 485–516.

Jenny, A. B. and Saper, C. B. (1987) Organization of the facial nucleus and corticofacial projection in the monkey: a reconsideration of the upper motor neuron facial palsy. *Neurology,* 37: 930–939.

Kish, S. J., Shannak, K. and Hornykiewicz, O. (1988) Uneven pattern of dopamine loss in the striatum of patients with idiopathic Parkinson's disease. *N. Engl. J. Med.,* 318: 876–880.

Kuypers, H. (1968) *The Anatomical Organization of the Descending Pathways and their Contributions to Motor Control, Especially in Primates,* Karger, Basel.

Lawrence, D. G. and Kuypers, H. (1968) Functional organization of the motor system in the monkey, I: effects of bilateral pyramidal lesions. *Brain,* 91: 1–14.

LeGros Clark, W. E., Beattie, J., Riddoch, G. and Dott, N. M. (1938) *The Hypothalamus,* Oliver and Boyd, Edinburgh.

MacLean, P. D. (1986) Ictal symptoms relating to affects and their cerebral substrate. In: R. Plutchick (Ed.), *Emotion: Theory, Research, and Experience,* Academic Press, Orlando, FL, pp. 61–90.

MacLean, P. D. (1987) The midline frontolimbic cortex and the evolution of crying and laughing. In: E. Perecman (Ed.), *The Frontal Lobes Revisited,* IRBN Press, New York, pp. 121–140.

Nathan, P. W. and Smith, M. C. (1969) Effects of two unilateral cordotomies on the motility of the lower limbs. *Brain,* 96: 471–494.

Parhon, C. J. and Minea, J. (1907) L'origine du facial supérieur. *Presse Med,* 15: 521–522.

Penfield, W. (1955) The twenty-ninth Maudsley lecture: the role of the temporal cortex in certain psychical phenomena. *J. Ment. Sci.,* 101: 451.

Poeck, K. (1969) *Pathophysiology of Emotional Disorders Associated With Brain Damage,* Elsevier, Amsterdam.

Porter, R. (1968) The corticomotoneuronal component of the pyramidal tract: corticomotoneuronal connections and functions in primates. *Brain Res. Rev.,* 10: 1–26.

Roger, J., Lob, H., Waltregny, A. and Gastaut, H. (1967) Attacks of epileptic laughter: on 5 cases. *Electroencephalogr. Clin. Neurophysiol.,* 22: 279.

Schiffer, R. B. (1985) Treatment of pathologic laughing and weeping with amitriptyline. *N. Engl. J. Med.,* 312: 1480–1482.

Trosch, R., Sze, G., Brass, L. M. and Waxman, S. G. (1990) Emotional facial paresis with striatocapsular infarction. *J. Neurol. Sci.,* 98: 195–202.

Twitchell, T. E. (1951) Restoration of motor function following hemiplegia in man. *Brain,* 74: 143–180.

van Gehuchten, A. (1898) L'origine du facial chez le lapin. *Rev. Neurol. (Paris),* 6: 553.

Waxman, S. G. (1985) Norman Geschwind. *J. Neurol. Sci.,* 69: 113–115.

Waxman, S. G. (1988) Nonpyramidal motor systems and functional recovery after damage to the central nervous system. *J. Neurol. Rehab.,* 2: 1–6.

Waxman, S. G. and Geschwind, N. (1975) The interictal behavior syndrome of temporal lobe epilepsy. *Arch. Gen. Psychiatry,* 32: 1580–1586.

Wilson, S. A. K. (1924) Some problems in neurology, 11: pathological laughing and crying. *J. Neurol. Psychopathol.,* 16: 299–316.

Wilson, S. A. K. (1935) The epilepsies. In: O. Bumke and O. Foerster (Eds.), *Handbuch der Neurologie,* Vol. 17, Springer, Berlin, p. 1.

XIV AN AMBIVALENT SEE-SAW

Stroke is the third most frequent killer, and spinal cord injury paralyzes 14,000 people in the United States, mostly young adults, every year. Paralysis and other disabilities in these catastrophic disorders are due to damage to nerve cells and nerve fibers and, until recently, it was accepted as dogma that, once the insult had occurred, there was nothing that could be done. We are now beginning to ask, however, how precious cells in the brain and spinal cord die following loss of oxygen-carrying blood supply in stroke and following physical trauma in spinal cord injury. Cardiologists began to learn, decades ago, about the death of heart cells and, having understood this process, they developed a series of medications which can keep people alive—and functional—by protecting cells so that they do not die after heart attacks. Can we use similar information to lessen the toll exacted by stroke and spinal cord injury?

Cell death does not occur immediately after loss of oxygen or trauma to the nervous system. Loss of nerve cells occurs after a latent period of a few hours to a few days in these disorders, and is produced by a self-destructive process of secondary cell injury, which is set into motion by the initial insult. Some of the molecular steps involved in secondary cell injury can be blocked with drugs, suggesting that it may be possible to interrupt the death cascade, thereby protecting precious nervous tissue so that cells within it do not degenerate. "Neuroprotection" has emerged as an important goal of contemporary neuroscience.

The brain and spinal cord can be grossly divided into gray matter and white matter. Gray matter comprises parts of the nervous system where synapses impinge on the cell bodies and branchlike dendrites of neurons; it is within the gray matter, therefore, that synaptic transmission occurs and, as a result of this, gray matter has attracted more interest than white matter. White matter, on the other hand, consists of tracts of myelinated nerve fibers (white matter is white, in fact, because the lipid-rich myelin gives it a glistening appearance). White matter includes the descending nerve fibers necessary for motor control and the ascending nerve fibers that carry sensory information within the spinal cord.

One of the most exciting advances in neuroscience over the past decade has been the discovery that, within gray matter, secondary cell death involves a molecular cascade, called "excitotoxicity" (Choi, 1998; Lee et al. 1999). Neurons communicate with each other by releasing specialized molecules, called neurotransmitters, at synapses. These neurotransmitters can be excitatory (increasing electrical activity in postsynaptic neurons) or inhibitory (decreasing electrical activity in postsynaptic neurons). Most excitatory synapses within the brain and spinal cord utilize a neurotransmitter called glutamate. Following trauma or loss of oxygen or the oxygen-carrying blood supply, neurons have been shown to release inappropriately large amounts of glutamate, which excites cells, causing them to be active when they should be silent. This can, in turn, lead to release of still more glutamate, producing a self-reinforcing cycle. As the high concentration of glutamate interacts with postsynaptic neurons, it opens up membrane pores that are permeable to calcium. These provide a route for the influx of large amounts of calcium, which can overwhelm the buffering capacity of the cell and activate self-destructive enzymes. The discovery of this excitotoxic pathway was important: it suggested that, by blocking inappropriate glutamate release, its interaction with postsynaptic neurons, or the ensuing avalanche of calcium or its effect on these self-destructive enzymes, it might be possible to develop neuroprotective strategies that protect gray matter, preserving nerve cells and thereby limiting loss of function following stroke, brain and spinal cord injury, and other insults.

By the late 1980s excitotoxicity had been carefully studied by Choi and others, and I felt that there was not much that I could add to the story. But my coworkers and I were interested in white matter, in part because of the importance of white matter for function of the spinal cord. Given the absence of synapses within white matter, one would not expect excitotoxicity to occur there. This raised several questions: Does secondary injury occur within white matter axons? If so, is it calcium-dependent? How, in the absence of excitotoxicity, does injurious calcium enter nerve fibers within white matter? And, perhaps most important, can secondary cell injury in white matter be slowed or halted? Beginning in 1989 Peter Stys, Bruce Ransom, and I did a series of experiments aimed at answering these questions. Bruce suggested the use of the optic nerve as an experimental model providing a representative piece of white matter which could be readily isolated from gray matter and studied within a single tract. Since the nerve fibers within white matter are small and fragile, intracellular recording or voltage-clamping for more than a few minutes were not practical. At Bruce's suggestion, Peter therefore used suction electrodes to record the activity of undissected nerve fibers within the optic nerve. Peter had just joined the laboratory as a postdoc and, having an engineering background, he was able to refine the suction electrode into a highly quantitative tool for recording electrical activity of the optic nerve so that we could monitor the functional integrity in its small nerve fibers (Stys et al. 1991, 1993).

Using these methods, we first asked: given the absence of receptors for glutamate on nerve fibers with axons within white matter, does calcium-mediated cell injury occur there? We tested this by exposing the isolated optic nerve to anoxia, or loss of oxygen, under highly controlled conditions in the laboratory, and monitoring its function (Stys et al. 1990). Under normal circumstances, with calcium present in the extracellular fluid, this resulted in severe loss of function within the optic nerve. But if we removed calcium from the extracellular fluid bathing the optic nerve, all of the nerve fibers within it survived and continued to function, even after an hour with no oxygen. This taught us that, even in the absence of excitotoxicity, irreversible injury of nerve fibers in white matter is dependent on the presence of calcium in the extracellular milieu (Stys et al. 1990). The calcium was presumably flooding cells during anoxia, but which cells? Using the electron microscope, our colleague Joel Black examined the anoxic optic nerve, and we found that axons are an important target of calcium-mediated injury within white matter (Waxman et al. 1992, 1993). We thus learned that, even in the absence of excitoxicity, calcium influx into axons constitutes part of the pathway leading to secondary cell injury of white matter.

The next step was to determine how calcium enters axons. These studies are described in Stys, Waxman, and Ransom (1992), which follows this chapter. In these experiments we again used suction electrodes, together with various channel-blocking drugs and manipulation of the ion concentrations in the fluid surrounding nerve fibers. These experiments, and observations on the optic nerve under various experimental conditions with the electron microscope (Waxman et al. 1994), suggested that two different molecules, sodium channels and the "sodium-calcium exchanger," collaborate to carry damaging amounts of calcium into axons. The sodium-calcium exchanger is an antiporter molecule, a see-saw which normally carries sodium into cells, exchanging it for calcium and thereby maintaining intracellular calcium at low levels which are optimal for cell function. The sodium-calcium exchanger operates as a thermodynamic machine and thus is an ambivalent see-saw. It can be driven to operate in a "reverse" mode when intracellular sodium is high and, when this occurs, it can carry calcium —even damaging concentrations of calcium—into axons. Our experiments showed us that, following damage to the optic nerve, sodium channels admit sodium ions into axons. Our results also indicated that this triggers reverse sodium-calcium exchange in the anoxic optic nerve, a mechanism of injurious calcium entry that does not require glutamate channels. Several years later, after establishing his own laboratory in Ottawa, Stys used electron probe microanalysis to more directly demonstrate reverse sodium-calcium exchange in the anoxic optic nerve (LoPachin and Stys 1995; Stys and LoPachin 1997).

Once we had learned that sodium channels and the sodium-calcium exchanger can collaborate to carry injurious calcium into axons within white matter, a next step was to ask whether blockade of these critical molecules, using drugs that bind specifically to them, might have a protective effect. This led to a series of experiments that showed that it is indeed possible to protect white matter from anoxic injury with drugs that block sodium channels or the sodium-calcium exchanger (Stys, Waxman, and Ransom 1992; Stys, Ransom, and Waxman 1992; Fern et al. 1993; Stys 1994).

Stys's replacement in our laboratory was Bob Fern, who had just completed his Ph.D. in physiology at University College London. He took this line of work a step farther, and showed that several neurotransmitters (gamma-amino-butyric acid, also called GABA; and adenosine) can modulate this injurious cascade, thereby having a protective effect on damaged white matter (Fern, Waxman, and Ransom 1994, 1995). Fern's experiments added a new dimension by showing that, following injury, cells within white matter release these protective substances, an endogenous action that limits subsequent cell injury. He termed this novel mechanism "autoprotection."

These results would at first blush appear to provide a basis for neuroprotection after stroke and spinal cord injury. But what, in fact, are the prospects? We know a lot about mechanisms of secondary cell injury in gray matter of the nervous system, and on this basis a series of compounds—drugs that block the effects of glutamate, for example—have been studied and shown to be neuroprotective in animal models of stroke. But clinical studies in humans have, to date, shown either no improvement in outcome or, at best, only very modest improvement. We do not know for sure why these clinical stroke trials have been so disappointing. One hopeful possibility is that the drugs that were tested do protect gray matter from stroke, but fail to provide clinical improvement because their beneficial effects are eclipsed by damage to unprotected white matter. If this conjecture is correct, combined neuroprotection of both gray and white matter might be expected to improve the outcome after stroke. Similar logic applies to spinal cord injury.

Research on neuroprotection is going on around the world, and if it continues at its current pace I can envision a scenario in which, at some time in the future, the victims of automobile accidents who have injured their spinal cords and patients who have suffered strokes will be cared for in special units similar to coronary care units. Because secondary cell injury progresses relatively quickly, neuroprotective medications would be administered to these patients on-site by trained emergency medical personnel or immediately upon arrival in the emergency room. Just as cardiologists use tools—drugs that preserve heart tissue—to help patients with heart attacks, neurologists would have new tools—medications that modulate the behavior of critical molecules along the pathway to cell damage—to protect precious brain and spinal cord tissue. This new therapeutic armamentarium would preserve not only the structure but also the function of our brains and spinal cords. This will not be easy, but there is an array of molecules like the ambivalent see-saw that may present opportunities to make this happen.

References

Choi, D. W. Calcium-mediated neurotoxicity: still center-stage in hypoxic-ischemic neuronal death. *Trends Neurosci.* 18: 58–60, 1995.

Fern, R., Ransom, B. R., Stys, P. K., and Waxman, S. G. Pharmacological protection of CNS white matter during anoxia: actions of phenytoin, carbamazepine and diazepam. *J. Pharmacol. Exper. Ther.* 266: 1549–1555, 1993.

Fern, R., Waxman, S. G., and Ransom, B. R. Modulation of anoxic injury in CNS white matter by adenosine, and interaction between adenosine and GABA. *J. Neurophysiol.* 72: 2609–2616, 1994.

Fern, R., Waxman, S. G., and Ransom, B. R. Endogenous GABA attenuates CNS white matter dysfunction following anoxia. *J. Neurosci.* 15: 699–708, 1995.

Lee, J. M., Zipfel, G. J., and Choi, D. W. The changing landscape of ischaemic brain injury. *Nature* 399: A7–A14, 1999.

LoPachin, R. M., and Stys, P. K. Elemental composition and water content of rat optic nerve myelinated axons and glial cells: effects of in vitro anoxia and reoxygenation. *J. Neurosci.* 15: 6735–6746, 1995.

Stys, P. K. Protective effects of antiarrhythmic agents against anoxic injury in CNS white matter. *J. Cereb. Blood Flow Metab.* 15: 425–432, 1994.

Stys, P. K., and LoPachin, R. M. Mechanisms of calcium and sodium fluxes in anoxic myelinated central nervous system axons. *Neuroscience* 82: 21–32, 1997.

Stys, P. K., Ransom, B. R., Waxman, S. G., and Davis, P. K. Role of extracellular calcium in anoxic injury of mammalian central white matter. *Proc. Natl. Acad. Sci. U.S.A.* 87: 4212–4216, 1990.

Stys, P. K., Ransom, B. R., and Waxman, S. G. Compound action potential of nerve recorded by suction electrode: A theoretical and experimental analysis. *Brain Res.* 546: 18–32, 1991.

Stys, P. K., Ransom, B. R., and Waxman, S. G. Tertiary and quaternary local anesthetics protect CNS white matter from anoxic injury at concentrations that do not block excitability. *J. Neurophysiol.* 67: 236–240, 1992.

Stys, P. K., Sontheimer, H., Ransom, B. R., and Waxman, S. G. Non-inactivating, TTX-sensitive Na^+ conductance in rat optic nerve axons. *Proc. Natl. Acad. Sci. U.S.A.* 90: 6976–6980, 1993.

Stys, P. K., Waxman, S. G., and Ransom, B. R. Ionic mechanisms of anoxic injury in mammalian CNS white matter: Role of Na^+ channels and Na^+-Ca^{2+} exchanger. *J. Neurosci.* 12: 430–439, 1992.

Waxman, S. G., Black, J. A., Stys, P. K., and Ransom, B. R. Ultrastructural concomitants of anoxic injury and early post-anoxic recovery in rat optic nerve. *Brain Res.* 574: 105–119, 1992.

Waxman, S. G., Black, J. A., Ransom, B. R., and Stys, P. K. Protection of the axonal cytoskeleton in anoxic optic nerve by decreased extracellular calcium. *Brain Res.* 614: 137–145, 1993.

Waxman, S. G., Black, J. A., Ransom, B. R., and Stys, P. K. Anoxic injury of rat optic nerve: ultrastructural evidence for coupling between Na^+ influx and Ca^{2+}-mediated injury in myelinated CNS axons. *Brain Res.* 644: 197–204, 1994.

22 Ionic Mechanisms of Anoxic Injury in Mammalian CNS White Matter: Role of Na$^+$ Channels and Na$^+$–Ca^{2+} Exchanger

Peter K. Stys, Stephen G. Waxman, and Bruce R. Ransom

Abstract White matter of the mammalian CNS suffers irreversible injury when subjected to anoxia/ischemia. However, the mechanisms of anoxic injury in central myelinated tracts are not well understood. Although white matter injury depends on the presence of extracellular Ca^{2+}, the mode of entry of Ca^{2+} into cells has not been fully characterized. We studied the mechanisms of anoxic injury using the in vitro rat optic nerve, a representative central white matter tract. Functional integrity of the nerves was monitored electrophysiologically by quantitatively measuring the area under the compound action potential, which recovered to 33.5 ± 9.3% of control after a standard 60 min anoxic insult. Reducing Na$^+$ influx through voltage-gated Na$^+$ channels during anoxia by applying Na$^+$ channel blockers (TTX, saxitoxin) substantially improved recovery; TTX was protective even at concentrations that had little effect on the control compound action potential. Conversely, increasing Na$^+$ channel permeability during anoxia with veratridine resulted in greater injury. Manipulating the transmembrane Na$^+$ gradient at various times before or during anoxia greatly affected the degree of resulting injury; applying zero-Na$^+$ solution (choline or Li$^+$ substituted) before anoxia significantly improved recovery; paradoxically, the same solution applied after the start of anoxia resulted in more injury than control. Thus, ionic conditions that favored reversal of the normal transmembrane Na$^+$ gradient during anoxia promoted injury, suggesting that Ca^{2+} loading might occur via reverse operation of the Na$^+$–Ca^{2+} exchanger. Na$^+$–Ca^{2+} exchanger blockers (bepridil, benzamil, dichlorobenzamil) significantly protected the optic nerve from anoxic injury. Together, these results suggest the following sequence of events leading to anoxic injury in the rat optic nerve: anoxia causes rapid depletion of ATP and membrane depolarization leading to Na$^+$ influx through incompletely inactivated Na$^+$ channels. The resulting rise in the intracellular [Na$^+$], coupled with membrane depolarization, causes damaging levels of Ca^{2+} to be admitted into the intracellular compartment through reverse operation of the Na$^+$–Ca^{2+} exchanger. These observations emphasize

that differences in the pathophysiology of gray and white matter anoxic injury are likely to necessitate multiple strategies for optimal CNS protection.

White matter (WM) of the CNS, a tissue composed exclusively of axons, myelin, and glial cells, is injured by anoxia and ischemia, although it is more resistant to such injury than gray matter (Ransom et al., 1990a). Damage to WM disrupts afferent and efferent axonal connections and can result in severe neurological disability. Clinically, anoxic/ischemic WM injury is commonly caused by focal or global disruption of cerebral blood flow, that is, stroke. In addition, traumatic spinal cord injury prominently involves WM, and damage to spinal tracts is due in part to vascular compromise leading to anoxia/ischemia (Young, 1987; Fehlings et al., 1989). The mechanisms of anoxic/ischemic injury in WM are known to be different from those operating in gray matter (for reviews, see Bengtsson and Siesjö, 1990; Ransom et al., 1990a), but have not yet been fully characterized. An understanding of these fundamental mechanisms in WM may lead the way to developing protective strategies against such injury.

Irreversible anoxic/ischemic injury in gray matter involves influx of Ca^{2+} across the membrane through excitotoxin-gated channels (Choi, 1985), and possibly via voltage-gated Ca^{2+} channels (Krieglstein et al., 1989; Weiss et al., 1990). Using the in vitro rat optic nerve model, we showed that influx of extracellular Ca^{2+} is also a critical mediator of anoxic injury in CNS WM (Stys et al., 1990a). In contrast to gray matter, however, this Ca^{2+} influx in WM does not occur via excitotoxin-gated or voltage-gated Ca^{2+} channels (Ransom et al., 1990b; Stys et al., 1990b). Here we report evidence suggesting that WM anoxic injury largely depends on a persistent membrane Na$^+$ conductance, which in turn allows intracellular [Na$^+$] to rise sufficiently to

Reprinted with permission from *The Journal of Neuroscience* 12: 430–439, 1992.

Table 22.1
Composition of perfusion solutions (in mM)

	Normal CSF	Zero-Na⁺ Choline	Zero-Na⁺ Li⁺
NaCl	126	—	—
KCl	3.0	1.75	1.75
LiCl	—	—	127
Choline Cl	—	127	—
MgSO₄	2.0	2.0	2.0
NaHCO₃	26	—	—
Choline bicarbonate	—	26	26
NaH₂PO₄	1.25	—	—
KH₂PO₄	—	1.25	1.25
CaCl₂	2.0	2.0	2.0
Dextrose	10	10	10

promote reverse operation of the Na^+–Ca^{2+} exchanger. We have found that a large part of the damaging Ca^{2+} influx occurs via reverse Na^+–Ca^{2+} exchange; blocking either Na^+ channels or the Na^+–Ca^{2+} exchanger significantly protects CNS WM against anoxic injury.

Materials and Methods

Long–Evans rats aged 50–70 d were anesthetized with an 80% CO_2, 20% O_2 gas mixture and decapitated. The rat optic nerve (RON) has developed mature physiological properties in animals of this age (Connors et al., 1982; Foster et al., 1982; Ransom et al., 1985). The RONs were dissected free, placed in a modified interface perfusion chamber (Medical Systems Corp., Greenvale, NY), and incubated for 60–90 min before measurements were begun. The tissue was maintained at 37°C, oxygenated in a 95% O_2, 5% CO_2 atmosphere (pH 7.45), and perfused with artificial cerebrospinal fluid (CSF). Compositions of normal CSF and, choline- and Li⁺-substituted zero-Na⁺ solutions are shown in table 22.1.

Orthodromic stimulation and recording from RONs were accomplished using suction electrodes (Stys et al., 1990a, 1991a). Square constant-voltage stimulus pulses (50 μsec duration) were delivered via an isolation unit at 30 sec intervals. Stimulus strength was set to 25% above the strength that was required to elicit a maximal compound action potential (CAP; typically 70–120 V). Evoked CAPs were digitized (Nicolet 310 digital oscilloscope, 200 kHz sampling rate, 12 bit vertical resolution) and transferred to a microcomputer (Apple Macintosh IIfx), where the records were stored and analyzed using custom software (Stys, 1991).

Functional integrity of the RONs was quantitated by computing the area under the CAP (calculated over the interval from 0.2 to 12 msec with respect to stimulus onset), since activities of individual axons within a myelinated nerve bundle sum linearly to form the compound response (Buchthal and Rosenfalck, 1966; Cummins et al., 1979; Wijesinghe et al., 1991). We believe the CAP area to be the most representative measure of overall functional integrity of the nerve, since it reflects the number of axons that are capable of conducting action potentials. Under some conditions, CAP area recovered almost fully but the shape of the response remained irreversibly altered. This suggests that, in these experiments, most axons recovered the ability to conduct action potentials, but some injury still occurred and resulted in a slowing of the conduction velocities of some constituent fibers. We did not attempt to study conduction velocity systematically. Stable and reproducible measurements of CAP area were obtained after correcting for drift inherent in suction electrode recording (Stys et al., 1991a).

Anoxia was achieved by switching to a 95% N_2, 5% CO_2 atmosphere. Following the switch to 95% N_2, 5% CO_2, the concentration of O_2 in the recording chamber fell from 95% to zero in approximately 2 min, as measured with an O_2 probe (World Precision Instruments, New Haven, CT). A standard 60 min period of anoxia was used. Unless otherwise stated, postanoxic activity was measured 60 min after the end of anoxia, since optic nerves attained their maximal recovery by the end of this 60 min reoxygenation period (Davis and Ransom, 1987; Stys et al., 1990a).

Tetrodotoxin (TTX; Sigma) and saxitoxin (STX; Calbiochem) were diluted from stock solutions in distilled water. Veratridine (Sigma) was first dissolved in ethanol. Benzamil (Research Biochemicals Inc.) and bepridil (Sigma) were dissolved in dimethylsulfoxide (DMSO). 3,4-Dichlorobenzamil (DCB) was a generous gift from Dr. G. Kaczorowski (Merck Sharp & Dohme Research Laboratories) and was prepared as a 20 mM stock solution in DMSO. The final concentration of DMSO never exceeded 0.2% v/v; this concentration of DMSO has no effect on either control or postanoxic CAPs.

Errors are reported as standard deviations, and statistical significance was calculated using the unpaired t test with pooled variance.

Results

The CAP in RON is rapidly attenuated under anoxic conditions. CAP area falls by 50% in approximately 4 min following the switch to a 95% N_2, 5% CO_2 atmosphere, and is virtually completely lost by 8–10 min (Stys et al., 1990a). Following a 60 min anoxic period, and 60 min of reoxygenation, CAP area recovered to a stable level of 33.5 ± 9.3% of control area (figure 22.1A).

Na$^+$ Channel Blockade Protects against Anoxic Injury

Na$^+$ influx during anoxia is responsible for some of the acute injury seen in gray matter (Rothman and Olney, 1986). To test whether voltage-gated Na$^+$ channels are involved in mediating irreversible anoxic injury in WM, the Na$^+$ channel blockers TTX and STX were applied at various times before the start of anoxia and continued until 10 min after the end of anoxia; both agents significantly improved postanoxic CAP recovery (figure 22.1A). CAP area recovered to 81.5 ± 11% in 1 μM TTX versus 33.5 ± 9.3% in normal CSF. Similar experiments with 1 μM STX also revealed significantly improved postanoxic recovery of CAP area (58.2 ± 14.3%), although not to the same extent as with TTX. Lower concentrations of TTX resulted in progressively less recovery in a dose-dependent fashion.

In order to test whether it was necessary to block electrogenesis with TTX to protect the optic nerve from anoxia, we studied the effects of lower concentrations of TTX on the response of the optic nerve to anoxia. Whereas excitability was completely abolished after 6 min of perfusion with 1 μM TTX, CAP area after 60 min exposure to 10 nM TTX in normal O_2 atmosphere was 107.1 ± 8% of control, although peak latencies in some nerves were prolonged by 10–20%. Such low concentrations of TTX, which had no effect on the control CAP area, were also protective against anoxia (postanoxic CAP area = 56.4 ± 14%).

Control experiments with 1 μM TTX and STX under normoxic conditions revealed that the effects of both agents were not completely reversible in our experimental system, even after

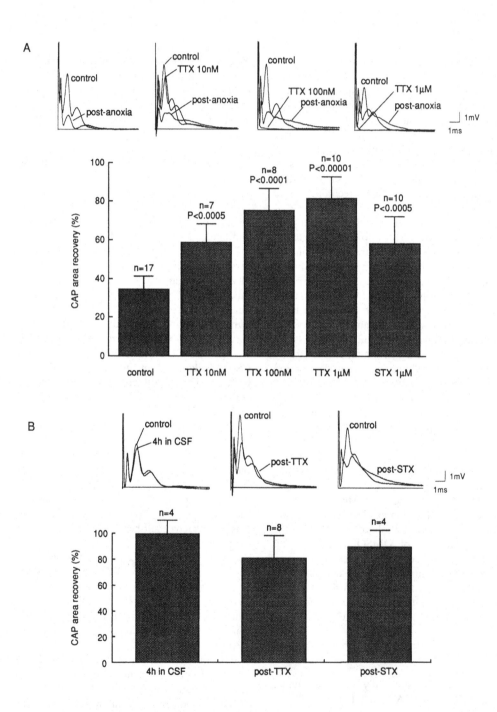

3 hr of wash. Figure 22.1*B* shows the results of exposing RONs to either TTX or STX at 1 μM for 1 hr, and then washing in normal CSF for 3 hr. Mean CAP area recovered incompletely to 80.8 ± 17% of control at TTX (to a level very near to that seen in anoxia experiments where RONs were exposed to TTX), and to 89.8 ± 13% after STX. Maintaining RONs in normal CSF for the same period of time (4 hr) resulted in a mean CAP area of 99.4 ± 11%, indicating that the incomplete recovery of the CAP following TTX or STX was due to incomplete washout of the blockers and not "rundown" of nerve excitability with prolonged incubation. Observations on the recovery from anoxia after TTX and STX exposure may therefore underestimate the true degree of protection.

If reducing Na^+ channel permeability with TTX or STX is protective during anoxia, increasing Na^+ permeability would be expected to result in more injury. This hypothesis was tested by treating the optic nerves with veratridine, an alkaloid that increases Na^+ permeability (Catterall, 1980). The agent was applied beginning 1 hr before anoxia and continued until 10 min after the end of anoxia. Recovery after a standard 60 min period of anoxia was reduced in the presence of veratridine (figure 22.2). After 1 hr of exposure to 1 μM veratridine, preanoxic

CAP area was reduced to 69.0 ± 15% of control, and postanoxic recovery was significantly reduced to 11.0 ± 12% as compared to recovery in normal CSF (33.5 ± 9.3%). The amount of additional injury with veratridine was dose dependent; 0.3 μM veratridine caused a modest increase in injury (21.1 ± 10%), whereas 0.1 μM had little effect (32.0 ± 17%). Control experiments in O_2 showed that the modest depression of the preanoxic CAP magnitude seen with 0.3 and 1 μM veratridine was completely reversible after 1 hr of wash. Veratridine also accelerated the rate of fall of CAP area at the onset of anoxia. At 1 μM, CAP area fell by 50% in about 1.5 min ($n = 2$) versus 3.9 min in normal CSF ($n = 5$; $p < 0.001$) (figure 22.2*B*).

Na^+ Influx through Na^+ Channels Is Required for Anoxic Injury

Because Na^+ channels are known to be permeable to other ions (Hille, 1984), experiments were performed to determine whether influx of Na^+ ions through the Na^+ channel contributes to irreversible anoxic injury, or if the presence of a finite Na^+ permeability (which might admit other ions such as Ca^{2+}) is sufficient. Figure 22.3*A* shows an experiment where Na^+ in the perfusing solution was replaced with equimolar

Figure 22.1
Effect of Na^+ channel blockers on CAP recovery after 60 min of anoxia. (*A*) Recovery of CAP area in normal CSF was 33.5% of control after a 60 min anoxic insult. TTX significantly improved recovery in a dose-dependent manner. Note that at 10 nM, TTX had virtually no effect on the area of the preanoxic CAP (*top tracings*) but was significantly protective against anoxic injury. Higher concentrations of TTX abolished the preanoxic CAP. *STX* 1 μM was also markedly protective. The difference in recovery between 1 μM TTX and 1 μM STX was significant (*p* < 0.001). *Top panels* show representative tracings of CAPs before and 1 hr after a 60 min anoxic period in normal CSF, and with exposure to TTX (10 nM to 1 μM). TTX was applied 60 min before the onset of anoxia at 10 and 100 nM, and 20 min before anoxia at 1 μM. TTX was continued until 15 min after reoxygenation when normal CSF was resumed. Up to 3 hr of wash was allowed before postanoxic readings were taken. (*B*) Optic nerves were exposed to either 1 μM TTX or STX for 90 min under normoxic conditions and then washed for 3 hr. Neither agent was completely reversible as evidenced by the incomplete recovery of CAP area and persistent alterations in the shape of the waveforms (not significantly different from CAP area after 4 hr in CSF). Nerves incubated for a similar period of time in normal CSF showed no change in shape or CAP area. Therefore, the results shown in *A* likely underestimate the true degree of recovery. *Top panels* show representative CAPs in normal CSF, and 3 hr after a 90 min exposure to 1 μM TTX or STX. Bars represent SD in this and all subsequent figures.

A

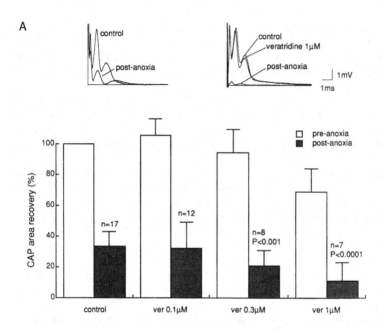

B

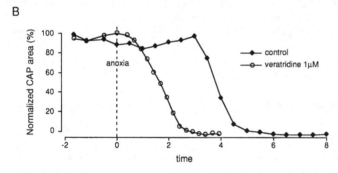

Figure 22.2
Effect of veratridine on CAP recovery after 60 min of anoxia. (*A*) As shown in the bar graph, veratridine had little effect on the pre- or postanoxic CAP at 0.1 μM. At higher concentrations (0.3 and 1 μM), veratridine modestly reduced the preanoxic CAP area in a reversible manner, and significantly increased the degree of anoxic injury. Tracings of CAPs before and 1 hr after 60 min of anoxia in normal CSF and with exposure to 1 μM veratridine. (*B*) CAP area diminished more rapidly with the onset of anoxia in the presence of 1 μM veratridine than in normal CSF.

choline, a cation that does not permeate the Na^+ channel, or with the permeable Li^+ ion. The zero-Na^+ solution was begun 20 min before anoxia and continued until 15 min after the end of anoxia. The rate at which extracellular $[Na^+]$ fell during zero-Na^+ perfusion was estimated by the rate of loss of the CAP (figure 22.3*C*). Recovery of CAP area was significantly improved $(88.0 \pm 5.4\%$ for choline-substituted solution, and $99.1 \pm 20\%$ for Li^+-substituted solution) after a 60 min anoxic challenge in the absence of extracellular Na^+. Perfusion with choline-substituted zero-Na^+ solution for 90 min under normoxic conditions, followed by 60 min in normal CSF, resulted in no diminution of CAP area $(102.0 \pm 17\%$; figure 22.3*B*) but subtly altered the shape of the waveform (not shown).

Na^+ Influx Continues throughout Anoxia

The above results suggested that irreversible anoxic injury in WM depends on Na^+ influx through voltage-gated Na^+ channels. Does this damaging Na^+ influx occur rapidly after the onset of anoxia, or more gradually throughout the anoxic period? To answer this question, experiments were performed where TTX (1 μM) was introduced at various times before or after the start of anoxia and continued until 10 min after the end of the anoxic period (figure 22.4). Thus, for example, time $t = -20$ min indicates that TTX was started 20 min before the onset of anoxia, and $t = +20$ min indicates that TTX was introduced 20 min after the start of anoxia. When TTX was started before anoxia (i.e., $t = -20$ min), CAP area recovery was enhanced to $81.5 \pm 11\%$. As the introduction of TTX solution was delayed with respect to the onset of anoxia, progressively less recovery occurred, so that with introduction at 60 min (i.e., at the time of reoxygenation), the degree of recovery $(38.1 \pm 12\%)$ approached the standard level $(33.5 \pm 9.3\%)$. Although the precise time course of Na^+ channel blockade with TTX perfusion is unknown, a rough estimate can be obtained

from the observation that the CAP was completely abolished about 6 min after exposure to 1 μM TTX. These results suggest that although Na^+ influx probably begins soon after the onset of anoxia, Na^+ movement that contributes to anoxia-induced injury continues throughout the anoxic period.

Reversing the Transmembrane Na^+ Gradient Increases Anoxic Injury

One way in which changes in $[Na^+]$ can influence anoxic injury is by modulating Ca^{2+} movements across cell membranes by altering the rate and direction of the Na^+–Ca^{2+} exchanger (Stys et al., 1991*b*). Changes in perfusion $[Na^+]$ will directly alter the transmembrane gradient of Na^+ and indirectly affect it by influencing $[Na^+]_i$. Perfusing the optic nerves with zero-Na^+ solution before anoxia will tend to deplete both the extracellular and the intracellular space of Na^+. Introducing zero-Na^+ after the start of anoxia, when presumably $[Na^+]_i$ has begun to rise above its resting level, will produce a reversed transmembrane Na^+ gradient. If the Na^+–Ca^{2+} exchanger plays a role in mediating Ca^{2+} influx during anoxia, altering the perfusing $[Na^+]$ in this way might influence the degree of anoxic injury. Figure 22.5 shows an experiment where zero-Na^+ solution (either choline or Li^+ substituted) was begun at various times before or after the start of anoxia. As the introduction of zero-Na^+ CSF was delayed with respect to the onset of anoxia, from $t = -20$ to $t = +20$ min (i.e., 20 min before anoxia and 20 min after the start of anoxia, respectively), progressively more injury occurred. Interestingly, when the choline-substituted zero-Na^+ CSF was introduced well into the anoxic period, at $t = +20$ or $+40$ min, significantly more injury occurred (CAP recovery at $t = +20$ was $16.1 \pm 8\%$ and at $t = +40$ was $13.7 \pm 6\%$) than with normal $[Na^+]$ maintained throughout (i.e., $33.5 \pm 9.3\%$). The degree of recovery returned to near normal $(38.4 \pm 6\%)$ with the introduction of zero-Na^+ for a brief

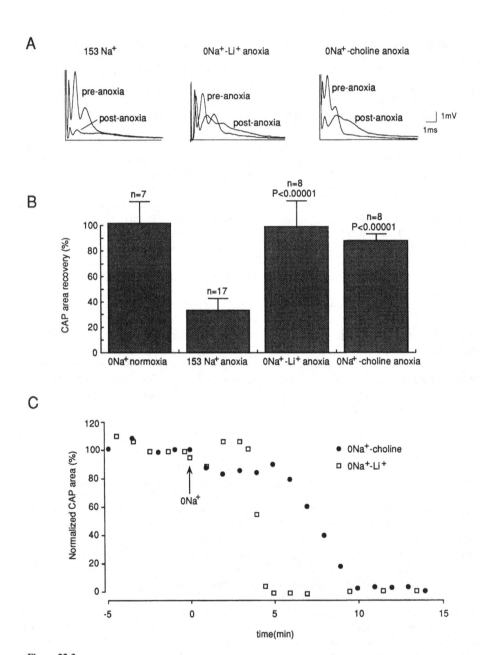

Figure 22.3
Effect of removing Na^+ from the perfusing solution on CAP recovery after 60 min of anoxia. (*A*) Representative CAPs pre- and postanoxia showing the protective effects of zero-Na^+ solution (Li^+ or choline substituted) when applied beginning 20 min before anoxia and continued until 15 min after reoxygenation. Recovery of CAP area

15 min period at the time of reoxygenation ($t = +60$ min). Li$^+$-substituted zero-Na$^+$ CSF displayed a similar profile.

Na$^+$–Ca^{2+} Exchange Blockers Protect against Anoxic Injury

We have previously shown that irreversible anoxic injury in the RON is dependent on extracellular Ca^{2+}, so that the omission of Ca^{2+} from the perfusing solution during 60 min of anoxia results in 100% recovery of CAP area (Stys et al., 1990a). Together with the present results, this suggests that both Na$^+$ and Ca^{2+} are critical for the production of anoxic injury and that movements of Na$^+$ and Ca^{2+} are closely interdependent. A major mechanism for coupling the fluxes of Na$^+$ and Ca^{2+} is via the Na$^+$–Ca^{2+} exchanger, and a preliminary study suggests that blocking this mechanism is protective in WM (Stys et al., 1991b).

Figure 22.6A shows the effects of three blockers of Na$^+$–Ca^{2+} exchange on the degree of recovery from anoxia; all three agents block the Na$^+$–Ca^{2+} exchanger by competitively inhibiting the Na$^+$ binding site. Bepridil (Kaczorowski et al., 1989), applied 60 min before until 15 min after 60 min of anoxia, was protective at concentrations of 10–100 μM, with optimal protection seen at 50 μM ($69.0 \pm 14\%$). Bepridil had no effect on preanoxic CAPs at these concentrations. Two derivatives of amiloride, benzamil and DCB (Kleyman and Cragoe, 1988), also displayed protective effects. Benzamil improved

recovery in a dose-dependent manner; at 500 μM it produced $71.0 \pm 15\%$ recovery. At this concentration, benzamil reduced the preanoxic CAP area to $61.1 \pm 20\%$ of control. However, protective effects were also seen at lower concentrations of benzamil (100 μM) where the preanoxic CAP area was not reduced. DCB (3 μM) also improved recovery ($49.9 \pm 17\%$), although to a lesser degree (figure 22.6A). No change in the control CAP was seen at this concentration. Higher concentrations could not be reliably tested due to the limited solubility of this compound.

Because these Na$^+$–Ca^{2+} exchange blockers did not fully protect the optic nerve from anoxia, we studied the combined effect of TTX plus exchange blockers to determine whether Na$^+$ conductance played an additive role in mediating anoxic injury. The addition of 1 μM TTX to either bepridil or benzamil further enhanced recovery by 5–10% to $73.7 \pm 10\%$ and $77.2 \pm 16\%$, respectively, close to the recovery seen with TTX alone (figure 22.6B). It should again be noted that results with TTX probably underestimate the true recovery due to the incomplete washout of this blocker.

Discussion

In the mammalian CNS, both gray and WM regions suffer irreversible injury when subjected to extended periods of anoxia/ischemia, and this injury appears to depend on Ca^{2+} in both tissues.

after a 60 min anoxic insult was significantly enhanced compared to normal CSF ([Na$^+$] = 153 mM). (B) Bar graph quantitatively illustrating the protective effects of zero-Na$^+$ solutions. Control experiments revealed that exposure of optic nerves to zero-Na$^+$ solution (choline substituted) under normoxic conditions for 90 min did not cause a reduction in CAP area (measured 1 hr after resuming normal CSF), although the shape of the response was altered: Perfusing the nerves with zero-Na$^+$ CSF significantly enhanced CAP area recovery in both choline- and Li$^+$-substituted solutions. Statistical differences were calculated with respect to the postanoxic recovery in normal CSF (153 Na$^+$ anoxia). (C) Graph of normalized CAP area versus time showing the time course of CAP attenuation with introduction of zero-Na$^+$ solution into the perfusion chamber. Both solutions completely abolished the evoked response, although Li$^+$-substituted solution had a more rapid effect.

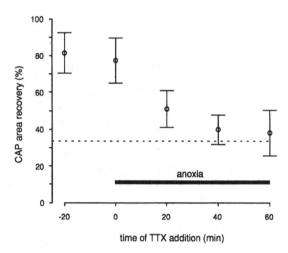

Figure 22.4

Effects of TTX 1 μM, applied at various times before or after a 60 min anoxic period, on CAP area recovery. Optic nerves were washed for 3 hr in normal CSF after anoxia to remove as much residual TTX as possible, before postanoxic readings were taken. Control experiments showed that TTX was not completely removed even after 3 hr of wash (see figure 22.1). Recovery diminished gradually as the introduction of TTX solution was delayed with respect to the onset of anoxia, suggesting that Na^+ influx begins soon after the onset of anoxia and continues throughout the anoxic period.

The route of the damaging Ca^{2+} entry into cells in WM during anoxia is not fully understood, but unlike gray matter (Choi, 1990), this is not mediated by voltage-sensitive Ca^{2+} channels (Stys et al., 1990b; Waxman et al., 1991) or by the excitotoxin receptors activated by glutamate and aspartate (Ransom et al., 1990b).

Na^+ Channels Play a Central Role in Anoxic Injury

Could other ion channels, known to be present in myelinated CNS axons, admit Ca^{2+} into the intracellular compartment under anoxic conditions in WM? Blocking Na^+ channels with TTX and STX had a marked protective effect, the magnitude of which is likely to be underestimated in these experiments due to persistent toxin binding. Even at 10 nM TTX, a concentra-

tion that had little effect on the control CAP, a significant protective effect was observed. Thus, there exists a "therapeutic window" where action potential electrogenesis need not be abolished in order to protect WM from anoxic injury.

If blocking Na^+ conductance improves recovery from anoxia, it would be expected that increasing Na^+ conductance would worsen outcome. Exposing nerves to veratridine, an alkaloid that increases Na^+ permeability by shifting Na^+ channel activation to more negative potentials and inhibiting inactivation (Catterall, 1980), increased the degree of irreversible anoxic injury in a dose-dependent manner. These results and previous observations (Stys et al., 1990a) indicate that both extracellular Ca^{2+} and a finite Na^+ permeability must be present to cause irreversible anoxic injury. Moreover, the degree of injury is proportional to both the level of Ca^{2+}

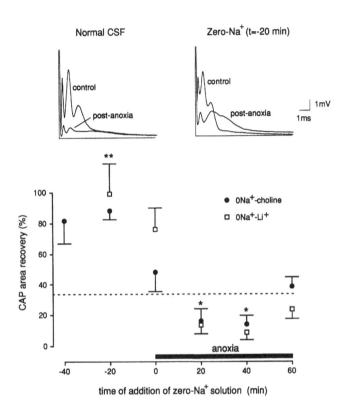

Figure 22.5

Effects of zero-Na$^+$ solution, applied at various times before or after anoxia, on CAP area recovery; graph showing CAP area recovery after 60 min of anoxia plotted against the time (in minutes) with respect to the onset of anoxia, when zero-Na$^+$ CSF (choline or Li$^+$ substituted) was applied. Normal CSF was resumed 15 min after the end of anoxia, and postanoxic readings were taken 1 hr after reoxygenation. Recovery was computed as the ratio of CAP area postanoxia to area preanoxia in CSF containing normal [Na$^+$] (153 mM). Recovery was greatly enhanced when zero-Na$^+$ CSF was started *before* anoxia. As the introduction of zero-Na$^+$ CSF was delayed with respect to the onset of anoxia, progressively less recovery was seen. When the zero-Na$^+$ solution was applied *after* the onset of anoxia ($t = +20$ or $+40$ min), significantly more injury occurred than with normal CSF ([Na$^+$] = 153 mM) maintained throughout the anoxic period (broken line). When zero-Na$^+$ CSF was briefly applied for 15 min at $t = 60$ min, the degree of injury approached the control value. *Top panels* show representative CAPs pre- and postanoxia in normal CSF and in choline-substituted zero-Na$^+$ CSF that was started 20 min before anoxia. Statistical differences were calculated with respect to the standard recovery in normal CSF (*, $p < 0.0001$; **, $p < 0.00001$).

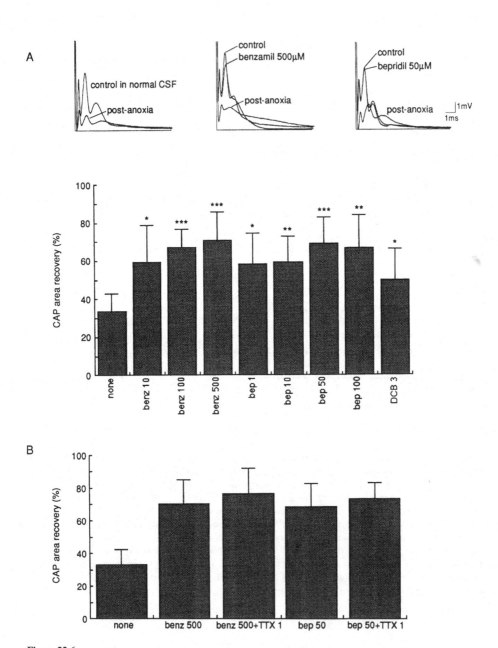

Figure 22.6
Effects of Na^+–Ca^+ exchange inhibitors on CAP recovery after anoxia. (*A*) Benzamil (benz), bepridil (bep), or DCB were applied 60 min before the start of anoxia and continued until 15 min after reoxygenation, when normal CSF was resumed. Postanoxic activity was measured 1 hr after reoxygenation. Benzamil significantly improved recovery

exposure (Stys et al., 1990a) and magnitude of Na^+ permeability.

Na^+ Gradient Collapses Gradually during Anoxia

The CAP is lost within minutes of the onset of anoxia (Stys et al., 1990a) paralleled by a rise in extracellular $[k^+]$ to about 15 mM (Walz et al., 1986), indicating that the optic nerve is heavily dependent on oxidative energy metabolism for the maintenance of ionic gradients. The results shown in figure 22.4 suggest that damaging Na^+ influx through Na^+ channels continues throughout the anoxic period. If Na^+ equilibrated completely across membranes within minutes of the onset of anoxia, introducing TTX at +20 min should not have further improved recovery.

Na^+ channels are not perfectly selective and are known to possess a finite permeability to other ions, including Ca^{2+}. The $Na^+ : Ca^{2+}$ permeability ratio has been estimated to be as low as 10 : 1 (Hille, 1984), although higher permeability ratios have been suggested (Lederer et al., 1991). Given that extracellular Ca^{2+} is necessary for anoxic injury in the optic nerve, a critical question is whether the injury related to the finite Na^+ permeability that exists during anoxia is primarily due to Na^+ or Ca^{2+} influx through these channels. Our results indicate that anoxia-induced Ca^{2+} entry does not occur through Na^+ channels, because perfusion with zero-Na^+ solution markedly improved recovery but would not prevent Ca^{2+} influx through this channel (figure 22.3). This result strongly suggests that influx of Na^+, and not Ca^{2+}, through voltage-gated Na^+

channels is an important step in the sequence of events leading to anoxic injury.

Does a Persistent Na^+ Conductance Mediate Na^+ Influx?

Under conditions of massive energy failure and membrane depolarization, as suggested by a rapid attenuation of the CAP and rise in $[K^+]_o$, it might be expected that Na^+ channels would be inactivated. Our results suggest, however, that there exists a finite, persistent Na^+ conductance at levels of membrane depolarization attained during anoxia. In some preparations, Na^+ conductance does not inactivate completely even with prolonged membrane depolarization (Stafstrom et al., 1982, 1985; Gilly and Brismar, 1989) and may even start to increase at more positive membrane potentials (Chandler and Meves, 1970; Bezanilla and Armstrong, 1977). In the optic nerve, it is not yet clear if the persistent Na^+ conductance represents incomplete inactivation of a homogeneous population of Na^+ channels, or a subpopulation of noninactivating channels. An intriguing possibility is that the conductance of a subpopulation of the latter channels might be dominant under pathological conditions such as anoxic depolarization. This raises the question whether these channels have distinct pharmacological sensitivity, allowing blockade of the noninactivating component while sparing normally inactivating fast Na^+ channels (those channels responsible for action potential electrogenesis), thus leaving normal axonal conduction relatively unaffected. There is evidence that slowly inactivating or persistent

of CAP area in a dose-dependent manner over a concentration range of 10–500 μM. Bepridil (1–100 μM) and DCB (3 μM) also significantly improved recovery. Benzamil had no effect on the preanoxic response at 10 and 100 μM, and reduced CAP area modestly to $61.1 \pm 20\%$ of control at 500 μM in a reversible manner. Bepridil and DCB had no effect on preanoxic responses at the concentrations shown. *, $p < 0.01$; **, $p < 0.001$; ***, $p < 0.0001$; $n = 7$–10 for each drug and concentration. (B) Addition of 1 μM TTX to solutions containing maximally protective concentrations of bepridil or benzamil further improved recovery by 5–10% (not statistically significant; see Results). n = 4–10 for each category.

Na$^+$ channels can be preferentially blocked by certain local anesthetics (Stafstrom et al., 1985; Schneider and Dubois, 1986).

The degree of protection from anoxia by TTX was dose dependent, even over a concentration range where measurable excitability was already completely abolished (figure 22.1A). Typically, Na$^+$ channels are blocked by TTX with high affinity (half-maximal inhibition, <10 nM) (Hille, 1968); at 100 nM TTX, evoked activity was already completely abolished. No difference in the degree of protection against anoxia would be expected between 100 nM and 1 μM TTX, since beyond 100 nM TTX normal Na$^+$ channels should be fully blocked. This raises the interesting possibility of a subpopulation of Na$^+$ channels that are partially resistant to TTX (Ransom and Holz, 1977; Roy and Narahashi, 1990), and with a differential sensitivity to TTX and STX. The difference in protection seen with TTX and STX, and the relatively high concentrations of TTX required for optimal protection suggest that the Na$^+$ channels most relevant to anoxic injury do not follow the pharmacological profile expected for normally inactivating Na$^+$ channels, and could represent a distinct subpopulation.

Magnitude and Direction of Na$^+$ Gradient Modulates Anoxic Injury

Both extracellular Ca^{2+} (Stys et al., 1990a) and Na$^+$ are required to produce irreversible anoxic injury in WM. One way in which fluxes of these ions could be coupled is via the Na$^+$–Ca^{2+} exchanger. This membrane protein, found in all excitable and many nonexcitable cells, functions to maintain cellular Ca^{2+} homeostasis by extruding Ca^{2+} in exchange for Na$^+$ (Baker et al., 1969; Allen et al., 1989). The stoichiometry is generally thought to be 3 Na$^+$: 1 Ca^{2+} (Blaustein and Santiago, 1977; Rasgado-Flores and Blaustein, 1987), resulting in a transport process that is electrogenic (one net inward charge per Ca^{2+} ion extruded); consequently, both the rate and

direction of Ca^{2+} transport will be influenced by membrane potential. Under normal conditions of membrane polarization and [Na$^+$]$_i$, the exchanger uses the energy stored in the transmembrane electrochemical gradient of Na$^+$ to transport Ca^{2+} out of the cell. However, with membrane depolarization and/or increasing [Na$^+$]$_i$, the Na$^+$–Ca^{2+} exchanger can operate in reverse, transporting Ca^{2+} into the intracellular compartment in exchange for Na$^+$ (Baker et al., 1969; Cervetto et al., 1989). Thus, reverse Na$^+$–Ca^{2+} exchange is a potential route of Ca^{2+} influx during anoxia, a time when membranes depolarize and [Na$^+$]$_i$ increases as a result of ATP depletion.

The results illustrated in figure 22.5 are consistent with the hypothesis that a significant portion of the damaging Ca^{2+} influx that occurs during anoxia is carried by reverse Na$^+$–Ca^{2+} exchange. When zero-Na$^+$ solution is introduced before anoxia (figure 22.5, $t = -20$ min), [Na$^+$]$_i$ will tend to decrease from its resting level of about 25 mM (Ballanyi et al., 1987; Erecińska and Silver, 1989; Erecińska et al., 1991). To operate in the reverse direction, that is, transport of Ca^{2+} into the cell in exchange for Na$^+$, the exchanger requires intracellular Na$^+$ [[Na$^+$]$_i$ $\approx$ 25 mM for half-maximal activation in squid giant axon (Requena et al., 1989)]. Reducing [Na$^+$]$_i$ by perfusing with zero-Na$^+$ CSF prior to and during anoxia would inhibit reverse operation of the exchanger, reduce Ca^{2+} influx, and protect the tissue from injury.

Interestingly, delaying the introduction of zero-Na$^+$ until well into the anoxic period results in more injury than seen with normal [Na$^+$] maintained throughout (figure 22.5, broken line). In normal [Na$^+$]$_o$ (i.e., 153 mM), [Na$^+$]$_i$ will increase during anoxia, to above its resting level. Introduction of zero-Na$^+$ solution after the start of anoxia is deleterious ($t = +20$ and $+40$ min, figure 22.5), because now a large *reverse* Na$^+$ gradient ([Na$^+$]$_i$ > [Na$^+$]$_o$) forces the exchanger to transport more Ca^{2+} into the cell. Under these circumstances, we postulate that even more Ca^{2+}

enters the intracellular space than during a normal anoxic period (with $[Na^+] = 153$ mM), where at worst the Na^+ gradient would collapse completely ($[Na^+]_i = [Na^+]_o$) but would never be reversed.

Perfusion with zero-Na^+ solution during normoxia would also result in a reversed Na^+ gradient (e.g., prior to anoxia in figure 22.5, $t = -40$ and -20 min). Nevertheless, in control experiments no decrease in CAP area is observed (though the shape of the CAP is irreversibly altered) following a 90 min exposure to zero-Na^+ CSF in an O_2 atmosphere (figure 22.3B). We hypothesize that this does not cause damage to the optic nerve because in a normal O_2 atmosphere the supply of ATP is not limited, and the Ca^{2+}-ATPase would be capable of extruding most of the excess Ca^{2+} admitted through reverse Na^+–Ca^{2+} exchange. Moreover, switching to zero-Na^+ under normoxic conditions (with $[Na^+]_i \approx 25$ mM) would not create a reverse gradient of the same magnitude as when zero-Na^+ is applied during anoxia, when $[Na^+]_i$ has already risen above its resting value.

Although it is clear that introducing zero-Na^+ CSF will, at least transiently, reverse the Na^+ gradient and cause reverse operation of the Na^+–Ca^{2+} exchanger, under realistic conditions of anoxia/ischemia, ion gradients would never reverse but merely collapse. Why then might the exchanger operate to raise $[Ca^{2+}]_i$ without artificial manipulation of ion gradients? Figure 22.7 shows equations and a graphical representation of the behavior of the Na^+–Ca^{2+} exchanger at thermodynamic equilibrium (Blaustein and Santiago, 1977; Sheu and Fozzard, 1982). Intracellular $[Ca^{2+}]$ at equilibrium is an exponential function of membrane potential (increasing with membrane depolarization) and a function of the cube of the ratio of intracellular to extracellular $[Na^+]$ (assuming a stoichiometry of $3\,Na^+$: $1\,Ca^{2+}$). Thus, membrane depolarization and/or an increase in $[Na^+]_i$ will result in an increased steady-state $[Ca^{2+}]_i$. This increased $[Ca^{2+}]_i$ could, in theory, occur either by true reversal of

the exchanger, or by attenuation of forward exchange, unmasking the effects of an alternate Ca^{2+} influx pathway. If the latter were true, pharmacological inhibition of the exchanger (see below) should result in more anoxic injury, since any beneficial effects of exchanger-mediated Ca^{2+} extrusion would be further attenuated by the inhibitors. Our results, which demonstrate significantly reduced anoxic injury in nerves treated with Na^+–Ca^{2+} exchanger blockers, are clearly inconsistent with this argument and support the notion that Ca^{2+} is admitted via reversal of the Na^+–Ca^{2+} exchanger. Moreover, the exchanger can operate in reverse without a *reversal* of the Na^+ gradient. If the starting $[Ca^{2+}]_i$ is at or below the exchanger equilibrium, a *diminution* of the Na^+ gradient will be sufficient to cause the exchanger to operate in reverse as it attempts to reach its new, more elevated steady state $[Ca^{2+}]_i$. It should be noted that a combination of membrane depolarization and an increase in $[Na^+]_i$ (both of which occur during anoxia) will have a synergistic effect, raising $[Ca^{2+}]_i$ to high levels if the exchanger is allowed to operate.

Interestingly, inhibition of Na^+–Ca^{2+} exchange activity has been reported to exacerbate glutamate neurotoxicity in cultured neurons (Mattson et al., 1989; Andreeva et al., 1991), suggesting that in model systems containing neuronal cell bodies and synapses, the exchanger functions to extrude rather than to admit Ca^{2+} under pathological conditions (it should be noted that the effects of extracellular K^+-induced depolarization on exchanger function cannot be studied in these systems). The surface-to-volume ratio in neuronal cell bodies is much smaller than in the small (mean diameter, ≈ 0.75 μm; Foster et al., 1982) axons that are present in the RON. When challenged, the rise in $[Na^+]_i$ in a neuron can thus be expected to be much less pronounced than in a small diameter axon, and therefore a favorable exchange equilibrium (i.e., tending toward a lower $[Ca^{2+}]_i$) would be maintained for a longer period of time. In contrast, a small axon

A

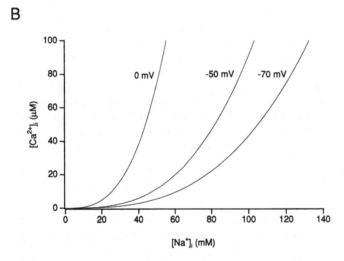

$$E_{NaCa} = \frac{n\,E_{Na} - 2\,E_{Ca}}{n - 2} \qquad \text{eq.1}$$

$$[Ca]_i = [Ca]_o \,\text{Exp}\left[\frac{F\,Vm\,(n-2)}{R\,T}\right]\left[\frac{[Na]_i}{[Na]_o}\right]^n \qquad \text{eq.2}$$

B

Figure 22.7
(A) Equations describing the behavior of the Na$^+$–Ca^{2+} exchanger (Blaustein and Santiago, 1977; Sheu and Fozzard, 1982). E_{NaCa}, E_{Na}, and E_{Ca} are reversal potentials of the exchanger, Na$^+$, and Ca^{2+} ions, respectively, and n represents the exchanger stoichiometry. The exchanger will operate in the direction required to bring its reversal potential closer to membrane potential, V_m. At thermodynamic equilibrium, $E_{NaCa} = V_m$. Substituting V_m into eq. 1, expanding the expressions for E_{Na} and E_{Ca}, and rearranging, we obtain an expression (eq. 2) for the intracellular [Ca^{2+}] that would be maintained by the Na$^+$–Ca^{2+} exchanger. F, Faraday's constant; R, gas constant; T, absolute temperature. (B) Graphical representation of eq. 2 at three values of membrane potential assuming a stoichiometry of 3 Na$^+$: 1 Ca^{2+}. With increasing [Na$^+$]$_i$ and/or membrane depolarization, both of which occur during anoxia, the Na$^+$–Ca^{2+} exchanger will tend to increase [Ca^{2+}]$_i$.

having a limited intracellular volume, a high density of Na^+ channels at the node of Ranvier, and possibly restricted ionic diffusion (see below) may suffer a rapid and pronounced rise in $[Na^+]_i$ with the Na^+–Ca^{2+} exchanger quickly recruited to operate in reverse. If surface-to-volume considerations significantly influence the behavior of the exchanger under pathological conditions, it is possible that this transporter may play opposite roles in different regions of the same neuron, transporting Ca^{2+} out of the soma, while admitting damaging quantities of Ca^{2+} into the axon and dendritic processes.

Pharmacological Blockers of Na^+–Ca^{2+} Exchange Are Protective

Further evidence implicating the Na^+–Ca^{2+} exchanger was obtained by demonstrating that direct pharmacological inhibition of this transporter offers significant protection against anoxic injury (figure 22.6A). These agents also block voltage-gated Ca^{2+} channels (Galizzi et al., 1986; Kleyman and Cragoe, 1988; Garcia et al., 1990); we have previously shown, however, that such channels do not play a role in WM anoxic injury (Stys et al., 1990b). Benzamil also possesses inhibitory effects on Na^+ channels (Kleyman and Cragoe, 1988); at a concentration of 500 μM in our experiments, benzamil reduced CAP area to 61.1% of control. Nevertheless, protective effects were seen at lower concentrations of 10 and 100 μM, where little if any change in the control CAP was evident, indicating minimal effects of benzamil on Na^+ channels. Similarly, DCB protected the optic nerves at a concentration where the control CAP was unchanged. The reduced efficacy of DCB, compared to the other two inhibitors, may be due to its limited solubility, preventing reliable experiments at higher concentrations. Although the absolute contribution of the Na^+–Ca^{2+} exchanger in isolation must await more specific inhibitors, we conclude that a large part of Ca^{2+} influx during anoxia is mediated by this system.

A similar mechanism has been proposed in ischemic myocardium (Renlund et al., 1984), and in reperfusion of heart following exposure to Ca^{2+}-free solution (Chapman and Tunstall, 1987).

Addition of 1 μM TTX to optimal concentrations of both bepridil or benzamil further improved recovery from anoxia by 5–10% (not statistically significant), approximately to the same degree as with TTX alone (figure 22.6B). This suggests either that bepridil or benzamil alone failed to block reverse exchange completely (requiring the additional effect of TTX to eliminate the rise in $[Na^+]_i$) or that a small portion of Ca^{2+} influx occurs directly through Na^+ channels. The near-complete recovery seen with Li^+-substituted zero-Na^+ solution introduced 20 min before anoxia suggests that little Ca^{2+} was admitted directly through the Na^+ channels, however.

Protective Effects Are Not Due to Energy Sparing

Although our results are consistent with Ca^{2+} influx via reverse operation of the Na^+–Ca^{2+} exchanger during anoxia in WM, it could be argued that blocking Na^+ channels or eliminating Na^+ from the perfusate is protective because it spares energy reserves. According to this argument, reducing the demand for ATP by preventing or slowing the collapse of the Na^+ gradient would allow residual ATP (generated perhaps from anaerobic metabolism) to fuel other Ca^{2+}-extruding mechanisms, such as the Ca^{2+}-ATPase, sufficiently to prevent significant cellular injury. The data shown in figure 22.5 strongly argue against a simple "energy-sparing" effect. If perfusion with zero-Na^+ was protective because of energy sparing, the relationship between recovery and duration of exposure to high $[Na^+]_o$ should be monotonic; that is, the longer the anoxic nerve is exposed to high $[Na^+]_o$, the greater should be the depletion of energy reserves, and the more injury should result. Fig-

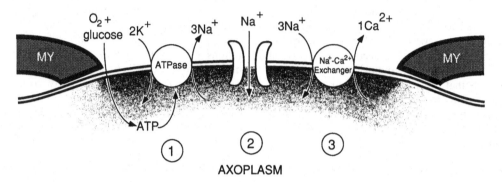

EXTRACELLULAR

AXOPLASM

Figure 22.8

Hypothetical sequence of events leading to anoxia-induced Ca^{2+} accumulation in myelinated (MY) CNS axons. Under conditions of anoxia/ischemia, reserves of ATP are rapidly depleted, leading to failure of the Na^+-K^+ ATPase and subsequent collapse of ionic gradients (*1*). Na^+ ions enter the axoplasmic space through incompletely inactivated Na^+ channels (*2*). This influx of Na^+ ions leads to a rise in $[Na^+]_i$, which may be exaggerated by restricted diffusion of ions under the nodal membrane. Both membrane depolarization and an increase in intracellular $[Na^+]$ cause reverse operation of the Na^+–Ca^{2+} exchanger, which admits damaging quantities of Ca^{2+} into the cell.

ure 22.5 clearly shows this not to be the case; intermediate exposure times ($t = +20$ or $+40$) are more injurious than maintaining the nerves in normal $[Na^+]_o$ solution for the full anoxic period. This observation is inconsistent with an energy-sparing action of zero-Na^+ solution but is readily explained if anoxic injury is primarily caused by Ca^{2+} influx via reverse operation of the Na^+–Ca^{2+} exchanger.

Although it is possible that maneuvers that reduce the consumption of ATP by Na^+-K^+ ATPase may play a protective role, our results suggest that this role is minor and that Ca^{2+} influx via reverse Na^+–Ca^{2+} exchange is a major mechanism of anoxic injury in CNS WM. A diagram of the sequence of events leading to anoxia-induced Ca^{2+} accumulation in WM is shown in figure 22.8. According to this hypothetical sequence, anoxic injury begins with ATP depletion and failure of Na^+-K^+ ATPase,

resulting in a breakdown of ionic gradients (1). Leakage of Na^+ through Na^+ channels (possibly a subpopulation of noninactivating channels; see above) causes $[Na^+]_i$ to rise (2), resulting in reverse operation of the Na^+–Ca^{2+} exchanger (3). Ca^{2+} admitted through reverse exchange accumulates in the intracellular space, rises to toxic levels, and produces irreversible injury, probably through activation of Ca^{2+}-dependent systems such as calpains, lipases, protein kinase C, and so on (Siesjö and Wieloch, 1985; Nicotera et al., 1986; Orrenius et al., 1988). Due to the serial nature of Na^+ and Ca^{2+} influx in the proposed cascade, blocking either Na^+ channels and/or the Na^+–Ca^{2+} exchanger should protect CNS myelinated axons against anoxic injury. This prediction is supported by the present results.

The very high density of Na^+ channels at the nodes of Ranvier (Waxman and Ritchie, 1985) may render this region especially vulnerable to anoxic injury. Moreover, ultrastructural studies of myelinated axons reveal a dense undercoating subjacent to the nodal membrane (Waxman et al., 1972). It has been suggested that this specialized region of axoplasm may restrict diffusion of ions and focally intensify disturbances in ion concentrations (Bergman, 1970). Localized increases in $[Na^+]_i$ would further drive reverse Na^+-Ca^{2+} exchange, admitting even more Ca^{2+} into a restricted intracellular compartment. Thus, it is possible that the specialized architecture of CNS myelinated axons may serve to enhance their susceptibility to anoxic injury.

Acknowledgments

This work was supported by grants from the National Institute of Neurological Disorders and Stroke (B.R.R.), the American Paralysis Association (S.G.W.), and by the Medical Research Service, Veterans Administration (S.G.W.). P.K.S. was supported by a fellowship from the Blinded Veterans Association and by a Centennial Fellowship from the Medical Research Council of Canada.

References

Allen TJA, Noble D, Reuter H (1989) Sodium-calcium exchange. New York: Oxford UP.

Andreeva N, Khodorov B, Stemashook E, Cragoe E Jr, Victorov I (1991) Inhibition of Na^+/Ca^{2+} exchange enhances delayed neuronal death elicited by glutamate in cerebellar granule cell cultures. Brain Res 548: 322–325.

Baker PF, Blaustein MP, Hodgkin AL, Steinhardt RA (1969) The influence of calcium on sodium efflux in squid axons. J Physiol (Lond) 200: 431–458.

Ballanyi K, Grafe P, ten Bruggencate G (1987) Ion activities and potassium uptake mechanisms of glial cells in guinea-pig olfactory cortex slices. J Physiol (Lond) 382: 159–174.

Bengtsson F, Siesjö BK (1990) Cell damage in cerebral ischemia: physiological, biochemical, and structural aspects. In: Cerebral ischemia and resuscitation (Schurr A, Rigor BM, eds), pp 215–233. Boca Raton, FL: CRC.

Bergman C (1970) Increase of sodium concentration near the inner surface of the nodal membrane. Pfluegers Arch 317: 287–302.

Bezanilla F, Armstrong CM (1977) Inactivation of the sodium channel. I. Sodium current experiments. J Gen Physiol 70: 549–566.

Blaustein MP, Santiago EM (1977) Effects of internal and external cations and of ATP on sodium–calcium and calcium–calcium exchange in squid axons. Biophys J 20: 79–111.

Buchthal F, Rosenfalck A (1966) Evoked action potentials and conduction velocity in human sensory nerves. Brain Res 3: 1–122.

Catterall WA (1980) Neurotoxins that act on voltage-sensitive sodium channels in excitable membranes. Annu Rev Pharmacol Toxicol 20: 15–43.

Cervetto L, Lagnado L, Perry RJ, Robinson DW, McNaughton PA (1989) Extrusion of calcium from rod outer segments is driven by both sodium and potassium gradients. Nature 337: 740–743.

Chandler WK, Meves H (1970) Evidence for two types of sodium conductance in axons perfused with sodium fluoride solution. J Physiol (Lond) 211: 653–678.

Chapman RA, Tunstall J (1987) The calcium paradox of the heart. Prog Biophys Mol Biol 50: 67–96.

Choi DW (1985) Glutamate neurotoxicity in cortical cell culture is calcium dependent. Neurosci Lett 58: 293–297.

Choi DW (1990) Cerebral hypoxia: some new approaches and unanswered questions. J Neurosci 10: 2493–2501.

Connors BW, Ransom BR, Kunis DM, Gutnick MJ (1982) Activity-dependent K^+ accumulation in the developing rat optic nerve. Science 216: 1341–1343.

Cummins KL, Perkel DH, Dorfman LJ (1979) Nerve fiber conduction velocity distributions. I. Estimation based on the single-fiber and compound action potentials. Electroencephalogr Clin Neurophysiol 46: 634–646.

Davis P, Ransom BR (1987) Anoxia and CNS white matter: in vitro studies using the rat optic nerve. Soc Neurosci Abstr 13: 1634.

Erecińska M, Silver IA (1989) ATP and brain function. J Cereb Blood Flow Metab 9: 2–19.

Erecińska M, Dagani F, Nelson D, Deas J, Silver IA (1991) Relations between intracellular ions and energy metabolism. A study with monensin in synaptosomes, neurons and C6 glioma cells. J Neurosci 11: 2410–2421.

Fehlings MG, Tator CH, Linden RD (1989) The relationships among the severity of spinal cord injury, motor and somatosensory evoked potentials and spinal cord blood flow. Electroencephalogr Clin Neurophysiol 74: 241–259.

Foster RE, Connors BW, Waxman SG (1982) Rat optic nerve: electrophysiological, pharmacological and anatomical studies during development. Dev Brain Res 3: 371–386.

Galizzi J-P, Borsotto M, Barhanin J, Fosset M, Lazdunski M (1986) Characterization and photo-affinity labeling of receptor sites for the Ca^{2+} channel inhibitors $d\text{-}cis$-diltiazem, $(\pm)$-bepridil, desmethoxyverapamil, and $(+)$-PN 200-110 in skeletal muscle transverse tubule membranes. J Biol Chem 261: 1393–1397.

Garcia ML, King VF, Shevell JL, Slaughter RS, Suarez KG, Winquist RJ, Kaczorowski GJ (1990) Amiloride analogs inhibit L-type calcium channels and display calcium entry blocker activity. J Biol Chem 265: 3763–3771.

Gilly WF, Brismar T (1989) Properties of appropriately and inappropriately expressed sodium channels in squid giant axon and its somata. J Neurosci 9: 1362–1374.

Hille B (1968) Pharmacological modifications of the sodium channels of frog nerve. J Gen Physiol 51: 199–219.

Hille B (1984) Ionic channels of excitable membranes, p. 240. Sunderland, MA: Sinauer.

Kaczorowski GJ, Slaughter RS, King VF, Garcia ML (1989) Inhibitors of sodium–calcium exchange: identification and development of probes of transport activity. Biochim Biophys Acta 988: 287–302.

Kleyman TR, Cragoe EJJ (1988) Amiloride and its analogs as tools in the study of ion transport. J Membr Biol 105: 1–21.

Krieglstein J, Sauer D, Nuglisch J, Karkoutly C, Beck T, Bielenberg GW, Rossberg C, Mennel HD (1989) Protective effects of calcium antagonists against brain damage caused by ischemia. In: Proceedings of the international workshop on cerebral ischemia and cal-cium (Hartmann G, Kuschinsky W, eds). Heidelberg: Springer.

Lederer WJ, Niggli E, Hadley RW (1991) Sodium–calcium exchange: response. Science 251: 1371.

Mattson MP, Guthrie PB, Kater SB (1989) A role for Na^+-dependent Ca^{2+} extrusion in protection against neuronal excitotoxicity. FASEB J 3: 2519–2526.

Nicotera P, Hartzell P, Davis G, Orrenius S (1986) The formation of plasma membrane blebs in hepatocytes exposed to agents that increase cytosolic Ca^{2+} is mediated by the activation of a non-lysomal proteolytic system. FEBS Lett 209: 139–144.

Orrenius S, McConkey DJ, Jones DP, Nicotera P (1988) Ca^{2+}-activated mechanisms in toxicity and programmed cell death. ISI Atlas Sci Pharmacol 2: 319–324.

Ransom BR, Holz RW (1977) Ionic determinants of excitability in cultured mouse dorsal root ganglion and spinal cord cells. Brain Res 136: 445–453.

Ransom BR, Yamate CL, Connors BW (1985) Activity-dependent shrinkage of extracellular space in rat optic nerve: a developmental study. J Neurosci 5: 532–535.

Ransom BR, Stys PK, Waxman SG (1990a) The pathophysiology of anoxia in mammalian white matter. Stroke [Suppl] 21: III-52-III-57.

Ransom BR, Waxman SG, Davis PK (1990b) Anoxic injury of CNS white matter: protective effect of ketamine. Neurology 40: 1399–1403.

Rasgado-Flores H, Blaustein MP (1987) Na/Ca exchange in barnacle muscle cells has a stoichiometry of $3 Na^+/1 Ca^{2+}$. Am J Physiol 252(5 Pt 1): C499–C504.

Renlund DG, Gerstenblith G, Lakatta EG, Jacobus WE, Kallman CH, Weisfeldt ML (1984) Perfusate sodium during ischemia modifes post-ischemic functional and metabolic recovery in the rabbit heart. Mol Cell Cardiol 16: 795–801.

Requena J, Whittembury J, Mullins LJ (1989) Calcium entry in squid axons during voltage clamp pulses. Cell Calcium 10: 413–423.

Rothman SM, Olney JW (1986) Glutamate and the pathophysiology of hypoxic-ischemic brain damage. Ann Neurol 19: 105–111.

Roy M-L, Narahashi T (1990) Differential properties of tetrodotoxin-sensitive and tetrodotoxin-resistant sodium channels in rat dorsal root ganglion neurons. Soc Neurosci Abstr 16: 181.

Schneider MF, Dubois JM (1986) Effects of benzocaine on the kinetics of normal and batrachotoxin-modified Na channels in frog node of Ranvier. Biophys J 50: 253–530.

Sheu S-S, Fozzard HA (1982) Transmembrane Na^+ and Ca^{2+} electro-chemical gradients in cardiac muscle and their relationship to force development. J Gen Physiol 80: 325–351.

Siesjö BK, Wieloch T (1985) Brain injury: neurochemical aspects. In: Central nervous system trauma status report (Becker DP, Povlishock JT, eds), pp 513–532. Bethesda, MD: National Institutes of Health.

Stafstrom CE, Schwindt PC, Crill WE (1982) Negative slope conductance due to a persistent subthreshold sodium current in cat neocortical neurons in vitro. Brain Res 236: 221–226.

Stafstrom CE, Schwindt PC, Chubb MC, Crill WE (1985) Properties of persistent sodium conductance and calcium conductance of layer V neurons from cat sensorimotor cortex. J Neurophysiol 53: 153–170.

Stys PK (1991) NEUROBASE: a general-purpose program for acquisition, storage and digital processing of transient signals using the Apple Macintosh II computer. J Neurosci Methods 37: 47–54.

Stys PK, Ransom BR, Waxman SG, Davis PK (1990a) Role of extracellular calcium in anoxic injury of mammalian central white matter. Proc Natl Acad Sci USA 87: 4212–4216.

Stys PK, Ransom BR, Waxman SG (1990b) Effects of polyvalent cations and dihydropyridine calcium channel blockers on recovery of CNS white matter from anoxia. Neurosci Lett 115: 293–299.

Stys PK, Ransom BR, Waxman SG (1991a) Compound action potential of nerve recorded by suction electrode: a theoretical and experimental analysis. Brain Res 546: 18–32.

Stys PK, Waxman SG, Ransom BR (1991b) Na^+–Ca^{2+} exchanger mediates Ca^{2+} influx during anoxia in mammalian CNS white matter. Ann Neurol 30: 375–380.

Walz W, Ransom BR, Carlini WG (1986) The effects of anoxia on extracellular ions and excitability in rat optic nerve: a developmental study. Soc Neurosci Abstr 12: 165.

Waxman SG, Ritchie JM (1985) Organization of ion channels in the myelinated nerve fiber. Science 228: 1502–1507.

Waxman SG, Pappas GD, Bennett MV (1972) Morphological correlates of functional differentiation of nodes of Ranvier along single fibers in the neurogenic electric organ of the knife fish *Sternarchus.* J Cell Biol 53: 210–224.

Waxman SG, Ransom BR, Stys PK (1991) Nonsynaptic mechanisms of calcium-mediated injury in CNS white matter. Trends Neurosci 14(10): 461–468.

Weiss JH, Hartley DM, Koh J, Choi DW (1990) The calcium channel blocker nifedipine attenuates slow excitatory amino acid neurotoxicity. Science 247: 1474–1477.

Wijesinghe RS, Gielen FLH, Wikswo JP Jr (1991) A model for compound action potentials and currents in a nerve bundle. I. The forward calculation. Ann Biomed Eng 19: 43–72.

Young W (1987) The post-injury responses in trauma and ischemia: secondary injury or protective mechanisms? Cent Nerv Syst Trauma 4: 27–51.

23 Modulation of Anoxic Injury in CNS White Matter by Adenosine and Interaction between Adenosine and GABA

Robert Fern, Stephen G. Waxman, and Bruce R. Ransom

Summary and Conclusions

1. We examined the role of adenosine in the development of anoxic injury in a CNS white matter tract, the rat optic nerve. Application of adenosine protected the rat optic nerve from anoxic injury; 2.5 µM adenosine increased compound action potential (CAP) recovery after a standard 60-min anoxic period from 28.6 ± 2.5%, mean ± SE, to 51.0 ± 3.1% ($P < 0001$). The protective effect of adenosine was abolished by the adenosine receptor antagonist theophylline (100 µM).

2. The protective effect of adenosine evolved slowly after adenosine application; maximum protection required 60 min of adenosine exposure before the onset of anoxia. The concentration dependence of the protective effect was parabolic, with maximum protection at 2.5 µM. Neither high nor very low adenosine concentrations protected against anoxia. These characteristics are similar to those previously found for the inhibitory neurotransmitter γ-aminobutyric acid (GABA) in the same preparation.

3. Inhibition of adenosine receptors (100 µM theophylline) reduced the level of recovery from that found under control conditions (24.3 ± 4.8% compared with 36.2 ± 2.5%, $P < 0.05$). The adenosine uptake inhibitor propentofylline, which potentiates release of endogenous adenosine during brain anoxia, significantly increased CAP recovery after anoxia. This effect was abolished by theophylline. It appeared therefore that release of endogenous adenosine limited injury in the optic nerve during anoxia.

4. The protective effect of adenosine was removed by pretreatment with the protein kinase C (PKC) inhibitor staurosporine (10 nM), indicating that activation of PKC was required for protection after exposure to adenosine.

5. Coadministration of low nanomolar concentrations of GABA shifted the concentration dependence of the protective effect of adenosine to lower concentrations. In the presence of 20 nM GABA, maximum protection was found at 2.5 µM adenosine; in 40 nM GABA, maximum protection was found at 1.5 µM adenosine; and in 100 nM GABA, maximum protection was observed at 900 nM adenosine.

6. The data suggest that adenosine and GABA can act synergistically at nanomolar concentrations to recruit a PKC-mediated protective mechanism during anoxia in white matter. Synergism between the two receptor types may be necessary to activate this autoprotective mechanism during small increases in the concentration of adenosine and GABA that occur in anoxic white matter.

Reprinted with permission from *Journal of Neurophysiology* 72: 2609–2616, 1994.

Introduction

Ischemia in the CNS is accompanied by a rapid accumulation of neuroactive substances in the extracellular space (Benveniste et al. 1984; Collis and Hourani 1993; Hagberg et al. 1985; Shimada et al. 1993; Van Wylen et al. 1986). Increases in the extracellular concentration of the neurotransmitters glutamate and γ-aminobutyric acid (GABA) and the neuromodulator adenosine may be of central importance in the development of the brain injury associated with ischemia (Choi 1988; Lyden and Lonzo 1994; Rothman and Olney 1987; Rudolphi et al. 1992; Saji and Reis 1987). Glutamate, in particular, is thought to be linked to pathophysiological changes in brain cells after calcium ion influx through glutamate-gated ion channels (Choi 1988; Choi et al. 1987; Rothman and Olney 1987). Adenosine, conversely, is proposed to act as a protective agent during ischemia (Rudolphi et al. 1992), dilating blood vessels in the brain when blood flow is compromised (Phillis et al. 1985) and acting directly to reduce release of excitotoxins, such as glutamate, from synaptic endings (Fredholm and Hedquist 1980).

The inhibitory neurotransmitter GABA can also act to limit injury during ischemia, probably by antagonizing the effects of glutamate (Saji and Reis 1987). GABA may also act in a neuroprotective fashion in certain anoxia-resistant species by shutting down brain function during anoxic stress and conserving energy (Lutz 1992). In white matter of the mammalian brain we have recently demonstrated that GABA is involved in an autoprotective feedback loop that reduces the degree of irreversible dysfunction during anoxia (Fern et al. 1994). GABA released from stores endogenous to white matter acts at GABA-B receptors to recruit a G-protein/protein kinase C (PKC)-mediated intracellular pathway that raises the resistance of optic nerve axons to anoxic injury. Block of this autoprotective mechanism significantly increases postanoxic compound action potential (CAP) recovery compared with control.

Adenosine is an ideal candidate as a neuroprotective agent in the brain because it is produced when there is a mismatch between oxygen supply and demand (Meghji et al. 1989; Rudolphi et al. 1992; Van Wylen et al. 1986). We have investigated the actions of adenosine on the development of anoxic injury in white matter and have focused on interactions between adenosine and GABA-B receptors. We report here that adenosine significantly protects white matter from anoxic injury in a fashion similar to GABA. Endogenous adenosine recruits a PKC-mediated intracellular mechanism that increases resistance to anoxia, whereas coadministration of low nanomolar concentrations of GABA shifts the concentration dependence of the protective effect of adenosine down to the nanomolar range. It seems, therefore, that the combined action of GABA and adenosine may allow recruitment of the protective mechanism during the small rises in extracellular concentration of adenosine and GABA that occur during ischemia in white matter in vivo.

Methods

The experimental protocol has been described previously (Fern et al. 1993; Stys et al. 1992). Female Long-Evans rats between 50 and 75 days old were anesthetized with an 80% CO_2–20% O_2 gas mixture and decapitated. The optic nerves were dissected free and placed in a modified interface perfusion chamber and incubated for a 60- to 90-min equilibration period. Nerves were maintained at $37\,^{\circ}C$, oxygenated in a 95% O_2–5% CO_2 atmosphere, and perfused at a rate of 1.4 ml/min with artificial cerebrospinal fluid (aCSF) containing (in mM) 153 Na^+, 3.0 K^+, 2.0 Mg^{2+}, 2.0 Ca^{2+}, 133 Cl^-, 26 HCO_3, 2.0 SO_4^{2-}, 1.0 H_2PO_4, and 10 dextrose, pH 7.45.

CAPs were evoked by a 125% supramaximal stimulus applied via a suction electrode to the distal nerve end. Recordings were made from a second suction electrode at the proximal nerve end, employing a method that compensates for instability inherent in the suction electrode technique (Stys et al. 1991). Anoxia was induced by changing to a 5% CO_2–95% N_2 atmosphere, which results in the effective exclusion of O_2 from the interface chamber within 60 s (Ransom et al. 1992). Anoxia was maintained for a 60-min period. CAP recovery after anoxia was determined by measuring CAP area after 60 min of reoxygenation, a time after which no further recovery occurs (Stys et al. 1992). Changes in the area under the CAP were calculated by computer and were assumed to correspond to changes in the number of functional optic nerve axons (Cummins et al. 1979; Wijesinghe et al. 1991).

To study the effects of a test solution on anoxic injury, we typically first perfused nerves in the solution for 60 min and took baseline readings. A 60-min anoxic period was then initiated. At the end of the anoxic period the nerves were reoxygenated for 60 min and a second reading taken. Control experiments were performed in aCSF and were interspersed between test experiments (a test experiment would typically be followed by a control experiment, or vice versa). Mean CAP recovery in control experiments was compared with that found under the test condition and significance was determined by analysis of variance (ANOVA)

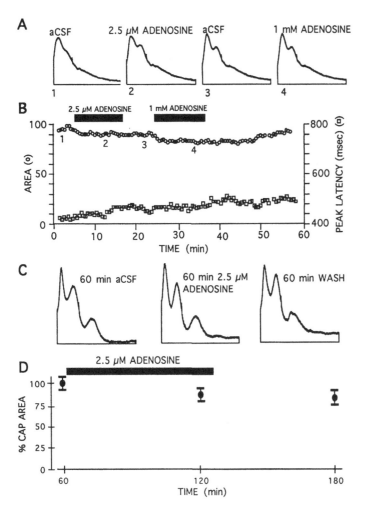

Figure 23.1
Adenosine did not influence nerve conduction in the normoxic rat optic nerve. (*A*) 4 compound action potentials (CAPs) recorded from an optic nerve before and during exposure to 2.5 µM and 1 mM adenosine. (*B*) CAP area (arbitrary units) and the latency between stimulation and the 1st peak of the CAP (peak latency) plotted against time. Filled bars: periods of exposure to 2.5 µM and 1 mM adenosine. These data are the complete set from which the CAPs in *A* are taken (numbers in *A* correspond to those in *B*). Similar data were found in a total of 4 optic nerves. (*C*) 3 CAPs recorded before, toward the end of, and subsequent to a 60-min exposure to 2.5 µM adenosine. (*D*) Change in mean CAP area before, during, and after a 60-min exposure to 2.5 µM adenosine, plotted against time (*n* = 6). There was no significant change in CAP area during perfusion with adenosine. aCSF, artificial cerebrospinal fluid.

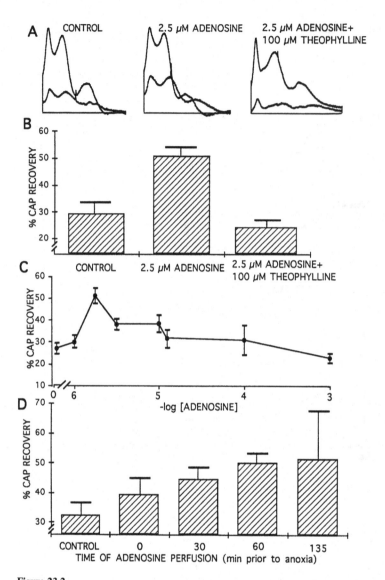

Figure 23.2
Adenosine (2.5 μM) improved the recovery of rat optic nerves after anoxia. (*A*) Pairs of pre- and postanoxic CAPs
are shown superimposed (the smaller of each pair is the postanoxic CAP). Under control conditions the CAP fell to
a low level after anoxia. In the presence of 2.5 μM adenosine the CAP recovered to a greater extent, an effect
abolished by the adenosine antagonist theophylline (100 μM). (*B*) Summary of the data showing that mean CAP
recovery was $28.6 \pm 2.5\%$ under control conditions ($n = 20$), $51.0 \pm 3.1\%$ in the presence of 2.5 μM adenosine
($n = 15$, $P < 0.0001$), and $24.5 \pm 5.0\%$ in the presence of both adenosine and theophylline ($n = 6$). (*C*) Concentration dependence of the protective effect of adenosine, showing that maximum protection was produced by 2.5 μM
adenosine. Each point is the mean CAP recovery found for between 4 and 15 optic nerves. Only 1 concentration was
tested on any single optic nerve. (*D*) Data summary showing the development of the protective effect of adenosine;
maximum protection was reached after ∼60 min of adenosine perfusion ($n = 8–15$).

or *t*-test, as appropriate. This technique was designed to minimize problems arising from variation in the degree of recovery found under control conditions, and accounts for the differences in control values used to assess the various test conditions. If all the control experiments were combined to produce a single massed control, and significance tested against this control using ANOVA, statistical significance would in all cases be greater than the significance obtained by comparing each test condition and its separate control. Results are presented as means $\pm$ SE. Only one test solution at one concentration was examined in any single optic nerve.

Results

To examine the possibility that adenosine receptors present in the rat optic nerve might influence nerve conduction, we perfused optic nerves with adenosine while recording the CAP at 1-min intervals. CAPs recorded during a 10-min exposure to 2.5 μM or 1 mM adenosine did not exhibit any significant changes in shape or area compared with those recorded before or subsequent to the adenosine exposure (specimen records are shown in figure 23.1*A*). The complete data set for one nerve is shown in figure 23.1*B*, where CAP area and peak latency are plotted against time (similar data were obtained in a total of 4 nerves). Longer periods of adenosine perfusion also failed to affect CAP shape or area (figure 23.1, *C* and *D*). Thus 60 min of 2.5 μM adenosine exposure did not change CAP area significantly ($n = 6$). The slight drift in CAP area evident in figure 23.1*D* was characteristic of the isolated rat optic nerve preparation.

Adenosine Protects Rat Optic Nerves from Anoxic Injury

GABA protects white matter by the direct recruitment of an intracellular pathway via a G-protein linked receptor (Fern et al. 1994). To examine the possibility that adenosine might have a similar action in CNS white matter, we perfused rat optic nerves with adenosine before the induction of anoxia. Three superimposed pairs of CAPs are shown in figure 23.2*A*. The larger of each pair is a CAP recorded before anoxia and the smaller is the postanoxic recovery. In control experiments, where nerves were perfused with aCSF throughout, mean postanoxic CAP recovery was $28.6 \pm 2.5\%$, mean $\pm$ SE ($n = 20$; figure 23.2, *A* and *B*). When 2.5 μM adenosine was added to the aCSF 60 min before anoxia, CAP recovery was significantly increased (mean CAP recovery $51.0 \pm 3.1\%$, $n = 15$; $P < 0.0001$; figure 23.2, *A* and *B*) compared with the control value. The adenosine receptor antagonist theophylline (100 μM), added to the aCSF 10 min before adenosine, removed the protective effect (figure 23.2, *A* and *B*).

The dose-response relationship for the protective effect of adenosine against anoxic injury was investigated by applying various adenosine concentrations 60 min before anoxia in separate experiments (data plotted in figure 23.2*C*). Maximum protection was afforded by 2.5 μM adenosine, with higher and lower concentrations being less effective. Significant protection was also found at higher concentrations, with 10 μM adenosine producing mean CAP recovery of $38.3 \pm 3.9\%$ ($n = 8$, $P < 0.05$). Reducing the adenosine concentration to 1 μM removed any protective effect, with postanoxic CAP recovery being similar to that under control conditions (mean CAP recovery $30.0 \pm 3.7\%$, $n = 8$).

Adenosine (2.5 μM) had no effect on the rate of conduction failure after the onset of anoxia, and no delay in the onset of conduction failure was observed. Thus CAP area fell to $23.0 \pm 6.0\%$ of preanoxic CAP area after 20 min of anoxia in the presence of 2.5 μM adenosine ($n = 4$), which was not significantly different from the $23.6 \pm 3.9\%$ of preanoxic CAP area found in aCSF after 20 min of anoxia ($n = 5$). These results suggest that adenosine does not act to protect optic nerves by delaying the early disruption of ionic homeostasis that occurs in the initial stages of anoxia in white matter (Ransom et al. 1992).

In the above experiments adenosine was applied to the nerves 60 min before anoxia to allow the steady-state effect of adenosine to be examined. To examine the temporal evolution of the protective effect, nerves were exposed to 2.5 μM adenosine over various time periods before anoxia. Data from a total of 42 experiments are summarized in figure 23.2D, where it can be seen that the protective effect of adenosine was fully developed after 60 min of pretreatment.

We have previously reported that activation of PKC mimics the protective effect of GABA, whereas block of PKC removes GABA-mediated protection (Fern et al. 1994). To test for the involvement of PKC in the protection produced by adenosine, the PKC inhibitor staurosporine was employed. In the absence of adenosine, perfusion with staurosporine (10 nM) resulted in lower postanoxic CAP recovery (mean CAP recovery 23.7 ± 3.0%, $n = 8$) than typically found under control conditions (mean CAP recovery 36.7 ± 2.9%, $n = 12$; figure 23.3). This finding is consistent with removal of autoprotection after PKC inhibition (Fern et al. 1994). Coapplication of 2.5 μM adenosine with staurosporine failed to significantly increase the degree of postanoxic CAP recovery from that found in staurosporine alone (26.9% ± 4.1, $n = 6$; figure 23.3). The protection provided by adenosine, therefore, was not found when PKC was inhibited. Because staurosporine has been demonstrated to be nontoxic during anoxia of white matter (Fern et al. 1994), this is strong evidence that PKC activation was essential for the protective effect of adenosine.

Interaction between GABA and Adenosine during Anoxia

Perfusion with 2.5 μM adenosine produced mean CAP recovery of 51.0 ± 2.5% in the experiments discussed above, whereas in a separate series of experiments, perfusion with 1 μM GABA produced mean CAP recovery of 47.7 ± 3% ($n = 12$), a degree of recovery not significantly different from that found with adenosine (figure 23.4C; $P > 0.5$). The shape of the dose-response relationship, the degree of protection produced, and the time of pretreatment necessary for protection are remarkably similar for GABA (Fern et al. 1994) and adenosine (this study). We therefore examined possible interactions between these two neuroactive substances.

We investigated the possibility that a high concentration of one agonist might desensitize the response to the second agonist. Coapplication of 1 mM GABA with 2.5 μM adenosine removed the protective effect normally produced by adenosine (mean CAP recovery 35.5 ± 4.2%, $n = 4$; figure 23.4, A and C). Furthermore, a high concentration of adenosine (100 μM) removed the protective effect of 1 μM GABA (mean CAP recovery 33.8 ± 9.8%, $n = 4$; figure 23.4, B and C). This suggests a common mechanism underlying the reduced protection found at high adenosine and GABA concentrations.

To further investigate interactions between GABA-B and adenosine receptors, we coadministered low concentrations of GABA to optic nerves with various adenosine concentrations. Adenosine and GABA were both applied for 60 min before anoxia. In the presence of 20 nM GABA, the dose-response relationship for the protection produced by adenosine was similar to that found in the absence of exogenous GABA, with maximum protection found at 2.5 μM adenosine (figure 23.5A). In a separate series of experiments performed in the presence of 40 nM GABA, no significant protection was found at this adenosine concentration (figure 23.5B). Significant protection was observed, however, at 1.5 μM adenosine. The concentration dependence of the protective action of adenosine was shifted to still lower concentrations in a series of experiments performed in 100 nM GABA (figure

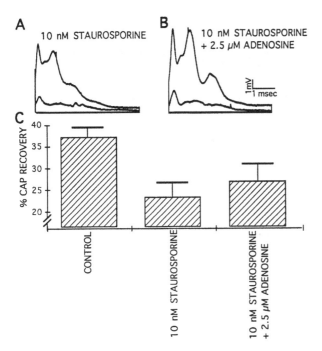

Figure 23.3
Protective effect of adenosine was absent during inhibition of protein kinase C (PKC). (*A*) Pre- and postanoxic CAPs from a nerve perfused with 10 nM staurosporine. A low level of postanoxic CAP recovery is apparent. (*B*) Typical data taken from an experiment where the nerve was perfused with both 10 nM staurosporine and 2.5 μM adenosine, illustrating a low level of postanoxic CAP recovery. (*C*) Data summary showing that the application of adenosine failed to significantly increase postanoxic CAP recovery when PKC was inhibited with staurosporine. Mean CAP recovery in 10 nM staurosporine was $23.7 \pm 3.0\%$ ($n = 8$); mean CAP recovery in 10 nM staurosporine plus 2.5 μM adenosine was $26.9 \pm 4.1\%$ ($n = 6$).

23.5*C*), with maximum protection found at 900 nM adenosine.

Endogenous Adenosine Protects against Anoxic Injury

We have recently reported that blocking the effects of endogenous GABA reduces the degree of postanoxic CAP recovery from that found in control conditions (Fern et al. 1994). In the current experiments, application of the GABA-B antagonist 5-amino valeric acid (5-AVA,

500 μM) reduced the degree of CAP recovery found after anoxia to ~70% of that found in the absence of the antagonist (mean CAP recovery in 5-AVA $25.2 \pm 4.5\%$, $n = 8$; mean recovery in aCSF $36.2 \pm 2.5\%$, $n = 20$, $P < 0.05$; figure 23.6*C*), similar to our previous results. The adenosine antagonist theophylline (100 μM) was applied using the same protocol to examine whether endogenous adenosine can also influence the degree of CAP recovery found after anoxia. Theophylline significantly reduced postanoxic CAP recovery, with a similar level of

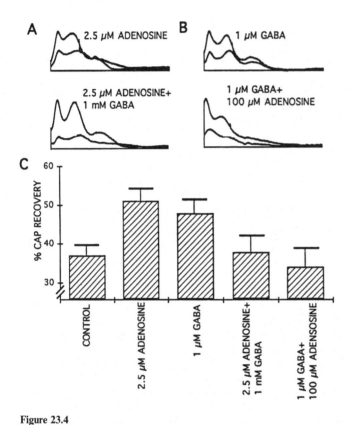

Figure 23.4

High concentration of γ-aminobutyric acid (GABA) desensitized the effect of adenosine, and vice versa. Pairs of pre- and postanoxic CAPs are shown (smaller CAPs are the postanoxic CAPs). (*A*) *Top pair* of CAPs demonstrates the typically high postanoxic recovery found in the presence of 2.5 μM adenosine. *Bottom pair* of CAPs shows a reduced level of CAP recovery when 1 mM GABA was coadministered with 2.5 μM adenosine. (*B*) *Top pair* of CAPs show high recovery found in 1 μM GABA. The protection produced by GABA was not evident when 100 μM adenosine was coadministered with 1 μM GABA. (*C*) Summary of experiments. Mean CAP recovery in the presence of 1 μM GABA was $47.7 \pm 3.0\%$ ($n = 8$), which was not significantly different from the value of $51.0 \pm 3.1\%$ found in the presence of 2.5 μM adenosine ($n = 15$). CAP recovery in the presence of 2.5 μM adenosine plus 1 mM GABA was $35.5 \pm 4.2\%$ ($n = 4$); in the presence of 1 μM GABA and 100 μM adenosine CAP recovery was $33.8 \pm 9.8\%$ ($n = 4$). Neither value is significantly greater than the $36.7 \pm 2.9\%$ mean CAP recovery found under control conditions ($n = 12$).

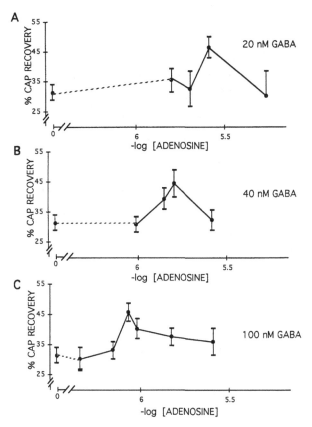

Figure 23.5

Low concentrations of GABA altered the adenosine dose-response relationship. (*A–C*) Protective effect of various adenosine concentrations applied in the presence of 20, 40, or 100 nM GABA, respectively. Note that the concentration of adenosine that produced maximum protection was shifted to the left at higher GABA concentrations (*n* = 4–16).

recovery found to that in the presence of 5-AVA (mean CAP recovery in theophylline 24.3 ± 4.8%, $n = 8$; $P < 0.05$; figure 23.6, $A–C$). The low level of CAP recovery produced by theophylline could not be explained by a toxic effect of the drug; the same period of theophylline application in the absence of anoxia did not significantly depress the CAP (figure 23.6D).

It appeared that both endogenous GABA and endogenous adenosine acted protectively during anoxia. It was surprising, therefore, that when GABA-B receptors and adenosine receptors were blocked simultaneously, the degree of postanoxic recovery was similar to that found when one species of receptor was blocked alone (mean CAP recovery in the presence of 100 μM theophylline plus 500 μM 5-AVA 24.7 ± 3.6%, $n = 15$; figure 23.6C). However, considering the degree of interaction found between adenosine and GABA in figure 23.4, it may be that inhibition of only one type of receptor is sufficient to effectively eliminate endogenous activation of the intracellular pathway that mediates autoprotection.

The results described above suggest the activation of adenosine receptors by endogenous adenosine during anoxia in the rat optic nerve. Manipulation of endogenous brain adenosine can be achieved via a number of pharmacological means, including blockade of adenosine uptake (Jacobson et al. 1992; Rudolphi et al. 1992). To this end we employed the adenosine uptake inhibitor propentofylline (HWA 285), a blood-brain barrier permeable drug with potential clinical utility (Andiné et al. 1990; DeLeo et al. 1988a,b; Fredholm and Linström 1986). Propentofylline was applied to the optic nerves 60 min before anoxia at 100-μM and 1-mM concentrations. Propentofylline (1 mM, but not 100 μM) significantly increased the degree of postanoxic CAP recovery from 32.6 ± 3.0% ($n = 11$) to 48.4 ± 9.1% ($n = 5$, $P < 0.05$; figure 23.7). This is consistent with the dose-response relationship for the effectiveness of propentofylline (Fredholm and Linström 1986). The protection provided by 1 mM propentophylline was blocked by 100 μM theophylline (mean CAP

recovery 30.45 ± 3.2%, $n = 4$), which indicated that the action of propentophylline was mediated by adenosine.

Variation between Groups of Control Experiments

In this and a previous study (Fern et al. 1994), a surprisingly similar degree of postanoxic recovery was found in single experiments under conditions that blocked the autoprotective mechanism (via interference with either GABA-B receptors, adenosine receptors, or PKC). The mean CAP recovery found under these various conditions was 25.7 ± 0.08%, with a range between 15.3 and 31.7% ($n = 24$). The variance about the mean CAP recovery found in control experiments performed side by side with these test experiments was larger than the variance around the mean CAP recovery in experimental groups where autoprotection was blocked: 32.7 ± 1.96%, with a larger range (15–62%, $n = 24$). An F test was performed to test for significance in the apparent difference in variance between the control experiments versus experiments where autoprotection was blocked. The F statistic was 5.88, which corresponds to $P < 0.0001$, indicating a significant difference in the variance between the two conditions. This suggests the presence of an uncontrolled factor generating variance in control experiments that was not present when the autoprotective mechanism was blocked. It is possible therefore that differences in the level of activity of the autoprotective mechanism may contribute to the variability that characterizes postanoxic CAP recovery between control experiments.

Discussion

The current experiments complement our recent findings, which implicate the inhibitory neurotransmitter GABA in the development of anoxic injury in the rat optic nerve (Fern et al. 1994). We here report that the neuromodulator adeno-

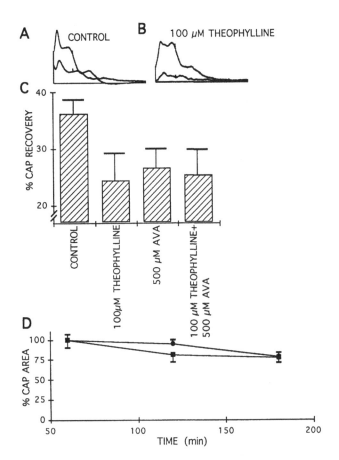

Figure 23.6
Block of endogenous adenosine reduced postanoxic CAP recovery. (*A*) Typical pre- and postanoxic CAPs in normal aCSF. (*B*) CAPs recorded in the presence of the adenosine receptor antagonist theophylline (100 μM). (*C*) Summary of data showing that mean CAP recovery was significantly reduced by both theophylline (mean CAP recovery $24.3 \pm 4.8\%$, $n = 8$, $P < 0.05$) and the GABA-B receptor antagonist amino valeric acid AVA (500 μM) (mean CAP recovery $25.2 \pm 4.5\%$, $n = 8$, $P < 0.05$). Coadministration of AVA and theophylline did not reduce mean CAP recovery to a greater extent than addition of AVA or theophylline alone (mean CAP recovery $24.7 \pm 3.6\%$, $n = 15$). (*D*) Theophylline was not toxic to the rat optic nerve. Mean CAP area plotted against time in aCSF (●, $n = 8$) and 100 μM theophylline (■, $n = 8$). Mean CAP areas were not significantly different from one another at either time point.

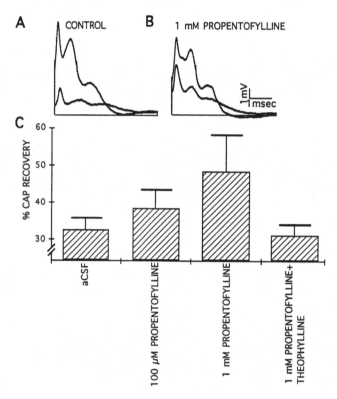

Figure 23.7
Potentiation of endogenous adenosine release mimicked the application of exogenous adenosine. (*A*) Typical CAP recovery found under control conditions. (*B*) Pre- and postanoxic CAPs in the presence of the adenosine uptake inhibitor propentofylline (1 mM). (*C*) Data summary showing that 1 mM propentofylline significantly increased mean postanoxic CAP recovery (48.4 ± 9.1%, $n = 5$, compared with 32.6 ± 3.0%, $n = 11$, P < 0.05). The protective effect of 1 mM propentophylline was blocked by 100 μM theophylline (mean recovery 30.45 ± 3.2%, $n = 4$).

sine mimicked the actions of GABA in this preparation. Application of 2.5 μM adenosine increased CAP recovery after anoxia to 51.0 ± 3.0%. Block of adenosine receptors with theophylline significantly reduced the level of recovery compared with the control value (24.3 ± 4.8% compared with 36.2 ± 2.5%), whereas block of adenosine uptake with propentofylline, which potentiates release of endogenous adenosine during anoxia (Jacobson et al. 1992; Rudolphi et al. 1992), resulted in significant protection during anoxia (48.4 ± 9.1% CAP recovery com-

pared with 32.6 ± 3.0%). Adenosine was therefore involved in an autoprotective mechanism that provided a degree of tolerance to anoxia in CNS white matter.

Interaction of GABA and Adenosine

The characteristics of the protection provided by GABA and adenosine were remarkably similar. The maximum protection produced by GABA and by adenosine was not significantly different (47.7% compared with 51.0%), and the protective effect of both substances developed over a 60-min time course, had a parabolic dose-response profile, and was removed by inhibition of PKC. The data indicate that GABA and adenosine may recruit the same intracellular pathway to increase tolerance to anoxia in the optic nerve. Thus low concentrations of GABA shifted the concentration dependence of the protective effect of adenosine to lower concentrations. This was not a simple addition of GABA protection to an unchanged level of adenosine protection. As can be seen from figure 23.5, addition of increasing GABA concentrations affected a translocation of the adenosine dose-response curve to the left. Thus adding GABA to optic nerves exposed to adenosine mimicked the effect of addition of a second dose of adenosine. Similar convergence between GABA-B and adenosine receptors has been reported in cerebral pyramidal neurons, where both receptor types are linked to the same hyperpolarizing potassium conductance (McCormick and Williamson 1989).

The protective effect of adenosine was apparently mediated by PKC. Thus inhibition of PKC prevented the increase in CAP recovery normally produced by exogenous adenosine and reduced CAP recovery to the level found during adenosine receptor blockade. PKC has been identified as the second messenger in a number of adenosine-mediated effects (e.g., Marala et al. 1993; Nishimura et al. 1992; Schwiebert et al. 1992), including a protective effect against anoxic injury in heart cells (e.g., Armstrong et al. 1994). The activation of PKC by adenosine has also been demonstrated to be G-protein mediated (Delumeau et al. 1991; Schwiebert et al. 1992). The presence of a G-protein/PKC-mediated intacellular protective pathway recuited by GABA-B receptors has recently been described in the rat optic nerve (Fern et al. 1994).

GABA and Adenosine in White Matter

The extracellular concentration of GABA in CNS white matter (internal capsule of the rat)

increases from ~10 nM in control conditions to 100 nM during 120 min of ischemia (Shimada et al. 1993). The free extracellular adenosine concentration in the normoxic rat brain lies between 40 nM and 1.3 µM and rises to between 1 and 40 µM during anoxia or ischemia (Ballarin et al. 1991; Hagberg et al. 1987; Van Wylen et al. 1986; Zetterström et al. 1982). The efflux of adenosine during anoxia follows an increase in intracellular adenosine production from ATP and adenosine transport into the extracellular space via a nucleoside transport protein (Meghji et al. 1989). Release of adenosine occurs from both CNS neurons and glia. Glia may account for significant endogenous adenosine release in the rat optic nerve, because this structure contains significant numbers of astrocytes (Black et al. 1985; Butt and Ransom 1989). White matter has a lower oxygen consumption than gray matter (Nishizaki et al. 1988) and may therefore have a low level of extracellular adenosine. However, the concentration of extracellular GABA reported during anoxia of white matter is ideal for potentiation of the effect of low adenosine concentrations. It therefore seems that interaction between GABA and adenosine may allow recruitment of the autoprotective mechanism during small rises in concentration of these substances during white matter anoxia.

Ablation of Protection at High Agonist Concentrations

High concentrations of adenosine did not protect against anoxia, and a similar effect was observed with high GABA concentrations (Fern et al. 1994). High concentrations of GABA also masked the protective effects of adenosine and vice versa. The current data therefore suggest interaction between GABA-B and adenosine receptors in receptor-mediated protection from anoxia in the optic nerve. Ablation of the effectiveness of an agonist at high concentrations can be the result of receptor desensitization, and has previously been observed for adenosine in hippocampal slices (Nishimura et al. 1992). Desensitization of receptors frequently follows PKC activation, both in general (Huganir and Greengard 1990) and specifically for GABA-B and adenosine receptors (Dutar and Nicoll 1988; Taniyama et al. 1992; Worley et al. 1987). The results demonstrate that both GABA-B and adenosine receptors are linked to activation of PKC in the optic nerve. It may be therefore that high levels of PKC activation at high agonist concentrations lead to receptor desensitization.

Possible Mechanism Underlying the Protective Effect of GABA and Adenosine

Anoxic damage in white matter and gray matter results from very different mechanisms. In gray matter it is believed that release of excitotoxins, such as glutamate, during membrane depolarization leads to opening of glutamate channels, calcium ion influx, and calcium-mediated cell damage (Choi 1988; Choi et al. 1987; Rothman and Olney 1987). In white matter, it appears that membrane depolarization leads to calcium ion influx through reverse action of the Na^+-Ca^{2+} exchanger subsequent to sodium ion influx through noninactivating sodium channels (Stys et al. 1992).

The neurotransmitter-mediated autoprotection we have described in white matter must depend on the modulation of some cellular element fundamental to the development of anoxic injury. We have previously suggested that this element may be the Na^+-Ca^{2+} exchanger (Fern et al. 1994). Thus activation of PKC is frequently linked to the downregulation of membrane transporters, including the Na^+-Ca^{2+} transporter (Mené et al. 1991). Downregulation of the Na^+-Ca^{2+} exchanger would lead to less calcium influx during anoxia and reduced injury (Stys et al. 1990a). Furthermore, downregulation of the exchanger would not be expected to have any significant influence on normoxic nerve conduction, because inhibition of Na^+-Ca^{2+} exchange in optic nerve axons with bepridil does not influence nerve conduction (unpublished observations). Our results are consistent, therefore, with the hypothesis that the Na^+-Ca^{2+} exchanger is downregulated by endogenous adenosine (Taglialatela et al. 1992). A second possible mechanism of adenosine's protective action could involve an inhibitory action on sodium channels, because a noninactivating sodium conductance is apparently a prerequisite for anoxic injury in the rat optic nerve (Stys et al. 1992).

Conclusions

Synaptic integration occurs in the gray matter of the brain, where incoming signals are processed and response signals are shaped; transmission of these signals, however, is performed by nerve fibers. It is not surprising, therefore, that infarcts in white matter, which represent ∼21% of strokes clinically, are associated with neurological disabilities (Bamford et al. 1987; Fisher 1982). Furthermore, the majority of strokes affect both gray and white matter, making the understanding of the pathophysiology of white matter anoxia an important goal.

The current findings, and previous results from this laboratory (Fern et al. 1994), have demonstrated a surprising new level of complexity to the pathophysiology of white matter anoxic injury. Extracellular accumulation of neurotransmitters does not underlie the development of anoxic injury in white matter; however, we now understand that the buildup of extracellular GABA and adenosine plays an important modulatory role in the pathophysiological process. These substances recruit a unique protective mechanism directed against axonal injury. This autoprotective mechanism in white matter is of clear utility, because nerve fiber tracts that are tolerant to anoxia must represent a significant survival characteristic (Bamford et al. 1987). Our results suggest, in fact, that variation in the degree of autoprotection may account for the variation observed between the degree of injury sustained by control (untreated) optic nerves exposed to anoxia. The potential for manipulating the autoprotective mechanism in white matter has yet to be examined in situ. However, the drugs we have employed to increase the level of endogenous GABA and adenosine in vitro are currently available for treatment of various neurological disorders. An examination of the utility of such drugs for reducing ischemic injury to white matter occurring within the CNS will require further studies.

Acknowledgments

This work was supported in part by grants from the National Institute of Neurological Disorders and Stroke to B. R. Ransom and the Medical Research Service, Department of Veterans Affairs to S. G. Waxman. R. Fern was supported in part by a grant from the Blinded Veterans Association and by a Spinal Cord Research Fellowship from the Eastern Paralyzed Veterans Association.

References

Andiné, P., Rudolphi, K. A., Fredholm, B. B., and Hagberg, H. Effect of propentofyyline (HWA 285) on extracellular purines and excitatory amino acids in CA1 of rat hippocampus during transient ischaemia. *Br. J. Pharmacol.* 100: 814–818, 1990.

Armstrong, S., Downey, J. M., and Ganote, C. E. Preconditioning of isolated rabbit cardiomyoctes: induction by metabolic stress and blockade by the adenosine antagonist SPT and calphostin C, a protein kinase C inhibitor. *Cadiovasc. Res.* 28: 72–77, 1994.

Ballarin, M., Fredholm, B. B., Ambrosio, S., and Mahy, N. Extracellular levels of adenosine and its metabolites in the striatum of awake rats: inhibition of uptake and metabolism. *Acta Physiol. Scand.* 142: 97–103, 1991.

Bamford, J., Sandercock, P., Jones, L., and Warlow, C. The natural history of lacunar infarction: the Oxfordshire community stroke project. *Stroke* 18: 545–551, 1987.

Benveniste, H., Drejer, J., Schousboe, A., and Diemer, N. H. Elevation of the extracellular concentrations of glutamate and aspartate in rat hippocamus during transient cerebral ischemia monitored by intracerebral microdialysis. *J. Neurochem.* 43: 1369–1374, 1984.

Black, A. A., Waxman, S. G., Ransom, B. R., and Feliciano, M. D. A quantitative study of developing axons and glia following altered gliogenesis in rat optic nerve. *Brain Res.* 380: 122–136. 1985.

Butt, A. M. and Ransom, B. R. Visualization of oligodendrocytes and astrocytes in the intact rat optic nerve by intracellular injection of lucifer yellow and horseradish peroxidase. *Glia* 2: 470–475, 1989.

Choi, D. W. Calcium-mediated neurotoxicity: relationship to specific channel types and role in ischemic damage. *Trends Neurosci.* 11: 465–469, 1988.

Choi, D. W., Maulucci-Gedde, M., and Kriegstein, A. R. Glutamate neurotoxicity in cortical cell culture. *J. Neurosci.* 7: 357–368, 1987.

Collis, M. G. and Hourani, S. M. O. Adenosine receptor subtypes. *Trends Pharmacol. Sci.* 14: 360–366, 1993.

Cummins, K. L., Perkel, D. H., and Dorfman, L. J. Nerve fibre conduction velocity distributions. I. estimation based on the single fibre and compound action potentials. *Electroencephalogr. Clin. Neurophysiol.* 46: 634–646, 1979.

DeLeo, J., Schubert, P., and Kreutzberg, G. W. Propentofylline (HWA285) protects hippocampal neurones of mongolian gerbils against ischemic damage in the presence of an adenosine antagonist. *Neurosci. Lett.* 84: 307–311, 1988a.

DeLeo, J., Schubert, P., and Kreutzberg, G. W. Protection against ischemic brain damage using propentofylline in gerbils. *Stroke* 19: 1535–1539, 1988b.

Delumeau, J. C., Petitet, F., Cordier, J., Glowinski, J., and Prémont, J. Synergistic regulation of cytosolic Ca^{2+} concentration in mouse astrocytes by NK1 tachykinin and adenosine agonists. *J. Neurochem.* 57: 2026–2035, 1991.

Dutar, P. and Nicoll, R. A. Pre- and postsynaptic GABA B receptors in the hippocampus have different pharmacological properties. *Neuron* 1: 585–591, 1988.

Dux, E., Fastbom, J., Ungerstedt, U., Rudolphi, K., and Fredholm, B. B. Protective effect of adenosine and a novel xanthine derivative propentofylline on the cell damage after bilateral carotid occlusion in the gerbil hippocampus. *Brain Res.* 516: 248–256, 1990.

Dux, E., Schubert, P., and Kreutzberg, G. W. Ultrastructural localization of calcium in ischemic hippocampal slices: the influence of adenosine and theophylline. *J. Cereb. Blood Flow Metab.* 12: 520–524, 1992.

Fern, R., Ransom, B. R., Stys, P. K., and Waxman, S. G. Pharmacological protection of CNS white matter during anoxia: actions of phenytoin, carbamazepine and diazepam. *J. Pharmacol. Exp. Ther.* 266: 1549–1555, 1993.

Fern, R., Waxman, S. G., and Ransom, B. R. Endogenous GABA attenuates CNS white matter dysfunction following anoxia. *J. Neurosci.* In press.

Fisher, C. M. Lacunar strokes and infarcts: a review. *Neurology* 32: 871–876, 1982.

Fredholm, B. B. and Hedquist, P. Modulation of neurotransmission by purine nucleotides and nucleosides (Abstract). *Biochemical Pharm.* 29: 1635–1643, 1980.

Fredholm, B. B. and Linström, K. The xanthine derivative 1-(5′-oxohexyl)-3-methyl-7-propyl xanthine (HWA 285) enhances the action of adenosine. *Acta Pharmacol. Toxicol.* 58: 187–192, 1986.

Hagberg, H., Andersson, P., Lacarewicz, J., Jacobson, I., Butcher, S., and Sanberg, M. Extracellular adenosine, inosine, hypoxanthine, and xanthine in relation to tissue nucleotides and purines in rat striatum during transient ischemia. *J. Neurochem.* 49: 227–231, 1987.

Hagberg, H., Lehmann, A., Sandberg, M., Nyström, B., Jacobson, I., and Hamberger, A. Ischemia-induced shift of inhibitory and excitatory amino acids from intra- to extracellular compartments. *J. Cereb. Blood Flow Metab.* 5: 413–419, 1985.

Huganir, R. L. and Greengard, P. Regulation of neurotransmitter receptor desensitization by protein phosphorylation. *Neuron* 5: 555–567, 1990.

Jacobson, K. A., van Galen, P. J. M., and Williams, M. Adenosine receptors: pharmacology, structure-activity relationships, and therapeutic potential. *J. Med. Chem.* 35: 407–422, 1992.

Lutz, P. L. Mechanisms for anoxic survival in the vertebrate brain. *Annu. Rev. Physiol.* 54: 601–618, 1992.

Lyden, P. D. and Lonzo, L. Combination therapy protects ischemic brain in rats. *Stroke* 25: 189–196, 1994.

Marala, R. B., Ways, K., and Mustafa, S. J. 2-Chloroadenosine prevents phorbol ester-induced depletion of protein kinase C in porcine coronary artery. *Am. J. Physiol.* 264 (*Heart Circ. Physiol.* 33): H1465–H1471, 1993.

McCormick, D. A. and Williamson, A. Convergence and divergence of neurotransmitter action in human cerebral cortex. *Proc. Natl. Acad. Sci. USA* 86: 8098–8102, 1989.

Meghji, P., Tuttle, J. B., and Rubio, R. Adenosine formation and release by embryonic chick neurones and glia in cell culture. *J. Neurochem.* 53: 1852–1860, 1989.

Mené, P., Pugliese, F., and Cinotti, G. A. Regulation of Na^+/Ca^{++} exchange in cultured human mesangial cells. *Am. J. Physiol.* 261 (*Renal Fluid Electrolyte Physiol.* 30): F466–F473, 1991.

Nishimura, S., Okada, Y., and Amatsu, M. Postinhibitory excitation of adenosine on neurotransmission in guinea pig hippocampal slices. *Neurosci. Lett.* 139: 126–129, 1992.

Nishizaki, T., Yamauchi, R., Tanimoto, M., and Okada, Y. Effects of temperature on the oxygen consumption in thin slices from different brain regions. *Neurosci. Lett.* 86: 301–305, 1988.

Phillis, J. W., DeLong, R. E., and Towner, J. K. Adenosine and the regulation of cerebral blood flow during anoxia. In: *Adenosine: Receptors and Modulation of Cell Function*, edited by V. Stefanovich, K. Rudolphi, and P. Schubert. Oxford, UK: IRL, 1985, p. 145–164.

Ransom, B. R., Walz, W., Davis, P. K., and Carlini, W. G. Anoxia-induced changes in extracellular K^+ and pH in mammalian central white matter. *J. Cereb. Blood Flow Metab.* 12: 593–602, 1992.

Rothman, S. M. and Olney, J. W. Excitotoxicity and the NMDA receptor. *Trends Neurosci.* 10: 299–302, 1987.

Rudolphi, K. A., Schubert, P., Parkinson, F. E., and Fredholm, B. B. Neuroprotective role of adenosine in cerebral ischaemia. *Trends Pharmacol. Sci.* 13: 439–445, 1992.

Saji, M. and Reis, D. J. Delayed transneuronal death of substantia nigra neurons prevented by γ-aminobutyric acid agonist. *Science Wash. DC* 235: 66–69, 1987.

Schwiebert, E. M., Karlson, K. H., Friedman, P. A., Dietl, P., Spielman, W. S., and Stanton, B. A. Adenosine regulates a chloride channel via protein kinase C and a G-protein in a rabbit cortical duct cell line. *J. Clin. Invest.* 89: 834–841, 1992.

Shimada, N., Graf, R., Rosner, G., and Heiss, W. D. Ischemia-induced accumulation of extracellular amino acids in cerebral cortex, white matter, and cerebrospinal fluid. *J. Neurochem.* 60: 66–71, 1993.

Stys, P. K., Ransom, B. R., and Waxman, S. G. Compound action potential of nerve recorded by suction electrode: a theoretical and experimental analysis. *Brain Res.* 546: 18–32, 1991.

Stys, P. K., Ransom, B. R., Waxman, S. G., and Davis, P. K. Role of extracellular calcium in anoxic injury of mammalian central white matter. *Proc. Natl. Acad. Sci. USA* 87: 4212–4216, 1990a.

Stys, P. K., Sontheimer, H., Ransom, B. R., and Waxman, S. G. Noninactivation, tetrodotoxin-sensitive Na$^+$ conductance in rat optic nerve axons. *Proc. Natl. Acad. Sci. USA* 90: 6976–6980, 1990b.

Stys, P. K., Waxman, S. G., and Ransom, B. R. Ionic mechanisms of anoxic injury in mammalian CNS white matter: role of Na$^+$ channels and Na$^+$-Ca^{++} exchanger. *J. Neurosci.* 12: 430–439, 1992.

Taglialatela, M., Canzoniero, L. M. T., Rossi, A. M., Mita, G., DiRenzo, G. F., and Annunziato, L. Adenosine receptors modulate the Na+/Ca++ exchanger in cerebral nerve endings. *Ann. NY Acad. Sci.* 639: 166–168, 1992.

Taniyama, K., Niwa, M., Kataoka, Y., and Yamashita, K. Activation of protein kinase C suppresses the γ-aminobutyric acid-B receptor-mediated inhibition of the vesicular release of noradrenaline and acetylcholine. *J. Neurochem.* 58: 1239–1245, 1992.

Van Wylen, D. G. L., Park, T. S., Rubio, R., and Berne, R. M. Increases in cerebral interstitial fluid adenosine concentration during hypoxia, local potassium infusion, and ischemia. *J. Cereb. Blood Flow Metab.* 6: 522–528, 1986.

Wijesinghe, R. S., Geilen, F. L. H., and Wikswo, J. P., Jr. A model for compound action potentials and currents in a nerve bundle. I. The forward calculation. *Ann. Biomed. Eng.* 19: 43–72, 1991.

Worley, P. F., Baraban, J. M., McCarren, M., Snyder, S. H., and Alger, B. E. Cholinergic phosphatidylinositol modulation of inhibitory, G protein linked, neurotransmitter actions: electrophysiological studies in rat hippocampus. *Proc. Natl. Acad. Sci. USA* 84: 3467–3471, 1987.

Zetterström, T., Vernet, L., Ungerstedt, U., Tossman, U., Jonzon, B., and Fredholm, B. B. Purine levels in the intact rat brain. Studies with an implanted perfused hollow fibre. *Neurosci. Lett.* 29: 111–115, 1982.

XV SYMPHONIA MOLECULARIS

The nervous system, of course, is unique among organs in being able to process sensory information, control motor activity, compute, and even think. Its ability to do this rests upon the capability of neurons to generate electrical impulses called action potentials. These occur when specialized molecules, called sodium channels, open up, allowing sodium ions to rush from the outside of the cell, across the membrane, generating electrical current in the process. Sodium channels thus provide the "molecular batteries" that enable neurons to produce electrical signals.

When I went to medical school, we learned about "the" sodium channel. The molecular structure of the channel had not been determined, but its presence was known, largely from the work of Sir Alan Hodgkin and Sir Andrew Huxley. These pioneering scientists, working at the University of Cambridge and at the Marine Biological Association in Plymouth, England, had exploited the fact that squids possess an unusually large axon, termed the "giant axon," which was larger than one millimeter across, so that they could insert tiny electrodes into it. Using these microelectrodes they were able to measure the electrical currents that flow across the membrane of the giant axon as it generates action potentials. From these recordings, these early neuroscientists discerned that there were tiny pores or channels within the axon membrane, selectively permeable to sodium ions, which acted as molecular batteries. Although they could not see the sodium channels or visualize them, Hodgkin and Huxley were able to infer some aspects of the structure of these channels and to predict that they possess "gates" that opened as the channels were stimulated, allowing sodium ions to pass through. For this research (see Hodgkin and Huxley 1952), they were awarded the Nobel prize in Physiology or Medicine in 1963.

In 1995, Andrew Huxley graciously wrote the first chapter of a book entitled *The Axon* that I edited together with Jeffery Kocsis and Peter Stys. In a concluding paragraph entitled "The Future as it Appeared in 1951," he stated that "any idea of analyzing the mode of operation of the channels by the methods of molecular genetics would have seemed to us in 1951 to be even further into the realms of science fiction."

Nearly forty years after Hodgkin and Huxley carried out their pioneering experiments, the revolution in molecular biology led to the cloning of the first sodium channel by Numa and his colleagues. Identification of the nucleotide sequence within the mRNA, which constitutes a blueprint for the channel, provided crucial information about its molecular structure (Noda et al. 1984). Like all proteins, the sodium channel consists of a chain of amino acids, much like a string of beads. In the case of the sodium channel, there were nearly eighteen hundred amino acids in the string. The structure of the sodium channel protein molecule suggested that it weaves through the cell membrane twenty-four times, six times each within four similar "domains." The fourth membrane-spanning segment, termed the S-4 segment in each domain, was different from the rest, containing a positively charged amino acid residue at every third position, which would be expected to cause it to move within an electrical field. The S-4 segments, in fact, appeared to act as "voltage sensors," reacting to stimulation by moving in and out of the membrane, and thereby opening or closing the gate. Molecular biology provided, for the first time, a picture of the molecular structure of sodium channels, and it was a beautiful structure indeed. And, notably, this structure was precisely as predicted by Hodgkin and Huxley.

In the years since the cloning of the first sodium channel, molecular biology has demonstrated that the concept of "the" sodium channel was a simplistic one. There were hints from electrophysiological and pharmacological experiments in the late 1970s and early 1980s that there might be more than one sodium channel. But the idea that there are multiple, diverse sodium channels had its formal birth when Numa and his colleagues demonstrated that, within the mammalian brain, there were three sodium channel genes, each encoding a related but different channel (Noda et al. 1986). Following this, other sodium channel genes encoding additional channels were discovered. We now know that there are, in fact, nearly a dozen genes, each encoding a sodium channel with a subtly different amino acid sequence.

Propelled by an interest in spinal cord injury, our studies on sodium channels emphasized spinal sensory neurons (also termed dorsal root ganglion neurons because their cell bodies are located within clusters called dorsal root ganglia). These neurons project their axons peripherally to the skin and muscles, and centrally to the brain; and they serve as sensory pathways, transmitting messages from sensory endings throughout the body upward, toward the brain. Compared to "higher" neurons that are located within the brain, these spinal sensory neurons serve a relatively simple function, encoding sensory information and carrying it upwards. In a sense, these neurons do not even think! Thus, one might have expected that they would have a simple organization in terms of sodium channels. Nothing could have been farther from the truth. Our early studies showed that even in spinal sensory neurons at least six different genes encode distinct sodium channels (Black et al. 1996). Different sodium channel genes were active, and thus the molecular machinery for impulse generation appeared to be different, in different types of spinal sensory neurons. Our research group added to this cornucopia by cloning an additional sodium channel, NaN, from spinal sensory neurons (Dib-Hajj et al. 1998). That story is told in part XVII.

What function does the multiplicity of sodium channels serve? Our early physiological studies in the "premolecular" era had provided some glimpses of the electrical activity in nerve fibers which suggested that they might possess multiple sodium channels with different roles. In 1983, using fine microelectrodes to penetrate single axons from the sciatic nerves of rats, we were able to observe that, following blockade of K^+ channels, some nerve fibers fired in inappropriate high-frequency bursts, with repetitive activity arising from a sustained depolarization that followed the primary impulse (Kocsis, Ruiz, and Waxman 1983). Sodium channels had classically been considered to open and close rapidly, and "fast" sodium channels with these traditional properties would not be expected to produce a sustained depolarization. The sustained depolarization provided an early hint that, together with "fast" sodium channels, "slow" sodium channels (which take longer to close) might be present in sensory neurons and their axons where they could contribute to the generation of trains of impulses. A few years later we observed similar bursting, and similar slow depolarizations, in human nerve fibers within nerve biopsies (Kocsis and Waxman 1987), and we talked about giving the slower sodium channel the nickname "pokey" because of its sluggish behavior.

It took nearly ten more years for us to definitively demonstrate the signatures of "fast" and "slow" sodium channels in different types of sensory neurons using patch clamp methods (Honmou et al. 1994). Connie Bowe, a pediatric neurologist who worked as a research fellow in our laboratories in the mid-1980s, made observations on impulse conduction that suggested that there were differences in the sodium channels in sensory and motor nerves (Bowe, Kocsis, and Waxman 1985; Bowe et al. 1987) and subsequently obtained recordings of impulse activity in different types of sensory axons, which again suggested that they might possess different types of sodium channels. In Honmou et al. (1994) we labeled different types of spinal sensory neurons and then studied their sodium currents. This permitted us to demonstrate that sodium channels in cutaneous afferent sensory neurons (which innervate and carry sensory information from the skin) are slower, opening and closing less rapidly, than sodium channels within muscle afferent neurons (which innervate and carry sensory information from muscle). This allows different types of sensory neurons to process information differently, some humming continuously in response to stimuli and others buzzing briefly in response to other stimuli.

Most spinal sensory neurons have several types of sodium channels in their membranes, and these channels can open simultaneously, making it difficult to discern the activity of each type. How, in view of this, can we learn about the contribution of each channel to the behavior of the neurons? Cummins, Howe, and Waxman (1998) provides an example, showing how we analyzed the contribution of a channel called PN1 known to be present in spinal sensory neurons. This paper first presents a "bottom-up" analysis of the PN1 sodium channel. For these experiments we used molecular biological techniques to insert the gene for PN1 in human embryonic kidney cells, which do not normally produce high levels of sodium channels. This permitted us to study the PN1 channels nearly in isolation. Using patch-clamp methods to record the activity of these channels, Ted Cummins, a young and very talented biophysicist, found that their recovery from inactivation is a very slow process; that is, following rapid opening and closing of these channels, they remain inactivated (unavailable for opening a second time) for a relatively long period of time. As a result of this slow repriming, PN1 channels would not be expected to support firing at high frequencies and, indeed, we found this to be the case.

What, then, do PN1 channels do? Our recordings showed that PN1 channels exhibit slow "closed-state inactivation"; that is, following stimulation that is not sufficient to open the channels, they inactivate, but do so slowly (Cummins, Howe, and Waxman 1998). The latter finding suggested to Cummins that the PN1 channels should remain available for activation during slow depolarizations such as the "generator" potentials produced by sensory neurons when they are stimulated, in contrast to most conventional or "fast" sodium channels which become unavailable because inactivation rapidly develops. To test this hypothesis, we slowly depolarized embryonic kidney cells containing PN1 channels with ramp-shaped stimuli. These experiments revealed that, indeed, these channels respond to these subtle perturbations, which are similar to the small generator potentials evoked in spinal sensory neurons by sensory stimuli, by opening and producing a current which further depolarizes the cell membrane. The PN1 channels in this model system thus have physiological properties that should permit them to amplify or boost sensory inputs.

Because PN1 channels normally are present within spinal sensory neurons, we next asked whether channels with similar physiological properties are present within these cells. Building upon our "bottom-up" approach, we did a "top-down" analysis, and using what we had learned from our studies on PN1 channels in kidney cells, we applied ramp-like stimuli to spinal sensory neurons. The results, shown in figures 8 and 9 of Cummins, Howe, and Waxman (1998), demonstrate that a sodium current, similar to that produced by the PN1 channels in isolation within human kidney cells, can be elicited in spinal sensory neurons by perturbations similar to receptor potentials. The currents produced by PN1 channels and by spinal sensory neurons in response to these stimuli are, in fact, almost identical. The "bottom-up" and "top-down" results thus converge, and show us that the PN1 channels in spinal sensory neurons can act as molecular amplifiers which boost sensory inputs, exciting other, "fast" sodium channels to produce the rapid depolarization necessary for nerve impulses. Here we have a physiological rationale, at least within one type of nerve cell, for the presence of multiple sodium channels.

Molecular analysis of the basis for electrical activity in the nervous system is now rapidly moving forward. It has shown us that molecules such as sodium channels can collaborate—like the different players that contribute to a symphony—to give nerve cells the unique patterns of firing that they use to process information and encode messages; and it has taught us that molecular diversity—the presence, for example, of multiple types of sodium channels deployed in different mixtures in different types of neurons—endows nerve cells with distinct functional properties. Where this explosion of knowledge will lead is not yet clear. I suspect that in the future we will find even more molecular diversity in the nervous system—introduced by tricks of the genome such as alternative splicing and RNA editing, and of the cell such as posttranslational modification—and that we will find an unexpected degree of variability in the physiological properties of molecules involved in neuronal computation. If this turns out to be true, the molecular underpinnings of nervous system function will be more complex than the first generations of cloners could have anticipated. Even if this additional diversity is not there, however, molecular biology will have helped us to understand how neurons integrate information and generate their messages, and it will have brought us closer to understanding the beautiful computer that resides in our brains and spinal cords. We are living through a molecular revolution. The science fiction that Huxley could only imagine in 1951 has become reality.

References

Black, J. A., Dib-Hajj, S. D., McNabola, K., Jeste, S., Rizzo, M. A., Kocsis, J. D., and Waxman, S. G. Spinal sensory neurons express multiple sodium channel α-subunit mRNAs. *Molec. Brain Res.* 43: 117–132, 1996.

Bowe, C. M., Kocsis, J. D., and Waxman, S. G. Differences between mammalian ventral and dorsal spinal roots in response to blockade of potassium channels during maturation. *Proc. Roy. Soc. Lond. B.* 224: 355–366, 1985.

Bowe, C. M., Kocsis, J. D., Targ, E. F., and Waxman, S. G. Physiological effects of 4-aminopyridine on demyelinated mammalian motor and sensory fibers. *Ann. Neurol.* 22: 264–268, 1987.

Cummins, T. R., Howe, J. R., and Waxman, S. G. Slow closed-state inactivation: a novel mechanism underlying ramp currents in cells expressing the hNE/PN1 sodium channel. *J. Neurosci.* 18: 9606–9619, 1998.

Dib-Hajj, S. D., Tyrrell, L., Black, J. A., and Waxman, S. G. NaN, a novel voltage-gated Na channel preferentially expressed in peripheral sensory neurons and down-regulated following axotomy. *Proc. Natl. Acad. Sci. U.S.A.* 95: 8963–8968, 1998.

Hodgkin, A. L., and Huxley, A. F. A quantitative description of membrane current and its application to conduction and excitation in nerve. *J. Physiol.* 117: 500–544, 1952.

Honmou, O., Utzschneider, D. A., Rizzo, M. A., Bowe, C. M., Waxman, S. G., and Kocsis, J. D. Delayed depolarization and slow sodium currents in cutaneous afferents. *J. Neurophysiol.* 71: 1627–1637, 1994.

Huxley, A. F. Electrical activity of nerve: the background up to 1952. In: *The Axon*, Waxman, S. G., Kocsis, J. D., and Stys, P. K. (eds.), New York, Oxford University Press, pp. 1–12, 1995.

Kocsis, J. D., Ruiz, J. A., and Waxman, S. G. Maturation of mammalian myelinated fibers: changes in action potential characteristics following 4-aminopyridine application. *J. Neurophysiol.* 50: 449–463, 1983.

Kocsis, J. D., and Waxman, S. G. Ionic channel organization of normal and regenerating mammalian axons. *Progress in Brain Research,* Vol. 71, *Neural Regeneration*, Seil, F. J., Herbert, E., and Carlson, B. (eds.), pp. 89–102, 1987.

Noda, M., Shimizu, S., Tanabe, T., Takai, T., Kayano, T., Ikeda, T., Takahashi, H., Nakayama, H., Kanaoka, Y., Minamino, N., Kangawa, K., Matsuo, H., Raftery, M. A., Hirose, T., Inayama, S., Hayashida, H., Miyata, T., and Numa, S. Primary structure of *Electrophorus electricus* sodium channel deduced from complementary DNA sequence. *Nature* 312: 121–127, 1984.

Noda, M., Ikeda, T., Kayano, T., Suzuki, H., Takeshima, H., Kurasaki, M., Takahashi, H., and Numa, S. Existence of distinct sodium channel messenger RNAs in rat brain. *Nature* 320: 188–192, 1986.

24 Spinal Sensory Neurons Express Multiple Sodium Channel α-Subunit mRNAs

J. A. Black, S. D. Dib-Hajj, K. McNabola, S. Jeste, M. A. Rizzo, J. D. Kocsis, and S. G. Waxman

Abstract The expression of sodium channel α-, β1- and β2-subunit mRNAs was examined in adult rat DRG neurons in dissociated culture at 1 day in vitro and within sections of intact ganglia by in situ hybridization and reverse transcription polymerase chain reaction (RT-PCR). The results demonstrate that sodium channel α-subunit mRNAs are differentially expressed in small (<25 μm diam.), medium (25–45 μm diam.) and large (>45 μm diam.) cultured DRG neurons at 1 day in vitro (div). Sodium channel mRNA I is expressed at higher levels in large neurons than small DRG neurons, while sodium channel mRNA II is variably expressed, with most cells lacking or exhibiting low levels of detectable signal of these mRNAs and limited numbers of neurons with moderate expression levels. DRG neurons generally exhibit negligible or low levels of hybridization signal for sodium channel mRNA III. Sodium channel mRNAs Na6 and NaG show similar patterns of expression, with most large and many medium DRG neurons exhibiting high levels of expression. The mRNA for the rat cognate of human sodium channel hNE-Na is detected in virtually every DRG neuron; most cells in all size classes exhibit moderate or high levels of hNE-Na expression. Sodium channel SNS mRNA is expressed in all size classes of DRG neurons, but shows greater expression in small and medium DRG neurons than in large neurons. The mRNA for the rat cognate of mouse sodium channel mNa$_v$2.3 is not detected, or is detected at low levels, in most DRG neurons, regardless of size, although moderate expression is detected in some neurons. Sodium channel β1- and β2-subunit mRNAs exhibit similar expression patterns; they are detected in most DRG neurons, although the level of expression tends to be greater in large neurons than in small neurons. RT-PCR and in situ hybridization of intact adult DRG showed a similar pattern of expression of sodium channel mRNAs to that observed in DRG neurons in vitro. These results demonstrate that adult DRG neurons express multiple sodium channel mRNAs in vitro and in situ and suggest a molecular basis for the biophysical heterogeneity of sodium currents observed in these cells.

Reprinted with permission from *Molecular Brain Research* 43: 117–131, 1996.

1. Introduction

Spinal sensory (dorsal root ganglion (DRG)) neurons constitute a heterogeneous population of cells, based on morphology, physiology and receptor innervation [9, 49, 70]. Multiple, distinct voltage-gated sodium currents have been described in these cells (table 24.1), including sodium currents that are sensitive to tetrodotoxin (TTX) at nanomolar concentrations, and distinct TTX-resistant sodium currents that require micromolar concentrations of TTX for block [10, 27, 36, 40, 54]. At least three distinct sodium currents in DRG neurons can also be distinguished on the basis of different kinetic and voltage-dependent characteristics [11, 45, 50, 60]. Although differences in sodium currents were originally described between DRG neurons in different size classes, it is now known that DRG neurons subserving different sensory roles within the same size class (e.g., large cutaneous vs. large muscle afferents) express distinct sodium currents [26]. Moreover, while some DRG neurons express only a single type of sodium current, other DRG neurons co-express multiple types of sodium currents [11, 40, 45, 51, 52, 54, 60]. It has recently been shown that substantial cell-to-cell heterogeneity in sodium currents exists in DRG neurons, even in neurons of similar sizes [50].

Neural sodium channels are trimeric complexes composed of α-, β1- and β2-subunits [12]. The α-subunit forms the voltage-sensitive and ion-selective pore and is structurally diverse, arising from multiple sodium channel genes and alternative splicing of the transcripts [1, 2, 19–23, 34, 35, 55–57]. Two subfamilies of sodium channel α-subunit genes have been described based on sequence homology. For neural tissue, subfamily 1 includes rat brain sodium channels I, II [42], IIA [2], III [34], rat sodium channel 6 (Na6) [57], human neuroendocrine sodium channel (hNE-Na [35]; rat peripheral nerve 1

Table 24.1
Sodium current properties of cultured rat DRG neurons

Age	Time in vitro	Sodium current characteristics	Reference
E-17	3–4 weeks	25% (30 μm diam.)—fast, TTX-S; 44% (16 μm diam.)—slow, TTX-R; 31% (23 μm diam.)—bimodal	[45]
1–2 days	3–4 weeks	19% (39 μm diam.)—fast, TTX-S; 44% (20 μm diam.)—slow, TTX-R; 37% (28 μm diam.)—bimodal	
Adult	3–4 weeks	26% (46 μm diam.)—fast, TTX-S; 35% (26 μm diam.)—slow, TTX-R; 39% (36 μm diam.)—bimodal	
1–3 days	2–6 h	23%—slow (S); 0%—neonatal-like fast (FN); 14%—adult-like fast (FA); 52%—S + FN; 10%—S + FA	[60]
5–8 days	2–6 h	10%—S; 0%—FN; 66%—FA; S + FN—22%; S + FA—2%	
5–10 days	<48 h	10–15% slow, TTX-S; 85–90% fast, TTX-R	[36]
3–4 days	<24 h	mostly small (<15 μm diam.) neurons; solely or mainly TTX-R	[54]
4–8 days	<24 h	mostly small (<15 μm diam.) neurons; mixtures of TTX-R and TTX-S	
Adult	<24 h	many larger (>20 μm diam.); solely or mainly TTX-S. Some small (<15 μm diam.); solely TTX-R	
Adult	2 weeks–6 months	small neurons—mostly TTX-R with small TTX-S component; large neurons—predominantly TTX-S	[40]
Adult	12–48 h	small (<30 μm diam.)—coexpress fast, TTX-S and slow, TTX-R medium (30–50 μm diam.)—either fast, TTX-S and slow, TTX-R; or only intermediate, TTX-S large (>50 μm diam.)—intermediate, TTX-S	[11]
Adult	16–28 h	small (13–25 μm diam.)—45% TTX-R, 55% TTX-S	[18]
Adult	18–48 h	small (18–25 μm diam.)—mostly slow, TTX-R large (44–50 μm diam.)—either fast, TTX-S; or fast, TTX-S and slow, TTX-R	[50]

TTX-S = tetrodotoxin-sensitive; TTX-R = tetrodotoxin-resistant.

(PN1) ([16, 20]; G. Mandel, personal communication) and rabbit Schwann cell (NaS) [5] are homologs in other species) and rat SNS [1], while subfamily 2 includes human $Na_v2.1$ [22], mouse $mNa_v2.3$ [19] and rat NaG [21]. The roles played by the auxiliary sodium channel β1- and β2-subunits are not completely understood; however, co-expression of α- and β1-subunits modulates sodium current characteristics [6, 28, 31, 38, 48] and the β2-subunit has been suggested to be an important regulator of functional sodium channel expression and localization in neurons [29, 30].

The molecular correlates underlying the sodium current diversity observed in DRG neurons have not been established. Transcripts for sodium channels I, II, SNS and NaG have been detected by Northern blot analyses in rat DRG tissue [1, 4, 21, 65], and recently in situ hybridization studies have shown that the mRNAs for sodium channels I, II, SNS and NaG are expressed in some DRG neurons in situ [1, 65, 66]. However, systematic observations comparing the levels of various sodium channel mRNAs in DRG neurons in situ have not been available. Moreover, detailed information has not been available about the sodium channel transcripts that are expressed in DRG neurons in vitro, which may underlie the sodium current heterogeneity observed in patch clamp studies on these cells, and it is not clear whether DRG neurons express multiple sodium channel a-subunit mRNAs. In this study, we use in situ hybridization and reverse transcription polymerase chain reaction (RT-PCR) to examine the pattern of expression of sodium channel a-subunits I, II, III, Na6, hNE-Na, SNS, $mNa_v2.3$ and NaG and $\beta1$- and $\beta2$-subunit mRNAs in DRG neurons from adult rats. Results presented here demonstrate that multiple sodium channel mRNAs are expressed in most, if not all, cultured DRG neurons at 1 day in vitro (div), and show that a similar pattern of sodium channel mRNA is expressed in DRG neurons in vitro and in situ.

---

2. Materials and Methods

2.1. In Situ Hybridization

2.1.1. Probes The RNA probes used here recognize nucleotide sequences 7385–7820, 6807–7302, 6325–6822, 6461–6761, 6003–6308, 1476–1989, 5239–5479, 871–1308, 457–790 and 140–669 (GenBank numbering) of sodium channel a-subunit types I, II, III, Na6, hNE-Na, SNS, $mNa_v2.3$ and NaG and sodium channel $\beta1$- and $\beta2$-subunits, respectively. The construction of the digoxigenin-substituted riboprobes has been previously described and these probes have been utilized to localize sodium channel mRNAs in rat CNS and PNS tissue and cultured astrocytes and Schwann cells [7, 8, 46, 47, 65, 66].

2.1.2. Culture Cultures of DRG neurons from adult rats were established as described previously [50]. Briefly, lumbar ganglia (L4, L5) from adult Sprague–Dawley female rats were freed from their connective sheaths and incubated sequentially in enzyme solutions containing collagenase and then papain. The tissue was

triturated in culture medium containing 1:1 Dulbecco's modified Eagle's medium (DMEM) and Hank's F12 medium and 10% fetal calf serum, 1.5 mg/ml trypsin inhibitor, 1.5 mg/ml bovine serum albumin, 100 U/ml penicillin and 0.1 mg/ml streptomycin and plated at a density of 500–1000 cells/mm^2 on polyornithine/laminin-coated coverslips. The cells were maintained at 37°C in a humidified 95% air/5% CO_2 incubator overnight and then processed for in situ hybridization cytochemistry as described previously [8, 73].

2.1.3. Tissue Preparation Adult female Sprague–Dawley rats were deeply anesthetized with chloral hydrate and perfused through the heart, first with a phosphate-buffered saline (PBS) solution and then with 4% paraformaldehyde in 0.14 M Sorensen's phosphate buffer, pH 7.4, at 4°C. Following perfusion fixation, dorsal root ganglia at levels L4 and L5 were collected and placed in fresh fixative at 4°C. After 2–4 h, the tissue was transferred to a solution containing 4% paraformaldehyde and 30% sucrose in 0.14 M phosphate buffer and stored overnight at 4°C. Fifteen μm sections were cut and placed on poly-L-lysine-coated slides. The slides were processed for in situ hybridization cytochemistry as previously described [7, 66]. Following in situ hybridization cytochemistry, the slides were dehydrated, cleared and mounted with Permount.

2.1.4. RT-PCR Brain and L4, L5 DRG were dissected from adult Sprague–Dawley rats and total cellular RNA was isolated by the single step guanidinum isothiocyanate-acid phenol procedure [14]. The quality and relative yield of the RNA was assessed by electrophoresis in a 1% agarose gel.

2.1.5. Reverse Transcription First strand cDNA was synthesized essentially as previously described [17]. Briefly, 5 μg total RNA was reverse transcribed in a 50 μl final volume using 1 μM random hexamer (Boehringer Mannheim) and 500 units Super-Script II reverse transcriptase (Life Technologies) in the presence of 100 units of RNase Inhibitor (Boehringer Mannheim). The reaction buffer consisted of 50 mM Tris-HCl (pH 8.3), 75 mM KCl, 3 mM MgCl$_2$, 10 mM DTT and 125 µM dNTP. The reaction was allowed to proceed at 37 °C for 90 min, 42 °C for 30 min, then terminated by heating to 65 °C for 10 min. A control reverse transcription reaction contained all components except for reverse transcriptase.

2.1.6. PCR We used primers designed against highly conserved sequences in domain 1 (D1) and domain 4 (D4) to amplify products from multiple α-subunits that may be present in the cDNA pool (table 24.2). In addition, primers were designed against the 3′ untranslated sequences (3′ UTR) to specifically amplify α-subunits II, III and SNS products, and also against specific sequences in β1- and β2-subunits (table 24.2). All subunit sequences are based on Genbank database (accession numbers: I: X03638; II: X03639; III: Y00766; Na6: L39018; hNE-Na: X82835; SNS: X92184; mNa$_v$2.3: L36179; NaG: M965778; β1: M91808; β2: U37026).

The region amplified in domain 1 spans most of the conserved transmembrane segment D1-S3 and extends into the first half of D1-SS1; the central portion of this region shows significant sequence and length polymorphism (see table 24.3). Due to codon degeneracy, three forward primers (F1, F2, F3) were designed to ensure efficient priming from all templates that may be present in the cDNA pool (table 24.2). The reverse primer (R1) has several mismatches compared to the sequences of αI and α-hNE-Na: G to A at position 3, A to G at position 4 and T to G at position 7 (αI); and T to C at position 1 and A to G at position 19 (αhNE-Na). The lengths of amplified products and restriction enzyme polymorphism from D1 are shown in table 24.3.

Nested primers were designed to amplify sequences in D4. Highly conserved sequences downstream from D4-S2 and within D4-S3 were selected for the upstream primers and sequences 3′ to D4-S6 were selected for downstream primers for primary and secondary PCR. Due to codon degeneracy, and to obtain maximal priming from all templates, we designed a pair of oligonucleotides for each primary (A1/B1, A2/B2) and secondary (C1/D1, C2/D2) upstream and downstream primer. Primers A1/B1 and C1/D1 amplify segments of α-subunits in subfamily 1 (αI, II, III, Na6 and hNE-Na), while primers A2/B2 and C2/D2 amplify regions of α-subunits in subfamily 2 (amNa$_v$2.3 and NaG). Corresponding primers (e.g., A1 and A2) have similar predicted thermal profiles under our PCR conditions and will therefore anneal to their respective templates with comparable efficiency. The lengths of amplified products and restriction enzyme polymorphism from D4 are shown in table 24.3.

Primers that are specific to α-subunits II, III and SNS were designed against their respective 3′ UTR (table 24.2). The expected product sizes for II, III and SNS are 262, 496 and 403 bp, respectively.

The locations of the primers specific for sodium channel β1- and β2-subunits are given in table 24.2. The expected product sizes for β1- and β2-subunits are 592 and 720 bp, respectively.

Rat β-actin sequences were amplified from the same cDNA pool, using commercial primers (Clontech), to determine the presence of contaminating genomic DNA in the RNA preparations. PCR from a cDNA template amplifies a 764 bp fragment, and from a genomic template amplifies a 1440 bp fragment. A single DNA fragment, comigrating with the 800 bp molecular weight marker, was detected in control PCR reactions which indicates the absence of appreciable genomic DNA contamination in the RNA samples (data not shown).

Amplification was typically performed in 60 µl volume using 1 µl of the first strand cDNA, 0.8 µM of each primer and 1.75 units of Expand Long Template DNA polymerase enzyme mixture (Boehringer Mannheim). Control PCR

Table 24.2
Sequence locations for primers used for RT-PCR

	Primary		Secondary	
	5′	3′	5′	3′
Domain 1				
	F1	R1		
aI	813–832	1347–1370		
aIII	975–994	1512–1535		
ahNE-Na	604–623	1081–1104		
	F2	R1		
aII	775–784	1312–1335		
	F3	R1		
aNa6	580–599	1063–1086		
Domain 4				
	A1	B1	C1	D1
aI	5044–5065	5691–5714	5078–5101	5650–5679
aII	4973–4994	5620–5643	5007–5030	5579–5599
aIII	5014–5035	5661–5684	5049–5071	5620–5640
aNa6	4724–4745	5368–5391	4758–4781	5327–5347
ahNE-Na	4730–4751	5377–5400	4764–4787	5336–5356
	A2	B2	C2	D2
aNaG	185–206	822–855	221–244	791–811
3′ Untranslated region				
	F1	R1		
aII	6290–6310	6530–6552		
aIII	6325–6344	6803–6822		
aSNS	6078–6098	6461–6481		
β-subunits				
	F1	R1		
β1	298–320	872–890		
β2	140–160	840–860		

A1, A2, C1, C2, F1, F2 and F3: forward (5′) primers. B1, B2, D1, D2, R1: reverse (3′) primers.

Table 24.3
Length and restriction enzyme polymorphism of a-subunit RT-PCR products

Domain 1	aI (558 bp)[a]	aII (561 bp)	aIII (561 bp)	aNa6 (507 bp)	ahNE (501 bp)		Product size (bp)
*Eco*RV	+	−	−	−	−		152,406
*Eco*NI	−	+	−	−	−		204,357
*Ava*I	−	−	+	−	−		137,424
*Sph*I	−	−	−	+	−		126,381
*Bam*HI	−	−	−	−	+		134,367
Domain 4	aI (592 bp)[a]	aII (592 bp)	aIII (592 bp)	aNa6 (592 bp)	ahNE-Na (592 bp)	aNaG (590 bp)	Product size (bp)
*Nci*I	+	−	−	−	−	−	176,416
*Dsa*I	+	−	+	−	−	−	140,452
*Bst*UI	−	+	−	−	−	−	37,555
*Eco*RV	−	−	−	+	−	−	55,535
*Pvu*II	−	−	−	−	−	+	28,560

[a] Size of the amplification product from the respective a-subunit.

reactions in which the template was substituted by water or an aliquot from a control reverse transcription reaction lacking reverse transcriptase produced no amplification products (data not shown). Compared to conventional and thermostable DNA polymerases, Expand Long Template enzyme mixture increases the yield of the PCR products without an increase in non-specific amplification [3, 13]. The PCR reaction buffer consisted of 50 mM Tris-HCl (pH 9.2), 16 mM $(NH4)_2SO_4$, 2.25 mM $MgCl_2$, 2% (v/v) DMSO and 0.1% Tween 20. As described previously [17], amplification was carried out in two stages using a programmable thermal cycler (PTC-100, MJ Research, Cambridge, MA). First, a denaturation step at 94 °C for 4 min, an annealing step at 58 °C for 2 min and an elongation step at 72 °C for 90 s. Second, a denaturation step at 94 °C for 1 min, an annealing step at 58 °C for 1 min and an elongation step at 72 °C for 90 s. The second stage was repeated 33 times for a total of 35 cycles, with the elongation step in the last cycle extended to 10 min.

Secondary PCR was performed essentially as described above except that the template was 1 μl of a 1 : 1000 dilution of the primary PCR product and amplification was carried out for 25 cycles.

The identity of the a-subunits expressed in DRG and brain were determined by restriction enzyme analysis of their PCR products and by the presence of amplification products from their 3′ UTRs. For restriction enzyme analysis, typically 1/20 of the PCR reaction is digested for 1 h at the recommended temperature and the products resolved by electrophoresis in a 1.75% agarose gel. A summary of the predicted results of such analyses is presented in table 24.3.

3. Results

To examine the pattern of sodium channel mRNAs expressed in DRG neurons cultured from adult rats at 1 day in vitro (div), we probed these cells with riboprobes specific for sodium channel mRNAs I, II, III, Na6, hNE-Na, SNS, mNa$_v$2.3, NaG, β1 and β2. Subsequently, to ascertain whether the same pattern of sodium channel mRNAs is expressed by DRG neurons in situ, sodium channel α- and β-subunit mRNAs were examined with RT-PCR and in situ hybridization in intact DRG from adult rats.

3.1. Sodium Channel mRNA Expression in vitro

Sodium channel I mRNA is expressed in DRG neurons in vitro, and the level of expression is related to the size of the neuron (figure 24.1, I). Large (>45 μm diam.) neurons tend to express higher levels of sodium channel I mRNA than medium (25–45 μm diam.) and small (<25 μm diam.) DRG neurons. The expression of sodium channel II mRNA is not size-dependent; rather, DRG neurons of all sizes generally express low levels (figure 24.1, II). Most DRG neurons in vitro express negligible or low levels of sodium channel III mRNA (figure 24.1, III), although some larger DRG neurons express this mRNA at moderate levels. Na6 and NaG mRNAs both exhibit a gradient of expression in DRG neurons. Large and medium DRG neurons generally express high levels of Na6 mRNA, while Na6 mRNA is not detectable, or detectable at low levels, in small DRG neurons (figure 24.1, Na6). Likewise, most large and many medium DRG neurons express high levels of NaG mRNA and small DRG neurons generally express low levels of NaG (figure 24.1, NaG). The rat cognate of sodium channel hNE-Na mRNA is detectable in virtually every DRG neuron, with moderate or high levels of expression apparent in all size classes (figure 24.1, hNE). SNS mRNA is expressed in all size classes of DRG neurons, with a tendency toward greater levels of expression in small and medium size neurons than large neurons (figure 24.1, SNS). The rat cognate of sodium channel mNa$_v$2.3 mRNA is not detectable, or is detectable at only low levels,

in most DRG neurons and is present at moderate levels in only a few neurons of all cell sizes (figure 24.1, m2.3).

Sodium channel β1 and β2 mRNAs are detectable at moderate or high levels in most DRG neurons. However, the greatest levels of expression are generally observed in large neurons; small neurons tend to have lower levels of expression of both β-subunits (figure 24.2a, b).

For quantification of the hybridization signal, we measured cell diameter with a calibrated ocular reticle and scored the level of hybridization signal from "o" to "+ + +" for each cell (see table 24.4 legend). The relative levels of hybridization signal of sodium channel mRNAs I, II, III, Na6, hNE-Na, SNS, mNa$_v$2.3, NaG, β1 and β2 in small (<25 μm diam.), medium (25–45 μm diam.) and large (>45 μm diam.) DRG neurons in vitro are presented in table 24.4. Consistent with the qualitative descriptions above, sodium channel I mRNA is more highly expressed in large than in medium or small DRG neurons. Sodium channel II mRNA is not expressed or expressed at low levels in >73% of neurons in each size class, with 10–25% of cells showing no signal in each size class and only 1.9% of large diameter cells (and no small or medium cells) exhibiting a high level of expression. Sodium channel III mRNA exhibits negligible-to-low levels of expression in >90% of small and medium DRG neurons; in the large size class, 82% of the cells show negligible-to-low levels of expression, while 18% of the cells show moderate levels of sodium channel III mRNA. For each size class, the levels of Na6 and NaG mRNA expression are similar; both mRNAs show a tendency for higher levels of expression in larger neurons, with >50% of large neurons displaying high levels. The rat cognate of hNE-Na mRNA is widely expressed in DRG neurons. For all size classes, >75% of the cells show moderate-to-high levels of expression; in addition, hNE-Na is the only α-subunit mRNA in which every cell shows some level of expression (i.e., no cells with

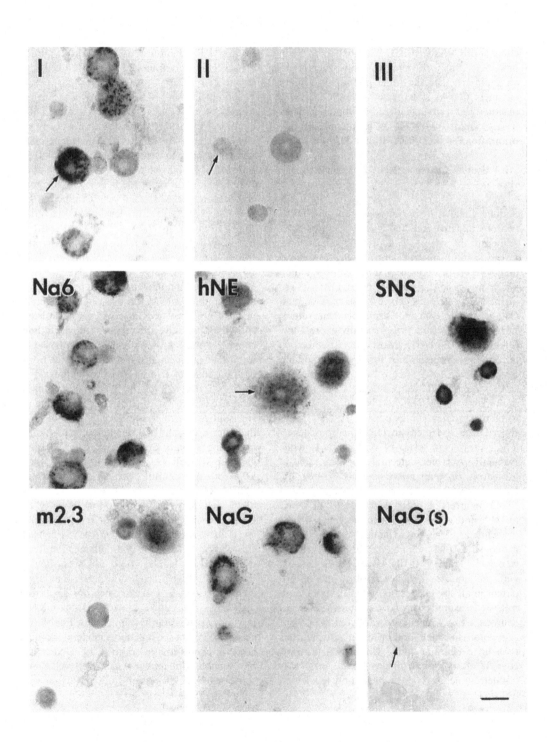

negligible signal). SNS mRNA is present at moderate-to-high levels in >50% of small and medium size DRG neurons, and in >30% of large neurons. In contrast, the rat cognate of $mNa_v2.3$ mRNA is not detectable, or is detectable at only low levels, in >75% of DRG neurons of each size class.

Sodium channel $\beta1$ and $\beta2$ mRNA are also detectable in most cells of all size classes; however, larger cell classes tend to show a greater percentage of cells with moderate-to-high levels of expression than smaller cells.

3.2. Sodium Channel mRNA Expression in situ

3.2.1. RT-PCR The restriction enzyme analysis of amplification products derived from cDNA derived from intact dorsal root ganglia, from domain 1 (D1) and domain (D4) and the amplification from the $3'$ UTR sequences, are shown in figure 24.3; the predicted sizes of restriction enzyme digestion of D1 and D4 are presented in table 24.3.

Lane 1 contains the amplification products using primers for D1. The appearance of two bands is consistent with the predicted results (table 24.3). Amplification products of *a*I (558 bp), *a*II and *a*III (561 bp) will migrate as a single band, while amplification products of *a*Na6 and *a*hNE-Na (507 bp and 501 bp, respectively) will migrate as a single lower molecular weight band. Lanes 2–6 show the result of cutting this DNA with *Eco*RV, *Eco*NI, *Ava*I, *Sph*I and *Bam*HI, respectively. Subunit *a*I product appears to constitute most of the higher molecular weight species in the input DNA (lane 2), suggesting that only a minor fraction is due to *a*II and/or *a*III products. Subunits *a*II (lane 3) and *a*III (lane 4) are not evident by this analysis; however, their presence could be inferred from the appearance of a residual band in lane 2. Restriction analysis also indicates the presence of subunits *a*Na6 and *a*hNE-Na in the amplified DNA pool (lanes 5 and 6, respectively). The restriction products for these *a*-subunits are in agreement with the predicted results shown in table 24.2.

Lane 8 contains the RT-PCR products from intact DRG RNA using primers for D4. These products migrate slightly faster than the 600 bp marker, in close agreement with the predicted sizes of 590 and 592 bp. Lanes 9–13 show the results of cutting this DNA with *Nci*I, *Dsa*I, *Bst*UI, *Eco*RV and *Pvu*II, respectively. These

Figure 24.1
Sodium channel *a*-subunit mRNAs in cultured DRG neurons 1 day in vitro. Hybridization with antisense riboprobes specific for sodium channel mRNAs I (*I*), II (*II*), III (*III*), Na6 (*Na6*), hNE-Na (*hNE*), SNS (*SNS*), $mNa_v2.3$ (*m2.3*) and NaG (*NaG*), and with a sense riboprobe for NaG (*NaG(s)*) are shown. Sodium channel mRNA I exhibits a gradient of expression, with greater levels of expression in larger neuons than in smaller neurons. The arrow indicates a neuron with a high ("+++") level of expression. Sodium channel mRNA II generally has low levels of hybridization signal in all size classes of DRG neurons. The arrow illustrates a neuron with a low ("+") level of expression. Most DRG neurons have negligible or low levels of sodium channel mRNA III expression. Na6 mRNA is highly expressed in most large and medium DRG neurons and has low expression in small DRG neurons. The rat cognate of sodium channel hNE-Na mRNA is detectable at moderate or high levels in most DRG neurons, regardless of size. The arrow indicates a neuron with moderate ("++") hybridization signal. The mRNA for SNS is highly expressed in many small and medium DRG neurons, and in some large neurons. The rat cognate of $mNa_v2.3$ mRNA exhibits a gradient of hybridization signal, with most neurons exhibiting low or non-detectable levels and some neurons expressing moderate levels. Most large and medium size DRG neurons express high levels of NaG mRNA. DRG neurons probed with sense probes (e.g., NaG(s)) generally exhibit non-detectable (arrow) or low levels of expression. These micrographs are shown at the same magnification as figure 24.5; the larger apparent cell diameter in vitro is due to spreading of the cells on the substrate and/or shrinkage of tissue sections during processing. ×200. Bar = 40 μm.

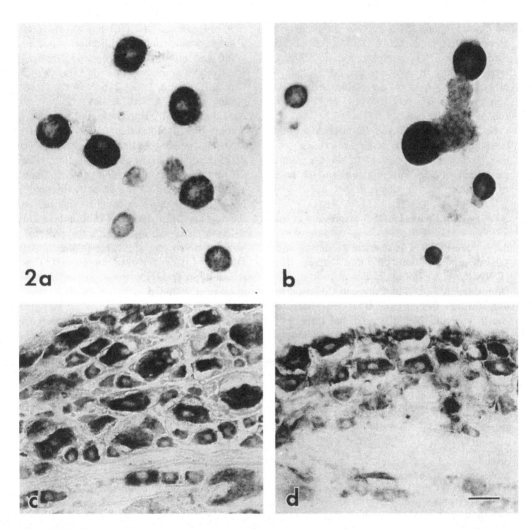

Figure 24.2
Sodium channel β1- and β2-subunit mRNAs in DRG neurons in vitro and in situ. (a) β1 mRNA is expressed at high levels in large DRG neurons in vitro and is expressed at lower levels in small DRG neurons. (b) β2 mRNA is highly expressed in many DRG neurons in vitro, regardless of size. (c) Most DRG neurons in situ express β1 mRNA, with greater hybridization signal present in large neurons compared to most small neurons. (d) β2 mRNA exhibits a similar pattern of expression as β1 mRNA in DRG neurons in situ, with many large neurons exhibiting high levels of hybridization signal. ×215. Bar = 40 μm.

Table 24.4
Expression of sodium channel subunit mRNAs in adult DRG neurons in vitro

mRNA	Small (<25 µm)					Medium (25–45 µm)					Large (>45 µm)				
	o	+	++	+++		o	+	++	+++		o	+	++	+++	
I	32.2	65.1	2.6	0.0	(152)	4.8	43.0	44.9	7.5	(107)	0.0	11.3	50.0	38.7	(142)
II	22.6	72.6	4.8	0.0	(84)	10.5	65.3	24.2	0.0	(95)	24.4	48.9	26.7	1.9	(90)
III	41.5	53.9	4.5	0.0	(89)	45.0	46.0	9.0	0.0	(100)	29.4	52.9	17.6	0.0	(85)
Na6	10.7	69.6	18.2	1.6	(253)	2.1	25.2	38.1	34.5	(139)	0.0	8.3	40.5	51.2	(84)
hNE-Na	0.0	20.9	58.6	20.5	(220)	0.0	3.2	50.8	45.9	(122)	0.0	11.1	61.1	27.8	(36)
SNS	11.2	24.2	58.0	6.0	(483)	24.6	19.4	44.4	11.6	(232)	13.2	50.0	30.5	6.3	(174)
NaG	13.9	65.8	18.8	1.5	(266)	5.2	25.2	35.6	34.1	(135)	0.0	9.4	39.6	50.9	(53)
mNa$_v$2.3	26.4	52.4	21.1	0.0	(208)	16.3	71.3	12.5	0.0	(160)	9.6	68.7	21.7	0.0	(83)
β1	0.3	55.8	32.0	10.4	(328)	0.9	16.2	41.0	41.9	(117)	0.0	0.0	21.3	78.7	(47)
β2	2.9	50.8	42.9	3.4	(524)	1.4	12.3	43.3	43.0	(349)	0.7	6.8	32.3	60.2	(266)

Numbers are percentages of DRG neurons that express: o = undetectable (e.g. figure 24.1, NaG(s)); + = low (e.g. figure 24.1, II); ++ = moderate (e.g. figure 24.1, hNE); +++ = high (e.g. figure 24.1, I) levels of mRNA for each size class. Numbers in parentheses are numbers of DRG neurons for each size class scored for expression of sodium channel mRNA from at least three separate experiments.

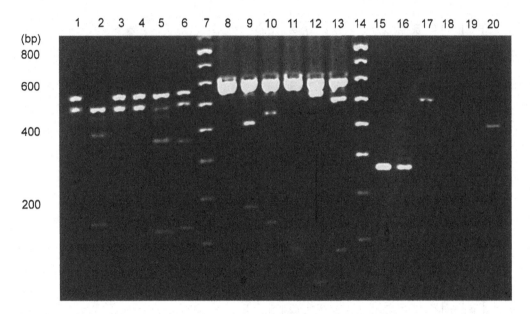

Figure 24.3
Analysis of RT-PCR products from adult rat DRG and brain. Lanes 7 and 14 contain the 100 bp marker (Pharmacia), lanes 1–6, 8–13, 16, 18 and 20 contain products from adult DRG and lanes 15, 17 and 19 contain products from adult brain. Lane 1 contains product from D1 and lanes 2–6 contain D1 RT-PCR product cut with *Eco*RV (*a*I-specific), *Eco*NI (*a*II-specific), *Ava*I (*a*III-specific), *Sph*I (*a*Na6-specific) and *Bam*HI (*a*hNE-Na-specific), respectively. Lane 8 contains RT-PCR product from D4 and lanes 9–13 contain D4 RT-PCR product cut with *Nci*I (*a*I-specific), *Dsa*I (*a*I- and *a*III-specific), *Bst*UI (*a*II-specific), *Eco*RV (*a*Na6-specific) and *Pvu*II (*a*NaG-specific), respectively. Lanes 15 and 16 contain *a*II-3′ UTR RT-PCR products from brain and DRG, respectively. Lanes 17 and 18 contain *a*III-3′ UTR RT-PCR products from brain and DRG, respectively. Lanes 19 and 20 contain *a*SNS-3′ UTR RT-PCR products from brain and DRG, respectively. The gel image was digitized using GelBase 7500 system (UVP, Inc.) and printed on a Fargo Primera Pro laser color printer (Fargo Electronics, Inc.) using their Black and White Dye sublimation technique.

results show the presence of *a*I (lane 9), *a*Na6 (lane 12) and *a*NaG (lane 13), but the absence of *a*II (lane 11), when compared with the predicted digestion sizes (table 24.3). The enzyme *Dsa*I cuts both *a*I and *a*III; there does not appear to be a decrease in the amount of uncut input DNA in lane 10 (*a*I and *a*III) compared to lane 9 (*a*I), suggesting a lack or low level of representation of *a*III in the mRNA derived from intact DRG.

RT-PCR performed with 3′ UTR primers specific for *a*II, *a*III and *a*SNS demonstrated the presence of *a*II and *a*SNS in DRG, but failed to detect *a*III in DRG. The *a*II amplification product derived from DRG (lane 16) comigrates with that produced from brain template (lane 15). No *a*III amplification product is produced from the DRG template (lane 18) under the same conditions that produce the expected low level of product from a brain template (lane 17). Also, *a*SNS is amplified from the DRG template (lane 20) but not the brain template (lane 19), in agreement with previous observations [1].

Figure 24.4 shows the amplification products of sodium channel β1- and β2-subunits from cDNA templates derived from DRG. The PCR product for β1 (lane 2) comigrated with the 600 bp size standard, in close agreement with the predicted size of 592 bp. The restriction enzyme profile of this DNA using *Pvu*II (lane 3) and *Acc*I (lane 4) digestion is consistent with the presence of β1 in the sample, based on sequence data [28]. The PCR product for β2 (lane 6) migrates slightly slower than the 700 bp size standard, in close agreement with the predicted size of 720 bp. The restriction enzyme profile of this DNA using *Bgl*II (lane 7), *Nco*I (lane 8) and *Pst*I (lane 9) is also consistent with the presence of β2 in the sample, based on sequence data [30].

3.3. In Situ Hybridization of Intact Dorsal Root Ganglia

In adult DRG in situ, sodium channel I mRNA is expressed at high levels in many of the larger DRG neurons, while smaller DRG neurons have negligible or low levels of expression (figure 24.5, I). In contrast, sodium channel II mRNA is detected at low levels in DRG neurons of all sizes (figure 24.5, II). Sodium channel III mRNA is not detected, or shows low levels of expression, in adult DRG neurons (figure 24.5, III). Na6 mRNA generally exhibits a moderate level of expression in all sizes of DRG neurons, though greater hybridization signal is observed in some medium and large DRG neurons (figure 24.5, Na6). The rat cognate of the mRNA for sodium channel hNE-Na is detected in most DRG neurons; however, the level of expression appears to be generally higher in larger DRG neurons than in smaller neurons (figure 24.5, hNE). Conversely, SNS mRNA is more prominently expressed in small and medium DRG neurons than large neurons (figure 24.5, SNS), although high levels of SNS mRNA expression are observed in some large DRG neurons (data not shown). The rat cognate for the mRNA for mNa$_v$2.3 is expressed in DRG neurons of all size

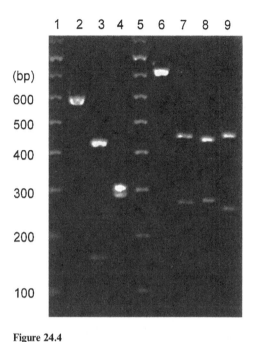

Figure 24.4

Analysis of RT-PCR products of sodium channel β1- and β2-subunit mRNAs from adult rat DRG. Lanes 1 and 5 contain the 100 bp size standard (Pharmacia). Lanes 2 and 6 contain PCR product of β1- and β2-subunit, respectively; the RT-PCR products migrate in the gel to positions in good agreement with their predicted sizes of 592 bp and 720 bp, respectively. Lane 3 shows *Pvu*II restriction enzyme products of the β1 fragment in close agreement with predicted sizes of 158 bp and 434 bp. Lane 4 shows *Acc*I restriction enzyme products of the β1 fragment in close agreement with predicted sizes of 298 bp and 303 bp. Lane 7 shows *Bgl*II restriction enzyme products of the β2 fragment in close agreement with predicted sizes of 272 bp and 448 bp. Lane 8 shows *Nco*I restriction enzyme products of the β2 fragment in close agreement with predicted sizes of 280 bp and 440 bp. Lane 9 shows *Pst*I restriction enzyme products of the β2 fragment in close agreement with predicted sizes of 260 bp and 460 bp.

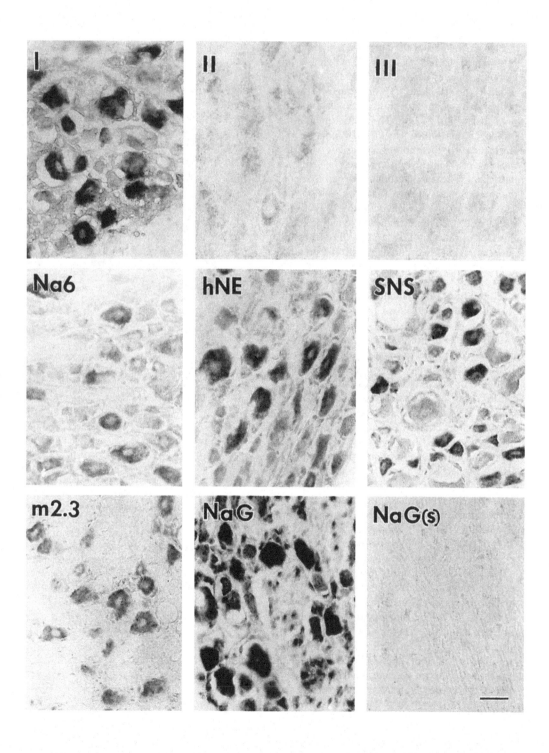

classes, but in general exhibits only low-to-moderate levels of expression in these cells (figure 24.5, m2.3). NaG mRNA is expressed by most adult DRG neurons, with the level of expression greatest in larger DRG neurons and more moderate in smaller neurons (figure 24.5, NaG).

Sodium channel β1 and β2 mRNAs are detected in virtually all DRG neurons (figure 24.2c, d). In general, larger DRG neurons appear to have greater levels of expression of β1 and β2 mRNAs than smaller DRG neurons, although some smaller DRG neurons also display high levels of expression.

4. Discussion

The results presented here demonstrate that: (1) adult DRG neurons in vitro express multiple sodium channel α-subunit mRNAs; (2) adult DRG neurons in vitro express sodium channel β1- and β2-subunit mRNAs; (3) large (>45 μm diam.) DRG neurons in vitro and in situ generally express higher levels of sodium channel transcripts for α-subunits I, NaG and Na6 than small (<25 μm diam.) DRG neurons; (4) SNS mRNA is detectable in some DRG neurons of all size classes, although generally the hybridization signal is greater in small and medium size neurons than large neurons; (5) hNE-Na is detectable in

every DRG neuron examined in vitro and in most DRG neurons in situ, and is present at moderate-to-high levels in most cells; and (6) the pattern of sodium channel mRNA expression in dissociated adult DRG neurons at 1 day in vitro (div) is similar to that exhibited by adult DRG neurons in situ.

4.1. Interpretation of In Situ Hybridization

To quantitate our in situ hybridization results, we scored cultured DRG neurons as showing "o" if no signal was apparent and as showing a "+" signal if any hybridization product was detectable (e.g. figure 24.1, NaG(s), II, arrows, respectively). No signal ("o") or "+" signals were observed with sense probes in DRG neurons in vitro. Thus, the significance of a "+" signal is not clear. In contrast, "++" (e.g. figure 24.1, hNE, arrow) and "+ + +" (e.g. figure 24.1, I, arrow) signals were not seen in neurons hybridized with sense probes. We have interpreted these levels of hybridization signals as indicating moderate or high levels of transcript expression that are biologically relevant.

4.2. Multiple α-Subunit mRNAs in DRG Neurons

DRG neurons are a heterogeneous population of cells. Classically, three major classes of DRG

Figure 24.5
Sodium channel α-subunit mRNAs in adult DRG neurons in situ. Fifteen μm sections of adult DRG, hybridized with antisense riboprobes specific for sodium channel mRNAs I (*I*), II (*II*), III (*III*), Na6 (*Na6*), hNE-Na (*hNE*), SNS (*SNS*), mNa_v2.3 (*m2.3*) and NaG (*NaG*), and with a sense riboprobe for NaG (*NaG(s)*) are shown. Sodium channel mRNA I is expressed in DRG neurons in situ, with higher levels of signal in large neurons than small neurons. Sodium channel mRNA II generally shows low levels of expression in all size classes of DRG neurons. Sodium channel mRNA III is not detectable in most DRG neurons. Na6 mRNA is generally expressed at moderate levels in all size classes of DRG neurons in situ, although some large neurons show high levels of expression. Most DRG neurons exhibit an hNE-Na mRNA hybridization signal. Large neurons tend to have greater signal than small neurons. SNS mRNA exhibits a gradient of hybridization signal in DRG neurons. High levels of expression are present in many small and medium DRG neurons, in addition to some large neurons, but is also not detectable, or is present at low levels, in other DRG neurons of all size classes. The rat cognate of the mRNA for mNa_v2.3 is expressed at low-to-moderate levels in DRG neurons. NaG mRNA exhibits a gradient of expression in DRG neurons, with high levels of expression in large neurons and lower levels in small neurons. ×210. Bar = 40 μm.

neurons are distinguished: A, B and C; the diameter of the cell soma for each class of neurons is well correlated with its axon size and, to a lesser extent, with different sensory modalities and the expression of different Trk receptors [25, 41]. Electrophysiological and pharmacological studies also demonstrate a diversity of sodium currents in DRG neurons (see table 24.1), including differential sensitivity to tetrodotoxin (TTX) and different kinetic and voltage-dependent properties. The sodium channels responsible for these inward currents are members of a supergene family, with two divergent subfamilies composed of at least eight distinct types in neural tissue [1, 2, 19, 21, 34, 35, 42, 57]. Alternative splicing of some sodium channel transcripts has also been reported [55, 56, 72], further increasing the potential for structural heterogeneity of the channels.

The in situ hybridization results presented here are consistent with the conclusion that most, if not all, DRG neurons in vitro express multiple sodium channel α-subunit mRNAs, in addition to β1- and β2-subunit mRNAs. Assuming that hNE-Na mRNA is present, at least at low levels, in all DRG neurons in vitro regardless of size, a *minimum* of 64% of small neurons and 72% of medium neurons express at least one additional sodium channel mRNA (see table 24.4). Moreover, 100% of large (>45 μm diam.) DRG neurons showed detectable levels of sodium channel α-subunit mRNAs I, NaG and Na6, and 88.7%, 90.5% and 91.7% of these cells expressed these transcripts at the "++" or "+ + +" level, in addition to hNE-Na, suggesting that each large DRG neuron expresses at least three sodium channel α-subunit transcripts.

A novel sodium channel α-subunit mRNA (SNS) has recently been cloned from adult rat DRG cDNA and, when expressed in *Xenopus* oocytes, is associated with a TTX-resistant sodium current [1]. Although SNS was originally reported to be present in small, but not large, DRG neurons [1], we detected this transcript in DRG neurons of all sizes in vitro and in situ.

Our observations are consistent with the presence of TTX-resistant currents which have been reported in large cutaneous afferent DRG neurons [51].

The low level of expression of sodium channel II mRNA in adult DRG neurons in vitro and in situ shown here is consistent with previous Northern blot analysis of DRG tissue [4]. The low level of sodium channel II mRNA in adult DRG neurons is also consistent with the expression in these cells of a silencing transcription factor (REST, RE1-silencing transcription factor [15, 37]; NRSF, neuron restrictive silencer factor [59]) that prevents the transcription of sodium channel II. Transcripts for REST have been demonstrated in Northern blots of neonatal DRG [15]. It has yet to be established whether similar silencer-type mechanisms regulate the expression and relative quantities of the other sodium channel α-subunits found in DRG neurons, or whether different regulatory mechanisms are utilized.

What are the functional consequences of multiple sodium channel mRNA expression in DRG neurons? If the full repertoire of sodium channel mRNAs observed in DRG neurons are translated, then the potentially diverse combinations of sodium channel mRNAs could contribute to the physiological heterogeneity of sodium currents present in DRG neurons. In this respect, neural sodium channel α-subunit mRNAs II [43], IIA [2, 28, 31, 58, 67, 71], III [33, 44, 62] and hNE-Na [35] have been expressed in *Xenopus* oocytes or mammalian cell lines, either alone or co-expressed with the β1- or β2-subunits. The sodium currents elicited in these model systems are generally characterized as kinetically fast and tetrodotoxin-sensitive, although there are substantial differences in gating properties and peak conductances of the sodium currents among these model systems. Of the sodium channel α-subunit mRNAs that have been expressed in model systems, only hNE-Na shows a high level of hybridization signal in all size classes of DRG neurons in vitro. Patch clamp methods to study cutaneous afferent DRG neurons after 1 day in vitro (div) have shown that, while nearly 50% of these cells expressed both fast, TTX-sensitive and slow, TTX-insensitive sodium currents, >50% expressed only the slow, TTX-insensitive sodium current [26, 51]. This raises the question of whether the hNE-Na gene can encode a channel which, under some circumstances, is TTX-insensitive; or, alternatively, whether hNE-Na mRNA is not translated in some cells. Post-translational modifications or interactions with *β*1- and/or *β*2-subunits could also modulate the sodium current characteristics of hNE-Na channels, yielding physiological differences. Alternatively, expression of SNS [1] could provide a basis for TTX-resistant sodium currents in these cells.

4.3. Sequence Polymorphism in DRG Neuron *a*-Subunit mRNA

We also used RT-PCR followed by restriction enzyme analysis to determine which sodium channel *a*-subunit(s) are expressed in adult rat DRG. This task is complicated by a lack of complete sequence for NaG [21], potential polymorphisms of published rat *a*-subunit sequences, and the derivation of the sequences of hNE-Na and mNa$_v$2.3 from human [35] and mouse [19] cDNAs, respectively. Therefore, to minimize the possibility of not detecting sodium channel transcripts that are expressed in DRG, we utilized, when possible, primers that were designed to amplify products from domains 1 and 4 (D1 and D4) and 3' untranslated regions (3' UTR) of cDNA from DRG. Our analyses show the presence of substantial levels of *a*-subunits I, Na6, hNE-Na, SNS and NaG and limited quantities of II in DRG; mRNA III was not detectable in the DRG samples.

Based on sequence homology, sodium channel *a*-subunits NaG and mNa$_v$2.3 have been grouped, together with human Na$_v$2.1 [22], in subfamily 2. While NaG has not been fully sequenced, the available sequence data supports

the suggestion that NaG and mNa$_v$2.3 are correlates in different species [19]. Sequences derived from cloning of additional portions of NaG are consistent with this interpretation (Dib-Hajj and Waxman, unpublished observations). In the present study, the primers and the restriction enzymes used could not distinguish between NaG and mNa$_v$2.3. It is interesting, however, that in situ hybridization studies with probes generated from NaG and mNa$_v$2.3 sequences showed differing levels of hybridization signal for these transcripts in DRG neurons in vitro and in situ. These differing patterns of hybridization signal may reflect the different lengths of the riboprobes (NaG: 437 bp, mNa$_v$2.3: 240 bp; the shorter probe would have fewer digoxigenin-conjugated UTP incorporated into it) and/or sequence differences between the mouse Na$_v$2.3 sequence used for generation of the riboprobe and the sequence of rat cognate in DRG resulting in inefficient hybridization. Alternatively, the Na$_v$2.3-derived riboprobe may be detecting an NaG-like transcript that has yet to be cloned and has low abundance in DRG.

4.4. Functional Implications

While DRG neurons exhibit similar patterns of multiple sodium channel mRNA expression in vitro and in situ, it is not clear whether all the transcripts are translated and, if translated, what is the cellular distribution of the sodium channel proteins. With regard to the first issue, there is evidence, in some neurons, for the expression of GABA$_A$ [24] and NMDARI [61] mRNAs with little translation of the transcripts. Thus, it is possible that not all the differing sodium channel transcripts expressed within a DRG neuron are translated. Assuming that multiple sodium channel mRNAs are translated, the cellular distribution of these sodium channel isoforms in DRG neurons is not clear. In CNS tissue, neurons have been suggested to exhibit a differential localization of sodium channel isotypes, with rat brain sodium channel I preferentially localized to neuronal somata and sodium channel II preferentially distributed to unmyelinated axons [68, 69]. Voltage-gated potassium channel isoforms have also been shown to exhibit differential cellular localization [39, 53, 64]. Multiple sodium channel isoforms in DRG neurons may show a spatially heterogeneous distribution, allowing subtle differences in sodium current properties between different regions of the neuron.

The pattern of sodium channel mRNA expression observed in DRG neurons in vitro is in general similar to that observed in DRG neurons in situ, indicating that the culturing process does not substantially alter, in the short term (<24 h), the expression of sodium channel mRNAs in these cells. It should be noted, however, that sodium channel mRNA III was not detected in DRG neurons in situ by either RT-PCR or in situ hybridization methods, while low levels of this transcript were detected in some DRG neurons in vitro by in situ hybridization. With the assumption that dissociation of DRG for culturing represents injury to the neurons, our observations in DRG neurons in vitro are consistent with previous reports of up-regulation of sodium channel III in axotomized DRG neurons [66] and facial nerve motor neurons [32]. In this regard, it has been shown that the mRNA for sodium channel PN1 [16] reaches maximal expression within 4 hours of induction with NGF [63]. The absence of substantial differences in sodium channel mRNA expression, other than a slight increase in type III a-subunit expression, between DRG neurons in vitro and in situ suggests that the up-regulation of type III mRNA following axotomy may represent a specific response of DRG neurons to axonal injury, and not a non-specific up-regulation of protein synthesis.

Acknowledgments

This work was supported in part by the Medical Research Service, Department of Veterans Affairs, and by a grant from the National Multiple Sclerosis Society. S.D.-H. was supported in part by an EPVA Spinal Cord Research Fellowship. M.A.R. was supported by a CIDA from the NINDS.

References

[1] Akopian, A. N., Sivilotti, L. and Wood, J. N., A tetrodotoxin-resistant voltage-gated sodium channel expressed by sensory neurons. *Nature*, 379 (1996) 258–262.

[2] Auld, V. J., Goldin, A. L., Krafte, D. S., Marshall, J., Dunn, J. M., Catterall, W. A., Lester, H. A., Davidson, N. and Dunn, R. J., A rat brain Na$^+$ channel a-subunit with novel gating properties, *Neuron*, 1 (1988) 449–461.

[3] Barnes, W. M., PCR amplification of up to 35-kb DNA with high fidelity and high yield from λ bacteriophage templates, *Proc. Natl. Acad. Sci. (USA)*, 91 (1994) 2216–2220.

[4] Beckh, S., Differential expression of sodium channel mRNAs in rat peripheral nervous system and innervated tissues, *FEBS Lett.*, 262 (1990) 317–322.

[5] Belcher, S. M., Zerillo, C. A., Levenson, R., Ritchie, J. M. and Howe, J. R., Cloning of a novel sodium channel a-subunit from rabbit Schwann cells, *Proc. Natl. Acad. Sci. USA*, 92 (1992) 11304–11308.

[6] Bennett, P. B., Makita, N. and George, Jr., A. L., A molecular basis for gating mode transitions in human skeletal muscle sodium channels, *FEBS Lett.*, 326 (1993) 21–24.

[7] Black, J. A., Yokoyama, S., Higashida, H., Ransom, B. R. and Waxman, S. G., Sodium channel mRNAs I, II and II in the CNS: cell-specific expression, *Mol. Brain Res.*, 22 (1994) 275–289.

[8] Black, J. A., Yokoyama, S., Waxman, S. G., Oh, Y., Zur, K. B., Sontheimer, H., Higashida, H. and Ransom, B. R., Sodium channel mRNAs in cultured spinal cord astrocytes: in situ hybridization in identified cell types, *Brain Res.*, 23 (1994) 235–245.

[9] Brown, A. G., *Organization in the Spinal Cord*, Springer, New York, 1981.

[10] Bossu, J.-L. and Feltz, A., Patch clamp study of the tetrodotoxin-resistant sodium current in group C sensory neurones, *Neurosci. Lett.*, 51 (1984) 241–246.

[11] Caffrey, J. M., Eng, D. L., Black, J. A., Waxman, S. G. and Kocsis, J. D., Three types of sodium channels in adult rat dorsal root ganglion neurons, *Brain Res.*, 592 (1992) 283–297.

[12] Catterall, W. A., Cellular and molecular biology of voltage-gated sodium channels, *Physiol. Rev.*, 72 (1992) S2–S47.

[13] Cheng, S., Fockler, C., Barnes, W. M. and Higuchi, R., Effective amplification of long targets from cloned inserts and human genomic DNA, *Proc. Natl. Acad. Sci. USA*, 91 (1992) 5695–5699.

[14] Chomczynski, P. and Sacchi, N., Single-step method of RNA isolation by acid guanidium thiocyanate-phenol-chloroform extraction, *Anal. Biochem.*, 162 (1987) 156–159.

[15] Chong, J. A., Tapia-Ramirez, J., Kim, S., Toledo-Aral, J. J., Zheng, Y., Boutros, M. C., Altshuller, Y. M., Frohman, M. A., Kraner, S. D. and Mandel, G., REST: a mammalian silencer protein that restricts sodium channel gene expression to neurons, *Cell*, 80 (1995) 949–957.

[16] D'Arcangelo, G., Pardiso, K., Shepherd, D., Brehm, P., Halegoua, S. and Mandel, G., Neuronal growth factor regulation of two different sodium channel types through distinct signal transduction pathways, *J. Cell Biol.*, 122 (1993) 915–921.

[17] Dib-Hajj, S. and Waxman, S. G., Genes encoding the β1 subunit of voltage-dependent Na$^+$ channel in rat, mouse and human contain conserved introns, *FEBS Lett.*, 377 (1995) 485–488.

[18] Elliott, A. A. and Elliott, J. R., Characterization of TTX-sensitive and TTX-resistant sodium currents in small cells from adult rat dorsal root ganglia, *J. Physiol.*, 463 (1993) 39–56.

[19] Felipe, A., Knittle, T. J., Doyle, K. L. and Tamkun, M. M., Primary structure and differential expression during development and pregnancy of a novel voltage-gated sodium channel in the mouse, *J. Biol. Chem.*, 269 (1994) 30125–30131.

[20] Fish, L. M., Sangameswaran, L., Delgado, S. G., Koch, B. D., Jakeman, L. B., Kwan, J. and Herman, R. C., Cloning of a sodium channel α-subunit (PN1) from rat dorsal root ganglia, *Soc. Neurosci. Abstr.*, 21 (1995) 1824.

[21] Gautron, S., Dos Santos, G., Pinto-Henrique, D., Koulakoff, A., Gros, F. and Berwald-Netter, Y., The glial voltage-gated sodium channel: cell- and tissue-specific mRNA expression, *Proc. Natl. Acad. Sci. USA*, 89 (1992) 7272–7276.

[22] George, Jr., A. L., Knittle, T. J. and Tamkun, M. M., Molecular cloning of an atypical voltage-gated sodium channel expressed in human heart and uterus: evidence for a distinct gene family, *Proc. Natl. Acad. Sci. USA*, 89 (1992) 4893–4897.

[23] Gustafson, T. A., Clevinger, E. C., O'Neill, T. J., Yarowsky, P. J. and Krueger, B. K., Mutually exclusive exon splicing of type III brain sodium channel alpha subunit RNA generates developmentally regulated isoforms in rat brain, *J. Biol. Chem.*, 268 (1993) 18648–18653.

[24] Hales, T. G. and Tyndale, R. G., Few cell lines with GABA$_A$ mRNA have functional receptors, *J. Neurosci.*, 14 (1994) 5429–5436.

[25] Harper, A. A. and Lawson, S. N., Conduction velocity is related to morphological cell type in rat dorsal root ganglion neurons, *J. Physiol.*, 359 (1985) 31–46.

[26] Honmou, O., Utzschneider, D. A., Rizzo, M. A., Bowe, C. M., Waxman, S. G. and Kocsis, J. D., Delayed depolarization and slow sodium currents in cutaneous afferents, *J. Neurophysiol.*, 71 (1994) 1627–1637.

[27] Ikeda, S. R. and Schofield, G. G., Tetrodotoxin-resistant sodium current of rat nodose neurones: monovalent cation selectivity and divalent cation block, *J. Physiol.*, 389 (1987) 255–270.

[28] Isom, L. L., De Jongh, K. S., Patton, D. E., Reber, B. F. X., Offord, J., Charbonneau, H., Walsh, K., Goldin, A. L. and Catterall, W. A., Primary structure and functional expression of the β1 subunit of the rat brain sodium channel, *Science*, 256 (1992) 839–842.

[29] Isom, L. L., De Jongh, K. S. and Catterall, W. A., Auxilliary subunits of voltage-gated ion channels, *Neuron*, 12 (1994) 1183–1194.

[30] Isom, L. L., Ragsdale, D. S., De Jongh, K. S., Westenbroek, R. E., Reber, B. F. X., Scheuer, T. and Catterall, W. A., Structure and function of the β2 subunit of brain sodium channels, a transmembrane glycoprotein with a CAM motif, *Cell*, 83 (1995) 433–442.

[31] Isom, L. L., Scheuer, T., Browstein, A. B., Ragsdale, D. S., Murphy, B. J. and Catterall, W. A., Functional co-expression of the β1 and type IIA α subunits of sodium channels in a mammalian cell line, *J. Biol. Chem.*, 270 (1995) 3306–3312.

[32] Iwahashi, Y., Furuyama, T., Inagaki, S., Morita, Y. and Takagi, H., Distinct regulation of sodium channel types I, II and III following nerve transection, *Mol. Brain Res.*, 22 (1994) 341–345.

[33] Joho, R. H., Moorman, J. R., Van Dongen, A. M. J., Kirsch, G. E., Silberberg, H., Schuster, G. and Brown, A. M., Toxin and kinetic profile of rat brain type III sodium channels expressed in *Xenopus* oocytes, *Mol. Brain Res.*, 7 (1990) 105–113.

[34] Kayano, T., Noda, M., Flockerzi, V., Takahashi, H. and Numa, S., Primary structure of rat brain sodium channel III deduced from the cDNA sequence, *FEBS Lett.*, 228 (1988) 187–194.

[35] Klugbauer, N., Lacinova, L., Flockerzi, V. and Hofmann, F., Structure and functional expression of a new member of the tetrodotoxininsensitive voltage-activated sodium channel family from human neuroendocrine cells, *EMBO J.*, 14 (1995) 1084–1090.

[36] Kostyuk, P. G., Veselovsky, N. S. and Tsyandryenko, A. Y., Ionic currents in the somatic membrane of rat dorsal root ganglion neurons. I. Sodium currents, *Neuroscience*, 6 (1981) 2423–2430.

[37] Kraner, S. D., Chong, J. A., Tsay, H.-J. and Mandel, G., Silencing the type II sodium channel gene: a model for neural-specific gene regulation, *Neuron*, 9 (1992) 37–44.

[38] Makita, N., Bennett, P. B. and George Jr., A. L., Voltage-gated β1-subunit mRNA expressed in adult human skeletal muscle, heart, and brain is encoded by a single gene, *J. Biol. Chem.*, 269 (1994) 7571–7578.

[39] Maletic-Savatic, M., Lenn, N. J. and Trimmer, J. S., Differential spatiotemporal expression of K$^+$ channel polypeptides in rat hippocampal neurons developing in situ and in vitro, *J. Neurosci.*, 15 (1995) 3840–3851.

[40] McLean, M. J., Bennett, P. B. and Thomas, R. M., Subtypes of dorsal root ganglion neurons based on different inward currents as measured by whole-cell voltage clamp, *Mol. Cell. Biochem.*, 80 (1988) 95–107.

[41] McMahon, S. G., Armanini, M. P., Ling, L. H. and Phillips, H. S., Expression and coexpression of Trk receptors in subpopulations of adult primary sensory neurons projecting to identified peripheral targets, *Neuron*, 12 (1994) 1161–1171.

[42] Noda, M., Ikeda, T., Kayano, T., Suzuki, H., Takeshima, H., Kurasaki, M., Takahashi, H. and Numa, S., Existence of distinct sodium channel messenger RNAs in rat brain, *Nature*, 320 (1986) 188–192.

[43] Noda, M., Ikeda, T., Kayano, T. Suzuki, H., Suzuki, T., Takeshima, H., Takahashi, H., Kuno, M. and Numa, S., Expression of functional sodium channels from cloned cDNA, *Nature*, 322 (1986) 826–828.

[44] Noda, M., Suzuki, H., Numa, S. and Stuhmer, W., A single point mutation confers tetrodotoxin and saxitoxin insensitivity on the sodium channel II, *FEBS Lett.*, 259 (1989) 213–216.

[45] Ogata, N. and Tatebayashi, H., Ontogenic development of the TTX-sensitive and TTX-insensitive Na$^+$ channels in neurons of the rat dorsal root ganglia, *Dev. Brain Res.*, 65 (1992) 93–100.

[46] Oh, Y., Black, J. A. and Waxman, S. G., Rat brain Na$^+$ channel mRNAs in non-excitable Schwann cells, *FEBS Lett.*, 350 (1994) 342–346.

[47] Oh, Y., Sashihara, S., Black, J. A. and Waxman, S. G., Na$^+$ channel β1 subunit mRNA: differential expression in rat spinal sensory neurons, *Mol. Brain Res.*, 30 (1995) 357–361.

[48] Patton, D. E., Isom, L. L., Catterall, W. A. and Golden, A. L., The adult rat brain β1 subunit modifies activation and inactivation gating of multiple sodium channel α subunits, *J. Biol. Chem.*, 269 (1994) 17649–17655.

[49] Perl, E. R., Function of dorsal root ganglion neurons: an overview. In: S. A. Scott (Ed.), *Sensory Neurons*, Oxford University Press, New York, 1992, pp. 3–23.

[50] Rizzo, M. A., Kocsis, J. D. and Waxman, S. G., Slow sodium conductances of dorsal root ganglion neurons: intraneuronal homogeneity and interneuronal heterogeneity, *J. Neurophysiol.*, 72 (1994) 2796–2815.

[51] Rizzo, M. A., Kocsis, J. D. and Waxman, S. G., Selective loss of slow and enhancement of fast Na$^+$ currents in cutaneous afferent dorsal root ganglion neurones following axotomy, *Neurobiol. Dis.*, 2 (1995) 87–96.

[52] Rizzo, M. A., Kocsis, J. D. and Waxman, S. G., Mechanisms of paraesthesiae, dyaesthesiae, and hyperaesthesiae: role of Na$^+$ channel heterogeneity, *Eur. Neurol.*, 36 (1996) 3–12.

[53] Rizzo, M. A. and Nonner, W., Transient K current in the somatic membrane of cultured central central neurons of embryonic rats, *J. Neurophysiol.*, 68 (1992) 1708–1719.

[54] Roy, M. L. and Narahashi, T., Differential properties of tetrodotoxin-sensitive and tetrodotoxin-resistant sodium channels in rat dorsal root ganglion neurons, *J. Neurosci.*, 12 (1992) 2104–2111.

[55] Sarao, R., Gupta, S. K., Auld, V. J. and Dunn, R. J., Developmentally regulated alternative RNA splicing of rat brain sodium channel mRNAs, *Nucleic Acids Res.*, 19 (1991) 5673–5679.

[56] Schaller, K. L., Krzemien, D. M., McKenna, N. M. and Caldwell, J. H., Alternatively spliced sodium channel transcripts in brain and muscle, *J. Neurosci.*, 12 (1992) 1370–1381.

[57] Schaller, K. L., Krzemien, D. M., Yarowsky, P. J., Krueger, B. K. and Caldwell, J. H., A novel, abundant sodium channel expressed in neurons and glia, *J. Neurosci.*, 15 (1995) 3231–3242.

[58] Scheuer, T., Auld, V. J., Boyd, S., Offord, J., Dunn, R. and Catterall, W. A., Functional properties of rat brain sodium channels expressed in a somatic cell line, *Science*, 247 (1990) 854–858.

[59] Schoenherr, C. J. and Anderson, D. J., The neuron-restrictive silencer factor (NRSF): a coordinate repressor of multiple neuron-specific genes, *Nature*, 267 (1995) 1360–1363.

[60] Schwartz, A., Palti, Y. and Meiri, H., Structural and developmental differences between three types of Na channels in dorsal root ganglion cells of newborn rats, *J. Membr. Biol.*, 116 (1990) 117–128.

[61] Sucher, N. J., Brose, N., Deitcher, D. L., Awobuluyi, M., Gasic, G. P., Bading, H., Cepko, C. L., Greenberg, M. E., Jahn, R., Heinemann, S. F. et al., Expression of endogenous NMDARI transcripts without receptor protein suggests post-transcriptional control in PC12 cells, *J. Biol. Chem.*, 268 (1993) 22299–22304.

[62] Suzuki, H., Beckh, S., Kubo, M., Yahagi, N., Ishida, H., Kayano, T., Noda, M. and Numa, S., Functional expression of cloned cDNA encoding sodium channel III, *FEBS Lett.*, 228 (1988) 195–200.

[63] Toledo-Aral, J. J., Brehm, P., Halegoua, S. and Mandel, G., A single pulse of nerve growth factor triggers long-term neuronal excitability through sodium channel gene induction, *Neuron*, 14 (1995) 607–611.

[64] Wang, H., Kunkel, D. D., Schwartzkroin, P. A. and Tempel, B. L., Localization of $K_v 1.1$ and $K_v 1.2$, two K channel proteins, to synaptic terminals, somata,

and dendrites in the mouse brain, *J. Neurosci.*, 14 (1994) 4588–4599.

[65] Waxman, S. G. and Black, J. A., Expression of mRNA for a sodium channel in subfamily 2 in spinal sensory neurons, *Neurochem. Res.*, 21 (1996) 395–402.

[66] Waxman, S. G., Kocsis, J. D. and Black, J. A., Type III sodium channel mRNA is expressed in embryonic but not adult spinal sensory neurons, and is reexpressed following axotomy, *J. Neurophysiol.*, 72 (1994) 466–470.

[67] West, J. W., Scheuer, T., Maechler, L. and Catterall, W. A., Efficient expression of rat brain type IIA Na^+ channel a subunits in a somatic cell line, *Neuron*, 8 (1992) 59–70.

[68] Westenbroek, R. E., Merrick, D. K. and Catterall, W. A., Differential subcellular localization of the RI and RII Na^+ channel subtypes in central axons, *Neuron*, 3 (1989) 695–704.

[69] Westenbroek, R. E., Noebels, J. L. and Catterall, W. A., Elevated expression of type II Na^+ channels in hypomyelinated axons of shiverer mouse brain, *J. Neurosci.*, 12 (1992) 2259–2267.

[70] Willis, W. D. and Coggeshall, R. E., *Sensory Mechanisms of the Spinal Cord*, Plenum, New York, 1991.

[71] Yang, X. C., Labarca, C., Nageot, J., Ho, B. Y., Elroy, S. O., Moss, B., Davidson, N. and Lester, H. A., Cell-specific posttranslational events affect functional expression at the plasma membrane but not tetrodotoxin sensitivity of the rat brain IIA sodium channel a-subunit expressed in mammalian cells, *J. Neurosci.*, 12 (1992) 268–277.

[72] Yarowsky, P. J., Kreuger, B. K., Olson, C. E., Clevinger, E. C. and Koos, R. D., Brain and heart sodium channel subtype mRNA expression in rat cerebral cortex, *Proc. Natl Acad. Sci. USA*, 88 (1991) 9453–9457.

[73] Zur, K. B., Oh, Y., Waxman, S. G. and Black, J. A., Differential up-regulation of sodium channel a- and $\beta 1$-subunit mRNAs in cultured embryonic DRG neurons following exposure to NGF, *Mol. Brain Res.*, 30 (1995) 97–103.

25 Delayed Depolarization and Slow Sodium Currents in Cutaneous Afferents

Osamu Honmou, David A. Utzschneider, Marco A. Rizzo, Constance M. Bowe, Stephen G. Waxman, and Jeffery D. Kocsis

Summary and Conclusions

1. Intraaxonal recordings were obtained in vitro from the sural nerve (SN), the muscle branch of the anterior tibial nerve (ATN), or the deefferented ATN (dATN) in 5- to 7-wk-old rats. Whole-nerve sucrose gap recordings were obtained from the SN and the ATN. This allowed study of cutaneous (SN), mixed motor and muscle afferent (ATN), and isolated muscle afferent (dATN) axons.

2. Application of the potassium channel blocking agent 4-aminopyridine (4-AP) to ATN or dATN resulted in a slight prolongation of the action potential. In contrast, a distinct delayed depolarization followed the axonal action potential in cutaneous afferents (SN) exposed to 4-AP. The delayed depolarization could be induced by a single whole-nerve stimulus or by injection of constant-current depolarizing pulses into individual axons. The delayed depolarization often gave rise to bursts of action potentials and was followed by a prominent afterhyperpolarization (AHP).

3. In paired-pulse experiments on single SN axons, the recovery time (half-amplitude of the action potential) was 3.06 ± 1.82 (SE) ms ($n = 12$). After exposure to 4-AP the recovery time of the delayed depolarization was considerably longer (half-recovery time: 99.0 ± 28.3 ms; $n = 15$) than that of the action potential (18.8 ± 9.1 ms; $n = 16$).

4. Application of tetraethylammonium (TEA) to cutaneous or muscle afferents alone had little effect on single action potential waveform. However, TEA reduced the amplitude of the AHP elicited by a single stimulus in cutaneous afferent axons after exposure to 4-AP and resulted in repetitive spike discharge.

5. The delayed depolarization and spike burst activity induced by 4-AP in SN was present in Ca^{2+}-free solutions containing 1 mM ethylene glycol-bis(β-aminoethyl ether)-N, N, N', N'-tetraacetic acid and was not blocked by Cd^{2+} (1.0 mM).

6. We obtained whole-cell patch-clamp recordings to study Na^+ currents from either randomly selected dorsal root ganglion neurons or cutaneous afferent neurons identified by retrograde labeling with Fluoro-Gold. The majority of the randomly selected neurons had a singular kinetically fast Na^+ current. In contrast, no identified cutaneous afferent neurons had a singular fast Na^+ current. Rather, they had a combination of kinetically separable fast and slow currents or a singular relatively slow Na^+ current.

7. These results demonstrate a difference in the sensitivity of myelinated cutaneous and muscle afferent axons to blockade of a 4-AP-sensitive K^+ channel. Cutaneous afferent axons give rise to a prominent depolarizing potential after the action potential, which is not present in the muscle afferent or motor axons. We propose that cutaneous afferent axons have kinetically slow Na^+ channels not present in muscle afferent and efferent fibers, whose activation underlies the delayed depolarization and multiple spike discharge. The results indicate a difference in the Na^+ channel organization of myelinated cutaneous versus muscle afferent axons and their cell bodies.

Introduction

Mammalian myelinated axons express a diversity of K^+ channel types that can be distinguished on the basis of kinetic and pharmacological properties (Baker et al. 1987; Kocsis et al. 1986, 1987). These include kinetically fast [4-aminopyridine (4-AP)-sensitive] and slow [tetraethylammonium (TEA-sensitive)] K^+ currents (Roper and Schwartz 1989) and an inward rectifier (Baker et al. 1987; Birch et al. 1991; Eng et al. 1990). It has been suggested that the organization of these channels on myelinated motor and sensory axons may differ because these two groups of axons exhibit different sensitivities to K^+ channel blockade (Bowe et al. 1985; Kocsis et al. 1986). Although blockade of the 4-AP-sensitive fast K^+ current in motor axons results in a modest broadening of the action potential, a similar pharmacological blockade of sensory

Reprinted with permission from *Journal of Neurophysiology* 71: 1627–1637, 1994.

axons produces a distinct depolarization on the falling phase of the action potential, termed the delayed depolarization (Bowe et al. 1985; Kocsis et al. 1983). The delayed depolarization, which can exceed 20 mV and last for tens of milliseconds, often gives rise to bursts of spikes. The absence of this prominent depolarizing potential in motor axons suggests a fundamental difference in the ionic channel organization of sensory versus motor myelinated axons. Although several lines of evidence suggest that the delayed depolarization of sensory axons is the result of a Na^+ channel that is kinetically distinct from the channel that gives rise to the action potential (Kocsis et al. 1983, 1987; Pongrácz et al. 1991), the electrophysiological origin of the delayed depolarization remains unresolved.

More recently, Bowe et al. (1992) demonstrated in regenerated nerves that the delayed depolarization is not present in all regenerated sensory myelinated axons and that it may be specific for cutaneous afferents. In the present study we examined the electrophysiological properties of normal myelinated cutaneous and muscle afferent axons using intraaxonal and sucrose gap recordings to determine the electrophysiological basis for these differences in cutaneous and muscle afferent axons. Our observations on these axons implicate a difference in Na^+ channel organization; therefore whole-cell patch-clamp techniques were used to assess the Na^+ channel properties of the dorsal root ganglion (DRG) cell bodies of origin for cutaneous and noncutaneous sensory axons.

Our results indicate that the delayed depolarization occurs in rapidly conducting cutaneous afferent axons and is virtually absent in muscle afferent and motor axons. Moreover, whole-cell voltage-clamp experiments on the cell bodies of cutaneous afferent fibers reveal a disproportionately large distribution of neurons that express slow Na^+ currents or both fast and slow Na^+ currents. In contrast, muscle afferent neurons displayed primarily a singular fast Na^+ current.

The presence of kinetically fast and slow Na^+ currents on the cell bodies of the cutaneous afferent neurons supports the hypothesis that the delayed depolarization results from the activation of a slow Na^+ current. The specificity of the delayed depolarization to cutaneous afferents and its association with burst firing further suggest a role of a slow Na^+ current in cutaneous signal transduction.

Methods

Female Wistar rats, ranging in age from 5 to 7 wk, were anesthetized with pentobarbital sodium (50 mg/kg) and exsanguinated by carotid section. Relatively young rats were selected because of the diminishing sensitivity to 4-AP that occurs in mammalian myelinated axons during maturation (Bowe et al. 1985; Kocsis et al. 1983). The sural nerve (SN) was selected to study myelinated cutaneous afferents because it contains >90% sensory and autonomic fibers (Peyronnard and Charron 1982) and nearly all of myelinated sensory fibers are cutaneous afferents. To permit selective examination of muscle afferent axons we studied the muscle branch of the anterior tibial nerve (ATN) after ventral rhizotomy of L_4–L_6 (performed 10–12 days before ATN excision); this deefferented nerve is abbreviated dATN. We exposed the SN and ATN and excised a 1.5- to 3.0-cm segment of nerve distal to the sciatic notch. The nerves were desheathed and placed in a modified Krebs solution referred to as a normal electrolyte solution (NS). Only nerves that could be removed and desheathed with no apparent disruption were studied.

Solutions and Drugs

The modified Krebs solution contained (in mM) 124 NaCl, 3.0 KCl, 1.3 NaH_2PO_4, 2.0 $MgCl_2$, 2.0 $CaCl_2$, 26.0 $NaHCO_3$, and 10.0 dextrose, saturated with 95% O_2-5% CO_2. Isotonic KCl solutions contained (in mM) 120 KCl, 7.0 NaCl, 1.3 NaH$_2$PO$_4$, 2.0 MgCl$_2$, 2.0 CaCl$_2$, 26.0 NaHCO$_3$, and 10.0 dextrose. The isotonic sucrose solution contained 320 mM sucrose. Test solutions containing TEA (10 mM), 4-AP (1 mM), or tetrodotoxin (TTX, 10 nM) were made by adding appropriate concentrations to the modified Krebs solution. The nerves were exposed to 4-AP and TEA for ≥20 min and no longer than 1 h.

Sucrose Gap Recording

Isolated SN and ATN segments were positioned across a sucrose gap chamber (Kocsis and Waxman 1983) partitioned into compartments by petroleum jelly seals. The center compartment was continuously washed with isotonic sucrose solution, the right compartment with modified Krebs solution to which blocking agents were added, and the left compartment with isotonic KCl solution. All solutions flowed at 1–2 ml/min. Experiments were carried out at 20 °C.

The nerve segments were oriented with the distal end within the test compartment. The two outer compartments were connected to the inputs of a high-impedance DC-coupled differential electrometer (Axoprobe 1A; Axon Instruments) with silver–silver chloride wires embedded in agar bridge electrodes (3% agar in 1 M NaCl). The nerve was stimulated with a bipolar Teflon-coated stainless steel electrode cut flush and placed directly on the nerve segment in the test compartment. Stimulation pulses were delivered through an isolation unit and the timing of the pulses was controlled by a digital timing device. The high extracellular resistance in the middle (isotonic sucrose) compartment limited signal conduction through the axon cylinder. To allow for relatively homogeneous membrane activation and to minimize temporal dispersion, the number of active nodes was reduced by limiting the length of nerve segment positioned in the test well to 2–4 mm.

Intraaxonal Recording

For intraaxonal recordings, nerves were placed in an in vitro submersion-type chamber. Intraaxonal recordings were performed with borosilicate electrodes pulled on a Brown-Flaming P-80 puller and filled with 4 M potassium acetate and 0.1 M KCl. The DC resistances of the microelectrodes ranged from 100 to 150 MΩ. Identification of intraaxonal recordings utilized criteria that have been discussed previously (Kocsis and Waxman 1982). Intraaxonal recordings with resting potentials larger than −50 mV and action potentials equal to or larger than resting potential were studied. Impalements were considered to be intracellular if passage of a constant hyperpolarizing current caused an increase in action potential amplitude compared with that recorded in the resting state (Barrett and Barrett 1982; Blight and Someya 1985; Kapoor et al. 1993; Kocsis and Waxman 1982). Whole-nerve stimulation pulses were delivered through a bipolar Teflon-coated stainless steel stimulation electrode cut flush and placed directly on the nerve segment. Single axon stimulation pulses were delivered through the recording microelectrode and consisted of constant-current pulses (≤0.5 nA) ≤100 ms in duration provided by the step current command of the recording amplifier and monitored on a separate channel. An active bridge circuit was used to compensate for electrode and preparation resistance. Action potential recovery properties were evaluated during the presentation of paired stimuli delivered at varying interstimulus intervals. The sharp electrodes selected for larger axons and the relatively fast conduction velocities indicated that all axons studied were myelinated.

Cell Culture

DRG cultures were prepared according to the methods of Birch et al. (1992), with slight modification. Lumbar (L$_4$–L$_5$) ganglia of 5- to

7-wk-old female Wistar rats were excised after exsanguination under pentobarbital anesthesia (50 mg/kg) and freed of both nerve trunks and connective tissue sheath. Pooled ganglia were incubated with gentle agitation for 25 min in a solution containing a mixture of complete saline solution (CSS) and 1 mg/ml collagenase (Boehringer Mannheim Biochemical), 0.2 mg/ml cysteine, 1.5 mM $CaCl_2$, 0.5 mM ethylenedinitrilotetraacetic acid, disodium slat. The CSS contained (in mM) 137 NaCl, 5.3 KCl, 1 $MgCl_2$, 25 sorbitol, 3 mM $CaCl_2$, and 10 N-2-hydroxyethylpiperazine-N'-2-ethanesulfonic acid (HEPES), titrated to pH 7.2 with NaOH. This was followed by a 10-min incubation with 30 U/ml papain (Worthington Biochemical), then a 25-min incubation in the above CSS mixture. Ganglia were then transfered to culture media containing 1:1 Dulbecco's Modified Eagles' Medium, and Ham's F12 medium containing 10% fetal calf serum, 1.5 mg/ml trypsin inhibitor, 1.5 mg/ml bovine serum albumin, 100 U/ml penicillin, and 0.1 mg/ml streptomycin (GIBCO). The ganglia were then gently triturated using a siliconized Pasteur pipette and plated on a polyornithine/laminin coated glass coverslip.

In whole-cell patch-clamp experiments, DRG cell bodies giving rise to cutaneous afferent fibers were identified by retrograde labeling with Fluoro-Gold (Schmued and Fallon 1986). A 4% solution of Fluoro-Gold mixed in distilled water was injected subcutaneously in the lateral plantar region 1 wk before sacrifice for culture preparation.

Solutions for Voltage-Clamp Experiments

Before electrical recording the coverslips containing cultured DRG were rinsed in a protein-free saline containing (in mM) 25 NaCl, 110 tetramethylammonium (TMA) chloride, 3.0 KCl, 1.0 $CaCl_2$, 1.0 $MgCl_2$, 0.1 $CdCl_2$, 1.0 4-AP, and 10 HEPES titrated to pH 7.4 with NaOH (this added an additional 5–6 mOsm of Na^+ ion). Cells placed in a recording chamber maintained

their morphological and electrical properties in this saline bath at 18–20 °C for ≥ 2 h. Recording pipettes were filled with (in mM) 140 CsCl, 2 $MgCl_2$, 1 ethylene glycol-bis(β-aminoethyl ether)-N, N, N', N'-tetraacetic acid (EGTA), and 10 HEPES titrated to pH 7.2 with CsOH.

Without external cadmium (0.1 mM) cells exhibited additional components of noninactivating inward current, presumably carried by Ca^{2+} ions. TMA was used as a nonpermeant monovalent cation to replace external Na^+ to reduce current amplitude and therefore errors caused by series resistance artifact. Cs^+ ions, known to be impermeant to most conventional K^+ channels, were used to replace internal K^+. In some experiments (figure 25.9, C and D) a small amount of sustained outward current remained at the end of a strong depolarizing pulse, indicating either that not all K^+ had been completely dialyzed from the internal milieu or that a Cs^+-resistant component was present.

Voltage-Clamp Recording Technique

The whole-cell patch-clamp method (Hamill et al. 1981) was used to record voltage-dependent Na^+ currents from the cultured DRG. Patch electrodes (Corning #7052 capillary glass) of 1.2–1.6 $M\Omega$ were constructed and fire-polished using a Narishige PP-83 vertical puller and MF-83 microforge. The electrodes were mounted on the headstage of a Medical Systems APC-8 patch-clamp amplifier using a 500-$M\Omega$ feedback resistor. The shunt capacitance between the pipette and bath was kept at a minimum by maintaining the bath level to ~10–20 μm above the cell being clamped. Capacity current was further reduced, along with linear leak currents, via P/4 pulse protocols (Bezanilla and Armstrong 1977).

The current was sampled and converted into (16 bit) digital form using an acquisition system (ITC-16, Instrutech) that interfaced the patch-clamp amplifier with an Apple Macintosh computer. The current was sampled at 50 kHz and low-pass filtered (4-pole Bessel filter) at 10 kHz.

Generally, four sweeps were averaged at each test pulse.

Results

Action Potential Waveforms of Cutaneous Afferent, Normal, and Deefferented Muscle Nerves Recorded in NS

The compound action potential (CAP) and single fiber action potentials were similar in shape and time course for cutaneous, muscle, and deefferented muscle nerves. The control CAPs of the SN and the ATN recorded in the sucrose gap (figure 25.1, A and B) were similar in shape and waveform. The average CAP half-width for SN was 0.64 ± 0.13 (SD) ms ($n = 14$); for ATN it was 0.64 ± 0.07 ms ($n = 8$). Similarly, mean spike half-width calculated from single axon recordings in SN ($n = 16$), ATN ($n = 4$), and dATN ($n = 10$) were relatively comparable: 0.81 ± 0.24, 0.75 ± 0.06, and 0.74 ± 0.24 ms, respectively. Rarely was spontaneous impulse activity observed in any of the axon populations during recording in NS. Low-amplitude depolarizing afterpotentials were occasionally observed but were not common features of the action potentials.

Effects of 4-AP on Action Potential Waveform of Cutaneous Afferents and Normal and Deefferented Muscle Nerves

Application of 4-AP led to different changes in muscle and sensory nerve responses. The ATN action potential was prolonged in duration, with a gradual and continuous return to baseline over several milliseconds (figure 25.1B). In contrast, the response recorded from the SN (figure 25.1A) displayed a delayed depolarization and characteristic "ripple" after the initial action potential waveform (Kocsis et al. 1983).

Intraaxonal recordings indicate that the differences in CAP waveforms are attributable to

differences in 4-AP-induced membrane potential and burst-firing patterns. After exposure to 4-AP, the action potentials recorded in axons from intact ATNs and dATNs were broadened (figure 25.1, D and F). In contrast, application of 4-AP to SN resulted in a pronounced depolarization after the initial action potential (the delayed depolarization) and individual axons responded to a single brief (100 µs) stimulus with bursts of action potentials arising from the delayed depolarization (figure 25.1C). Although some axons in SNs bathed in NS showed isolated "spontaneous" action potentials, a single stimulus never evoked spike burst activity.

A temporal correspondence was noted between the late component of the whole-nerve response (figure 25.1A, arrowhead) and the delayed depolarization with superimposed spike burst activity recorded intraaxonally (figure 25.1C) from the same SN. The initial action potential was more reliably elicited than the late spikes and the late spikes varied in latency and amplitude from sweep to sweep. The delayed depolarization often terminated in an afterhyperpolarization (AHP), as shown in figure 25.2C; both the delayed depolarization and AHP occurred after whole-nerve or single axon stimulation. In figure 25.1E, the fiber was activated by passage of a constant-current depolarizing pulse through the recording microelectrode. Note the distinct hump (delayed depolarization) after the action potential.

Comparison of Effects of 4-AP and TEA

To examine the role of TEA-sensitive K^+ current in muscle afferents and cutaneous afferents we studied SN and dATN before and after exposure to TEA. Application of TEA alone to either type of nerve had a relatively negligible effect on single action potential waveform (figure 25.2, A and B). However, striking effects were observed when TEA was applied to 4-AP-treated sensory nerves. In the presence of 4-AP a prominent AHP followed the delayed depolarization elic-

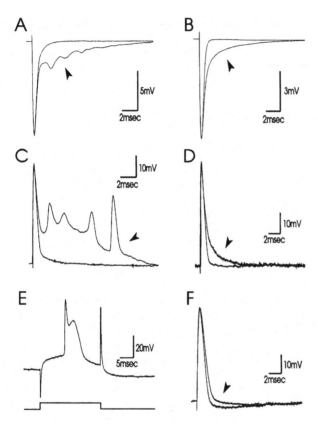

Figure 25.1
Superimposed action potentials recorded from the sural nerve (SN), anterior tibial nerve (ATN), and deefferented
ATN (dATN) before and after superfusion with 4-aminopyridine (4-AP) (1 mM). Compound action potential
recorded in the sucrose gap chamber from SN (*A*) and ATN (*B*). Intraaxonal recordings from SN (*C*), ATN (*D*),
and dATN (*F*) are also shown. An action potential elicited by long depolarization pulse applied into a single axon
in the SN through the recording microelectrode after 1 mM 4-AP application (*E*). Arrowheads: response after 4-AP
application.

ited by a single stimulus in SN (figure 25.2, C and E). The peak amplitude of the AHP shown in figure 25.2E is 5 mV and the duration is ~ 100 ms. Application of 10 mM TEA reduced the 4-AP-induced AHP (figure 25.2, D and F) and resulted in repetitive spike discharge. The combination of 4-AP and TEA led to increased spontaneous action potential activity.

These results are in agreement with previous studies that demonstrated a TEA-sensitive AHP that is enhanced in the presence of 4-AP (Eng et al. 1988).

Recovery Time of the Action Potential and the Delayed Depolarization in SN

We used paired stimuli, presented at varying interstimulus intervals, to examine the refractory period of the initial action potential and the delayed depolarization in the SN after 4-AP application. The refractory period of the delayed depolarization, as measured by the time course of amplitude recovery, was significantly greater than that of the initial action potential. The time courses of recovery of the action potential before and after 4-AP application are presented in figure 25.3, A and B, respectively. When a conditioning stimulus was presented at an interstimulus interval of 30 ms, the action potential was elicited, but the delayed depolarization was not observed (figure 25.3C). However, the delayed depolarization appeared with a longer interstimulus interval (200 ms) (figure 25.3D). The amplitudes of the test action potential and delayed depolarization in a SN were evaluated separately as a function of interstimulus interval (figure 25.4A); the increased recovery time of the delayed depolarization is evident. A discrepancy between the recovery times of the action potential and the delayed depolarization was also noted in assessments of the interstimulus interval required to attain 50% recovery of the amplitude compared with the control action potential (figure 25.4B). The half-recovery time was 3.06 ± 1.82 ms ($n = 12$) for control SN action potentials,

18.84 ± 9.13 ms ($n = 16$) for the initial SN action potential after exposure to 4-AP, and 99.06 ± 28.27 ms ($n = 15$) for the delayed depolarization.

Effects of Membrane Potential on Delayed Depolarization

The magnitude of the delayed depolarization is affected by membrane potential. Shifts in the holding potential in the depolarizing direction were accompanied by a comparable amplitude decrement in the delayed depolarization in the SN (figure 25.5). Conversely, when the holding potential was shifted in the hyperpolarizing direction the delayed depolarization became larger. Holding potentials positive to -40 mV eliminated the response. These data suggest that the mechanism underlying the delayed depolarization is an active, voltage-dependent process that is sensitive to the membrane potential before stimulation.

Effects of Ca^{2+} and Na^+ Channel Blockade on the 4-AP-Induced Delayed Depolarization of Cutaneous Afferents

The effects of 4-AP on cutaneous sensory nerves were not dependent on the presence of extracellular Ca^{2+}. Nerves were bathed for 1 h in a superfusion solution in which $CaCl_2$ was removed and replaced by a solution containing 2.0 mM $MgCl_2$ and 1 mM EGTA. Introduction of 4-AP in this Ca^{2+}-free environment was still effective in eliciting a delayed depolarization (figure 25.6A). Application of Cd^{2+} (1 mM), a Ca^{2+} channel blocker (Hagiwara and Byerly 1981), to the superfusate did not significantly alter the action potential waveform. It also did not block the 4-AP-induced burst activity (figure 25.6B) or the delayed depolarization and AHP (figure 25.6C). Phosphates were excluded from the solutions to prevent Cd^{2+} precipitation. The Na^+ channel blocking toxin TTX (10 nM) completely blocked both the early and late depolar-

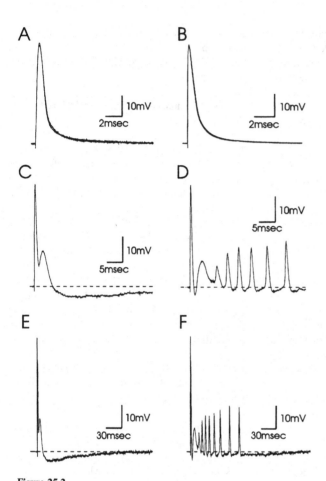

Figure 25.2
Intraaxonal recordings of action potentials from SN and dATN with and without tetraethylammonium (TEA) (10 mM). Superimposed action potentials recorded from SN (*A*) and dATN (*B*) before and after 10 mM TEA superfusion. (*C*) In the presence of 4-AP a single whole-nerve stimulus leads to a delayed depolarization in SN. A prominent afterhyperpolarization (AHP) follows the delayed depolarization, as shown in (*C*) and (*E*) (longer time base). (*D*) When TEA is applied in combination with 4-AP (*D*, and at a longer time base in *F*) the AHP is eliminated and a single stimulus induces repetitive firing.

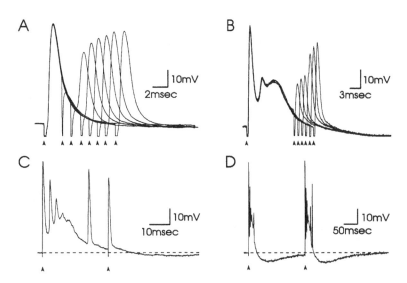

Figure 25.3
Single fiber action potentials recorded from SN. (*A*) Series of action potential responses to double shock stimulation at varying interstimulus intervals before (*A*) and after (*B–D*) superfusion with 4-AP. When conditioned by another stimulus (interstimulus interval, 30 ms) the delayed depolarization is obliterated but the initial spike is not (*C*). However, the delayed depolarization appears with a longer interstimulus interval (200 ms) (*D*).

ization induced by 4-AP after whole-nerve stimulation (figure 25.7*A*). Responses to intraaxonal passage of a constant-current depolarizing pulse were also inhibited by TTX (figure 25.7*B*). The delayed depolarization appeared to require the preceding strong depolarization of the initial spike for activation.

Na$^+$ Currents on DRG Neuronal Cell Bodies

Whole-cell patch-clamp recordings were obtained from either randomly selected DRG neurons 44–50 μm diam or those of the same size range identified by retrograde labeling with Fluoro-Gold (see Methods). Only neurons without neurites were selected to minimize problems associated with space clamp. An example of a Fluoro-Gold-labeled DRG neuron is shown in figure 25.8. Of the two neurons observed with bright field microscopy (figure 25.8*A*), only one

is retrogradely labeled by subcutaneous injection of Fluoro-Gold, indicating that it is a cutaneous afferent neuron. Of the population of 27 randomly selected size-matched neurons (i.e., a group containing muscle and cutaneous afferents), 18 (67%) had a singular fast Na$^+$ current of the form seen in the neuron of figure 25.9, *C* and *D*; 2 had kinetically separable (fast and slow) Na$^+$ currents, 5 had only a single slow current, and 2 were indeterminate.

The Na$^+$ currents shown in figure 25.9, *C* and *D*, were recorded from a nonlabeled, randomly selected 48-μm-diam neuron. In figure 25.9*C* the neuron was held at −60 mV, preconditioned at −120 mV for 150 ms, then depolarized to test potentials from −40 to +20 mV in steps of 10 mV as shown in figure 25.9*A*. The inward current, which follows after a variable delay, exhibits voltage-dependent kinetics, spontaneous decrease in the current after a maximum,

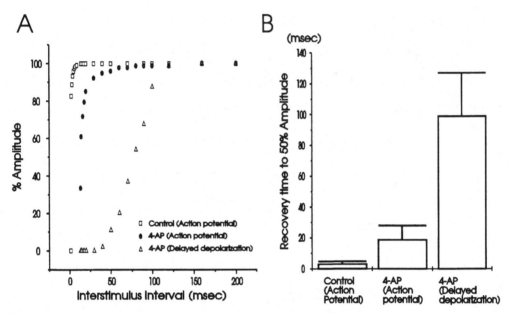

Figure 25.4

Graphic presentation of amplitude recovery vs. interstimulus interval in single fiber examined under various conditions as described above in figure 25.3. Peak amplitude (percent of control value) of initial spike and the delayed depolarization of single fiber action potential response plotted vs. interstimulus interval before and after 4-AP application (*A*). Note the increased refractoriness of the delayed depolarization. (*B*) Comparison of the interstimulus interval required to attain 50% recovery of the amplitude for each group. Error bars: SD.

and reversal near that expected for Na^+ ion (+50 mV under these conditions). The current traces in figure 25.9*D* were recorded from the same cell but using the protocol shown in figure 25.9*B*. In this protocol the 150-ms conditioning potential was varied between −140 and −40 mV in steps of 10 mV and followed by a test potential to +20 mV (to simplify the figure, not all sweeps are shown). The kinetics of each trace are the same, but the peak amplitude decreases as the conditioning potentials become more positive and eventually approaches 0 at −40 mV. Thus this neuron had a uniform population of Na^+-selective channels that exhibited rapid, voltage-dependent activation and inactivation, and steady-state inactivation properties.

In 14 Fluoro-Gold-identified cutaneous afferent neurons in the same size range, 6 had kinetically separable (fast and slow) Na^+ currents, another 6 had a single relatively slow current, and the remaining 2 were relatively slow but indeterminate as to whether or not more than one current was present. Although it might be argued that Fluoro-Gold labeling could have affected channel expression and/or current kinetics, neurons with either an isolated slow variety or with multiple current components were present in unlabeled preparations. Figure 25.9, *E* and *F*, shows voltage-dependent inward currents recorded from a neuron that had kinetically separable currents. Using the same stimulation protocols as in figure 25.9, *C* and *D*, the identified

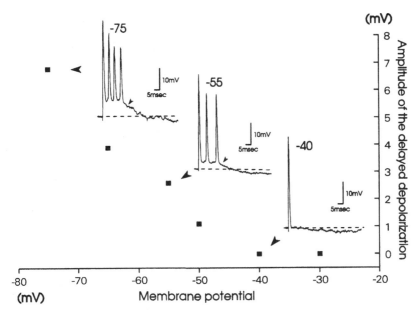

Figure 25.5
Relationship between the magnitude of the delayed depolarization and the resting membrane potential. When spikes arose from the delayed depolarization the peak was measured from an extrapolated waveform without spikes. Data were recorded at various resting membrane potentials (−80 to −20 mV). Selected responses (−40, −55, and −75 mV) are shown.

cutaneous afferents revealed a more complex inward current that appeared to be the result of activation of two types of Na^+ selective channels. In figure 25.9E, weak depolarizations elicited a prolonged, inward current that showed little sign of inactivation after 12 ms. At −20 mV a small bump in the record (*) indicates the emergence of a faster kinetic component. The peak of this faster component was best observed at strong depolarizations of +10 to +20 mV (figure 25.9E) and occurred at ∼1.5 ms. The singular fast current of figure 25.9C had a peak current at 0.9–1.0 ms at the same depolarization. At +20 mV the net current of figure 25.9E takes the form of a sharp peak followed by a ramplike decay that does not conform to a simple exponential decay, as would occur if a uniform population of channels were inactivating. Taken

together, the slow component of current, when compared to the fast component, appeared to activate at test potentials 10–20 mV more negative.

It is unlikely that the slow currents we identified on DRG cell bodies are a result of artifact related to unfavorable space-clamp conditions for two reasons. First, the neurons recorded from were 44–50 µm diam with a corresponding surface area of 6,000–8,000 µm^2 and a theoretical capacitance of 60–80 pF. Neurons without neurites were selected for these studies and the measured capacitances tended to confirm the absence of neurites. The capacitive currents we observed had time constants of 0.1–0.3 ms, corresponding to series resistance, in the worst case, of ∼4 MΩ. This would tend to impose a lower limit on the kinetic measurements of the faster

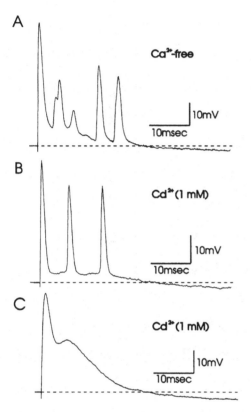

Figure 25.6
Effects of Ca^{2+}-free and Cd^{2+} solutions on 4-AP-induced delayed depolarization and bursting activity. Intraaxonal recordings of action potentials recorded from SN without Ca^{2+} [with 1 mM ethylene glycol-bis(β-aminoethyl ether)-N,N,N',N'-tetraacetic acid (EGTA)] generate both a delayed depolarization and burst activity (A). Cd^{2+} (1 mM) did not block burst activity (B) or the delayed depolarization (C). ($A-C$) were obtained from different axons.

variety of current such as that shown in figure 25.9, C and D. Second, the presence of a combination of fast and slow currents in cells of equivalent size and therefore capacitance favors the idea that two separate channel families underlie these currents. The current plots depicted in figure 25.9E indicate the presence in a single cell of kinetically separable components. It is not clear whether the faster component, which occurs in combination with a slow component, corresponds to the fast Na^+ channel that was observed in isolation in other sensory neurons (figure 25.9, C and D). The fast current that occurs in isolation peaks earlier than the fast Na^+ current that occurs in combination with a slower one in other cells under the same stimulating conditions. The presence of multiple types of Na^+ channels in 44- to 50-μm DRG neurons is consistent with previous observations (Caffrey et al. 1992; Roy and Narahashi 1992).

In figure 25.9F, the two kinetic components show different sensitivity to the conditioning potential. At -140 mV conditioning potential the current reaches a peak (*) and then follows a ramplike decay. With progressively more positive conditioning potentials, the sharp peak gives way to a more smoothly contoured peak whose maximum amplitude (#) occurs later than the sharp peak. This result conforms with those of Caffrey et al. (1992) and of Roy and Narahashi (1992), and with our data (not shown) in which the steady-state inactivation of the slower form of Na^+ conductance, when studied in isolation, is incomplete and is shifted to more positive potentials (Rizzo et al. 1993).

Discussion

Mammalian myelinated axons express several pharmacologically and kinetically distinct ion channel types that influence the shape and patterning of action potentials (Baker et al. 1987; Eng et al. 1988; Kocsis et al. 1986, 1987; Roper and Schwartz 1989). It is now appreciated that individual channel types are regionally distributed along the myelinated axon in a nonuniform fashion. Sodium channels cluster in high density at the node of Ranvier (Black et al. 1990; Brismar 1980; Chiu and Ritchie 1981; Chiu et al. 1979; Waxman 1977; Waxman and Ritchie 1993). The distribution of K^+ channels in mam-

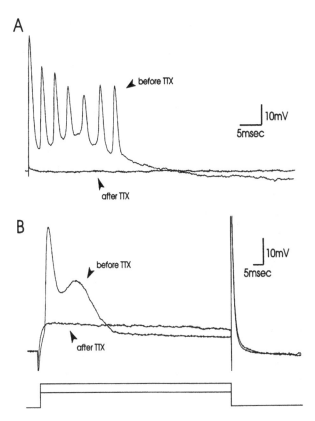

Figure 25.7
10 nM tetrodotoxin (TTX) blocks the delayed depolarization and bursting activity as well as initial spike. Super-imposed intraaxonal recordings after presentation of a single stimuli in SN before and after TTX application (*A*). (*B*) Both the initial spike and the delayed depolarization elicited by long depolarization pulse applied into the axon through the recording microelectrode are also blocked by 10 nM TTX. The initial action potential and the delayed depolarization do not recover even if stronger depolarizing pulse is applied after TTX application.

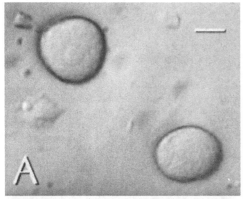

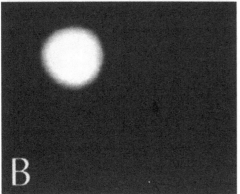

Figure 25.8
Bright field (*A*) and fluorescence images of dorsal root ganglion (DRG) neurons selected for voltage-clamp experiments. The labeled neuron in (*B*) was identified after subcutaneous injection of Fluoro-Gold and therefore considered to be a cutaneous afferent neuron. Calibration in *A* is 20 μm.

malian axons is more complex in that at least two types of K^+ currents have been identified: a fast 4-AP-sensitive current and a slower TEA-sensitive K^+ current (Baker et al. 1987; Kocsis et al. 1986; Roper and Schwartz 1989; see Black et al. 1990 for review). Recent work suggests that the TEA-sensitive current is present at the node and that the 4-AP-sensitive current has a greater representation in the paranodal or internodal

axon membrane (Baker et al. 1987; Eng et al. 1988). Additionally, an inwardly rectifying current, which utilizes both Na^+ and K^+ as charge carriers, is present on both peripheral (Baker et al. 1987; Birch et al. 1991) and CNS axons (Eng et al. 1990).

Despite generally similar morphological features at both the light and electron microcopic level (Bowe et al. 1992; Fields et al. 1986), different types of mammalian myelinated axons subserve specialized physiological functions and it is reasonable to suspect that their selective physiological properties may be subserved by distinctive distributions of various ion channels. It has been suggested that sensory fibers may have kinetically fast and slow Na^+ channels. This possibility was recognized in studies using intraaxonal recording techniques on sciatic nerve fibers (Kocsis et al. 1983). A subpopulation of axons gave rise to a prominent, Ca^{2+}-independent, delayed depolarization after the action potential after application of 4-AP (Bowe et al. 1985). This potential was present on sensory (dorsal root) and not motor (ventral root) fibers (Bowe et al. 1985, 1992; Kocsis et al. 1986). It should be pointed out that relatively young animals were used in the present study because the effects of 4-AP on axons attenuate during maturation (Kocsis et al. 1983). However, on demyelination of adult nerves 4-AP elicits effects on sensory and motor axons similar to those of immature rats, including the delayed depolarization (Targ and Kocsis 1986). The results of the present study further demonstrate that the delayed depolarization is not a general property of sensory axons, as has been previously suggested, but rather is specific for cutaneous afferents.

Mechanism Underlying the Delayed Depolarization

The delayed depolarization we described in cutaneous afferents is distinct from the depolarizing afterpotential previously reported (Barrett and

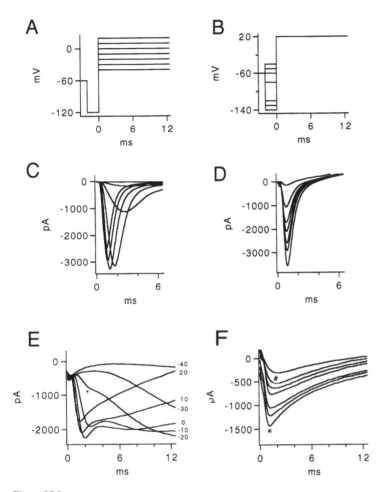

Figure 25.9
Whole-cell patch-clamp recordings from 2 DRG neurons after 24 h in culture. Two stimulus protocols were applied.
(*A*) From a holding potential of −60 mV the cells were conditioned at −120 mV for 100 ms, then depolarized to
−40 to +20 mV in steps of 10 mV. (*B*) Cells were conditioned for 150 ms at −140 to −40 mV in steps of 10 mV,
then depolarized to +20 mV. (*C* and *D*) Voltage-dependent Na⁺ currents recorded from a randomly chosen
medium-sized neuron using protocols from (*A*) and (*B*), respectively. (*D*) Not all current records are displayed for
clarity. Note that a small amount of sustained outward current remained during the test pulse indicating that internal cesium had not adequately diffused into the cell from the pipette. (*E* and *F*) Currents were recorded from a
cutaneous afferent neuron identified via retrograde Fluoro-Gold labeling. Stimulus protocols from (*A*) and (*B*) were
applied to (*E*) and (*F*), respectively. External and internal solutions and recording techniques are described in
Methods. Temperature: 19 °C. (*F*) Record obtained from a holding potential of −20 mV was subtracted from each
record. Traces in (*E*) are marked with test potential for clarity.

Barrett 1982; Blight and Someya 1985; Bowe et al. 1987). The latter can be explained on the basis of passive discharge of the internodal capacitance through the myelin resistance. The delayed depolarization in cutaneous afferent axons was observed only after blockade of the 4-AP-sensitive K^+ channel. Several lines of evidence have been presented that indicate that the delayed depolarization results from activation of a Na^+-selective channel that is distinct from the channel that underlies the action potential. First, the delayed depolarization can be selectively inactivated and its amplitude is directly dependent on the holding potential (figure 25.5). These observations support the idea that the delayed depolarization is due to membrane permeability changes to an ion whose reversal potential is positive to the resting potential. An alternative candidate to Na^+ would be Ca^{2+}, but this is unlikely to be the charge carrier because the delayed depolarization is present in the absence of external Ca^{2+} and could not be inhibited by Cd^{2+}.

It is well established that both TTX-sensitive and TTX-resistant Na^+ channels are present on mammalian DRG neurons (Caffrey et al. 1992; Elliot and Elliot 1993; Kostyuk et al. 1981; McLean et al. 1988; Roy and Narahashi 1992). Such a demonstration has not been made for mammalian axons. In our experiments on axons both the action potential and the delayed depolarization were blocked by TTX. This does not, however, prove that the delayed depolarization results from the activation of a TTX-sensitive current because with our recording configuration the delayed depolarization may be activated by the action potential. Definitive characterization of the kinetics and pharmacology of the current underlying the delayed depolarization will require a voltage-clamp analysis of the nodal and possibly paranodal axonal membranes in cutaneous afferent fibers. To date, such an analysis of these relatively small myelinated axons has not been carried out. However, our patch-clamp studies on the cell bodies of identified cutaneous

afferents indicate that a relatively large proportion of these neurons express on their membranes at least two populations of Na^+ channels distinguishable both by kinetics and sensitivity to the conditioning potential. Taken together these results are consistent with the idea that the slow Na^+ channels are present on the axons of cutaneous afferents.

An alternative and more traditional explanation to account for the delayed depolarization is that a single Na^+ channel type can support late currents over a narrow voltage domain in which neither of the steady-state activation (m_∞) and inactivation (h_∞) parameters are 0 (Hodgkin and Huxley 1952; McAllister et al. 1975). If the m_∞-h_∞ overlap occurred after a single action potential, this could account for a prolonged, weakly depolarizing inward current. However, the presence of kinetically fast Na^+ spikes generated by and superimposed on the delayed depolarization make this explanation unlikely. Furthermore, this rationale cannot account for the amplitude in the delayed response during strong depolarizations when the membrane potential is positive to the overlapping voltage domain.

Another possibility is that a fraction of a single population of Na^+ channels enters a gating mode, which allows delayed openings and slower inactivation kinetics (Alzheimer et al. 1993; Armstrong and Bezanilla 1977; Patlak and Ortiz 1986; Sigworth 1981). These descriptions generally do not apply to what in our case would correspond to a significant fraction (>50%) of the channels, and the slow inactivation time constants are 1 order of magnitude faster than what we observed in our preparations. The ratio of the amplitude of slow versus fast components of Na^+ channel inactivation (Neumcke and Stämpfli 1982) in large rat sciatic nerve fiber was found to be <0.4 for depolarizations positive to -50 mV (in the presence of 6 nM TTX). For weak depolarizations (-38 mV) the slow inactivation time constant was 1.23 ms, ≥ 1 order of magnitude faster then the delayed

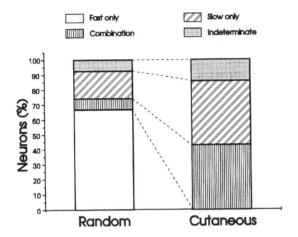

Figure 25.10
The relative distribution of "singular fast," "combination of fast and slow," "singular slow," and "indeterminate" currents in randomly selected DRG neurons 44–50 μm diam and cutaneous afferent neurons of the same size range identified by retrograde labeling with Fluoro-Gold. Note that randomly selected neurons utilize a large population of singular fast Na$^+$ current. In contrast, cutaneous afferent neurons have a greater representation of kinetically slower Na$^+$ current, often with multiple types.

depolarization observed in our preparation. These early studies were performed on large myelinated nerve fibers, and it appears unlikely that the fast Na$^+$ currents of our sensory axons are capable of an as yet undiscovered kinetically slow gating mode that could support such a large and prolonged inward current.

Unique Na$^+$ Current on Cutaneous Afferent Neurons

The present results support the idea that DRG neurons corresponding to cutaneous afferent neurons have a population of Na$^+$ channels that is unique and distinguishes them from afferents that arise from noncutaneous receptors. DRG cells giving rise to the cutaneous afferents are more likely to have a relatively slow Na$^+$ channel or more than one population of Na$^+$ channels when compared to all size-matched, randomly selected neurons. Moreover, when cutaneous afferents were selectively examined,

none had rapidly activating and inactivating channels. In contrast, in a randomly chosen population of DRG cells containing muscle as well as cutaneous afferent neurons, 67% of the cells exhibited a singular "fast" current. The relative distribution of these currents in randomly selected and identified cutaneous afferent neurons is summarized in figure 25.10. These data suggest that most noncutaneous afferent neurons express a uniform population of rapidly activating and inactivating Na$^+$ channels. In contrast, cutaneous afferent neurons have a greater representation of kinetically slower Na$^+$ channels, often with multiple types on the same neuron. These results are consistent with the idea that cutaneous afferent axons may have kinetically distinct and multiple Na$^+$ channels.

Functional Role of the Delayed Depolarization

The functional role of the delayed depolarization on cutaneous afferents is not certain. Similar responses have been suggested to be associated with pathological responses, i.e., abnormal repetitive impulse generation after blockade of fast K^+ channels (Kocsis and Waxman 1987; Kocsis et al. 1983). One possibility is that slow Na^+ channels along the trunks of cutaneous afferent axons play a role in high-frequency discharge. Alternatively, it is possible that the functionally relevant site for a kinetically slow Na^+ channel on cutaneous afferents is at the sensory ending in the periphery, where this channel may participate in transduction or regulation of incoming sensory impulse activity. The deposition of slow Na channels along the axonal trunk, i.e., along the course of their transport from the site of synthesis in the cell body to peripheral sensory endings, may be unimportant for normal impulse activity. The localization of fast K^+ currents at the paranodal and internodal region would prevent activation of the ectopic Na^+ currents under normal conditions, thereby minimizing evolutionary pressure for the development of a more selective targeting mechanism to route these channels exclusively to the sensory ending.

We propose that blockade of the 4-AP-sensitive K^+ current allows the delayed activation of the kinetically slower Na^+ current that underlies the delayed depolarization. The delayed depolarization was not generated when the 4-AP-sensitive K^+ current was not blocked. This observation suggests that a possible functional role of the 4-AP-sensitive K^+ current in cutaneous afferents is to limit generation of the delayed depolarization and the associated spike burst activity.

The use of ionic channel blocking agents in the treatment of patients with a variety of neurological disorders has further elucidated the potential functional importance of specific ionic conductances. Potassium channel blockade with 4-AP has been examined in clinical studies in patients with Eaton-Lambert syndrome (Lundh et al. 1977; Murray and Newsom-Davis 1981) and multiple sclerosis (Davis et al. 1990; Jones et al. 1983; Stefoski et al. 1987) in an attempt to

enhance the release of synaptic transmitters and to overcome conduction block, respectively. Paresthesias and dysesthesias have been reported as side effects of 4-AP, whereas distinctive motor afferent or efferent complications have not been noted (Lundh et al. 1979; Murray and Newsom-Davis 1981). These observations further emphasize the specificity of 4-AP action with regard to the induction of burst firing in cutaneous sensory fibers.

In conclusion, the results reported here demonstrate a fundamental difference in the electrophysiological organization of cutaneous versus muscle afferent myelinated axons. In particular, cutaneous afferent axons give rise to a prolonged depolarizing potential after the action potential after blockade of fast 4-AP-sensitive K^+ channels. Several lines of evidence, including whole-cell patch-clamp experiments on the cell bodies of the cutaneous afferent axons, suggest that a kinetically slow Na^+ channel underlies the depolarizing afterpotential. These properties of cutaneous afferent axons provide a basis for pharmacologically distinguishing them from motor fibers and from muscle afferent fibers. Moreover, the expression of the delayed depolarization on cutaneous afferents predicts a plausible mechanism for the generation of ectopic impulse activity that may be specific for cutaneous afferents.

Acknowledgments

This work was supported in part by grants from the National Multiple Sclerosis Society (RG 2135 and RG 1231); the National Institute of Neurological Disorders and Stroke (NS-10174), and The Medical Research Service of the Department of Veterans Affairs. D. Utzschneider was supported in part by a Spinal Cord Research Fellowship from the EPVA, O. Honmou was supported in part by a gift from the Heumann Fund, and M. A. Rizzo was supported by a C.I.D.A. (NS01606).

References

Alzheimer, C., Schwindt, P. C., and Crill, W. E. Modal gating of Na⁺ channels as a mechanism of persistent Na⁺ current in pyramidal neurons from rat and cat sensorimotor cortex. *J. Neurosci.* 13: 660–673, 1993.

Armstrong, C. M. and Bezanilla, F. Inactivation of the sodium channel. II. Gating experiments. *J. Gen. Physiol.* 70: 567–590, 1977.

Baker, M., Bostock, P., Grafe, P., and Martius, P. Function and distribution of three types of rectifying channel in rat spinal root myelinated axons. *J. Physiol. Lond.* 383: 45–67, 1987.

Barrett, E. F. and Barrett, J. N. Intracellular recording from vertebrate myelinated axons: mechanism of the depolarizing afterpotential. *J. Physiol. Lond.* 323: 117–144, 1982.

Benzanilla, F. and Armstrong, C. M. Inactivation of the sodium channel. I. Sodium current experiments. *J. Gen. Physiol.* 70: 549–566, 1977.

Birch, B. D., Eng, D. L., and Kocsis, J. D. Intranuclear Ca²⁺ transients during neurite regeneration of an adult mammalian neuron. *Proc. Natl. Acad. Sci. USA* 89: 7978–7982, 1992.

Birch, B. D., Kocsis, J. D., DiGregorio, F., Bhisitkul, R. B., and Waxman, S. G. A voltage- and time-dependent rectification in rat dorsal spinal root axons. *J. Neurophysiol.* 66: 719–728, 1991.

Black, J. A., Kocsis, J. D., and Waxman, S. G. Ion channel organization of the myelinated fiber. *Trends Neurosci.* 13: 48–54, 1990.

Blight, A. R. and Someya, S. Depolarizing afterpotentials in myelinated axons of mammalian spinal cord. *Neuroscience* 15: 1–12, 1985.

Bowe, C. M., Evans, N. H., and Hildebrand, C. Distinctive abnormalities in regenerated rat cutaneous and muscle nerves after nerve crush injury. *Soc. Neurosci. Abstr.* 18: 1320, 1992.

Bowe, C. M., Kocsis, J. D., and Waxman, S. G. Differences between mammalian ventral and dorsal spinal roots in response to blockade of potassium channels during maturation. *Proc. R. Soc. Lond. B Biol. Sci.* 224: 355–366, 1985.

Bowe, C. M., Kocsis, J. D., and Waxman, S. G. The association of the supernormal period and the depolarizing afterpotential in myelinated frog and rat sciatic nerve. *Neuroscience* 21: 585–593, 1987.

Brismar, T. Potential clamp analysis of membrane currents in rat myelinated nerve fibers. *J. Physiol. Lond.* 298: 171–184, 1980.

Caffrey, J. M., Eng, D. L., Black, J. A., Waxman, S. G., and Kocsis, J. D. Three types of sodium channels in adult rat dorsal root ganglion neurons. *Brain Res.* 592: 283–297, 1992.

Chiu, S. Y. and Ritchie, J. M. Evidence for the presence of potassium channels in the paranodal region of acutely demyelinated mammalian nerve fibres. *J. Physiol. Lond.* 313: 415–437, 1981.

Chiu, S. Y., Ritchie, J. M., Rogart, R. B., and Stagg, D. A quantitative description of membrane currents in rabbit myelinated nerve. *J. Physiol. Lond.* 292: 149–166, 1979.

Davis, F. A., Stefoski, D., and Rush, J. Orally administered 4-aminopyridine improves clinical signs in multiple sclerosis. *Ann. Neurol.* 27: 186–192, 1990.

Elliott, A. A. and Elliott, J. R. Characterization of TTX-sensitive and TTX-resistant sodium currents in small cells from adult rat dorsal root ganglia. *J. Physiol. Lond.* 463: 39–56, 1993.

Eng, D. L., Gordon, T. R., Kocsis, J. D., and Waxman, S. G. Development of 4-AP and TEA sensitivities in mammalian myelinated nerve fibers. *J. Neurophysiol.* 60: 2168–2179, 1988.

Eng, D. L., Gordon, T. R., Kocsis, J. D., and Waxman, S. G. Current-clamp analysis of a time-dependent rectification in rat optic nerve. *J. Physiol. Lond.* 421: 185–202, 1990.

Fields, R. D., Black, J. A., Bowe, C. M., Kocsis, J. D., and Waxman, S. G. Differences in intramembranous particle distribution in the paranodal axolemma are not associated with functional differences of dorsal and ventral roots. *Neurosci. Lett.* 67: 13–18, 1986.

Hagiwara, S. and Byerly, L. Calcium channel. *Annu. Rev. Neurosci.* 4: 69–125, 1981.

Hamill, O. P., Marty, A., Neher, E., Sakmann, B., and Sigworth, F. V. Improved patch-clamp techniques for high-resolution current recording from cells and cell-free membrane patches. *Pfluegers Arch.* 391: 85–100, 1981.

Hodgkin, A. L. and Huxley, A. F. A quantitative description of membrane current and its application to conduction and excitation in nerve. *J. Physiol. Lond.* 117: 500–544, 1952.

Jones, R. E., Heron, J. R., Foster, D. H., Snelgar, R. S., and Mason, R. J. Effects of 4-aminopyridine in patients with multiple sclerosis. *J. Neurol. Sci.* 60: 353–362, 1983.

Kapoor, R., Smith, K. J., Felts, P. A., and Davies, M. Internodal potassium currents can generate ectopic impulses in mammalian myelinated axons. *Brain Res.* 611: 165–169, 1993.

Kocsis, J. D., Bowe, C. M., and Waxman, S. G. Different effects of 4-aminopyridine on sensory and motor fibers: pathogenesis of paresthesias. *Neurology* 36: 117–120, 1986.

Kocsis, J. D., Eng, D. L., Gordon, T. R., and Waxman, S. G. Functional differences between 4-aminopyridine and tetraethylammonium-sensitive potassium channels in myelinated axons. *Neurosci. Lett.* 75: 193–198, 1987.

Kocsis, J. D., Ruiz, J. A., and Waxman, S. G. Maturation of mammalian myelinated fibers: changes in action-potential characteristics following 4-aminopyridine application. *J. Neurophysiol.* 50: 449–463, 1983.

Kocsis, J. D. and Waxman, S. G. Intra-axonal recordings in rat dorsal column axons: membrane hyperpolarization and decreased excitability precede the primary afferent depolarization. *Brain Res.* 238: 222–227, 1982.

Kocsis, J. D. and Waxman, S. G. Long-term regenerated nerve fibres retain sensitivity to potassium channel blocking agents. *Nature Lond.* 304: 640–642, 1983.

Kocsis, J. D. and Waxman, S. G. Ion channel organization of normal and regenerating mammalian axons. In: *Progress in Brain Research. Neural Regeneration,* edited by Seil, F. J., Herbert, E., and Carlson, B. Amsterdam: Elsevier, 1987, vol. 71, p. 89–101.

Kostyuk, P. G., Veselovsky, N. S., and Tsyndrenko, A. Y. Ionic currents in the somatic membrane of rat dorsal root ganglion neurons. I. Sodium currents. *Neuroscience* 6: 2423–2430, 1981.

Lundh, H., Nilsson, O., and Rosen, I. 4-Aminopyridine: a new drug tested in the treatment of Eaton-Lambert syndrome. *J. Neurol. Neurosurg. Psychiatry* 40: 1109–1112, 1977.

McAllister, R. E., Noble, D., and Tsien, R. W. Reconstruction of the electrical activity of cardiac Purkinje fibers. *J. Physiol. Lond.* 251: 1–59, 1975.

McLean, M. J., Bennett, P. B., and Thomas, R. M. Subtypes of dorsal root ganglion neurons based on different inward currents as measured by whole-cell voltage clamp. *Mol. Cell. Biochem.* 80: 95–107, 1988.

Murray, N. M. and Newsom-Davis, J. Treatment with oral 4-aminopyridine in disorders of neuromuscular transmission. *Neurology* 31: 265–271, 1981.

Neumcke, B. and Stämpfli, R. Sodium currents and sodium-current fluctuations in rat myelinated nerve fibres. *J. Physiol. Lond.* 329: 163–184, 1982.

Patlak, J. B. and Ortiz, M. Two modes of gating during late Na+ channel currents in frog sartorius muscle. *J. Gen. Physiol.* 87: 305–326, 1986.

Peyronnard, J. M. and Charron, L. Motor and sensory neurons of the rat sural nerve: a horseradish peroxidase study. *Muscle & Nerve* 5: 654–660, 1982.

Pongrácz, F., Waxman, S. G., Shepherd, G. M., and Kocsis, J. D. Slow sodium conductance in ionic control of conduction in myelinated axon: a computational model. *Soc. Neurosci. Abstr.* 17: 954, 1991.

Rizzo, M. A., Waxman, S. G., and Kocsis, J. D. Heterogeneity of voltage-dependent Na^+ conductance in dorsal root ganglion neurons of adult rat. *Soc. Neurosci. Abstr.* 19: 1528, 1993.

Roper, J. and Schwarz, J. R. Heterogeneous distribution of fast and slow potassium channels in myelinated rat nerve fibers. *J. Physiol. Lond.* 416: 93–110, 1989.

Roy, M. L. and Narahashi, T. Differential properties of tetrodotoxin-sensitive and tetrodotoxin-resistant sodium channels in rat dorsal root ganglion neurons. *J. Neurosci.* 12: 2104–2111, 1992.

Schmued, L. and Fallon, J. Fluoro-Gold: a new fluorescent retrograde axonal tracer with numerous unique properties. *Brain Res.* 377: 147–154, 1986.

Sigworth, F. J. Covariance of nonstationary sodium current fluctuations at the node of Ranvier. *Biophys. J.* 34: 111–133, 1981.

Stefoski, D., Davis, F. A., Faut, M., and Schauf, C. L. 4-Aminopyridine improves clinical signs in multiple sclerosis. *Ann. Neurol.* 21: 71–77, 1987.

Targ, E. F. and Kocsis, J. D. Action potential characteristics of demyelinated rat sciatic nerve following application of 4-aminopyridine. *Brain Res.* 363: 1–9, 1986.

Waxman, S. G. Conduction in myelinated, unmyelinated, and demyelinated fibers. *Arch. Neurol.* 34: 585–590, 1977.

Waxman, S. G. and Ritchie, J. M. Molecular dissection of the myelinated axon. *Ann. Neurol.* 33: 121–136, 1993.

26 Slow Closed-State Inactivation: A Novel Mechanism Underlying Ramp Currents in Cells Expressing the hNE/PN1 Sodium Channel

Theodore R. Cummins, James R. Howe, and Stephen G. Waxman

Abstract To better understand why sensory neurons express voltage-gated Na$^+$ channel isoforms that are different from those expressed in other types of excitable cells, we compared the properties of the hNE sodium channel [a human homolog of PN1, which is selectively expressed in dorsal root ganglion (DRG) neurons] with that of the skeletal muscle Na$^+$ channel (hSkM1) [both expressed in human embryonic kidney (HEK293) cells]. Although the voltage dependence of activation was similar, the inactivation properties were different. The V$_{1/2}$ for steady-state inactivation was slightly more negative, and the rate of open-state inactivation was ~50% slower for hNE. However, the greatest difference was that closed-state inactivation and recovery from inactivation were up to fivefold slower for hNE than for hSkM1 channels. TTX-sensitive (TTX-S) currents in small DRG neurons also have slow closed-state inactivation, suggesting that hNE/PN1 contributes to this TTX-S current. Slow ramp depolarizations (0.25 mV/msec) elicited TTX-S persistent currents in cells expressing hNE channels, and in DRG neurons, but not in cells expressing hSkM1 channels. We propose that slow closed-state inactivation underlies these ramp currents. This conclusion is supported by data showing that divalent cations such as Cd^{2+} and Zn^{2+} (50–200 μM) slowed closed-state inactivation and also dramatically increased the ramp currents for DRG TTX-S currents and hNE channels but not for hSkM1 channels. The hNE and DRG TTX-S ramp currents activated near −65 mV and therefore could play an important role in boosting stimulus depolarizations in sensory neurons. These results suggest that differences in the kinetics of closed-state inactivation may confer distinct integrative properties on different Na$^+$ channel isoforms.

One of the hallmarks of most excitable cells is the presence of voltage-gated sodium currents, which underlie the rapid action potentials characteristic of neurons and muscle cells. Nearly a dozen distinct voltage-gated sodium channels have been cloned from mammals (Black and

Reprinted with permission from *The Journal of Neuroscience* 18: 9607–9619, 1998.

Waxman, 1996). Many of these channels have specific developmental, tissue, or cellular distributions. Rat brain type III neuronal channels are primarily expressed early during development (Felts et al., 1997). Immunocytochemical experiments indicate that although rat brain type I (rbI) channels are concentrated in cell bodies, rat brain type II (rbII) channels may be preferentially targeted to neurites (Westenbroek et al., 1989). Other neuronal isoforms are predominantly expressed in peripheral tissues (Akopian et al., 1996; Felts et al., 1997; Toledo-Aral et al., 1997; Dib-Hajj et al., 1998).

It is becoming apparent that the different isoforms may also have distinct functional properties. For example, Smith and Goldin (1998) have shown that although rbI and rbII channels both encode fast sodium currents, the voltage dependence of activation and steady-state inactivation is significantly more positive for the rbI channels. Recent evidence indicates that the Na6 isoform underlies resurgent and subthreshold persistent sodium currents in cerebellar Purkinje cells (Raman and Bean, 1997). One of the isoforms primarily expressed in peripheral neurons such as dorsal root ganglion (DRG) neurons, SNS or PN3, encodes a TTX-resistant channel that has slow inactivation kinetics when expressed in *Xenopus* oocytes (Akopian et al., 1996; Sangameswaran et al., 1996). Another isoform that is also highly expressed in DRG neurons (hNE, NaS, or PN1) has been cloned from human (Klugbauer et al., 1995), rabbit (Belcher et al., 1995) and rat (Sangameswaran et al., 1997; Toledo-Aral et al., 1997) and encodes a TTX-sensitive (TTX-S) channel (Klugbauer et al., 1995).

The human homolog of this isoform, hNE, has been expressed in the mammalian human embryonic kidney cell line HEK293, but the initial characterization did not demonstrate any exceptional differences between hNE and other

TTX-S isoforms (Klugbauer et al., 1995). This isoform is particularly interesting because it is expressed in a majority of small DRG neurons (Black et al., 1996) and may be the predominant TTX-S channel in these sensory neurons. We (Cummins and Waxman, 1997) and others (Elliott and Elliott, 1993) have shown that the predominant TTX-S current in small DRG neurons from adult rats has slow repriming (recovery from inactivation) kinetics, much slower than those observed in adult CNS neurons (Costa, 1996) and axotomized DRG neurons (Cummins and Waxman, 1997). Therefore we were interested in determining whether the hNE sodium channel had slow repriming kinetics or other unique properties.

Materials and Methods

Transfection and Preparation of Stably Transfected Cell Lines

Transfections were performed using the calcium phosphate precipitation technique. HEK293 cells are grown under standard tissue culture conditions (5% CO_2; 37 °C) in DMEM supplemented with 10% fetal bovine serum. The calcium phosphate–DNA mixture was added to the cell culture medium and left for 15–20 hr, after which time the cells were washed with fresh medium. After 48 hr, antibiotic (G418, Geneticin; Life Technologies, Gaithersburg, MD) was added to select for neomycin-resistant cells. After 2–3 weeks in G418, colonies were picked, split, and subsequently tested for channel expression using whole-cell patch-clamp recording techniques.

Culture of Dorsal Root Ganglion Neurons

DRG cells were studied after short-term culture (12–24 hr). The culture was performed as previously described (Caffrey et al., 1992). Briefly, the L4 and L5 DRG ganglia were harvested from adult female Sprague Dawley rats. The DRG were treated with collagenase and papain, dissociated in DMEM and Ham's F12 medium supplemented with 10% fetal bovine serum, and plated on glass coverslips. Recordings were made within 24 hr of dissociation.

Whole-cell Patch-clamp Recordings

Whole-cell patch-clamp recordings were conducted at room temperature (~21 °C) using an EPC-9 amplifier. Data were acquired on a Macintosh Quadra 950 computer using the Pulse program (version 7.89; HEKA Electronic). Fire-polished electrodes (0.8–1.5 MΩ) were fabricated from 1.65 mm Corning 7052 capillary glass using a Sutter P-97 puller (Novato, CA). To minimize space-clamp problems, we selected for recording only isolated cells with a soma diameter of <25 μm. Cells were not considered for analysis if the initial seal resistance was <5 GΩ or if they had high leakage currents (holding current >0.1 nA at −80 mV), membrane blebs, or an access resistance >4 MΩ. The average access resistance was 2.3 ± 0.6 MΩ (mean ± SD; $n = 116$) for cells expressing hNE channels and 2.3 ± 0.6 MΩ ($n = 52$) for cells expressing hSkM1 channels. Voltage errors were minimized using 80% series resistance compensation, and the capacitance artifact was canceled using the computer-controlled circuitry of the patch-clamp amplifier. Linear leak subtraction, based on resistance estimates from four to five hyperpolarizing pulses applied before the depolarizing test potential, was used for all voltage-clamp recordings. Membrane currents were usually filtered at 2.5 kHz and sampled at 10 kHz. The pipette solution contained (in mM): 140 CsF, 1 EGTA, 10 NaCl, and 10 HEPES, pH 7.3. The standard bathing solution was (in mM): 140 NaCl, 3 KCl, 1 $MgCl_2$, 1 $CaCl_2$, and 10 HEPES, pH 7.3. The liquid junction potential for these solutions was <8 mV; data were not corrected to account for this offset. The osmolarity of all solutions was adjusted to 310 mOsm (Wescor 5500 osmometer, Logan, UT). The offset potential was zeroed before patching the cells and checked after each recording for drift; if the drift was >10 mV per hour, the recording was discarded.

Data Analysis

Data were analyzed using the Pulsefit (HEKA Electronic) and Origin (Microcal Software, Northampton, MA) software programs. Unless otherwise noted, statistical significance was determined by $p < 0.05$ using an unpaired t test. Results are presented as mean $\pm$ SEM, and error bars in the figures represent SEs. The curves in the figures are drawn to guide the eye unless otherwise noted. Time course data were fitted with single-exponential functions. Although in some instances fitting to a dual exponential would improve the overall fit, the second component was typically small (<10%), and the predominant component was not much different from that estimated with the single-exponential fits.

Results

Sodium Current Activation

To compare the properties of the hNE (Klugbauer et al., 1995) and hSkM1 (George et al., 1992) sodium channels, we created HEK293 cell lines that stably expressed the hNE and hSkM1 channels. Fast-inactivating TTX-S sodium currents were observed in cells transfected with hNE and hSkM1 channels (figure 26.1A). Figure 26.1B shows that the current–voltage (I–V) curve for the peak sodium current was similar for hNE and hSkM1 channels. The midpoint of activation was -25.8 ± 0.8 mV (mean $\pm$ SE; $n = 45$) for hNE currents and -27.0 ± 0.8 mV ($n = 31$) for hSkM1 currents.

Other parameters relating to activation were also examined. The time course of activation, estimated using a Hodgkin and Huxley fit of currents elicited with a step depolarization to -30 mV, was similar for hNE channels ($\tau_m =$

303 ± 17 μsec; $n = 25$) and hSkM1 channels ($\tau_m = 289 \pm 23$ μsec; $n = 20$). Deactivation kinetics was examined at potentials ranging from -120 to -50 mV after a short (0.5 msec) activating pulse (see figure 26.1C, *current traces*). Figure 26.1C shows that the time constants for deactivation were also similar for hNE and hSkM1 channels. Resurgent currents such as those reported by Raman et al. (1997) in Purkinje neurons were not observed in HEK293 cells expressing either hNE or hSkM1 channels. Noninactivating currents, defined as the residual current measured at 100 msec during a step depolarization to 0 mV, were small for both hNE channels ($0.1 \pm 0.1\%$ of peak; $n = 23$) and hSkM1 channels ($0.1 \pm 0.1\%$ of peak; $n = 17$).

Steady-state Inactivation and Inactivation Kinetics

Although the activation kinetics is similar for hNE and hSkM1 currents, figure 26.2A shows that the decay phase is slower for the hNE current. The rate of inactivation was quantified by fitting the decay phase of the macroscopic current with a single-exponential function. The time constants estimated from these fits are plotted as a function of the test potentials in figure 26.2B. The time constants were greater for hNE currents than for hSkM1 channels over the entire voltage range from -50 to $+30$ mV. At 0 mV, for example, hNE currents inactivated with a time constant of 0.77 ± 0.03 msec ($n = 10$), and hSkM1 channels inactivated with a time constant of 0.51 ± 0.05 msec ($n = 10$). This difference was statistically significant ($p < 0.01$).

The voltage dependence of steady-state inactivation (h_∞) was examined by holding the cells at prepulse potentials between -130 and -10 mV for 500 msec before stepping to the test potential (-10 mV) for 20 msec. The h_∞ curves are plotted in figure 26.2C. The midpoint of the h_∞ curve was significantly ($p < 0.001$) more negative for hNE channels (-78 ± 1 mV; $n = 45$) than for hSkM1 channels (-72 ± 1 mV; $n = 31$).

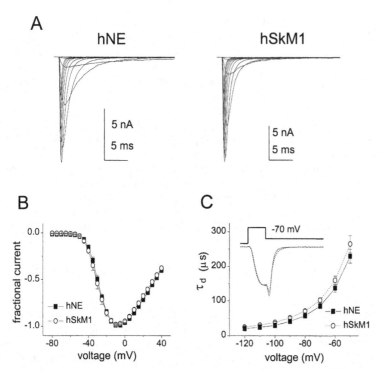

Figure 26.1

hNE and hSkM1 channels have similar activation properties. (*A*) Family of *traces* from representative HEK293 cells expressing either hNE channels (*left*) or hSkM1 channels (*right*). The currents were elicited by 40 msec test pulses to various potentials from −60 to 30 mV. Cells were held at −100 mV. (*B*) Normalized peak current-voltage relationship for hNE (filled squares; n = 14) and hSkM1 (open circles; n = 12). (*C*) The deactivation time course of hNE and hSkM1 channels examined at potentials ranging from −120 to −50 mV after a 0.5 msec activation pre-pulse to 0 mV. Deactivation time constants were obtained from single-exponential fits to the tail currents for hNE (filled squares; n = 16) or hSkM1 (open circles; n = 12) channels. Inset. Traces showing representative hNE (solid line) and hSkM1 (dotted line) deactivation tail currents at −70 mV.

Because TTX-S currents in DRG neurons recover relatively slowly from inactivation and because hNE transcripts are detected in the majority of DRG neurons (Black et al., 1996), we wanted to compare the time course for recovery from inactivation for hNE and hSkM1 channels. Recovery was examined after 20 msec inactivating pulses at −20 mV (protocol shown in figure 26.3*A*). We used 20 msec inactivating prepulses to allow complete fast inactivation without inducing slow inactivation. Similar

results were also obtained with 5 and 100 msec inactivating prepulses (data not shown). Figure 26.3*A* shows currents from a representative hNE cell and hSkM1 cell illustrating recovery at −80 mV. Although only ∼50% of the hNE current has recovered after 100 msec at −80 mV, virtually all of the hSkM1 current has recovered at this time. In general, the time course for recovery from inactivation for both hNE and hSkM1 currents could be fitted well with a single-exponential function. The average recovery time course at −80 mV for hNE and hSkM1 currents is shown in figure 26.3*B*. The time constant for recovery of hNE channels ($\tau = 104 \pm 8$ msec; $n = 12$) was more than sixfold greater than the corresponding time constant for hSkM1 channels ($\tau = 16 \pm 4$ msec; $n = 11$).

We also compared the time course for the development of inactivation of hNE and hSkM1 channels. The protocol for these experiments is shown at the *top* of figure 26.3*C*. Cells were stepped to the inactivation potential (from a holding potential of −100 mV) for increasing durations and then steeped to the test potential (−20 mV) to measure the fraction of current remaining available. Figure 26.3*C* shows representative currents illustrating the development of inactivation at −80 mV for hNE and hSkM1 channels. Although less than one-half of the hNE inactivation has occurred after the 100 msec inactivating pulse (at −80 mV), hSkM1 inactivation is nearly complete at this time point. The average time course for development of inactivation at −80 mV from 12 hNE and 11 hSkM1 cells is shown in figure 26.3*D*. The data from these cells were fitted well with a single-exponential function, and the time constant was almost five-

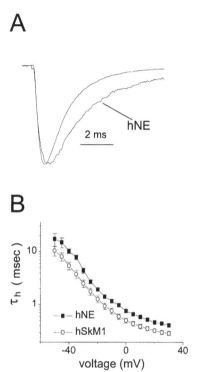

A

hNE

2 ms

B

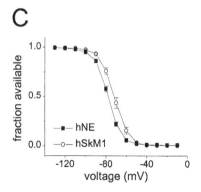

τ_h (msec)

10

1

—■— hNE

—○— hSkM1

-40   0   40

voltage (mV)

C

fraction available

1.0

0.5

0.0

—■— hNE

—○— hSkM1

-120   -80   -40   0

voltage (mV)

Figure 26.2
hNE and hSkM1 channels have distinct inactivation properties. (*A*) Representative currents from whole-cell recordings of a cell expressing hNE channels (trace labeled *hNE*) and a cell expressing hSkM1 channels (unlabeled trace). Currents were elicited by a step de-

polarization to −30 mV from a holding potential of −100 mV and were scaled for comparison. The hNE current decays more slowly than does the hSkM1 current. (*B*) Inactivation kinetics as a function of voltage. The macroscopic decay time constant is greater for hNE currents filled squares; n = 10) than for hSkM1 currents (open circles; n = 10) at each voltage. Time constants were estimated from single-exponential fits to the decay phase of currents elicited by 100 msec step depolarizations to the indicated potential. (*C*) Comparison of hNE (filled squares; n = 13) and hSkM1 (open circles; n = 12) steady-state inactivation. Steady-state inactivation was estimated by measuring the peak current amplitude elicited by 20 msec test pulses to −10 mV after 500 msec prepulses to potentials over the range of −130 to −10 mV. Current is plotted as a fraction of the maximum peak current.

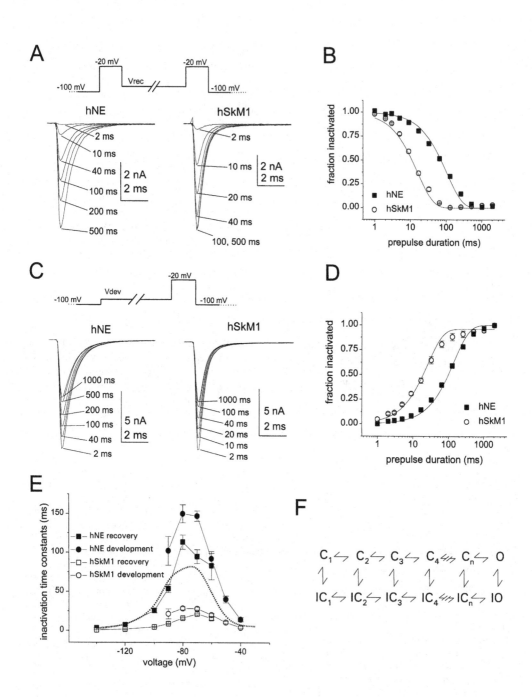

fold greater for hNE channels ($\tau = 144 \pm$ 11 msec; $n = 12$) than for hSkM1 channels ($\tau = 26 \pm 7$ msec; $n = 11$).

The time course for recovery from inactivation was measured at voltages ranging from -140 to -60 mV, and the time course for development of inactivation was measured from -90 to -40 mV for both hNE and hSkM1. At most voltages both the rate of recovery from inactivation and the development of inactivation were much slower for hNE channels (figure 26.3E). The time constants for inactivation of hNE currents are similar to those measured for the TTX-S currents in small DRG neurons (figure 26.3E, *dotted curve*) (Cummins and Waxman, 1997). By contrast, the predominant time constants measured for cloned rbII channels (Sakar et al., 1995) and the sodium currents in adult hippocampal neurons (Costa, 1996) are similar to those for the hSkM1 channels.

The difference between hNE and hSkM1 inactivation kinetics can be considered in the context of a simple multistate sodium channel gating scheme (Vandenberg and Bezanilla, 1991; Kuo and Bean, 1994) such as that shown in figure 26.3F. This model has multiple closed states leading to the open state. Channels progress through these closed states during depolarization. In this model, inactivation can occur from any of the closed states as well as from the open state. The rate of macroscopic inactivation at potentials positive to -20 mV is thought primarily to reflect inactivation of channels in the open state. The results shown in figure 26.2B thus suggest that open-state inactivation is $\sim$50% slower for hNE channels than it is for hSkM1 channels. At potentials less than -60 mV, at which the probability of channel opening is very low, inactivation would occur primarily from the closed states. The time course for the develop-

Figure 26.3
Recovery from inactivation and development of inactivation are slower for hNE channels than for hSkM1 channels. (*A*) Family of current traces from cells expressing hNE or hSkM1 currents showing the rate of recovery from inactivation at -80 mV. The standard recovery from inactivation voltage protocol is shown above the current traces. The cells were prepulsed to -20 mV for 20 msec to inactivate all of the current and then brought back to -80 mV for increasing recovery durations before the test pulse to -20 mV. The maximum pulse rate was 0.5 Hz. (*B*) Time course for recovery from inactivation of peak currents at -80 mV. Recovery is much slower for hNE (filled squares; $n = 12$) than for hSkM1 (open circles; $n = 11$) currents. The solid curves show single-exponential functions fitted to the data, with time constants of 104 msec (hNE) and 16 msec (hSkM1). The data are plotted on a logarithmic time axis to allow comparison of the disparate time courses. (*C*) Family of current traces from cells expressing hNE and hSkM1 currents showing the rate of development of inactivation at -80 mV. The standard development of inactivation voltage protocol is shown above the current traces. From a holding potential of -100 mV, the cells were prepulsed to -80 mV for increasing durations and then stepped to -20 mV to determine the fraction of current inactivated during the prepulse. (*D*) Time course for development of inactivation for the peak current. Inactivation develops more slowly at -80 mV for hNE channels (filled squares; $n = 12$) than for hSkM1 channels (open circles; $n = 11$). The solid curves are single-exponential functions fitted to the data, with time constants of 144 msec (hNE) and 26 msec (hSkM1). (*E*) The time constants for recovery from inactivation (squares) and development of inactivation (circles) plotted as a function of voltage. Time constants were estimated from single-exponential fits to time courses measured with the protocols shown in (*A*) and (*C*) for cells expressing hNE channels (filled symbols; $n = 15$) and hSkM1 channels (open symbols; $n = 11$). For comparison the inactivation time constants for the TTX-S current in small DRG neurons are shown (dotted curve). (*F*) Basic multistate gating scheme for sodium channel activation and fast inactivation. Closed states are indicated by Cs, inactivated closed states are indicated by ICs, the open state is indicated by O, and the inactivated open state is indicated by IO. At very negative potentials, channels reside in the leftmost closed state, and with depolarization the channels progress toward the open state. Channels can inactivate from any state.

ment of inactivation between −90 to −60 mV was much slower for hNE than for hSkM1 channels, and therefore our data indicate that closed-state inactivation is relatively slow for hNE channels.

Recovery from inactivation was also relatively slow for hNE currents compared with hSkM1 currents. However, although the inactivation time constants were dramatically different for hNE and hSkM1 currents, we observed a discrepancy between the rate for development of inactivation and the rate for recovery from inactivation when measured at the same potential (from −90 to −60 mV). This discrepancy was observed for both hNE and hSkM1 currents (figure 26.3E). At −80 mV, for example, recovery from inactivation was ~30% faster than was development of inactivation for hNE channels. Similarly, for hSkM1 channels recovery from inactivation at −80 mV was ~40% faster than was development of inactivation at −80 mV. This discrepancy is not completely unexpected, because the development of inactivation and recovery from inactivation protocols examine distinct processes. Although development of inactivation at −80 mV exclusively involves closed-state inactivation, recovery from inactivation, also measured at −80 mV, follows a 20 msec depolarizing step, during which a significant proportion of the channels inactivate from the open state. Thus recovery involves both open-state and closed-state inactivation (Aldrich et al., 1983). Interestingly, although the values for development of inactivation and for recovery from inactivation differed, the values did not differ markedly, and both processes could be reasonably well fit with a single exponential (figure 26.3B, D). Kuo and Bean (1994) reported that most sodium channels probably must close (i.e., make the IO to IC transition) before recovering from inactivation. Thus the rate of recovery from inactivation also probably reflects primarily the rate of channel transition between the closed-inactivated and closed states.

Functional Significance of Slow Recovery from Inactivation

The slow rate for development of closed-state inactivation and recovery from inactivation in hNE channels is intriguing, especially because it is so pronounced at voltages near the typical resting potential for neurons. Slower recovery from inactivation should decrease the maximum firing frequency. Figure 26.4 shows that during a 50 Hz pulse train the current amplitude remains much higher for cells expressing hSkM1 channels (figure 26.4A) than for cells expressing hNE channels (figure 26.4B). Although 45 ± 16% of the peak current remains available for the second pulse and 36 ± 17% remains for the 50th pulse for hSkM1 channels ($n = 8$), only 23 ± 8 and 10 ± 5% remain available for the second and 50th pulses, respectively, for hNE channels ($n = 12$). The lower availability for hNE channels occurs even though macroscopic inactivation is ~50% slower for hNE channels and more hSkM1 channels presumably inactivate during the 2 msec step depolarizations. Thus, because hNE channels reprime more slowly than do hSkM1 channels, a cell expressing a pure population of hNE channels should not be capable of the high firing frequencies that might be expected in a cell expressing hSkM1 channels. The firing rate is limited by the repriming rate, which probably reflects the frequency of transitions between the closed-inactivated and closed states.

Functional Significance of Slow Development of Inactivation

The slow rate for the development of closed-state inactivation in hNE channels can also have important consequences. Because closed-state inactivation occurs so slowly, especially at voltages from −90 to −50 mV, short prepulses are not sufficient to reach steady-state conditions for hNE channels. For example, a 50 msec prepulse to −80 mV only allows 30% of the channels to

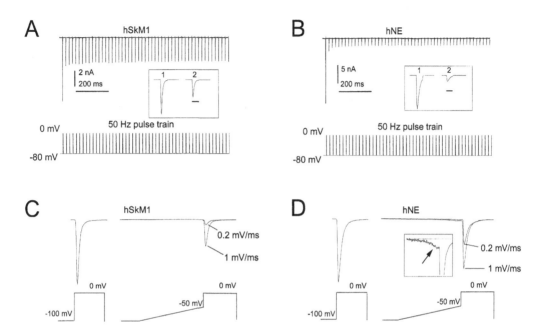

Figure 26.4

Functional consequences of slow closed-state inactivation. (*A*) The sodium currents elicited in a cell expressing hSkM1 channels by a 50 Hz pulse train. The cell, held at −80 mV, was depolarized to 0 mV for 2 msec every 20 msec during the 1 sec pulse train. (*Inset*) Currents elicited by the first and second depolarizations on an expanded time scale (calibration bar, 2 msec). The current elicited by the second pulse is approximately one-half the amplitude of the current elicited by the first pulse. (*B*) The sodium currents elicited in a cell expressing hNE channels by a 50 Hz pulse train. Details are as described in (*A*). The current elicited by the second pulse is much smaller than that elicited by the first pulse. (*C*) Comparison of hSkM1 current elicited by a step depolarization to 0 mV from −100 mV (left trace) with the hSkM1 current elicited by a step depolarization from −50 mV that was preceded by a slow ramp depolarization from −100 to −50 mV (right traces). The voltage protocol is shown below the current traces. Two different ramp speeds were used: 1 mV/msec (50 msec total duration) and 0.2 mV/msec (250 msec total duration). After the 50 msec ramp, less than one-half of the current remains available for activation, and after the 250 msec ramp, only ~10% of the current is available. (*D*) Currents elicited by the voltage protocols detailed in *C* in a cell expressing hNE channels. After the 50 msec ramp, much of the hNE current remains available for activation, and after the 250 msec ramp, more than one-third of the current is still available. (*Inset*) The end of the 50 msec ramp depolarization at higher gain. The arrow indicates a region where the ramp depolarization elicits an inward current before the step depolarization.

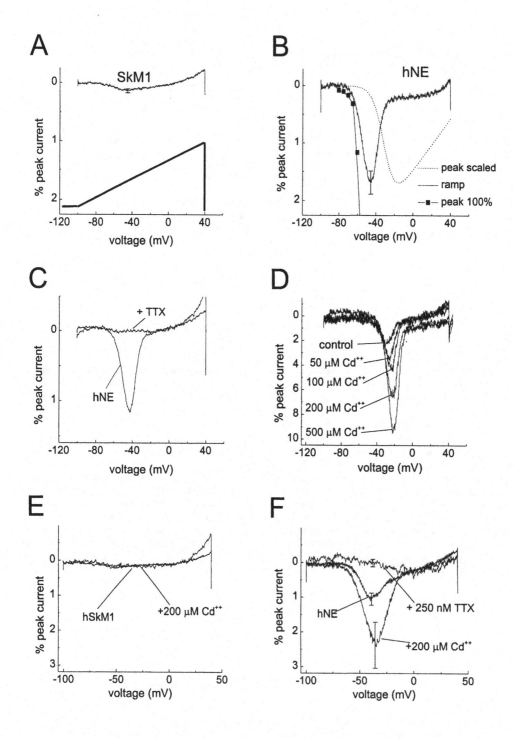

inactivate, compared with 97% for a 500 msec prepulse. As a consequence of this, if "steady-state inactivation" is measured using 50 msec prepulses, the estimated midpoint of the h_∞ curve is significantly more positive for hNE channels (-56 ± 2 mV) than for hSkM1 channels (-70 ± 1 mV).

Based on this observation, we predicted that a large fraction of hNE channels, but not hSkM1 channels, would remain available for activation during slow ramp depolarizations. To test this, cells were slowly depolarized from -100 to -50 mV and then stepped to 0 mV to determine how much current remained available for activation. For hSkM1 channels (figure 26.4C), $37 \pm 19\%$ ($n = 9$) of the current remained available after a 50 msec (1 mV/msec) ramp, and only $10 \pm 12\%$ remained after a 250 msec (0.2 mV/msec) ramp. In contrast, significantly more current remained available for hNE channels (figure 26.4D), with $76 \pm 10\%$ ($n = 14$) of the current available after the 50 msec ramp and $36 \pm 13\%$ still available after the 250 msec ramp. Thus, although neurons expressing faster re-priming channels may be capable of firing at higher frequencies, neurons expressing hNE channels should be able to generate action potentials in response to slowly rising inputs that do not elicit a regenerative response in neurons expressing channels with fast closed-state inactivation.

Slow Ramp Currents Can Be Evoked in hNE Channels

As can be seen in the inset in figure 26.4D, during some of the ramp and step experiments on cells expressing hNE channels, a small inward current was observed during the slow ramp. This was further examined using extended ramp depolarizations that ranged from -100 to 40 mV. These slow ramps (0.23 mV/msec) elicited little or no current in cells expressing hSkM1 channels (figure 26.5A), but prominent currents were evoked in cells expressing hNE channels (figure 26.5B). The hNE ramp currents were $1.7 \pm 0.2\%$ ($n = 11$) of the peak current amplitude (obtained in response to stimulation with step depolariza-

Figure 26.5
Characterization of ramp currents. Ramp currents were examined using 600 msec voltage ramps from -100 to $+40$ mV ($\sim$0.23 mV/msec). (A) The average ramp current recorded in cells expressing hSkM1 channels (n = 12). The *thick solid line* at the *bottom* illustrates the ramp voltage protocol. The ramp current is plotted as a percentage of the peak sodium current elicited with step depolarizations from -100 mV. The error bar indicates the SE at -45 mV. (B) The average ramp current recorded in cells expressing hNE channels (n = 11). The ramp current is plotted as a percentage of the peak sodium current elicited with step depolarizations from -100 mV. The error bar indicates the SE at -45 mV. The *dotted curve* shows the averaged current-voltage (I–V) relationship for the peak current elicited with step depolarizations in these cells scaled to the amplitude of the ramp current. The filled squares show the peak I–V data at full scale. Only the foot of the curve can be seen at this scale. The step depolarizations to -60 mV elicited $\sim$1.2% of the current elicited by the step depolarizations to -15 mV. (C) Current traces elicited in an hNE cell by 600 msec ramps. The current (plotted as a percentage of peak current) is shown before and after the addition of 250 nM TTX to the extracellular solution. TTX blocks the ramp current. (D) Current *traces* elicited in an hNE cell by 600 msec ramps shown before and after the addition of increasing concentrations of cadmium (50–500 μM Cd^{2+}) to the extracellular solution. Cadmium increases the amplitude of the ramp current in hNE cells. (E) The average currents elicited by 600 msec ramps in cells expressing hSkM1 channels shown before and after addition of 200 μM cadmium to the extracellular solution (n = 4). Cadmium does not induce hSkM1 ramp currents. (F) The average currents elicited by 600 msec ramps in cells expressing hNE channels shown before and after addition of 200 μM cadmium to the extracellular solution (n = 5). Cadmium increased the amplitude of the ramp current by $\sim$150%, and all of the ramp current in cadmium was blocked by 250 nM TTX. Error bars indicate SE at -40 mV.

tions to −10 mV) and, when compared with the scaled peak current–voltage relationship, reach maximal amplitude at potentials ∼20 mV more negative than the peak currents (figure 26.5B). This type of ramp current, often referred to as "subthreshold" or persistent current, has been recorded in several different types of neurons (Stafstrom et al., 1985; Brown et al., 1994; Cepeda et al., 1995; Chao and Alzheimer, 1995; Fleidervish and Gutnick, 1996; Pennartz et al., 1997; Raman and Bean, 1997; Feigenspan et al., 1998; Parri and Crunelli, 1998). It has been proposed that, because neuronal ramp currents occur near resting potentials and are often larger than other voltage-gated currents at these potentials, ramp currents may significantly influence excitability (Crill, 1996). Indeed, it has been shown that persistent sodium currents in the dendrites of neocortical neurons can help boost transmission of synaptic depolarizations (Schwindt and Crill, 1995).

The narrow voltage range in which hNE ramp currents are recorded is very similar to that for ramp currents recorded in neurons. The mechanism underlying the distinct voltage dependence of neuronal ramp currents has not been completely understood. Because ramp currents seem to be activated at more negative potentials than the currents elicited with step depolarizations, it has been suggested that distinct channel populations might underlie ramp currents and transient currents in neurons. In the HEK293 cells the ramp and transient currents are probably generated by the same channel isoform. Indeed, the apparent difference in voltage dependence, at least for hNE channels, is an artifact that results from the scaling of the peak current–voltage curve to the size of the ramp current. The ramp current at −55 mV and the peak current elicited with a step depolarization to −55 mV are both ∼1% of the maximum peak current (measured with step depolarizations). When the peak current data are plotted at full scale (figure 26.5B, solid squares), it is clear that the foot of the peak

current–voltage relationship closely matches the voltage dependence of the onset of the ramp current.

Our data indicate that the ramp currents are observed at −60 mV because hNE channels, with slow closed-state inactivation kinetics, do not all inactivate during slow ramps and therefore some remain available for activation. Conversely, although a step depolarization to −55 mV activates $1.9 \pm 0.6\%$ ($n = 10$) of the peak current for hSkM1 channels, almost no hSkM1 current is observed during slow ramp depolarizations because the hSkM1 channels undergo rapid closed-state inactivation and are inactivated during slow depolarizations before reaching the open state. The decay of the ramp currents at more depolarized voltages probably reflects channels undergoing open-state inactivation, which is still relatively fast in hNE channels. Therefore, our results suggest that the distinct voltage dependence of ramp currents does not necessarily arise from unique activation properties of the underlying sodium channels but rather from their distinctive inactivation kinetics.

hNE Ramp Currents Are Differentially Sensitive to TTX and Cadmium

To confirm that the ramp currents recorded in hNE cells were sodium currents, we tested the pharmacology of the ramp currents with nanomolar concentrations of TTX, which blocks hNE channels, and micromolar concentrations of cadmium, which does not block hNE channels (Klugbauer et al., 1995) but does block voltage-gated calcium channels. Figure 26.5C shows that the hNE ramp currents were blocked by 250 nM TTX. The effect of cadmium on hNE ramp currents is illustrated in figure 26.5D. Surprisingly, cadmium increased the size of the ramp currents, at concentrations that are equal to or lower than those routinely used in the isolation of sodium currents (Brown et al., 1994; Cepeda et al., 1995; Fleidervish and Gutnick, 1996; Pennartz et al.,

1997; Raman and Bean, 1997; Parri and Cru-nelli, 1998). In five cells expressing hNE chan-nels, 200 μM cadmium increased the size of the ramp currents by 160 ± 17%, and the total ramp current was also blocked by TTX (figure 26.5F). By contrast, cadmium did not induce ramp cur-rents in cells expressing hSkM1 channels (figure 26.5E).

To understand how cadmium increased ramp currents, we examined the effect of cadmium on the other properties of hNE and hSkM1 currents. Cadmium (200 μM) had little effect on hNE peak current amplitude, which was de-creased by 5 ± 5% (n = 8). Cadmium also did not significantly alter noninactivating hNE cur-rents (0.35 ± 0.16% of peak, control; 0.29 ± 0.14% in 200 μM Cd^{2+}; n = 6), measured at 100 msec during a step depolarization to 0 mV. The midpoints of activation (−27 ± 2 mV, control; −27 ± 3 mV, cadmium; n = 8) and steady-state inactivation (−77 ± 3 mV, control; −74 ± 4 mV, cadmium; n = 8) for hNE currents were not significantly altered by 200 μM cad-mium. Similarly, cadmium did not alter these properties in hSkM1 channels (data not shown).

However, as can be seen in figure 26.6A, 200 μM cadmium did prolong the time course for the development of closed-state inactivation in hNE channels. In seven cells, 200 μM cadmium increased the time constant for the development of inactivation at −80 mV by 61 ± 17% and increased by time constant for recovery from inactivation at −80 mV by 46 ± 12%. These differences were significant (paired t test, p < 0.005). In contrast, 200 μM cadmium did not affect the time course for development of closed-state inactivation in hSkM1 channels (figure 26.6B). Even at higher concentrations (500 μM), cadmium had little effect on hSkM1 channels, increasing the time constant for the development of inactivation at −80 mV by only 7 ± 6% and the time constant for recovery from inactivation at −80 mV by only 6 ± 4%. Although figure 26.6C shows that even 100 μM cadmium greatly increased the inactivation time constants for

hNE channels at voltages ranging from −100 to −50 mV, figure 26.6D demonstrates that 500 μM cadmium had little effect on the inactivation time constants of hSkM1 channels in this voltage range. This demonstrates that the lack of effect of cadmium on hSkM1 channels was not simply a slight difference in sensitivity to cadmium. Interestingly, cadmium had no effect on the rate of decay of macroscopic currents (evoked by step depolarizations ranging from −30 to +30 mV) for either hNE channels (200 μM; figure 26.6E) or hSkM1 channels (500 μM; figure 26.6F). This indicates that cadmium primarily slows closed-state inactivation but not opens-state inac-tivation of hNE channels. This also provides additional evidence to support the hypothesis that slow closed-state inactivation of hNE chan-nels underlies the generation of ramp currents.

Some, but not all, divalent cations modulate hNE channels, and this is illustrated in figure 26.7. Zinc, like cadmium, increased hNE ramp currents (figure 26.7A) and also increased the in-activation time constants for closed-state inacti-vation at negative potentials (figure 26.7B). Cobalt (200 μM) had a slightly less pronounced effect (data not shown) than did cadmium and zinc, whereas barium (200 μM) had virtually no effect on hNE ramp currents (figure 26.7C) and on hNE inactivation time constants (figure 26.7D). These data also support the link between slow closed-state inactivation and the generation of ramp currents.

Ramp Currents and Slow Closed-state Inactivation in DRG Neurons

Because hNE is expressed in a majority of small DRG neurons (Black et al., 1996) and the TTX-S sodium current in small DRG neurons has slow closed-state inactivation kinetics (Elliott and Elliott, 1993; Cummins and Waxman, 1997), we tested whether cadmium also modu-lated DRG TTX-S currents. We used 100 μM cadmium for these experiments because this concentration was used in studies by others

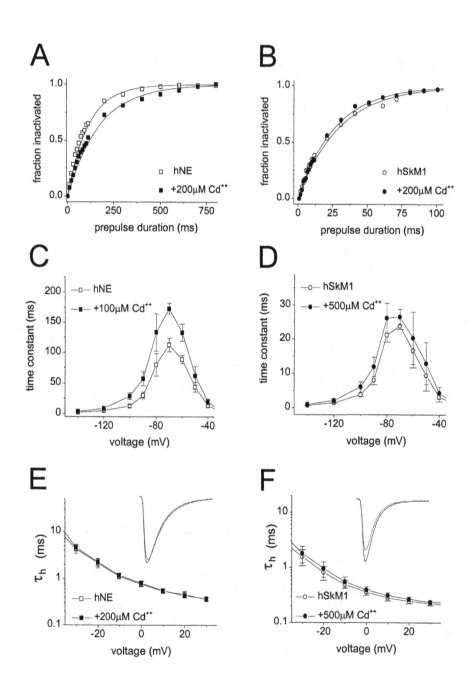

(Parri and Crunelli, 1998) and in our previous studies on repriming kinetics in small DRG neurons (Cummins and Waxman, 1997). Figure 26.8, *A* and *B*, shows that cadmium slowed the development of inactivation for the TTX-S current in small DRG neurons. Cadmium had a dramatic effect on the time constants of inactivation for DRG TTX-S channels at potentials ranging from −100 to −60 mV (figure 26.8*C*). Small DRG neurons also displayed ramp currents that were increased by cadmium and blocked by TTX (figure 27.8*D*). In four cells, 100 µM cadmium increased the amplitude of the ramp current by 45 ± 6%. The ramp current recorded in 100 µM cadmium was 1.9 ± 0.3% (*n* = 6) of the peak TTX-S fast sodium current in small DRG neurons, compared with 1.7 ± 0.2% (*n* = 9) for hNE ramp currents in 100 µM cadmium.

There is an apparent difference between the voltage dependence of DRG TTX-S peak current elicited with step depolarizations and that of the ramp current (figure 26.9*A*). However, as was shown for hNE currents in figure 26.5*B*, this apparent difference is an artifact that results from the scaling of the peak current curve to the size of the ramp currents. The *solid squares* in figure 26.9*A* show that when the peak current data are plotted at full scale, the threshold for activation of DRG TTX-S currents elicited with step depolarizations is similar to that for the DRG TTX-S ramp current. Although multiple sodium channels probably contribute to the excitability of DRG neurons, these data support the hypothesis that a single sodium channel isoform can underlie both a peak transient TTX-S current and a TTX-S ramp current and argue against the need to invoke multiple channel populations to account for these currents. Figure 26.9*B* shows that the voltage dependences of the TTX-S ramp and peak currents in small DRG neurons were nearly identical to those of the hNE currents recorded in HEK293 cells under the same conditions. This is consistent with the

Figure 26.6
Cadmium modulates closed-state inactivation in hNE but not in hSkM1 channels. (*A*) Cadmium slows the development of sodium current inactivation in a cell expressing hNE channels. The time course for development of inactivation at −80 mV is shown before (open squares) and after (filled squares) addition of 200 µM Cd^{2+} to the extracellular solution. The solid curves are single-exponential functions fit to the hNE data before ($\tau = 96$ msec) and after ($\tau = 155$ msec) cadmium. (*B*) Cadmium does not slow the development of sodium current inactivation in a cell expressing hSkM1 channels. The time course for development of inactivation at −80 mV is shown before (open circles; $\tau = 29$ msec) and after (filled circles; $\tau = 26$ msec) addition of 200 µM Cd^{2+} to the extracellular solution. Please note the difference in the *x*-axis scales between (*A*) and (*B*). (*C*) The inactivation time constants between −140 and −40 mV for Na^+ currents in cells expressing hNE cells (*n* = 5) are shown before (open squares) and after (filled squares) addition of 100 µM Cd^{2+} to the extracellular solution. At voltages at which both development of inactivation and recovery from inactivation were measured (i.e., between −60 and −90 mV), the inactivation time constant was estimated by averaging the development of inactivation and recovery from inactivation time constants. (*D*) The inactivation time constants between −140 and −40 mV for Na^+ currents in cells expressing hSkM1 cells (n = 4) are shown before (open circles) and after (filled circles) addition of 500 µM Cd^{2+} to the extracellular solution. Note the difference in the *y*-axis scales between (*C*) and (*D*). (*E*) The inactivation time constants for open-state inactivation (τ_h) measured from single-exponential fits to the decay of currents elicited by step depolarizations to voltages between −30 and +30 mV for Na^+ currents in cells expressing hNE channels (*n* = 6) are shown before (open squares) and after (filled squares) addition of 200 µM Cd^{2+} to the extracellular solution. (*Inset*) Current traces are from a representative hNE cell before (solid trace) and after (dashed trace) cadmium. (*F*) Plots of τ_h measured at voltages between −30 and +30 mV for Na^+ currents in cells expressing hSkM1 channels (n = 4) are shown before (open circles) and after (filled circles) addition of 500 µM Cd^{2+} to the extracellular solution. *Inset*, Current *traces* are from a representative hSkM1 cell before (solid trace) and after (dashed trace) cadmium.

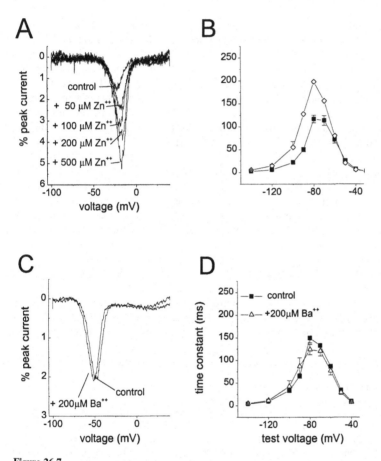

Figure 26.7

Zinc, but not barium, also modulates hNE closed-state inactivation and increases hNE ramp currents. (*A*) Current traces elicited in an hNE cell by 600 msec ramps are shown before and after the addition of increasing concentrations of zinc (50–500 μM) to the extracellular solution. Zinc increases the amplitude of the ramp current in hNE cells. (*B*) The inactivation time constants between −140 and −40 mV for Na⁺ currents in cells expressing hNE cells (n = 4) are shown before (filled squares) and after (open diamonds) addition of 100 μM Zn^{2+} to the extracellular solution. (*C*) Currents elicited by 600 msec ramps in an hNE cell are shown before and after addition of 200 μM barium to the extracellular solution. Barium does not increase hNE ramp currents (n = 4). (*D*) The inactivation time constants between −140 and −40 mV for Na⁺ currents in cells expressing hNE (n = 6) are shown before (filled squares) and after (open triangles) addition of 200 μM Ba^{2+} to the extracellular solution.

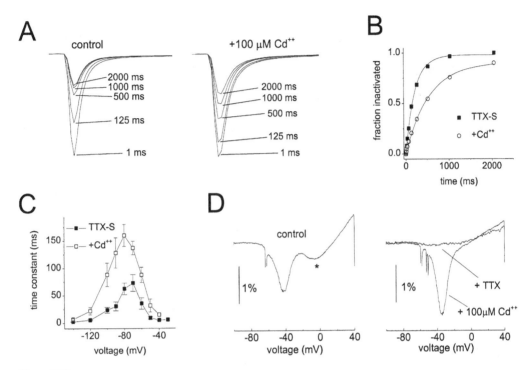

Figure 26.8
Cadmium modulates closed-state inactivation and ramp currents in DRG neurons. (*A*) Families of current *traces* from a small DRG neuron (21 μm in diameter) before (*left*) and after (*right*) application of 100 μM Cd^{2+} to the extracellular solution show that the rate of development of inactivation at −80 mV is slowed by Cd^{2+}. The TTX-S peak current amplitude was 98% of the total peak current amplitude in this cell. (*B*) Time course for development of inactivation of the peak current before (filled squares) and after (open circles) application of 100 μM Cd^{2+}. Data are from the currents shown in (*A*). (*C*) The inactivation time constants between −140 and −40 mV for TTX-S Na^+ currents in small (18–25 μm) DRG neurons from adult rats (n = 6) are shown before (filled squares) and after (*open squares*) addition of 100 μM Cd^{2+} to the extracellular solution. Data were obtained with the same two-pulse protocol described in figure 26.3*C*. The TTX-S peak current amplitude was 75 ± 4% (n = 6) of the total peak current amplitude for these cells. (*D*) Ramp current recorded in a small DRG neuron before (*left*) and after (*right*) addition of 100 μM Cd^{2+} to the extracellular solution. Cd^{2+} increases the ramp current component that peaks near −40 mV. This component is blocked by 250 nM TTX (*right*). A second component (*left*; marked by the asterisk) is apparently blocked by Cd^{2+} and may therefore be a calcium current. The ramp, which extended from −100 to +40 mV, was 600 msec long. The scale bar indicates the percentage of the peak current amplitude measured with a step depolarization to −10 mV.

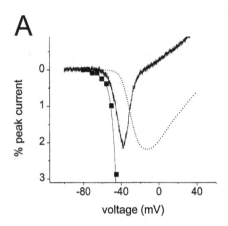

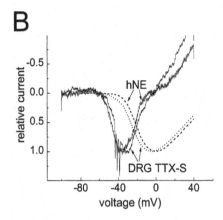

Figure 26.9
The thresholds for activation of ramp currents and peak transient currents are similar. (*A*) The ramp current recorded in a small DRG neuron expressing predominantly TTX-S sodium current. The ramp current is plotted as a percentage of the peak sodium current elicited with step depolarizations from −100 mV. The dotted curve shows the current-voltage (*I–V*) relationship for the peak current elicited with step depolarizations in this cell scaled to the amplitude of the ramp current. The filled squares show the peak *I–V* data at full scale; only the foot of the curve can be seen at this scale. The ramp, which extended from −100 to +40 mV, was 600 msec long. The access resistance for this cell was 2 MΩ, and 80% series resistance compen-

data indicating that the hNE transcript is expressed in a majority of small neurons. Because hNE channels and DRG TTX-S currents both exhibit slow closed-state inactivation and because cadmium can modulate closed-state inactivation and increase ramp currents in both DRG neurons and in HEK293 cells expressing hNE channels, a similar mechanism probably underlies the ramp currents in both preparations.

Discussion

We have compared the functional properties of hNE and hSkM1 sodium channels expressed in HEK293 cells. Our data show that although the voltage dependences of activation and steady-state inactivation are similar for hNE and hSkM1 channels, hNE channels display slower open-state inactivation, slower closed-state inactivation, and slower recovery from inactivation than do hSkM1 channels. We also observed relatively large TTX-sensitive currents during ramp depolarizations in cells expressing hNE, but not hSkM1, channels.

Mechanism Underlying hNE Ramp Currents

Our results indicate that ramp currents arise in hNE channels because the hNE channels have slow closed-state inactivation. Closed-state inactivation and recovery from inactivation were up

sation was used. (*B*) Comparison of ramp currents in small DRG neurons that expressed predominantly TTX-S currents (n = 5) and in HEK293 cells expressing hNE channels (n = 9). The currents, elicited with 600 msec ramps that extended from −100 to +40 mV, were normalized for comparison of voltage dependence. The peak current-voltage curves (dotted and dashed lines) for the cells from which the ramp currents were recorded are also shown. Note that both the DRG TTX-S and the hNE ramp currents reach maximum amplitude ∼20 mV more negative than did the peak currents.

to 500% slower for hNE channels than for hSkM1 channels. Because closed-state inactivation develops much more slowly for hNE than for hSkM1 channels, hNE channels are less likely to inactivate during slow subthreshold depolarizations and are more likely to be available to open when the voltage reaches threshold. This mechanism is consistent with the voltage dependence of the ramp currents. As figure 26.5B shows, the ramp currents and the currents elicited with step depolarizations have similar thresholds.

Although the generation of ramp currents by slow closed-state inactivation can be described by a model such as that shown in figure 26.3F, it should be noted that this model is probably incomplete. For example, hNE channels also display slow inactivation (data not shown), a kinetically and functionally distinct process from fast inactivation. TTX-S currents in rabbit Schwann cells (from which NaS, the rabbit ortholog of hNE, was cloned) exhibit at least three kinetically distinct types of inactivation (Howe and Ritchie, 1992). Therefore it is likely that hNE, PN1, and NaS exhibit complex inactivation characteristics in addition to the distinctive closed-state inactivation properties described here.

Our data do not eliminate the possibility that persistent currents can also arise from other sodium channel isoforms or from different mechanisms. Several mechanisms have been proposed to underlie persistent sodium currents in neurons: (1) window currents, (2) modal gating, and (3) distinct channel isoforms (Crill, 1996). Indeed, in DRG neurons persistent window currents can arise from TTX-resistant channels (Cummins and Waxman, 1997), and Alzheimer et al. (1993) demonstrated with single-channel recordings that CNS sodium channels can generate persistent currents by switching between different gating modes. Although these previously described mechanisms may provide an explanation for some of the persistent sodium current in neurons, our results show that persistent threshold currents can be generated by a fourth mechanism, slow closed-state inactivation. Indeed, this mechanism can account for the threshold ramp currents that have been observed in many neuronal preparations without invoking distinct channel populations.

It is not clear which channel structures are responsible for the slow closed-state inactivation in hNE. Several studies (Ji et al., 1996; Dib-Hajj et al., 1997; Chen et al., 1998) have implicated the S3–S4 linker of domain 4 as being important in repriming kinetics. Interestingly, there is a threonine (T1590) in the domain 4 S3–S4 linker of hNE (and NaS) at a position where most of the other sodium channel isoforms, including hSkM1 and rBII, have a lysine. However, rat PN1 (Sangameswaran et al., 1997; Toledo-Aral et al., 1997) also has a lysine at this position, suggesting that other parts of the channel might determine the slow closed-state inactivation of hNE channels. The only consistent difference between the hNE, NaS, and PN1 clones and hSkM1 and rBII in a region previously identified as playing a prominent role in inactivation is in the S4–S5 linker of domain 3 (Yang et al., 1994). Although hNE, NaS, and PN1 have an isoleucine at position 1304, hSkM1 and rBII have a leucine. This is a conservative substitution, but Smith and Goldin (1997) recently published compelling evidence indicating that the nearby alanine at position 1302 (hNE numbering) interacts directly with the putative inactivation particle for rBII.

Divalent Modulation of Closed-state Inactivation and Ramp Currents

The hypothesis that slow closed-state inactivation underlies ramp currents is supported by our data demonstrating that hNE currents are modulated by cadmium and zinc. These data show that cadmium and zinc increase the time constants for closed-state inactivation of the hNE sodium channels and increase the amplitude hNE ramp currents but have little effect on other channel properties. Although cadmium had no significant effect on hSkM1 currents, cadmium and zinc may modulate the development of inactivation and recovery from inactivation for other neuronal sodium channel isoforms. Indeed we have seen similar effects on rbII channels expressed in Chinese hamster ovary cells (T. R. Cummins, J. R. Howe, and S. G. Waxman, unpublished observations). Cadmium is commonly used in studies of sodium currents because at 0.1–0.5 mM concentrations it blocks calcium channels but not neuronal sodium currents (Klugbauer et al., 1995; Fozzard and Hanck, 1996). Virtually all of the previous studies on TTX-sensitive ramp currents in neurons used cadmium in the extracellular solution. Our results show that cadmium should be used cautiously when studying sodium currents.

In addition to the mechanistic implications of the cadmium and zinc modulation, these effects might also have physiological relevance. Cadmium has been shown to induce pathological changes in the CNS (Wong and Klaassen, 1982) and in sensory ganglia and peripheral nerve (Gabbiani et al., 1967; Sato et al., 1978). Although there is evidence suggesting that the Cd^{2+}-induced injury of white matter may result from disruption of mitochondrial function (Fern et al., 1996), our data raise the possibility that the enhancement of threshold sodium currents [which are known to contribute to white matter injury (Stys et al., 1993)] by cadmium might also contribute to the toxicity of cadmium. The modulation of sodium currents by zinc is intriguing for several reasons. Zinc can be coreleased with neurotransmitters at synapses (Frederickson and Moncrieff, 1994), raising the possibility that zinc could act as a modulator of dendritic sodium currents. It has also been reported that zinc can affect susceptibility to epileptic seizures (Fukahori and Itoh, 1990) and can modulate nociceptive impulse trafficking (Izumi et al., 1995), which involves small DRG neurons.

Functional Consequences of Slow Closed-state Inactivation and Ramp Currents

We have shown that hNE currents are similar to the TTX-S current in small DRG neurons, particularly with respect to the slow rate of closed-state inactivation and the properties of the ramp currents. The distinct properties of hNE sodium channels are expected to have important consequences for cellular excitability. For example, a cell expressing only hNE sodium channels would not be expected to be able to sustain high repetitive firing rates that might be sustained by a cell expressing hSkM1 channels. Conversely, the hNE cell would be expected to respond to slow depolarizing inputs that the hSkM1 cell could not respond to. Gilly and Armstrong (1984) proposed that threshold sodium currents could play an important role in impulse initiation and pacemaking. Because DRG TTX-S and hNE ramp currents can be evoked at potentials close to the resting potential of DRG neurons, they might contribute to the TTX-sensitive oscillations in resting membrane potential that have been observed in these cells (Study and Kral, 1996; Kapoor et al., 1997). Baker and Bostock (1997) proposed that persistent threshold sodium currents in DRG neurons might alternatively play an important role in amplifying depolarizing inputs. This is an intriguing possibility, especially because hNE transcripts (in contrast to other sodium channel transcripts) can be detected in virtually all DRG neurons (Black et al., 1996) and PN1 (the rat ortholog of hNE) immunoreactivity is reportedly highest in the growth cones of cultured rat DRG neurons (Toledo-Aral et al., 1997), suggesting that hNE/PN1/NaS is targeted to nerve terminals. This would situate it ideally for amplifying excitatory inputs.

Belcher et al. (1995) and Sangameswaran et al. (1997) reported that hNE/PN1/NaS mRNA can also be detected in CNS tissues, raising the possibility that this isoform could underlie threshold currents in other neuronal populations. Slow ramp depolarizations have been shown to induce TTX-sensitive ramp currents in many CNS neurons, including neocortical neurons (Stafstrom et al., 1985; Brown et al., 1994; Fleidervish and Gutnick, 1996), thalamocortical neurons (Parri and Crunelli, 1998), suprachiasmatic neurons (Pennartz et al., 1997), neostriatal neurons (Cepeda et al., 1995; Chao and Alzheimer, 1995), cerebellar Purkinje cells (Raman and Bean, 1997), and retinal amacrine cells (Feigenspan et al., 1998). Although CNS sodium currents seem to have predominantly fast repriming kinetics, slowly repriming sodium currents have been recorded in CNS neurons (Martina and Jonas, 1997). Sodium currents with slow repriming may be especially important in dendrites of CNS neurons (Colbert et al., 1997; Jung et al., 1997). However, some studies indicate that hNE or PN1 expression is restricted to the peripheral nervous system (Felts et al., 1997; Toledo-Aral et al., 1997), and it is likely that other isoforms can contribute to the ramp currents in CNS neurons. Indeed, recent evidence has indicated that Na6 underlies a large proportion of the ramp current in cerebellar Purkinje cells (Raman et al., 1997). It is not known whether Na6 channels, or any of the other channels isolated from brain, also have slow closed-state inactivation.

Conclusion

We have studied Na^+ currents produced by the hNE or PN1 sodium channel and have shown that hNE channels have slow closed-state inactivation. Our data show that this provides a previously unrecognized mechanism for the generation of threshold ramp currents and that these ramp currents are subject to modulation. Our results also demonstrate the presence of ramp currents, with voltage dependence and pharmacological characteristics very similar to those of hNE currents, in DRG neurons, which

express PN1. Because threshold ramp currents might play a role in the amplification of synaptic inputs, impulse initiation or the generation of pacemaker potentials in neurons, expression of PN1 and this novel modulation could influence the excitability of DRG neurons. Based on these observations, we propose that the kinetics of sodium channel closed-state inactivation may be an important factor in determining the integrative and firing properties of neurons.

Acknowledgments

This work was supported in part by the Medical Research Service, Department of Veterans Affairs, and by a grant from the National Multiple Sclerosis Society. T.R.C. was supported in part by a fellowship from the Paralyzed Veterans of America Spinal Cord Research Foundation.

References

Akopian AN, Sivilotti L, Wood JN (1996) A tetrodotoxin-resistant voltage-gated sodium channel expressed by sensory neurons. Nature 379: 257–262.

Aldrich RW, Corey DP, Stevens CF (1983) A reinterpretation of mammalian sodium channel gating based on single channel recording. Nature 306: 436–441.

Alzheimer C, Schwindt PC, Crill WE (1993) Modal gating of persistent Na^+ current in pyramidal neurons from rat and cat sensorimotor cortex. J Neurosci 13: 660–673.

Baker MD, Bostock H (1997) Low-threshold persistent sodium current in rat large dorsal root ganglion neurons in culture. J Neurophysiol 77: 1503–1513.

Belcher SM, Zerillo CA, Levenson R, Ritchie JM, Howe JR (1995) Cloning of a sodium channel a subunit from rabbit Schwann cells. Proc Natl Acad Sci USA 92: 11034–11038.

Black JA, Waxman SG (1996) Sodium channel expression: a dynamic process in neurons and non-neuronal cells. Dev Neurosci 18: 139–152.

Black JA, Dib-Hajj S, McNabola K, Jeste S, Rizzo MA, Kocsis JD, Waxman SG (1996) Spinal sensory neurons express multiple sodium channel α-subunit mRNAs. Mol Brain Res 43: 117–132.

Brown AM, Schwindt PC, Crill WE (1994) Different voltage dependence of transient and persistent Na+ currents is compatible with modal-gating hypothesis for sodium channels. J Neurophysiol 71: 2562–2565.

Caffrey JM, Eng DL, Black JA, Waxman SG, Kocsis JD (1992) Three types of sodium channels in adult rat dorsal root ganglion neurons. Brain Res 592: 283–297.

Cepeda C, Chandler SH, Shumate LW, Levine MS (1995) Persistent Na+ conductance in medium-sized neostriatal neurons: characterization using infrared videomicroscopy and whole cell patch-clamp recordings. J Neurophysiol 74: 1343–1348.

Chao TI, Alzheimer C (1995) Do neurons from rat neostriatum express both TTX-sensitive and a TTX-insensitive slow Na+ current? J Neurophysiol 74: 934–941.

Chen QY, Kirsch GE, Zhang DM, Brugada R, Brugada J, Brugada P, Potenza D, Moya A, Borggrefe M, Breithardt G, Ortizlopez R, Wang Z, Antzelevitch C, Obrien RE, Schulzebahr E, Keating MT, Towbin JA, Wang Q (1998) Genetic basis and molecular mechanism for idiopathic-ventricular fibrillation. Nature 392: 293–296.

Colbert CM, Magee JC, Hoffman DA, Johnston D (1997) Slow recovery from inactivation of Na+ channels underlies the activity-dependent attenuation of dendritic action potentials in hippocampal CA1 pyramidal neurons. J Neurosci 17: 6512–6521.

Costa PF (1996) The kinetic parameters of sodium currents in maturing acutely isolated rat hippocampal CA1 neurones. Dev Brain Res 91: 29–40.

Crill WE (1996) Persistent sodium currents in mammalian central neurons. Annu Rev Physiol 58: 349–362.

Cummins TR, Waxman SG (1997) Downregulation of TTX-resistant sodium currents and upregulation of a rapidly repriming TTX-sensitive sodium current in small spinal sensory neurons after nerve injury. J Neurosci 17: 3503–3514.

Dib-Hajj SD, Ishikawa K, Cummins TR, Waxman SG (1997) Insertion of a SNS-specific tetrapeptide in S3–S4 linker of D4 accelerates recovery from inactivation of skeletal muscle voltage-gated Na channel μ1 in HEK293 cells. FEBS Lett 416: 11–14.

Dib-Hajj SD, Tyrrell L, Black JA, Waxman SG (1998) NaN, a novel voltage-gated Na channel, is expressed preferentially in peripheral sensory neurons and downregulated after axotomy. Proc Natl Acad Sci USA 95: 8963–8968.

Elliott AA, Elliott JR (1993) Characterization of TTX-sensitive and TTX-resistant sodium currents in small cells from adult rat dorsal root ganglia. J Physiol (Lond) 463: 39–56.

Feigenspan A, Gustincich S, Bean BP, Raviola E (1998) Spontaneous activity of solitary dopaminergic cells of the retina. J Neurosci 18: 6776–6789.

Felts PA, Yokoyama S, Dib-Hajj S, Black JA, Waxman SG (1997) Sodium channel α-subunit mRNAs I, II, III, NaG, Na6 and hNE (PN1): different expression patterns in developing rat nervous system. Mol Brain Res 45: 71–82.

Fern R, Black JA, Ransom BR, Waxman SG (1996) Cd2+-induced injury in CNS white matter. J Neurophysiol 76: 3264–3273.

Fleidervish IA, Gutnick MJ (1996) Kinetics of slow inactivation of persistent sodium current in layer V neurons of mouse neocortical slices. J Neurophysiol 76: 2125–2130.

Fozzard HA, Hanck DA (1996) Structure and function of voltage-dependent sodium channels: comparison of brain II and cardiac isoforms. Physiol Rev 76: 887–926.

Frederickson CJ, Moncrieff DW (1994) Zinc-containing neurons. Biol Signals 3: 127–139.

Fukahori M, Itoh M (1990) Effects of dietary zinc status on seizure susceptibility and hippocampal zinc content in the El (epilepsy) mouse. Brain Res 529: 16–22.

Gabbiani G, Gregory A, Biac D (1967) Cadmium-induced selective lesions of sensory ganglia. J Neuropathol Exp Neurol 26: 498–506.

George Jr AL, Komisarof J, Kallen RG, Barchi RL (1992) Primary structure of the adult human skeletal muscle voltage-dependent sodium channel. Ann Neurol 31: 131–137.

Gilly WF, Armstrong CM (1984) Threshold channels—a novel type of sodium channel in squid giant axons. Nature 309: 449–450.

Howe JR, Ritchie JM (1992) Multiple kinetic components of sodium channel inactivation in rabbit Schwann cells. J Physiol (Lond) 455: 529–566.

Izumi H, Mori H, Uchiyama T, Kuwazuru S, Ozima Y, Nakamura I, Taguchi S (1995) Sensitization of nociceptive C-fibers in zinc-deficient rats. Am J Physiol 268: R1423–R1428.

Ji S, George AL, Horn R, Barchi RL (1996) Paramyotonia congenita mutations reveal different roles for segments S3 and S4 of domain D4 in hSkM1 sodium channel gating. J Gen Physiol 107: 183–194.

Jung H-Y, Mickus T, Spruston N (1997) Prolonged sodium channel inactivation contributes to dendritic action potential attenuation in hippocampal pyramidal neurons. J Neurosci 17: 6639–6646.

Kapoor R, Li YG, Smith KJ (1997) Slow sodium-dependent potential oscillations contribute to ectopic firing in mammalian demyelinated axons. Brain 120: 647–652.

Klugbauer N, Lacinova L, Flockerzi V, Hofmann F (1995) Structure and functional expression of a new member of the tetrodotoxin-sensitive voltage-activated sodium channel family from human neuroendocrine cells. EMBO J 14: 1084–1090.

Kuo C, Bean BP (1994) Na$^+$ channels must deactivate to recover from inactivation. Neuron 12: 819–829.

Martina M, Jonas P (1997) Functional differences in Na$^+$ channel gating between fast-spiking interneurones and principal neurones of rat hippocampus. J Physiol (Lond) 505: 593–603.

Parri HR, Crunelli V (1998) Sodium current in rat and cat thalamocortical neurons: role of a non-inactivating component in tonic and burst firing. J Neurosci 18: 854–867.

Pennartz CMA, Bierlaagh MA, Guersten AMS (1997) Cellular mechanisms underlying spontaneous firing in rat suprachiasmatic nucleus: involvement of a slowly inactivating component of sodium current. J Neurophysiol 78: 1811–1825.

Raman IM, Bean BP (1997) Resurgent sodium current and action potential formation in dissociated cerebellar Purkinje neurons. J Neurosci 17: 4517–4526.

Raman IM, Sprunger LK, Meisler MH, Bean BP (1997) Altered sub-threshold sodium currents and disrupted firing patterns in Purkinje neurons of Scn8a mutant mice. Neuron 19: 881–891.

Sakar SN, Adhikari A, Sikdar SK (1995) Kinetic characterization of rat brain type IIA sodium channel a-subunit stably expressed in a somatic cell line. J Physiol (Lond) 488: 633–645.

Sangameswaran L, Delgado SG, Fish LM, Koch BD, Jakeman LB, Stewart GR, Sze P, Hunter JC, Eglen RM, Herman RC (1996) Structure and function of a novel voltage-gated tetrodotoxin-resistant sodium channel specific to sensory neurons. J Biol Chem 271: 5953–5956.

Sangameswaran L, Fish LM, Koch BD, Rabert DK, Delgado SG, Ilnicka M, Jakeman LB, Novakovic S, Wong K, Sze P, Tzoumaka E, Stewart GR, Herman RC, Eglen RM, Hunter JC (1997) A novel tetrodotoxin-sensitive voltage-gated sodium channel expressed in rat and human dorsal root ganglia. J Biol Chem 272: 14805–14809.

Sato K, Iwamasa T, Tsuru T, Takeuchi T (1978) An ultrastructural study of chronic cadmium chloride-induced neuropathy. Acta Neuropathol (Berl) 41: 185–190.

Schwindt PC, Crill WE (1995) Amplification of synaptic current by persistent sodium conductance in apical dendrite of neocortical neurons. J Neurophysiol 74: 2220–2224.

Smith MR, Goldin AL (1997) Interaction between the sodium channel inactivation linker and domain III S4–S5. Biophys J 73: 1885–1895.

Smith RD, Goldin AL (1998) Functional analysis of rat I sodium channel in *Xenopus* oocytes. J Neurosci 18: 811–820.

Stafstrom CF, Schwindt PC, Chubb MC, Crill WE (1985) Properties of persistent sodium conductance and calcium conductance of layer V neurons from cat sensorimotor cortex in vitro. J Neurophysiol 53: 153–170.

Study RE, Kral MG (1996) Spontaneous action potential activity in isolated dorsal root ganglion neurons from rats with a painful neuropathy. Pain 65: 235–249.

Stys PK, Sontheimer H, Ransom BR, Waxman SG (1993) Noninactivating, tetrodotoxin-sensitive Na$^+$ conductance in rat optic nerve axons. Proc Natl Acad Sci USA 90: 6976–6980.

Toledo-Aral JJ, Moss BL, He Z-J, Koszowski AG, Whisenand T, Levinson SR, Wolf JJ, Silos-Santiago I, Halegoua S, Mandel G (1997) Identification of PN1, a predominant voltage-dependent sodium channel expressed principally in peripheral neurons. Proc Natl Acad Sci USA 94: 1527–1532.

Vandenberg CA, Bezanilla F (1991) A sodium channel gating model based on single channel, macroscopic and gating currents in the squid giant axon. Biophys J 60: 1511–1533.

Westenbroek RE, Merrick DK, Catterall WA (1989) Differential subcellular localization of the R_I and R_{II} Na^+ channel subtypes in central neurons. Neuron 3: 695–700.

Wong KL, Klaassen CD (1982) Neurotoxic effects of cadmium in young rats. Toxicol Appl Pharmacol 63: 330–337.

Yang N, Ji S, Zhou M, Ptacek LJ, Barchi RL, Horn R, George AL (1994) Sodium channel mutations in paramyotonia congenita exhibit similar biophysical phenotypes in vitro. Proc Natl Acad Sci USA 91: 12785–12789.

XVI   MESSENGERS OF PATHOS

Pain is a sensation that is, at one time or another, experienced by every person. Pain can be physiological, that is, a response to an external and injurious stimulus such as a pinprick or a hot object; when this happens, it alerts the organism and may trigger adaptive responses that include withdrawal of the body part that is threatened. In this case pain occurs for a good reason and has a protective purpose. Pain can also occur, however, in the absence of an external stimulus, without a good reason. *Neuropathic pain* can be persistent and can occur long after the initial insult, as a result of injury to nerve cells along the pain pathway. In these instances the pain-signaling system goes awry and no longer protects us. How does this happen? What can be done about it? Answers to these questions might help patients who experience pain, sometimes unremitting and severe, following nerve or spinal cord injuries. Answers might also help individuals who suffer from *inflammatory pain*, which occurs as a response to inflammation in disorders such as rheumatoid arthritis.

The message telling the brain that there is pain usually begins with electrical activity in a pain-signaling, or nociceptive, spinal sensory neuron that sends one branch of its nerve fiber peripherally to the skin, viscera, or muscles, and the other centrally to the spinal cord. Neuropathic and inflammatory pain are thought to arise, at least in part, from hyperexcitability of neurons along the pain pathway, that is, spontaneous firing of these cells when there is no noxious stimulus there to excite them, or firing in inappropriately long bursts that continue even after a painful stimulus ends. Where does this hyperexcitability come from? Can we identify molecules that cause pain-signaling nerve cells to fire without good reason? And, if so, can we silence these messengers of pathos?

I had worked on injury-evoked discharge in nerves as a student with Patrick Wall (Wall, Waxman, and Basbaum 1974) but did not, until recently, consider myself a "pain researcher," and I did not attend scientific meetings on pain or apply for grants for research on it. But science can go in unexpected directions. In 1994 we did a simple experiment: we injured the axons of spinal sensory neurons by cutting the sciatic nerve in rats, and asked whether, as a result of transection of sensory axons, there were changes in the production of sodium channels within the cell bodies of the neurons that give rise to them (Waxman, Kocsis, and Black 1994). Subtype-specific antibodies for the known sodium channels were not at that time available to us, but the nucleotide sequences for several channels were known, so we were able to design probes for in situ hybridization which visualizes the mRNAs that serve as blueprints for protein synthesis. We were interested in knowing how sodium channel expression in neurons changed in response to various injuries and we decided to first study the response to a "clean," well-defined injury—transecting of nerve fibers, simply severing them. Axons can regenerate briskly after they are injured within a peripheral nerve such as the sciatic, and we expected the neurons to turn up the rate of synthesis of the sodium channels that they needed as part of the process of regeneration.

When we did the experiment we saw, as expected, a modest up-regulation or turning-up of synthesis of several types of sodium channel genes (types I and II) which are usually present in these cells. We also, however, saw a dramatic turning-on of the synthesis of the previously undetectable type III sodium channel gene in spinal sensory neurons including C-type neurons (which include pain-signaling neurons) following axonal injury. These experiments showed us that, as a result of injury to their axons, there was a change in the pattern of gene activation within spinal sensory neurons which could result in the production of a new and different ensemble of sodium channels; we had observed the misexpression, of the wrong types of sodium channels, in injured pain-signaling neurons. These results turned our attention to the possibility that sodium channels, expressed in abnormal patterns after nerve injury, might contribute to neuropathic pain.

The apparent up-regulation of the type I and type II sodium channel genes had been modest, so as a next step we decided to focus (Dib-Hajj et al. 1996) on the type III gene, and on an additional sodium channel called SNS/PN3, which had just been discovered (Akopian, Sivilotti, and Wood 1996; Sangameswaran et al. 1996). SNS/PN3 was of special interest, since it was known to be present in spinal sensory neurons and trigeminal neurons (the counterparts of spinal sensory neurons which carry sensory information from the face), but it is not normally present in other types of nerve cells. In this study we confirmed that, after injury to their axons within the sciatic nerve, there is a turning-on (also called an up-regulation) of the type III sodium channel gene within spinal sensory neurons. We also found a strong down-regulation of the SNS/PN3 sodium channel (Dib-Hajj et al. 1996).

To understand the physiological effects of these changes in sodium channel gene expression, Ted Cummins and I next used patch-clamp methods and recorded electrical currents from C-type neurons after their axons had been injured (Cummins and Waxman 1997). In this study we asked: are there changes in sodium currents (the currents produced by sodium channels) after injury to the axons of C-type neurons? We knew, from earlier studies (Rizzo, Kocsis, and Waxman 1995) that, in spinal sensory neurons whose axons had been transected, there was a reduction in sodium current that was resistant to a neurotoxin called tetrodotoxin. Since Akopian, Sivilotti, and Wood (1996) and Sangameswaran et al. (1996) had shown that the SNS/PN3 sodium channel was tetrodotoxin-resistant, and because we knew that the SNS/PN3 gene was down-regulated in spinal sensory neurons following axonal injury, these patch-clamp results made sense. We also, however, observed the emergence of a new sodium current with unexpected and interesting properties.

Following the opening of a sodium channel (which permits it to generate electrical current), the channel becomes "inactivated" and is not available to open again for a period of time. Repriming is the recovery of sodium channels from inactivation. Cummins suggested that we study repriming and our recordings showed us that a "rapidly repriming" sodium current, which was not detectable before injury, emerged in C-type neurons after injury to their axons. Rapidly repriming sodium channels can respond to stimuli at rapid rates, thereby supporting the generation of nerve impulses at high frequencies. The most likely explanation for the emergence of this new current was that a previously silent channel had reared its head following injury. We speculated that abnormal expression of the type III sodium channel gene resulted in production of rapidly repriming channels which contribute to hyperexcitability of injured C-type neurons and to neuropathic pain.

Having become interested in repriming, particularly rapid repriming, we wanted to understand its molecular basis. Since the full amino acid sequence of the SNS/PN3 channel was known, and since SNS/PN3 was also known to reprime rapidly, we decided to study it as a model channel. Sodium channels are peptide molecules, chains of about eighteen hundred amino acids. We were particularly interested in the part of the molecule called the S-4 segment and the "linker" that attaches it like a hinge to the previous segment (S-3), because we knew that S-4 acts as a voltage-sensor, helping the channel to gate its current. We used informatics, examining the amino acid sequences of all known sodium channels and comparing them to SNS/PN3 to ask whether there was anything special about S-4 or the linker in the SNS/PN1 channel. As shown in figure 1 of Dib-Hajj et al. (1997) our search showed that SNS/PN3 contains three extra amino acids in the linker next to S-4. On this basis we hypothesized that the insertion of the three amino acids—three out of eighteen hundred—might affect the rate of repriming of the channel.

To learn more directly whether the three amino acid insertion affects repriming, we next used the technique of in situ mutagenesis. In these experiments we took a slowly repriming muscle sodium channel and inserted the three amino acids in the site predicted from SNS/PN3, in the linker next to S-4. If our hypothesis was correct, the speed of repriming of the mutant channel would be changed. To test this hypothesis we expressed the channel in a cell line, and Ted Cummins then used patch-clamp to study the kinetics of the currents in cells bearing the chimeric channel. The results, shown in figure 3 of Dib-Hajj et al. (1997), revealed a distinct acceleration of channel repriming as a result of the insertion of these three amino acids. Other physiological properties of the channel, however, were not changed. These experiments taught us that a small part of the channel, within the linker close to S-4, is important for repriming; and they showed that even small changes in the molecular structure of the channel, focused on this region, could alter recovery from inactivation.

By this time our work had been noticed by the pain research community and we, in turn, wanted to learn more about the pathophysiology of pain. In April of 1998 I traveled to the Spring Pain Meeting at Grand Cayman Island together with Joel Black, the senior cell biologist in our research group. Some important things happened at the meeting. Joel and I had time to walk the beach, sheltered from telephone calls, e-mail, and the day-to-day details of experiments, to reflect on the overall direction of our research, "retreat"-style. It was at the Cayman Island meeting that we decided, for example, to do studies on the "chronic constriction injury" model of neuropathic pain (Dib-Hajj et al. 1999). We each met new people and made new friendships. I began a friendship with John Wood, who had established a leading molecular pain research laboratory at University College London. This friendship was to blossom into a collaboration aimed at analyzing the role of sodium channels in pain using "knock-out" mice in which specific genes had been deleted; these experiments are described in part XVII. And we obtained antibodies produced by a pain research group in Stevenage, England, which helped us to localize abnormal collections of type III sodium channels within neuromas, the tangled webs of abortively regenerating nerve fibers that can generate abnormal impulse barrages after nerve injury (Black et al. 1999); parallels in the pattern of expression of type III channels and of rapidly repriming current provided us with additional evidence linking the emergence of rapidly repriming sodium current with the up-regulation of type III sodium channels in injured neurons.

Partly as a result of serendipitous observations, my coworkers and I joined the community of pain researchers—opening up a new set of scientific challenges and a new array of friendships. We have become part of an effort going on in laboratories around the world, dissecting the pain pathway molecule by molecule. While we and a few other laboratories are pursuing sodium channels, other research groups are characterizing the roles of different molecular targets such as substance P receptors, glutamate receptors, and vanilloid receptors in pain signaling (see, e.g., Levine 1998). One of these molecules may hold the key to the discovery of channel-altering medicines that will dampen the activity of pain-signaling neurons while sparing the functions of other kinds of nerve cells.

In some ways this multinational research effort is like a marathon. Hopefully, however, at the finish there will be quietude rather than applause. If science can harness the messengers of pathos, pain-signaling neurons may not have to fire when they should not. This would be a gift for patients with chronic pain. Silence of the messengers of pathos would mean that people would no longer have to feel pain without a good reason.

References

Akopian, A. N., Sivilotti, L., and Wood, J. N. A tetrodotoxin-resistant voltage-gated sodium channel expressed by sensory neurons. *Nature* 379: 257–262, 1996.

Black, J. A., Cummins, T. R., Plumpton, C., Chen, Y. H., Hormuzdiar, W., Clare, J. J., and Waxman, S. G. Upregulation of a silent sodium channel following peripheral, but not central, nerve injury in DRG neurons. *J. Neurophysiol.* 82: 2776–2786, 1999.

Cummins, T. R., and Waxman, S. G. Down-regulation of tetrodotoxin-resistant sodium currents and up-regulation of a rapidly repriming tetrodotoxin-sensitive sodium current in small spinal sensory neurons following nerve injury. *J. Neurosci.* 17: 3503–3514, 1997.

Dib-Hajj, S., Black, J. A., Felts, P., and Waxman, S. G. Down-regulation of transcripts for Na channel α-SNS in spinal sensory neurons following axotomy. *Proc. Natl. Acad. Sci. U.S.A.* 93: 14950–14954, 1996.

Dib-Hajj, S. D., Fjell, J., Cummins, T. R., Zheng, Z., Fried, K., LaMotte, R., Black, J. A., and Waxman, S. G. Plasticity of sodium channel expression in DRG neurons in the chronic constriction injury model of neuropathic pain. *Pain*, 83: 591–600, 1999.

Dib-Hajj, S. D., Ishikawa, I., Cummins, T. R., and Waxman, S. G. Insertion of a SNS-specific tetrapeptide in the S3–S4 linker of D4 accelerates recovery from inactivation of skeletal muscle voltage-gated Na channel μ1 in HEK293 cells. *FEBS Letts.* 416: 11–14, 1997.

Levine, J. D. New directions in pain research: Molecules to maladies. *Neuron* 20: 649–654, 1998.

Rizzo, M. A., Kocsis, J. D., and Waxman, S. G. Selective loss of slow and enhancement of fast Na^+ currents in cutaneous afferent DRG neurons following axotomy. *Neurobiol. Dis.* 2: 87–97, 1995.

Sangameswaran, L., Delgado, S. G., Fish, L. M., Koch, B. D., Jakeman, L. B., Stewart, G. R., Sze, P., Hunter, J. C., Eglen, R. M., and Herman, R. C. Structure and function of a novel voltage-gated, tetrodotoxin-resistant sodium channel specific to sensory neurons. *J. Biol. Chem.* 271: 5953–5956, 1996.

Wall, P. D., Waxman, S. G., and Basbaum, A. I. Ongoing activity in peripheral nerve: injury discharge. *Exper. Neurol.* 45: 576–589, 1974.

Waxman, S. G., Kocsis, J. D., and Black, J. A. Type III sodium channel mRNA is expressed in embryonic but not adult spinal sensory neurons, and is reexpressed following axotomy. *J. Neurophysiol.* 72: 466–471, 1994.

27 Down-Regulation of Transcripts for Na Channel α-SNS in Spinal Sensory Neurons Following Axotomy

S. Dib-Hajj, J. A. Black, P. Felts, and S. G. Waxman

Abstract Spinal sensory (dorsal root ganglion; DRG) neurons display slowly inactivating, tetrodotoxin-resistant (TTX-R), and rapidly inactivating, TTX-sensitive (TTX-S) Na currents. Attenuation of the TTX-R Na current and enhancement of TTX-S Na current have been demonstrated in cutaneous afferent DRG neurons in the adult rat after axotomy and may underlie abnormal bursting. We show here that steady-state levels of transcripts encoding the α-SNS subunit, which is associated with a slowly inactivating, TTX-R current when expressed in oocytes, are reduced significantly 5 days following axotomy of DRG neurons, and continue to be expressed at reduced levels, even after 210 days. Steady-state levels of α-III transcripts, which are present at low levels in control DRG neurons, show a pattern of transiently increased expression. In situ hybridization using α-SNS- and α-III-specific riboprobes showed a decreased signal for α-SNS, and an increased signal for α-III, in both large and small DRG neurons following axotomy. Reduced levels of α-SNS may explain the selective loss of slowly inactivating, TTX-R current. The abnormal electrophysiological properties of DRG neurons following axonal injury thus appear to reflect a switch in Na channel gene expression.

Multiple voltage-gated Na currents with different kinetics and voltage dependence have been observed in spinal sensory (dorsal root ganglion; DRG) neurons, which relay signals from peripheral receptors into the central nervous system. These include rapidly inactivating, TTX-sensitive (TTX-S) currents, and slowly inactivating, TTX-resistant (TTX-R) Na currents (1–4). Interplay of the currents influences the firing properties of DRG neurons (5–8) and may contribute to ectopic generation of action potentials in these cells following injury to their axons within peripheral nerves (9).

Neural Na channels are heterotrimers composed of an α subunit and two β subunits, β1 and

Reprinted with permission from *Proceedings of the National Academy of Sciences USA* 93: 14950–14954, 1996.

β2 (10–12). Nucleotide sequence variation allows identification of α subunits within single neurons by in situ hybridization (ISH) or in a cDNA pool using reverse transcriptase–PCR (RT-PCR) and restriction enzyme polymorphism (REP). ISH and RT-PCR/REP analyses have demonstrated that transcripts of multiple channel α subunits, including α-I, α-II, NaG, Na6, and hNE (PN1), are expressed in single DRG neurons (13). The expression of these transcripts may explain the diversity of Na currents in these cells. Recently, a novel α subunit [α-SNS (14), also termed PN3 (15)] was identified and found to be restricted to peripheral sensory neurons. α-SNS contains a serine at a site within domain I which has been shown, by site-directed mutagenesis, to confer resistance to TTX in the cardiac muscle Na channel (16). Expression of α-SNS cRNA produces a slowly inactivating, TTX-R current in *Xenopus* oocytes, suggesting that α-SNS is responsible for a TTX-R Na current in DRG neurons (14, 15).

Altered neuronal excitability has been demonstrated following axonal transection (17–19) and may underlie abnormal DRG bursting associated with pain syndromes (9, 20). Abnormal somatodendritic excitability following axotomy is Na dependent (21, 22), and it has been suggested that this is due to a shift, following axotomy, in vectorial transport of Na channels (23, 24). Recent experiments, however, demonstrated an attenuation of slowly inactivating, TTX-R currents and simultaneous enhancement of rapidly inactivating, TTX-S Na currents in large cutaneous afferent neurons following axotomy (25). This suggests an alternative mechanism, which could alter neuronal excitability—i.e., a switch in the types of Na channels that are expressed. Consistent with a switch in Na channel synthesis, transcripts encoding the α-III subunit, which are present at only very low levels in control DRG neurons, are expressed at moderate-to-high levels in axotomized DRG neurons together with elevated levels of a-I and a-II mRNAs (26). However, the effect of axotomy on other Na channel transcripts has not been examined, and a correlate for the reduced TTX-R currents following axonal injury has not been identified.

On the basis of our electrophysiological observations (25), we hypothesized that levels of a-SNS would decrease following axotomy of DRG neurons. To test this hypothesis, we used RT-PCR and ISH to study steady-state levels of a-SNS and a-III at specific time points following axotomy. Here we report a reduction in a-SNS transcripts that appears to explain the loss of the slowly inactivating, TTX-R Na currents in cutaneous afferent DRG neurons following axotomy. Further, we show that a-SNS levels are decreased in small, as well as large, DRG neurons following axotomy, suggesting that a reduction in slow, TTX-R currents may contribute to abnormal excitability of nociceptive neurons following axonal injury.

Materials and Methods

Surgical Techniques

Adult female Sprague–Dawley rats were anesthetized with ketamine/xylazine; sciatic nerves were exposed at mid-thigh level on the lesioned (A) side, ligated with 4–0 silk sutures, transected, and placed in a silicon cuff to prevent regeneration (27). The contralateral sciatic nerve served as control (C). Two rats were prepared for time points 1, 3, 14, 58, and 210 days post axotomy (dpa); four rats were prepared for time points 5, 7, and 21 dpa. Following CO_2 narcosis and decapitation, axotomized and control L4 and L5 DRGs were collected in separate Microcentrifuge tubes.

RNA Extraction

Total cellular RNA was isolated by the single-step guanidinium isothiocyanate/acid phenol procedure (28). Extraction buffer was used at 25 µl/mg of tissue (the two DRG pairs averaged 10 mg of wet weight). RNA concentration was determined by absorbance measurements at 230, 260, and 280 nm. The quality of the RNA was assessed by electrophoresis in a 1% agarose/2.2 M formaldehyde gel. First-strand cDNA was reverse-transcribed in a 50-ml final volume using 2 µg of total RNA, 1 mM random hexamer (Boehringer Mannheim), 500 units of SuperScript II reverse transcriptase (Life Technologies), and 100 units of RNase Inhibitor (Boehringer Mannheim). The buffer consisted of 50 mM Tris · HCl (pH 8.3), 75 mM KCl, 3 mM $MgCl_2$, 10 mM DTT, and 5 mM dNTP. The reaction was allowed to proceed at 37 °C for 90 min, then 42 °C for 30 min, and finally terminated by heating to 65 °C for 10 min.

PCR

We used primers described by Akopian et al. (14) for amplification of the a-SNS sequence from the total cDNA pool. These primers amplify a 572-bp fragment corresponding to nucleotides 2111–2683 (GenBank accession no. X92184). For subunit a-III, we used primers that amplify a 420-bp fragment in domain 1, including an alternatively spliced exon (29). The forward primer (5′-GACCCATGGAATTGGTTGGA-3′) corresponds to nucleotides 975–994; the reverse primer (5′-GACATAAAAGTGACTGTCATCTGC-3′) corresponds to nucleotides 1371–1394 (accession no. Y00766).

Rat β-actin sequences were coamplified using commercial primers (CLONTECH) for comparison to a-subunit transcripts. PCR from a cDNA template results in a 764-bp fragment, while a genomic template results in a 1440-bp fragment. A single DNA fragment, comigrating with the 800-bp marker, was detected in all PCR reactions, which indicates the absence of appreciable genomic DNA contamination (see figures 27.1A and 27.3A).

Amplification was typically performed in a 60-µl volume using 1 µl of first-strand cDNA, 1.85 µM (a-SNS) and 2.25 µM (a-III) primer, and 1.75 units of Expand Long Template (Boehringer Mannheim) DNA polymerase enzyme mixture (30, 31). The reaction mixture contained β-actin primers (0.66 μM). Control PCR with template replaced by water produced no amplification products (data not shown). The PCR buffer consisted of 50 mM Tris · HCl (pH 9.2), 16 mM $(NH_4)_2SO_4$, 2.25 mM $MgCl_2$, 2% (vol/vol) dimethylsulfoxide, and 0.1% Tween 20. Amplification was carried out in two stages (32): First, denaturation at 94 °C for 4 min, annealing at 58 °C for 2 min, and elongation at 72 °C for 90 sec. Second, denaturation at 94 °C for 1 min, annealing at 58 °C for 1 min, and elongation at 72 °C for 90 sec. The second stage was repeated 24 times (α-SNS) or 34 times (α-III) with the last elongation step extended to 10 min. Primer concentration and number of amplification cycles were empirically determined to ensure that amplification did not reach the plateau phase. Multiple amplifications were performed for every time point.

Amplification products were separated on a 1.6% agarose gel supplemented with 0.25 μg/ml ethidium bromide. Gel images were digitized using a GelBase 7500 system (Ultraviolet Products, San Gabriel, CA) with the gray scale converted to false colors. Gel tracks were scanned, and peaks corresponding to β-actin and α-subunits were quantified in autoanalysis mode. The level of α-subunit cDNAs in the cDNA pool was expressed as $a/(a + b)$, where a and b are the areas under the peaks of α-subunit and β-actin, to minimize the effect of variations in quantity of input RNA, efficiency of reverse transcription, and/or amplification among the samples. The level of the respective α-subunit in the axotomized (A) side was expressed as a ratio, comparing it to the level on the contralateral side (A/C ± SE). ORIGIN (Microcal, MA) software was used for statistical analyses.

In Situ Hybridization

Axotomized rats were deeply anesthetized with chloral hydrate and perfused with PBS and then with 4% paraformaldehyde in 0.14 M Sorensen's phosphate buffer, pH 7.4, at 4 °C. Control and axotomized L4 and L5 DRG were collected, placed in fixative at 4 °C for 2–4 hr, and immersed in 4% paraformaldehyde/30% sucrose in 0.14 M phosphate buffer, pH 7.4, at 4 °C. Sections (15 μm) were placed on poly-(L-lysine)-coated slides and processed for ISH cytochemistry with sense and antisense riboprobes as previously described (26, 33).

Results

RT-PCR

Comparison of the α-SNS amplification product, which migrates slightly faster than the 600-bp size marker for axotomized (A) and unlesioned contralateral (C) DRG consistent with its predicted length of 572 bp (14), indicates that there is an initial brief (1 dpa) up-regulation of steady-state α-SNS transcripts followed by a more sustained down-regulation that is most pronounced in the first week post axotomy (figure 27.1). A single amplification product was observed for each template, showing that there is no appreciable genomic DNA contamination in the samples. Using identical experimental conditions, we found comparable levels of transcripts for both α-SNS and α-III in control and sham-operated DRG tissues (data not shown).

The down-regulation of α-SNS transcripts was observed using two different primer sets: the α-SNS-specific primer set described by Akopian et al. (14) (figure 27.1) for all time points discussed below and α-SNS-specific primers that amplify sequences of the loop joining domains 1 and 2 (residues 1476–2129) for 7 dpa (data not shown). A similar pattern of α-SNS reduction was observed when templates from a more proximal dorsal root lesion were analyzed at 3, 7, and 21 dpa (data not shown).

Levels of α-SNS transcripts in the axotomized DRG were compared with those of the control contralateral DRG at 1, 3, 5, 7, 14, 21, 58, and

A

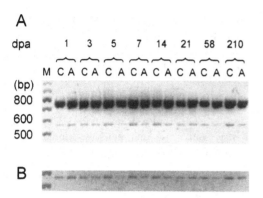

B

Figure 27.1
RT-PCR coamplification of a-SNS and β-actin transcripts from DRG following unilateral sciatic axotomy. (*A*) RT-PCR products from control (C) and axotomized (A) DRG at various dpa. Two products can be observed migrating slightly slower than the 800-bp marker (predicted β-actin product: 764 bp) and the 600-bp marker (predicted a-SNS product: 572 bp), respectively. Lane M contains a 100-bp standard. The gel image was digitized, inverted, and printed in black and white sublimation mode. (*B*) Computer enhancement for photographic purposes of the section of *A* containing the a-SNS amplification product.

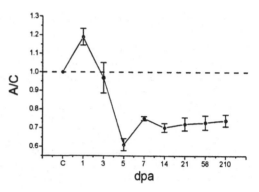

Figure 27.2
a-SNS transcript levels following axotomy. Levels of a-SNS transcripts in axotomized (A) and control (C) DRG were normalized to the coamplified β-actin transcripts. The A/C ratio is shown at various dpa. The A/C ratio of a-SNS transcripts in uninjured animals (indicated by C on the abscissa) is set at 1 and indicated by the dashed line. Four animals were used in the analysis at 5, 7, and 21 dpa, while two animals were used for each of the remaining time points. Mean ± SE from at least three independent amplifications was used to calculate each point, employing the ORIGIN program.

210 dpa. At least three independent amplification reactions were performed for each time point, with a-SNS amplification product normalized to the coamplified β-actin product. a-SNS levels were reduced in axotomized DRG at all postaxotomy times after 3 dpa (figure 27.2). The same pattern of down-regulation of a-SNS transcripts was observed with and without normalization to the β-actin coamplification product at all time points; the 21-dpa result shown in figure 27.1*B* is an exception and is probably due to more input RNA in the A sample (note that there is more β-actin coamplification product in A for this experiment).

The level of a-SNS transcripts appeared to increase slightly at 1 dpa (A/C: 1.18 ± 0.04). Levels of a-SNS transcripts then significantly decrease and fall below control levels, with an A/C

ratio of 0.6 ± 0.03 at 5 dpa (on a single-cell basis, this may represent an underestimate of the reduction in levels of transcript, since the ligation procedure does not result in transection of all axons within the nerve). Analysis of samples at 58 and 210 dpa indicates that a-SNS transcript levels in the axotomized DRG remain reduced compared with their preaxotomy levels even at these long postaxotomy times (figure 27.2).

The a-III subunit is expressed at low steady-state levels in adult DRG (refs. 13 and 26 and this study); therefore, quantification by RT-PCR was not attempted in this study. Qualitative analysis of the effect of axotomy on a-III transcripts was performed using a-III-specific primers (figure 27.3). As for a-SNS, a-III sequences were coamplified with β-actin (figure 27.3*A*). These experiments show that a-III transcript levels are up-regulated in the axotomized DRG tissue at 3 dpa, peak between 7 and 14 dpa, then

A

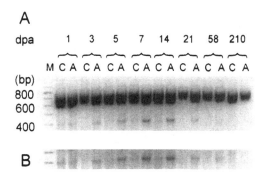

Figure 27.3
RT-PCR coamplification of a-III and β-actin transcripts. (*A*) RT-PCR products of transcripts from control (C) and axotomized (A) DRG at various dpa. Two products can be observed, one migrating slower than the 800-bp marker (predicted β-actin product: 764 bp) and another comigrating with the 400-bp marker (predicted a-III product: 412 bp). Lane M, 100-bp standard. (*B*) Computer enhancement of a-III amplification product.

decline by 21 dpa (figure 27.3*A*). The same pattern of up-regulation is observed when the amplification products are not normalized to those of β-actin (figure 27.3*B*). A similar result was observed using a generic primer set and REP with *Dra*I to detect a-III (data not shown).

In Situ Hybridization

Sections of DRG hybridized with a-SNS and a-III sense riboprobes showed no specific labeling (not shown). In control DRG hybridized with a-SNS antisense riboprobe, a-SNS signal was present in most small (<30-μm diameter) DRG neurons; in contrast, most large (>30-μm diameter) DRG neurons did not exhibit a-SNS hybridization signal (figure 27.4*a*). At 5 dpa (figure 27.4*b*), a-SNS hybridization signal was not detectable, or was detectable at low levels, in most DRG neurons of all sizes.

In control DRG sections hybridized with a-III antisense riboprobe, most neurons did not dis-

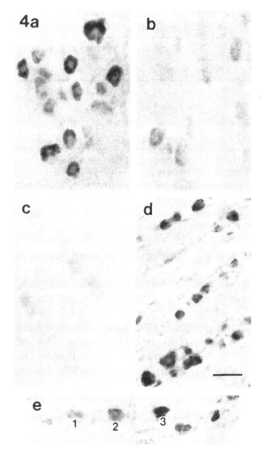

Figure 27.4
Sodium channel mRNA a-SNS and a-III expression in control and axotomized DRG neurons. (*a*) a-SNS is expressed in most small DRG neurons and in some large neurons in control DRG. (*b*) At 5 dpa, the a-SNS hybridization signal is attenuated. (*c*) a-III, control DRG. (*d*) a-III, 5 dpa. (*e*) Representative field from control DRG hybridized with a-SNS probe, to show + (1), ++ (2), and +++ (3) signals. (×215; bar = 40 μm.)

Table 27.1

Expression of sodium channel a-subunit mRNAs SNS and III in control and axotomized DRG neurons in situ

mRNA	Tissue	% small neurons (<30-µm diameter)					% large neurons (>30-µm diameter)				
		0	+	++	+++	(n)	0	+	++	+++	(n)
SNS	Control	3.1	13.2	42.2	41.5	(258)	44.2	33.7	19.6	2.5	(163)
SNS	Axotomized	40.4	31.6	23.6	4.4	(225)	58.3	25.9	14.4	1.4	(139)
III	Control	44.4	50.0	5.6	0.0	(144)	63.3	32.5	4.2	0.0	(121)
III	Axotomized	29.1	38.3	23.3	9.2	(120)	27.5	46.1	17.6	7.8	(102)

Numbers are percentage of DRG neurons that express 0, undetectable; +, marginal/low; ++, moderate; and +++, high levels of hybridization signal for each size class. Numbers in parentheses, number of DRG neurons for each size class scored for expression of sodium channel mRNA from at least two separate experiments.

play signal above background levels (figure 27.4c). At 5 dpa, however, moderate-to-high levels of a-III hybridization signal were present in DRG neurons of all sizes (figure 27.4d).

To confirm that a-SNS was decreased in both small and large DRG neurons, and that a-III was elevated in both groups of cells, we subdivided neurons into small (<30-µm diameter) and large (>30-µm diameter) subgroups (table 27.1). We observed a decrease in the percentage of large (control, 22%; postaxotomy, 16%) and small (control, 84%; postaxotomy, 28%) DRG neurons displaying moderate or high levels of a-SNS hybridization signal following axotomy. We also confirmed the increase in the percentage of large (control, 4%; postaxotomy, 25%) and small (control, 6%; postaxotomy, 33%) DRG neurons expressing moderate or high levels of a-III following axotomy.

Discussion

The major findings of this study are that: (*i*) transcript levels for Na channel a-SNS are downregulated in DRG neurons following axotomy; (*ii*) there is a concomitant up-regulation of the Na channel a-III transcript following axotomy; and (*iii*) these changes occur in both large and small DRG neurons.

Following axonal transection, the neuronal cell body displays retrograde changes that reflect disconnection from postsynaptic targets (34, 35), changes in axo–glial interactions (36), or an intrinsic reaction of the neuron to injury (37, 38). These changes include altered excitability of the soma-dendritic compartment and axon initial segment (17, 19), which involves Na-dependent electrogenesis (22, 23). While these early experiments were interpreted as suggesting a shift in vectorial transport of channels in axotomized neurons (21, 24), our results indicate that an altered pattern of gene expression contributes to the electrophysiological changes.

When studied at 18 dpa, large cutaneous afferent DRG neurons display a selective attenuation of slow, TTX-R Na currents and an enhancement of the fast, TTX-S Na currents (25). An ISH study on a-I, -II, and -III mRNAs in axotomized DRG neurons demonstrated an upregulation of Na channel mRNA a-I and -II, and the expression at moderate-to-high levels of a-III, which is present in embryonic DRG neurons but is barely detectable in adult nonlesioned DRG neurons (26). The present results demonstrate that the up-regulation of a-III mRNA in DRG neurons peaks at 7–14 days following axotomy and then declines. Assuming that a-III corresponds to a fast, TTX-S Na current, these observations suggest that the expression of this

Na current in DRG neurons following axotomy should show a similar time course.

In contrast to α-III, our results show a decrease in α-SNS transcripts in axotomized DRG. Comparison of α-SNS and α-III amplification products shows reciprocal changes in the transcripts of these two Na channels, possibly because they are influenced by opposing regulatory mechanisms. It is not clear how axotomy affects the expression of β-actin in DRG. mRNA encoding one form of β-tubulin is significantly increased, while neurofilament NF68 mRNA decreases following sciatic nerve axotomy (39). The fact that steady-state levels of α-SNS transcripts are down-regulated, while α-III transcript levels are up-regulated in axotomized DRG, indicates that these effects do not represent a nonspecific increase in channel expression following axonal injury, and it suggests that normalization with respect to β-actin levels does not introduce a large systematic error. Indeed, while the fast, TTX-S Na current (25) and a delayed tetraethylammonium-sensitive K current (40) increase in DRG neurons following axonal injury, inward rectification decreases (19, 41) together with the slow, TTX-R Na current, consistent with down-regulation of the appropriate transcripts.

Our findings demonstrate a down-regulation of transcripts for α-SNS and an up-regulation of transcripts for α-III in both large and small DRG neurons. On the basis of these results, we are led to predict that, in addition to the attenuation of slow, TTX-R Na current that has been observed in axotomized cutaneous afferent DRG neurons (25), an altered pattern of Na channel gene expression and a loss of slow, TTX-R sodium current should occur in small DRG neurons. Since these include nociceptive cells (42), our observations may be relevant to the pathogenesis of neuropathic pain, which results from abnormal burst activity following axonal injury (43, 44). Na currents in some DRG neurons display weak voltage dependence, with the open probability increasing over a large voltage domain (45). In DRG neurons which express abnormal combinations of Na channels following axonal injury, window currents can overlap, and activation of weakly voltage-dependent Na channels can produce subthreshold voltage excursions that trigger regenerative activity in steeply voltage-dependent channels, generating inappropriate burst activity that is associated with pain and paresthesia (9). On the basis of the present findings, we suggest that abnormal expression of Na channels encoded by α-III and α-SNS mRNA participates in this pathophysiologic process.

Acknowledgments

We thank B. R. Toftness for technical assistance. This work was supported in part by grants from the National Multiple Sclerosis Society and Medical Research Service, Department of Veterans Affairs.

References

1. Kostyuk, P. G., Veselovsky, N. and Tsyandryenko, A. (1981) *Neuroscience* 6: 2423–2430.

2. Yoshida, S., Matsuda, Y. and Samejima, A. (1978) *J. Neurophysiol.* 639: 125–134.

3. Roy, M. L. and Narahashi, T. (1992) *J. Neurosci.* 12: 2104–2111.

4. Caffrey, J. M., Eng, D. L., Black, J. A., Waxman, S. G. and Kocsis, J. D. (1992) *Brain Res.* 592: 283–297.

5. Elliott, A. A. and Elliott, J. R. (1993) *J. Physiol. (London)* 463: 39–56.

6. Honmou, O., Utzschneider, D. A., Rizzo, M. A., Bowe, C. M., Waxman, S. G. and Kocsis, J. D. (1994) *J. Neurophysiol.* 71: 1627–1638.

7. Jeftinija, S. (1994) *Brain Res.* 639: 125–134.

8. Schild, J. H., Clark, J. W., Hay, M., Medelowitz, D., Andresen, M. C. and Kunze, D. L. (1994) *J. Neurophysiol.* 71: 2338–2358.

9. Rizzo, M. A., Kocsis. J. D. and Waxman, S. G. (1996) *Eur. Neurol.* 36: 3–12.

10. Catterall, W. A. (1993) *Trends Neurosci.* 16: 500–506.

11. Isom, L. L., De Jongh, K. S. and Catterall, W. A. (1994) *Neuron* 12: 1183–1194

12. Isom, L. L., Ragsdale, D. S., De Jongh, K. S., Westenbroek, R. E., Reber, B. F. X., Scheuer, T. and Catterall, W. A. (1995) *Cell* 83: 433–442.

13. Black, J. A., Dib-Hajj, S., McNabola, K., Jeste, S., Rizzo, M. A., Kocsis, J. D. and Waxman, S. G. (1996) *Mol. Brain Res.*, 43: 117–131.

14. Akopian, A. N., Sivilotti, L. and Wood, J. N. (1996) *Nature (London)* 379: 258–262.

15. Sangameswaran, L., Delgado, S. G., Fish, L. M., Koch, B. D., Jakeman, L. B., Stewart, G. R., Sze, P., Hunter, J. C., Eglen, R. M. and Herman, R. C. (1996) *J. Biol. Chem.* 271: 5953–5956.

16. Satin, J., Kyle, J. W., Chen, M., Bell, P., Cribbs, L. L., Fozzard, H. A. and Rogart, R. B. (1992) *Science* 256: 1202–1205.

17. Eccles, J. C., Libet, B. and Young, R. R. (1958) *J. Physiol. (London)* 143: 11–40.

18. Kuno, M. and Llinas, R. (1970) *J. Physiol. (London)* 210: 807–821.

19. Gallego, R., Ivorra, I. and Morales, A. (1987) *J. Physiol. (London)* 391: 39–56.

20. Matzner, O. and Devor, M. (1992) *Brain Res.* 597: 92–98.

21. Dodge, F. A., Jr. and Cooley, J. (1973) *IBM J. Res. Dev.* 17: 219–229.

22. Sernagor, E., Yarom, Y. and Werman, R. (1986) *Proc. Natl. Acad. Sci. USA* 83: 7966–7970.

23. Titmus, M. J. and Faber, D. S. (1986) *J. Neurophysiol.* 55: 1440–1454.

24. Titmus, M. J. and Faber, D. S. (1990) *Prog. Neurobiol. (Oxford)* 35: 1–51.

25. Rizzo, M. A., Kocsis, J. D. and Waxman, S. G. (1995) *Neurobiol. Dis.* 2: 87–96.

26. Waxman, S. G., Kocsis, J. D. and Black, J. A. (1994) *J. Neurophysiol.* 72: 466–470.

27. Fitzgerald, M., Wall, P. D., Geodert, M. and Emson, P. C. (1985) *Brain Res.* 332: 131–141.

28. Chomczynski, P. and Sacchi, N. (1987) *Ann. Biochem.* 162: 156–159.

29. Gustafson, T. A., Clevinger, E. C., O'Neill, T. J., Yarowsky, P. J. and Krueger, B. K. (1993) *J. Biol. Chem.* 268: 18648–18653.

30. Barnes, W. M. (1994) *Proc. Natl. Acad. Sci. USA* 91: 2216–2220.

31. Cheng, S., Fockler, C., Barnes, W. M. and Higuchi, R. (1994) *Proc. Natl. Acad. Sci. USA* 91: 5695–5699.

32. Dib-Hajj, S. D., and Waxman, S. G. (1995) *FEBS Lett.* 377: 485–488.

33. Black, J. A., Yokoyama, S., Higashida, H., Ransom, B. R. and Waxman, S. G. (1994) *Mol. Brain Res.* 22: 275–290.

34. Foehring, R., Sypert, G. W. and Munson, J. (1986) *J. Neurophysiol.* 55: 947–965.

35. Purves, D. and Nja, A. (1978) in *Neuronal Plasticity*, ed. Cotman, C. W. (Raven, New York), pp. 27–47.

36. Bhisitkul, R., Kocsis, J. D., Gordon, T. and Waxman, S. G. (1990) *Exp. Neurol.* 109: 273–278.

37. Grafstein, B. (1986) in *The Retina, Part II*, eds. Adler, R. and Farber, D. B. (Academic, New York), pp. 275–335.

38. Waxman, S. G. and Anderson, M. J. (1982) *Cell Tissue Res.* 223: 487–492.

39. Hoffman, P. N. and Cleveland, D. W. (1988) *Proc. Natl. Acad. Sci. USA* 85: 4530–4533.

40. Utzschneider, D., Bhisitkul, R. and Kocsis, J. D. (1993) *Muscle Nerve* 16: 958–963.

41. Czeh, G., Kudo, N. and Kuno, M. (1977) *J. Physiol. (London)* 270: 165–180.

42. Perl, E. R. (1992) in *Sensory Neurons*, ed. Scott, S. (Oxford Univ. Press, New York), pp. 3–23.

43. Wall, P. D. and Devor, M. (1983) *Pain* 17: 321–339.

44. Kajander, K. C., Wakisaka, S. and Bennett, G. J. (1992) *Neurosci. Lett.* 138: 225–228.

45. Rizzo, M. A., Kocsis, J. D. and Waxman, S. G. (1994) *J. Neurophysiol.* 72: 2796–2816.

28 Down-Regulation of Tetrodotoxin-Resistant Sodium Currents and Up-Regulation of a Rapidly Repriming Tetrodotoxin-Sensitive Sodium Current in Small Spinal Sensory Neurons after Nerve Injury

Theodore R. Cummins and Stephen G. Waxman

Abstract Clinical and experimental studies have shown that spinal sensory neurons become hyperexcitable after axonal injury, and electrophysiological changes have suggested that this may be attributable to changes in sodium current expression. We have demonstrated previously that sodium channel α-III mRNA levels are elevated and sodium channel α-SNS mRNA levels are reduced in rat spinal sensory neurons after axotomy. In this study we show that small (C-type) rat spinal sensory neurons express sodium currents with dramatically different kinetics after axotomy produced by sciatic nerve ligation. Uninjured C-type neurons express both slowly inactivating tetrodotoxin-resistant (TTX-R) sodium current and a fast-inactivating tetrodotoxin-sensitive (TTX-S) current that reprimes (recovers from inactivation) slowly. After axotomy, the TTX-R current density was greatly reduced. No difference was observed in the density of TTX-S currents after axotomy, and their voltage dependence was not different from controls. However, TTX-S currents in axotomized neurons reprimed four times faster than control TTX-S currents. These data indicate that axotomy of spinal neurons is followed by downregulation of TTX-R current and by the emergence of a rapidly repriming TTX-S current and suggest that this may be attributable to the upregulation of a sodium channel isoform that was unexpressed previously in these cells. These axotomy-induced changes in sodium currents are expected to alter excitability substantially and could underlie the molecular pathogenesis of some chronic pain syndromes associated with injury to the axons of spinal sensory neurons.

Although chronic pain affects >60% of spinal cord injury patients (Knutsdottir, 1993; Levi et al., 1995; Subbarao et al., 1995), its pathophysiology is not well understood. One possibility is that nociceptive spinal sensory neurons generate inappropriate activity after injury. Spinal sensory neurons become hyperexcitable and generate spontaneous impulses after injury in

Reprinted with permission from *The Journal of Neuroscience* 17: 3503–3514, 1997.

experimental animals (Wall and Gutnick, 1974; Lisney and Devor, 1987; Matzner and Devor, 1994) and humans (Nystrom and Hagbarth, 1981; Nordin et al., 1984). Interestingly, anticonvulsants and local anesthetics have been used at concentrations known to act on sodium channels to manage chronic pain in humans (Boas et al., 1982; Chabal et al., 1989a; Chabal et al., 1992; Galer et al., 1993; Appelgren et al., 1996). Matzner and Devor (1992, 1994) proposed that the hyperexcitability associated with chronic pain results from an increase in sodium channel density at the site of injury. It also has been hypothesized that changes in the kinetics and voltage-dependent characteristics of sodium currents, possibly because of changes in the expression of sodium channel genes, contribute to the ectopic impulse generation and hyperexcitability of spinal sensory (dorsal root ganglion, DRG) neurons after nerve injury (Waxman et al., 1994; Rizzo et al., 1995, 1996).

DRG neurons possess a complicated mix of sodium currents (Caffrey et al., 1992; Black et al., 1996). Kostyuk et al. (1981) first reported that DRG neurons produced at least two types of sodium currents, including a fast TTX-sensitive (TTX-S) current and a slow TTX-resistant (TTX-R) current. Two groups recently cloned a sodium channel isoform (SNS) that is resistant to TTX and is proposed to underlie the TTX-R current in small neurons (Akopian et al., 1996; Sangameswaran et al., 1996). It is not clear which sodium channel isoform or isoforms underlie the TTX-S current. We have shown that normal DRG neurons can express as many as seven different sodium channel α-subunit mRNAs in situ and in vitro (Black et al., 1996), and, therefore, more than one sodium channel isoform might contribute to the TTX-S or the TTX-R component. However, it is not known what the physiological importance of the different isoforms is or if they have distinct kinetics.

Recently we demonstrated that axotomy induces an increase in the level of the type III and a decrease in SNS sodium channel mRNA in DRG C-type neurons (Waxman et al., 1994; Dib-Hajj et al., 1996), indicating that sodium current properties might be altered by axotomy. We hypothesized that axotomy increases a TTX-S current and decreases the TTX-R current in C-type DRG neurons, as previously demonstrated in large cutaneous afferent DRG neurons (Rizzo et al., 1995).

In this study we examined the effects of axonal injury on sodium current properties in small (18–25 μm) DRG C-type neurons (which include nociceptive and temperature-sensitive neurons) to determine whether the sodium currents of these neurons indeed do change after axotomy. Surprisingly, we found that axotomy is followed by the expression of a TTX-S current with different kinetic properties, especially recovery from inactivation, as well as downregulation of the TTX-R current in these cells. The axotomy-induced emergence of a sodium channel characterized by rapid repriming may provide a basis for hyperexcitability in injured DRG neurons.

Materials and Methods

Sciatic Nerve Injury

Axotomy of the sciatic nerve was performed as previously described (Waxman et al., 1994). Under anesthetic, the right sciatic nerve of adult Sprague–Dawley female rats was exposed, and a tight ligature was placed around the sciatic nerve near the sciatic notch proximal to the pyriform ligament. The nerve was sectioned with fine surgical scissors immediately distal to the ligature site, and the proximal nerve stump was fit into a silicone cuff. In some experiments the cuff contained 2 μl of an 8% Fluoro-gold solution for retrograde labeling, which facilitated definitive identification of axotomized neurons (Schmued

and Fallon, 1986). The incision was closed, and the animals were allowed to recover.

Culture of Spinal Sensory Neurons

DRG cells were studied after short-term culture (12–24 hr). The short-term culture (1) provided cells with truncated axonal processes that can be voltage-clamped readily and reliably, (2) allowed the cells sufficient time to adhere to the glass coverslip, and (3) was short enough to minimize changes in electrical properties that can occur in long-term cultures. The spontaneous electrical activity characteristic of DRG neurons after nerve injury can be observed in isolated injured neurons, but not in isolated control neurons (Study and Kral, 1996), demonstrating that the isolation procedure does not drastically alter the electrophysiological properties of the DRG neurons. Furthermore, adult rat DRG neurons maintained in vitro for 24 hr display a profile of sodium channel mRNA expression similar to that for DRG neurons in situ, indicating that short-term culture does not alter substantially the expression of sodium channel mRNAs in these cells (Black et al., 1996). It should be noted, however, that changes in both sodium currents and mRNA expression can be seen after 7 d in vitro. The culture was performed as previously described (Caffrey et al., 1992). L4–L5 DRG neurons were cultured between 2 and 60 d postaxotomy (DPA). Only the right sciatic nerve was ligated, and the left L4–L5 DRG neurons were used as controls.

Whole-Cell Patch-clamp Recordings

Whole-cell patch-clamp recordings were conducted at room temperature (∼21 °C) with an EPC-9 amplifier. Data were acquired on an Macintosh Quadra 950 computer with the Pulse program (v 7.89, HEKA Electronic, Germany). Fire-polished electrodes (0.8–1.5 MΩ) were fabricated from 1.5 mm Drummond capillary glass by using a Sutter P-97 puller (Sutter Instruments, Novato, CA). To minimize space clamp problems, we selected only isolated cells with a soma size of 18–25 μm for recording. Cells were not considered for analysis if the initial seal resistance was <5 GΩ or if they had high leakage currents (holding current >1.0 nA at −80 mV), membrane blebs, or an access resistance >4 MΩ. Access resistance was monitored throughout the experiment, and data were not used if resistance changes of >20% occurred. The average access resistance was 2.1 ± 0.6 MΩ (mean ± SD, $n =$ 113) for control cells and 2.0 ± 0.7 MΩ ($n =$ 187) for axotomized cells. Voltage errors were minimized by using 70–80% series resistance compensation, and the capacitance artifact was canceled by using the computer-controlled circuitry of the patch-clamp amplifier. Linear leak subtraction, based on resistance estimates from four to five hyperpolarizing pulses applied before the depolarizing test potential, was used for all voltage-clamp recordings. Membrane currents usually were filtered at 5 kHz and sampled at 20 kHz. The pipette solution contained (in mM): 140 CsF, 1 EGTA, 10 NaCl, and 10 HEPES, pH 7.3. The standard bathing solution was (in mM): 140 NaCl, 3 KCl, 1 $MgCl_2$, 1 $CaCl_2$, 0.1 $CdCl_2$, and 10 HEPES, pH 7.3. The liquid junction potential for these solutions was <8 mV; data were not corrected to account for this offset. The osmolarity of all solutions was adjusted to 310 mOsm (Wescor 5500 osmometer, Logan, UT). The offset potential was zeroed before patching the cells and checked after each recording for drift; if the drift was >10 mV/hr, the recording was discarded.

In situ Hybridization

To compare the patch-clamp results with the expression of SNS mRNA in DRG neurons, we used in situ hybridization results from adult rat DRG neurons at DPA5 (Dib-Hajj et al., 1996); this time point was chosen to correspond to electrophysiological recordings at DPA6, allowing for a 1 d lag between mRNA expression and the appearance of functional channels. The hybridization signal in small (<30 μm in diameter) DRG neurons was scored from 0 to +++, as described by Dib-Hajj et al. (1996).

Results

Sodium currents were recorded from small (18–25 μm) DRG neurons with whole-cell patch-clamp techniques. Control neurons were cultured from the uninjured left L4–L5 DRG of each rat (116 cells were studied from 14 different cultures). To examine the effects of injury on sodium currents, we cultured neurons from the axotomized right L4–L5 DRGs of rats at 2, 6, 22, and 60 d postaxotomy (DPA2, DPA6, DPA22, DPA60). For each time point, 10–15 cells per culture were recorded from at least three different cultures. Because not all of the L4–L5 axons are transected at the level of sciatic nerve ligation (because of branching of the nerve proximal to the ligation site), it is estimated that only ~70% of the neurons cultured actually were axotomized (Yip et al., 1984; Devor et al., 1985). In most experiments we did not use retrograde labeling and recorded from randomly chosen small C-type neurons. This provided a comparison with the previous study on mRNA expression (Dib-Hajj et al., 1996) in which it was not possible to identify axotomized neurons unequivocally. For some experiments (specified below), we studied fluorescently labeled axotomized neurons, which we could identify positively as axotomized neurons. Because the labeling was weak at DPA2 and DPA60, results on labeled cells are reported only for DPA6 and DPA22.

Sodium Currents Are Altered after Axotomy

Axotomy had a dramatic effect on the sodium currents of C-type neurons. Figure 28.1 shows

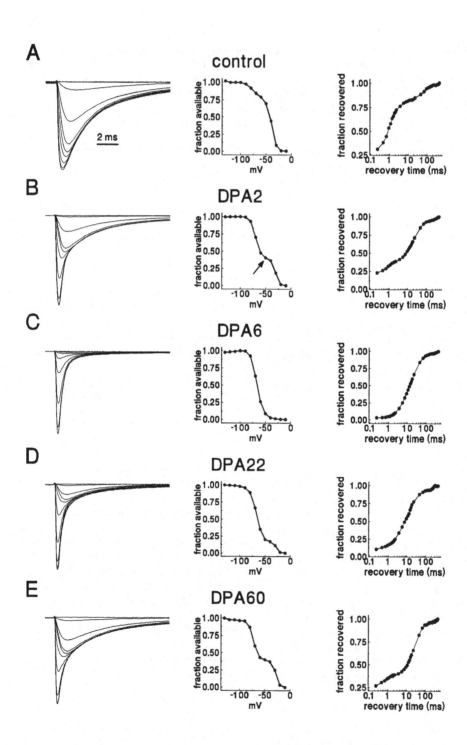

recordings from a typical cell at each time point. The sodium currents in control neurons were similar to those previously described in small DRG neurons (Caffrey et al., 1992; Roy and Narahashi, 1992; Elliott and Elliott, 1993; Rizzo et al., 1994). Most control neurons expressed both fast-inactivating and slow-inactivating sodium currents (table 28.1), which we refer to as "fast" and "slow," respectively. Axotomy decreased the number of cells expressing predominantly (>70% of total) slow currents and increased the number expressing predominantly (>70% of total) fast currents (table 28.1) in which the relative contributions were estimated by using the inflection point in the steady-state inactivation curves (figure 28.1).

As has been shown by others, in control neurons the fast-inactivating current was sensitive to nanomolar concentrations of TTX, but the slow-inactivating current was resistant (figure 28.2A, B). The relative TTX sensitivity of the fast and slow currents also was measured at DPA22 ($n = 7$) and DPA60 ($n = 5$) by using 100 nM TTX (figure 28.2C–F). For all cells in both groups the fast current was always sensitive and the slow current insensitive to TTX. As has been done in previous studies on DRG sodium currents (Roy and Narahashi, 1992; Elliott and Elliott, 1993; Jeftinija, 1994), we will refer to the fast-inactivating TTX-sensitive cur-

rents as the TTX-S component and the slow-inactivating TTX-resistant currents as the TTX-R component, although we did not always test the TTX sensitivity.

For the majority of experiments, prepulse inactivation was used to separate the TTX-R and TTX-S current components (McLean et al., 1988; Roy and Narahashi, 1992). Prepulse inactivation takes advantage of the differences in the inactivation properties of the TTX-S and TTX-R currents and is simpler than TTX subtraction. TTX subtraction and prepulse inactivation give essentially the same results (figure 28.3).

Inactivation Kinetics and Steady-state Inactivation

The rate of sodium current inactivation was measured in control neurons and after axotomy. The inactivating phase for both the TTX-S and TTX-R component was well fit with a single decaying exponential. In control neurons the time constant for fast inactivation (test potential = 0 mV), using the prepulse inactivation protocol, was estimated to be 10-fold slower for the TTX-R current than for the TTX-S current (table 28.2). Similar values were obtained for the TTX-S and TTX-R components, respectively, in DRG neurons after axotomy (table 28.2). However, because DRG neurons expressed predom-

Figure 28.1

Axotomy alters the inactivation kinetics and voltage dependence of inactivation of C-type DRG neurons. (*Left column*) Families of traces from representative control and axotomized C-type neurons are shown. Faster inactivation kinetics are observed for the total sodium current in axotomized neurons. The currents were elicited by 20 msec test pulses to −10 mV after 500 msec prepulses to potentials over the range of −130 mV to −10 mV. (*Middle column*) The corresponding steady-state inactivation curves are shown for each cell. Current is plotted as a fraction of peak current. In the control neuron the midpoint for steady-state inactivation (V_h) is −38 mV. At *DPA2* V_h is −62 mV, and at *DPA6* and *DPA22* V_h is −65 mV. At *DPA60* V_h is −50 mV. However, two current components can be resolved easily in the control, *DPA2*, *DPA22*, and *DPA60* cells: a slowly inactivating component that has a relatively depolarized voltage dependence of inactivation and a fast-inactivating component that has a more negative V_h. The steady-state inactivation curves for these cells are bimodal because of the different inactivation properties of the two components (arrow in *B* indicates point of inflection). The *DPA6* cell, on the other hand, appears to exhibit only fast-inactivating currents, and the steady-state inactivation is not inflected. (*Right column*) Repriming (recovery from inactivation) is shown for each cell. Changes in repriming are described in detail in the text and in figure 28.8.

Table 28.1
Effect of axotomy on sodium current kinetics

Cell type[a]	Current type (% of total)			Number of cells
	Fast	Mixed	Slow	
Control	15	39	46	113
Axotomized				
PDA2	32	48	20	40
PDA6	71	29	0	31
PDA22	73	21	6	33
PDA60	50	35	15	54

[a] Cells were categorized as displaying fast current if fast current constituted >70% of the total current and were categorized as displaying slow current if slow current constituted >70% of total current. Numbers are percentages of DRG neurons.

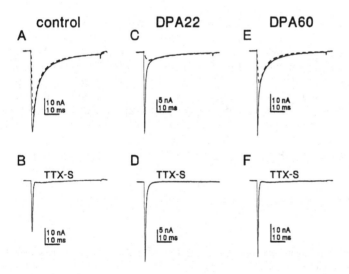

Figure 28.2
Tetrodotoxin (TTX) sensitivity of fast-inactivating and slowly inactivating currents in control neurons and neurons after axotomy. Representative current traces are shown for a *control* neuron (*A, B*) and neurons at *DPA22* (*C, D*) and *DPA60* (*E, F*). C-type neurons were held at −100 mV and stepped to 0 mV for 50 msec. Current traces are shown before (*solid trace*) and after (*dashed trace*) 100 nM TTX (*A, C, E*). The *TTX-S* component, obtained by using digital subtraction of the traces in *A, C,* and *E*, is shown in *B, D,* and *F*. The slow component is TTX-resistant, and the fast component is TTX-sensitive in all three groups.

inantly the TTX-S current after axotomy, the total current inactivated faster in these neurons than in control neurons (see figure 28.1).

Similarly, although a striking difference was observed between control neurons and neurons after axotomy in terms of the voltage dependence of steady-state inactivation (see figure 28.1), this difference was attributable primarily to the downregulation of the TTX-R component after axotomy. In control neurons the midpoint of steady-state inactivation (V_h; 500 msec inactivating prepulses) was significantly different for TTX-S currents and TTX-R currents (table 28.2, figure 28.3). Similar values were observed for the TTX-S and TTX-R currents, respectively, after axotomy (table 28.2). Thus the TTX-S and TTX-R components showed similar voltage dependencies of inactivation in control neurons and neurons after axotomy. It should be noted, however, that interneuronal variation, as previously described for small DRG neurons by Rizzo et al. (1994), was observed in the midpoint of steady-state inactivation for all of the groups.

Sodium Current Activation

Prepulse inactivation/subtraction was used to separate the TTX-R and TTX-S components. In control neurons the TTX-S component activated at potentials ~10 mV more negative than the TTX-R component (table 28.3). The midpoints of activation (V_m) estimated with TTX (100 nM) subtraction also showed that the TTX-S component in control neurons activated ~13 mV more negative than the TTX-R component.

We measured the voltage dependence of activation for the TTX-S current after axotomy at DPA6 and DPA22 (table 28.3). The V_m for the TTX-S currents from these neurons after axotomy was within 6 mV of the V_m for the TTX-S currents from control neurons. Similarly, the V_m for the TTX-R currents after axotomy was very close to the V_m for the TTX-R currents from control neurons. In all of the groups, cell-to-cell

variability, as originally reported by Rizzo et al. (1995), was observed for the voltage dependence of activation for TTX-R and TTX-S currents. It should be noted that precise measurements of activation in C-type DRG neurons are difficult because they have a high sodium current density. We used low-resistance patch pipettes and 70–80% series resistance compensation to minimize voltage errors. Our data on the voltage dependence of TTX-R and TTX-S current activation are similar to those reported by others (Roy and Narahashi, 1992; Elliott and Elliott, 1993; Ogata and Tatebayashi, 1993).

The TTX-R Current Is Downregulated after Axotomy

To quantitate the amount of TTX-R and TTX-S currents expressed in each cell, we used prepulse inactivation (McLean et al., 1988; Roy and Narahashi, 1992) to separate the TTX-S and TTX-R current components (figure 28.3). The estimates of the TTX-S and TTX-R current amplitudes obtained with prepulse inactivation were nearly identical to estimates obtained by using TTX subtraction from control and axotomized neurons (table 28.4).

The TTX-R current amplitude and current density (amplitude normalized to cell capacitance) were significantly lower than control at all postaxotomy time points (figure 28.4A). The lowest TTX-R current density (22% of control density) was observed at DPA6, with a gradual increase at DPA22 and DPA60, when it reached 46% of control levels. Surprisingly, axotomy had little effect on the current density of the TTX-S component (figure 28.4B). Cell capacitance, which provides an electrical estimate of surface area, essentially was unaffected by axotomy (figure 28.4C).

Under the conditions used in this study, both TTX-S and TTX-R currents were detected in most (95%) of the control neurons. Only 5 of 113 control cells expressed the TTX-S component alone, and only one expressed the TTX-R com-

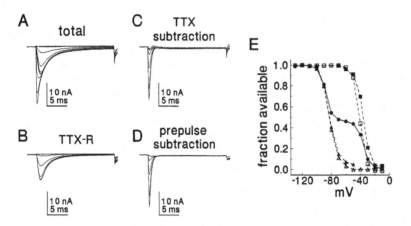

Figure 28.3
Separation of TTX-S and TTX-R currents. Current traces were recorded from a control neuron before (*A*) and after (*B*) addition of 100 nM TTX to the bath solution. The currents were elicited by 20 msec test pulses to −10 mV after 500 msec prepulses to potentials over the range of −130 mV to −10 mV. (*C*) The TTX-S component was obtained by digitally subtracting the data in (*B*) from (*A*). (*D*) The TTX-S currents were obtained by subtracting the data in *A* obtained with the −50 mV prepulse from the data in *A* obtained with more hyperpolarized prepulses. (*E*) The steady-state inactivation (h_∞) curve for the total current in *A* is shown (●). The h_∞ curves for the TTX-S and TTX-R components estimated with either TTX subtraction (□, TTX-R; △, TTX-S) or prepulse subtraction (■, TTX-R; ▲, TTX-S) also are shown in (*E*). Data were normalized to unity.

Table 28.2
Inactivation of Na^+ currents in C-type neurons

	Inactivation					
	TTX-R			TTX-S		
	k (mV/e-fold)	V_h (mV)	τh (at 0 mV) (msec)	k (mV/e-fold)	V_h (mV)	τh (at 0 mV) (msec)
Control (29)	7.5 ± 2.4	−30.9 ± 8.6	4.7 ± 1.9	6.4 ± 1.3	−69.3 ± 6.6	0.48 ± 0.14
Axotomized						
DPA2 (11)	8.7 ± 2.7	−32.7 ± 5.3	4.5 ± 1.4	6.7 ± 1.6	−68.4 ± 6.3	0.44 ± 0.13
DPA6 (13)	7.9 ± 2.6	−30.3 ± 6.8	4.8 ± 0.9	6.1 ± 0.7	−67.2 ± 4.1	0.55 ± 0.23
DPA22 (15)	6.4 ± 2.5	−31.3 ± 6.7	4.7 ± 1.3	6.9 ± 1.3	−66.6 ± 6.9	0.46 ± 0.12
DPA60 (15)	8.7 ± 2.7	−32.7 ± 5.3	4.7 ± 1.5	6.5 ± 1.4	−67.7 ± 5.1	0.53 ± 0.17

Numbers in parentheses indicate number of cells. Data are expressed as mean ± SD.

Table 28.3
Activation of Na$^+$ currents in C-type neurons

	Activation			
	TTX-R		TTX-S	
	k (mV/e-fold)	V_m (mV)	k (mV/e-fold)	V_m (mV)
Control	6.4 ± 1.5	−15.7 ± 2.6	6.4 ± 1.5	−27.6 ± 4.9
Axotomized				
DPA6 (9)	7.9 ± 1.2	−16.9 ± 6.9	6.3 ± 1.7	−21.8 ± 6.6
DPA22 (14)	6.8 ± 1.9	−16.2 ± 4.0	4.8 ± 1.8	−24.6 ± 5.5

Numbers in parentheses indicate number of cells. Data are expressed as mean ± SD.

Table 28.4
Current amplitude: comparison of prepulse inactivation and TTX subtraction

	TTX-R		TTX-S		
	Prepulse inactivation	TTX subtraction	Prepulse inactivation	TTX subtraction	n
Control	24.7 nA	22.1 nA	26.8 nA	28.7 nA	11
	±3.5	±3.0	±4.7	±4.8	
DPA22	4.5 nA	4.0 nA	29.1 nA	29.8 nA	7
	±1.8	±1.4	±3.4	±3.9	
DPA60	15.1 nA	15.1 nA	21.1 nA	22.7 nA	
	±4.8	±5.0	±2.8	±3.3	5

Data are expressed as mean ± SEM.

ponent in isolation. The ratio of the TTX-R amplitude to the TTX-S amplitude was 1.1 ± 0.8 (mean ± SD, $n = 113$) in control neurons. By contrast, the ratio of the TTX-R amplitude to TTX-S amplitude fell to 0.65 ± 0.09 ($n = 40$), 0.22 ± 0.05 ($n = 31$), 0.27 ± 0.06 ($n = 33$), and 0.45 ± 0.06 ($n = 54$) in neurons after axotomy at DPA2, DPA6, DPA22, and DPA60, respectively.

These patch-clamp data may be compared with the results of our previous study, which examined the expression of SNS and III mRNAs in DRG neurons after axotomy (Dib-Hajj et al., 1996). In that study the level of SNS mRNA expression in small DRG neurons was scored as undetectable, marginal/low, moderate, or high after nonisotopic in situ hybridization (ISH). The ISH data are shown in figure 28.5A. To compare the ISH results with changes in TTX-R current expression, we classified small DRG neurons as having a TTX-R/TTX-S current ratio of <0.1, 0.1–0.5, 0.5–1.0, or >1.0 (figure 28.5B) or as having a TTX-R current density of <100, 100–200, 200–500, or >500 pA/pF (figure 28.5C). The patterns for SNS mRNA expression (figure 28.5A) and TTX-R current levels (figure 28.5B, C) in control neurons are similar; that is, a large percentage of the cells express moderate or high levels of SNS mRNA and also have

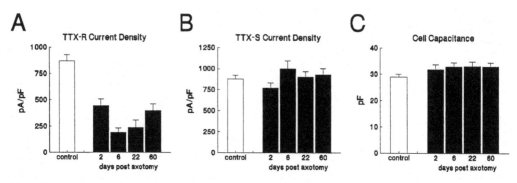

Figure 28.4

Axotomy decreases TTX-R current density. The TTX-S and TTX-R current densities were estimated in control ($n = 113$), DPA2 ($n = 40$), DPA6 ($n = 30$), DPA22 ($n = 33$), and DPA60 ($n = 47$) C-type neurons by using prepulse inactivation (500 msec prepulses) and a 0 mV test pulse. The TTX-R (*A*) and TTX-S (*B*) current densities were obtained by dividing the estimated peak current by the whole-cell capacitance. The TTX-R current density was significantly lower for the axotomized neurons at each time point (*A*). The TTX-S current density was not affected significantly by axotomy (*B*). Axotomy also did not alter cell capacitance significantly (*C*). Error bars indicate mean $\pm$ SD.

>200 pA/pF TTX-R current. Conversely, at DPA5 a high percentage of the DRG neurons have undetectable or low/moderate levels of SNS hybridization signal and at DPA6 a vast majority of DRG neurons show <200 pA/pF TTX-R current. At DPA60, on the other hand, approximately one-half of the cells expressed moderate to high levels of TTX-R current, which is consistent with an observed partial recovery of SNS mRNA levels at DPA58 (Dib-Hajj et al., 1996).

The TTX-R Current Is Downregulated in Labeled Axotomized Cells

Although the majority of cells at DPA6 and DPA22 exhibited predominantly TTX-S current (table 28.1), five cells at DPA6 and six cells at DPA22 had a relatively high TTX-R current density (>500 pA/pF). It has been estimated that only 70% of L4–L5 neurons are axotomized when the sciatic nerve is transected at the mid-thigh level (Yip et al., 1984; Devor et al., 1985), and therefore the cells that expressed high densities of TTX-R current might be DRG neurons

with axons that were not transected. To confirm that the TTX-R current was downregulated in axotomized cells, we did additional experiments in which axotomized neurons were identified unequivocally by selectively labeling with a fluorescent indicator (see Materials and Methods). Neurons were cultured at days 6 and 22 (DPA6 and DPA22). In these experiments all of the labeled cells expressed predominantly TTX-S currents. None of the labeled cells expressed >500 pA/pF of TTX-R current at either DPA6 ($n = 16$) or DPA22 ($n = 14$). The TTX-R to TTX-S ratio in labeled cells was 0.17 ± 0.04 ($n = 16$) at DPA6 and 0.15 ± 0.06 ($n = 14$) at DPA22. This clearly demonstrates that the TTX-R current is downregulated in axotomized C-type neurons.

Persistent Currents Are Decreased after Axotomy

Persistent currents (defined as the current remaining at the end of a 40 msec test depolarization) often were observed in small C-type

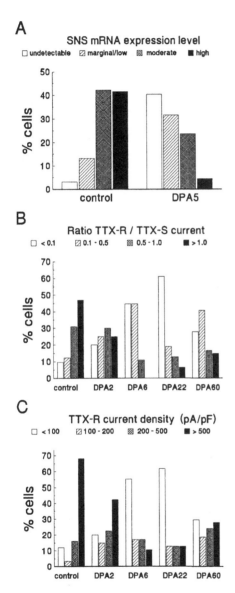

A

SNS mRNA expression level

□ undetectable ▨ marginal/low ▧ moderate ■ high

B

Ratio TTX-R / TTX-S current

□ < 0.1 ▨ 0.1 - 0.5 ▧ 0.5 - 1.0 ■ > 1.0

C

TTX-R current density (pA/pF)

□ < 100 ▨ 100 - 200 ▧ 200 - 500 ■ > 500

Figure 28.5

Axotomy has a similar effect on SNS mRNA expression and on TTX-R current expression. (*A*) The relative magnitude of SNS expression was measured in cultured control and *DPA5* C-type neurons by in situ hybridization (Dib-Hajj et al., 1996). Expression was

neurons. Figure 28.6 shows persistent current expressed as a fraction of the peak current for control neurons and Fluoro-gold-labeled DPA6 and DPA22 axotomized neurons. Persistent currents in control neurons were large, often >10% of the peak current (figure 28.6*A, B*). Even when measured at the end of a 200 msec test pulse, the persistent current still averaged almost 10% of the peak current in control neurons (figure 28.6*A*). In contrast, persistent currents after axotomy were small, typically <2% of the peak current (figure 28.6*B*). We believe that the large persistent currents in control neurons were generated by TTX-R channels because (1) the persistent currents in control neurons were not sensitive to nanomolar concentrations of TTX, and large persistent currents were not observed in control neurons that expressed primarily TTX-S current (figure 28.6*C*); and (2) the persistent currents occurred in a fairly narrow, negative voltage region, where TTX-R window currents, resulting from overlap between steady-state activation and inactivation processes, might occur. On the other hand, the voltage dependence is also consistent with what has been reported for low-voltage-activated T-type calcium currents in newborn DRG neurons (Ogata and Tatebayashi, 1992). We do not believe that these persistent currents are calcium currents because (1) our bath solution contains 100 μM Cd^{2+} and our pipette solution contained fluoride, which should block calcium currents; and (2) in a previous study we were unable to detect low-voltage-activated calcium currents in small adult DRG neurons (Caffrey et al., 1992).

classified as either undetectable, marginal/low, moderate, or high. (*B*) The ratio of the TTX-R current density to TTX-S current density is shown for control and axotomized neurons at *DPA2, DPA6, DPA22,* and *DPA60.* Cells were classified according to the ratio. (*C*) Shown is the TTX-R current density for *control* and axotomized neurons at *DPA2, DPA6, DPA22,* and *DPA60.* Cells were assigned to one of four groups for each time point on the basis of TTX-R current density.

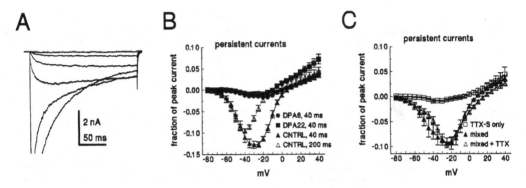

Figure 28.6

Axotomy decreases persistent currents in C-type neurons. (A) Family of currents recorded from a control small DRG neuron. Current was elicited by test potentials from −75 to −25 in 10 mV steps. The peak current in this cell was 47 nA. (B) Current-voltage relationship for the persistent current in small DRG neurons. Cells were held at −100 mV and stepped to step voltages from −80 to 40 mV for 40 msec. The average current measured from 38 to 40 msec was normalized to the maximum peak current for each cell and is plotted against the test voltage. Data are shown for control (▲, $n = 12$), DPA6 (●, $n = 14$), and DPA22 (■, $n = 14$). Axotomized cells in the DPA6 and DPA22 groups were identified with a fluorescent label. For the control neurons the persistent current also was measured by using 200 msec test depolarizations (△, $n = 11$). (C) The persistent current in control neurons ($n = 4$) that express both TTX-S and TTX-R currents is shown before (▲) and after (△) 100 nM TTX. In control neurons that express only TTX-S currents ($n = 5$), the persistent currents were small (□). Persistent currents were measured at 38–40 msec, as in (A).

Axotomy Upregulates a TTX-S Current with Rapid Recovery from Inactivation

Elliott and Elliott (1993) reported that in uninjured DRG neurons the TTX-R current recovered rapidly from inactivation and the TTX-S current recovered very slowly. We studied repriming in both control and axotomized small DRG neurons (figure 28.1, *right column*). We observed repriming kinetics similar to those reported by Elliott and Elliott (1993) in control neurons. The repriming kinetics in a typical control neuron are shown in figure 28.7, A and B. The time course was well fit with two exponentials. TTX was used to confirm that the slowly inactivating, rapidly repriming component was TTX-insensitive and that the fast-inactivating, slowly repriming component was TTX-sensitive ($n = 10$; figure 28.7C). In control

neurons that expressed both TTX-R and TTX-S currents, the TTX-R current recovered with a time constant of 1.0 ± 0.3 msec, and the TTX-S current recovered with a time constant of 60.5 ± 29.0 msec (mean $\pm$ SD, $n = 45$; recovery potential set at −100 mV). In some of the cells a small, ultraslow recovery component also was observed ($\tau \sim 150$–250 msec).

Figure 28.8A shows the averaged recovery time course for 45 control neurons that displayed both TTX-S and TTX-R currents, with the rapid and the slow repriming components also shown separately for clarity. For the five control neurons that only expressed TTX-S current, the time constant for recovery from inactivation was intermediate (13.9 ± 9.9 msec, mean $\pm$ SD, $n = 5$) between the rapid and slow time constants described above (data not shown). Only 3 of the 45 cells that expressed both TTX-S and TTX-R

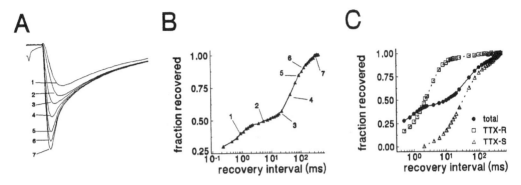

Figure 28.7
Recovery from inactivation has multiple components in control neurons. (*A*) Data from a typical control C-type neuron are shown. The cell was held at −100 mV, stepped to 0 mV for 20 msec to inactivate channels, and then brought back to −100 mV for increasing durations before the test potential of 0 mV. Current traces shown in (*A*) correspond to specific time points in the recovery time course shown in (*B*). The time course of recovery exhibited at least two components. The TTX-R component (traces 1 and 2) recovered rapidly, with a time constant of 0.7 msec. The TTX-S component recovered slowly (traces 5–7), with a time constant of 87 msec. (*C*) Data from another control neuron are shown. The time course of recovery is shown for the total current (●) and for the separated TTX-R (□) and TTX-S components (△). The TTX-R time course was obtained in the presence of 100 nM TTX. The TTX-S time course was obtained by subtracting the currents recorded with TTX from the data obtained without TTX.

currents exhibited a TTX-S component that recovered with a time course that might be considered as intermediate rather than slow.

The repriming kinetics were measured in DRG neurons at all time points after axotomy. The TTX-R component recovered rapidly in all of the cells from rats with ligated nerves. However, in only 2 of the 30 Fluoro-gold-labeled axotomized neurons was the TTX-R component large enough to measure accurately the repriming kinetics (figure 28.8*B*). In both of these cells, the TTX-R time constant for recovery from inactivation was near 0.9 msec, i.e., it remained close to control values.

In contrast, axotomy was followed by the emergence of a distinct TTX-S current, which we term the "rapidly repriming TTX-S" current. The time constant for recovery from inactivation for the rapidly repriming TTX-S current was shifted to dramatically shorter values. In all of the Fluoro-gold-labeled cells the TTX-S current

reprimed with an intermediate time course (figure 28.8*C, D*), with a time constant of 14.3 ± 6.3 msec (mean $\pm$ SD, $n = 16$) measured at DPA6 and 15.8 ± 5.1 msec ($n = 12$) at DPA22. This time constant in axotomized neurons is much shorter than the slow recovery time constant measured for the TTX-S current in the majority of control cells that expressed both TTX-R and TTX-S currents.

In recordings from randomly chosen DPA6 neurons from experiments in which Fluoro-gold labeling was not used, the TTX-S current dominated in 21 of 30 cells, and again the repriming time course was well fit with a single intermediate exponential ($\tau = 14.9 \pm 7.6$ msec). Of the other nine DPA6 neurons in these experiments, six fit the pattern observed in control neurons with rapid ($\tau = 1.3$ msec) and slow ($\tau = 72$ msec) repriming kinetics corresponding to TTX-R and TTX-S components, and three had both fast ($\tau = 1$ msec) and intermediate ($\tau = 20$ msec)

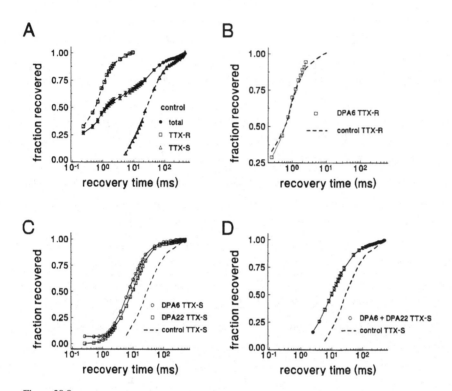

Figure 28.8

The kinetics of recovery from inactivation for TTX-S current, but not for TTX-R current, are different in axotomized neurons. (*A*) The averaged time course of recovery from inactivation for total current from control C-type neurons that expressed both TTX-S and TTX-R currents is shown (●, $n = 45$). At least two components can be distinguished. The time course of the rapid repriming component from control neurons with predominantly TTX-R (>75%) current is plotted separately (□, $n = 11$). The time course for the slow component (obtained by digitally subtracting the current recovered after 6 msec) in control cells expressing large TTX-S (>1 nA/pF) currents also is shown (△, $n = 12$). (*B*) The repriming time course of the TTX-R component in an axotomized neuron (*DPA6*) is shown (□). For comparison, the averaged repriming time course of the TTX-R components from control neurons also is shown (dashed curve). Recovery from inactivation for the TTX-R current does not shift after axotomy. (*C*) The time course of recovery from inactivation for injured DPA6 (○) and DPA22 (□) C-type neurons that expressed predominantly TTX-S currents is shown. For comparison, the repriming time course for the TTX-S current of control neurons also is shown (dashed curve). Note the leftward shift in the time course for recovery from inactivation for the TTX-S current after axotomy. (*D*) The averaged time course for recovery of the TTX-S current from inactivation in Fluoro-gold-identified axotomized DPA6 and DPA22 neurons ($n = 30$) is shown (○). For comparison, the repriming time course for the TTX-S current of control neurons also is shown (dashed curve).

kinetics corresponding to TTX-R and TTX-S components. In the DPA22 experiments in rats in which Fluoro-gold labeling was not used, the TTX-S component dominated in 22 of 29 cells, and 21 of these had an intermediate time course for repriming (16.2 ± 6.8 msec). In the remaining predominantly TTX-S cell, repriming had a slow time constant of 58 msec. For the seven DPA22 cells in these experiments with TTX-S and TTX-R currents, five had both fast ($\tau =$ 1.0 msec) and slow ($\tau = 85$ msec) recovery components, and two had fast ($\tau = 0.9$ msec) and intermediate ($\tau = 16$ msec) recovery components.

At DPA60, repriming kinetics was examined in 48 randomly chosen cells from experiments in which Fluoro-gold labeling was not attempted. Almost one-half of the cells exhibited predominantly TTX-S current. For these 21 TTX-S cells the time course showed intermediate kinetics ($\tau = 17.9 \pm 6.6$ msec). The other 27 DPA60 cells possessed both TTX-S and TTX-R currents. Sixteen of these cells displayed fast ($\tau = 1.3$ msec) and slow ($\tau = 69$ msec) components of repriming, six displayed fast ($\tau = 1.0$ msec) and intermediate ($\tau = 19$ msec) components, and five had multiple components. The repriming data indicate that axotomy results in the expression of TTX-S current with different properties, as well as downregulating the TTX-R current, and show that these changes persist for at least 60 d after axotomy.

TTX-S Currents in Normal and Axotomized Neurons Display Lidocaine Sensitivity

Previous studies have indicated that lidocaine and other sodium channel inhibitors can block ectopic impulses in injured neurons at concentrations that are not sufficient to block normal nociception (Yaari and Devor, 1985; Chabal et al., 1989b; Devor et al., 1992). Roy and Narahashi (1992) reported that TTX-R currents were less sensitive to lidocaine than TTX-S currents (K_D values of 200 μM and 50 μM, respectively). Therefore, we wanted to test the relative

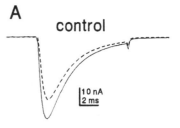

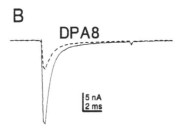

Figure 28.9

Axotomy increases the relative sensitivity of C-type neurons to frequency-dependent inhibition by lidocaine. Representative traces from a *control* (A) and *DPA8* (B) neuron are shown. Cells were exposed to 50 μM lidocaine. After 5 min, the cells were stimulated with a 10 Hz train of 20 depolarizations (to 0 mV for 10 msec). The currents elicited by the first (solid trace) and 20th (dashed trace) depolarizations are shown.

sensitivity of TTX-S currents in axotomized neurons. We applied 50 μM lidocaine to control and axotomized (labeled DPA8) neurons. Use-dependent lidocaine inhibition was measured by comparing the amplitude of the first and 20th pulse in a 10 Hz pulse train (10 msec, 0 mV depolarizations). Although the TTX-S component was inhibited by 62 ± 22%, the TTX-R component in control neurons was inhibited by only 11 ± 6% ($n = 4$). In the labeled DPA8 neurons the TTX-S current was inhibited by 53 ± 16% ($n = 4$). Thus the TTX-S components in both control and injured neurons were significantly more sensitive to therapeutic concentrations of lidocaine than the TTX-R component in control neurons. The sensitivity of the TTX-R current was not measured in DPA8 cells, because they exhibited only small TTX-R currents. Because the TTX-S current dominates in axotomized neurons, the total sodium current in axotomized neurons is relatively more sensitive to lidocaine than the current in uninjured neurons (figure 28.9).

Discussion

We have studied the effects of axotomy on sodium currents in small C-type DRG neurons. Axotomy results in dramatic and complex changes in the sodium currents expressed in these neurons. Axotomy decreased the amount of slowly inactivating TTX-R current and resulted in increased expression of a distinct fast-inactivating/rapidly repriming TTX-S current. These changes were still evident 60 d after axotomy. The results presented here, in conjunction with our previous studies that examined sodium channel mRNA expression in axotomized DRG neurons, provide new insights into the molecular pathophysiology of peripheral nerve injury and may have implications for understanding chronic pain syndromes.

Axotomy Downregulates TTX-R Current and SNS mRNA Levels

One striking effect of axotomy was the downregulation of TTX-R current density. It has been proposed that the TTX-R current is encoded by the SNS transcript (Akopian et al., 1996; Sangameswaran et al., 1996). Our data support this proposal. ISH demonstrated that ~90% of small neurons express SNS α-subunit mRNA (Black et al., 1996). This closely correlates with the observation presented here that 101 of 113 control neurons expressed significant levels (>50 pA/pF) of TTX-R current. Furthermore, the effect of axotomy on SNS mRNA levels at DPA5 is similar to the effect on TTX-R current density at

DPA6 (figure 28.5). With the use of RT-PCR of the whole ganglion, it has been demonstrated that SNS mRNA partially recovers toward control levels by 58 d after axotomy (Dib-Hajj et al., 1996). In agreement with the recovery of SNS levels at later times postaxotomy, we observed an increase in TTX-R current density between DPA6 and DPA60.

It has been suggested that axotomy might cause a reversion to an embryonic mode of sodium channel expression (Iwahashi et al., 1994; Waxman et al., 1994). The loss of TTX-R current is consistent with an embryonic mode of sodium channel expression. Fedulova et al. (1994) reported that only 24% of embryonic (E17) DRG neurons express TTX-R currents and observed a TTX-R current density in E17 cells that was comparable to our results from DPA6 and DPA22 axotomized neurons.

Axotomy Upregulates Rapidly Repriming TTX-S Current and Type III mRNA Levels

In contrast to the effect on SNS mRNA levels, axotomy induces expression of type III mRNA in DRG neurons (Waxman et al., 1994). Surprisingly, we did not see a significant change in the TTX-S current density after axotomy. However, the TTX-S current components in control and injured neurons displayed significantly different rates of recovery from inactivation. Axotomized neurons express a TTX-S current that recovers much faster than in control neurons (figure 28.8). The emergence of a TTX-S current with different repriming kinetics could result from upregulation of type III channels and downregulation of a TTX-S channel that is expressed in uninjured neurons. This axotomy-induced change in repriming kinetics is also consistent with a reversion to an earlier developmental mode of sodium channel expression (Ogata and Tatebayashi, 1992).

Our data raise the intriguing possibility that different channel isoforms may show important differences in terms of repriming kinetics. Surprisingly little electrophysiological difference has been observed to date among the different brain sodium channel isoforms, leading some to ask why so many channel isoforms exist. Differences in repriming kinetics could have important implications for excitability and repetitive firing properties. Changes in repriming kinetics also could have pathophysiological importance. Indeed, some of the skeletal muscle sodium channel mutations associated with hereditary forms of paramyotonia congenita increase the rate of recovery from inactivation (Yang et al., 1994), which can contribute to hyperexcitability of affected skeletal muscle by reducing the refractory period (Chahine et al., 1994).

If the slow- and fast-recovering TTX-S currents are encoded by distinct isoforms, then our results predict that other mRNAs besides SNS are downregulated by axotomy. If so, what α-subunit produces the TTX-S current in control neurons? We found that all but 1 of 113 control neurons expressed >50 pA/pF of TTX-S current. Using ISH, Black et al. (1996) found that virtually all small neurons express an mRNA that hybridized to the hNE-Na probe. Except for the SNS probe, no other transcript was nearly so abundant in uninjured small neurons. Recombinant hNE-Na channels expressed in HEK-293 cells seem to have fast inactivation decay kinetics and are TTX-sensitive (Klugbauer et al., 1995), but the repriming kinetics have not yet been characterized. Thus, the hNE-Na isotype is a candidate for encoding the TTX-S current with slow recovery from inactivation.

Physiological Implications

We show in figure 28.3 that control neurons express approximately the same amount of TTX-S and TTX-R current when held at -100 mV for prolonged periods. However, the resting potential of DRG neurons is reported to be approximately -60 mV (Caffrey et al., 1992; Jeftinija, 1994). At this potential much of the TTX-S current in C-type neurons (V_h approximately equal

to -69 mV; see table 28.2) might be inactivated. Indeed, Rizzo et al. (1994) studied C-type DRG neurons, using -60 mV as the holding potential, and observe virtually no TTX-S currents. This seems to indicate that control neurons produce high densities of TTX-S channels that are not available for activation. An alternative explanation is that small DRG neurons have a bistable resting potential, as has been reported for other types of excitable cells (Gola and Niel, 1993; O'Donnell and Grace, 1995). TTX-R persistent currents might play a role in setting the resting potential, as demonstrated in optic nerve axons (Stys et al., 1993). Under some circumstances the C-type neurons may reside at more negative potentials from which the TTX-S currents are available for activation. However, because the TTX-S current reprimes very slowly in control neurons, the TTX-S currents probably would be involved only in the initial response to a given stimulus. After the initial response the TTX-R currents probably dictate the repetitive firing properties.

Our results suggest that the situation in injured neurons is significantly different. In the labeled neurons at DPA6 and DPA22, the predominant sodium current was a TTX-S current with intermediate repriming kinetics. Downregulation of the TTX-R current should result in relatively rapid inactivation during spike electrogenesis, which would produce narrow action potentials. Axotomy also greatly reduces the TTX-R persistent currents, which could affect resting potential and thus might increase the relative amount of TTX-S current that is available for activation. Because the TTX-S current after axotomy reprimes relatively rapidly, the injured neurons would be expected to sustain higher firing frequencies.

Chronic Pain

This study, in conjunction with our previous studies on mRNA expression (Dib-Hajj et al., 1996), shows that axotomy causes a decrease in expression of the SNS channel and the TTX-R sodium current in small spinal sensory neurons. Thus the hyperexcitability observed in these cells after axotomy, which is believed to underlie some chronic pain syndromes, is not attributable to an increase in SNS/TTX-R current expression. On the other hand, our data show the emergence of a TTX-S current with rapid recovery from inactivation after axotomy (figure 28.8) and suggest that rapidly repriming TTX-S currents contribute to inappropriate firing in C-type neurons. Our results also show that type III mRNA expression is upregulated after axotomy (Waxman et al., 1994; Dib-Hajj et al., 1996).

Lidocaine and other sodium channel blockers have been used in the treatment of chronic pain (Boas et al., 1982; Chabal et al., 1989a). An expanding body of evidence suggests that it is possible pharmacologically to block some types of sodium channels while leaving other types unblocked; for example, it is possible pharmacologically to block the persistent sodium current that mediates damaging sodium influx in the anoxic optic nerve while leaving the fast sodium current, which underlies action potential electrogenesis, unblocked (Stys et al., 1992). Similarly, some sodium channel blockers inhibit ectopic activity in peripheral nerves at concentrations that do not block nociception (Yaari and Devor, 1985; Burchiel, 1988; Chabal et al., 1989b; Devor et al., 1992). Matzner and Devor (1994) found that high concentrations (3–300 μM) of TTX blocked ectopic impulses in chronically injured DRG neurons, providing additional evidence that sodium channels underlie hyperexcitability after nerve injury, although their results did not identify the channel subtype or subtypes involved. Interestingly, the recombinant SNS channel expressed in *Xenopus* oocytes is only weakly sensitive to lidocaine and phenytoin (Akopian et al., 1996). Consistent with this, Roy and Narahashi (1992) reported that the TTX-R channel is relatively insensitive to lidocaine ($K_D \sim 0.2$ mM), and we have confirmed that result. Our data (figure 28.9), on the other hand,

show that the predominant TTX-S current in axotomized neurons is sensitive to lidocaine.

Our data on sodium current (this study) and mRNA expression levels (Waxman et al., 1994; Dib-Hajj et al., 1996) indicate that altered expression of TTX-S sodium channel isoforms, in addition to or rather than an alteration in SNS and TTX-R currents, plays a predominant role in generating hyperexcitability, which underlies pain after injury to DRG neurons. Moreover, our results demonstrate that the TTX-S sodium channel that is expressed in spinal sensory neurons after axotomy exhibits rapid recovery from inactivation and suggest that this rapid repriming predisposes these cells to abnormal firing, which underlies chronic pain. Drugs targeted at the sodium channel isoforms producing rapidly repriming currents (possibly type III isoform) therefore may be appropriate for the treatment of some types of chronic pain.

Acknowledgments

This work was supported in part by the Medical Research Service, Department of Veterans Affairs. T.R.C. was supported in part by a fellowship from the Eastern Paralyzed Veterans Association and by a grant from the Paralyzed Veterans of America Spinal Cord Research Foundation. We thank Drs. Joel Black, Sulayman Dib-Hajj, and Marco Rizzo for helpful discussions.

References

Akopian AN, Sivilotti L, Wood JN (1996) A tetrodotoxin-resistant voltage-gated sodium channel expressed by sensory neurons. Science 379: 257–262.

Appelgren L, Janson M, Nitescu P, Curelaru I (1996) Continuous intracisternal and high cervical intrathecal bupivacaine analgesia in refractory head and neck pain. Anesthesiology 84: 256–272.

Black JA, Dib-Hajj S, McNabola K, Jeste S, Rizzo MA, Kocsis JD, Waxman SG (1996) Spinal sensory neurons express multiple sodium channel a-subunit mRNAs. Mol Brain Res 43: 117–132.

Boas RA, Covino BG, Shahnarian A (1982) Analgesic responses to i.v. lignocaine. Br J Anaesth 54: 501–505.

Burchiel KJ (1988) Carbamazepine inhibits spontaneous activity in experimental neuromas. Exp Neurol 102: 249–253.

Caffrey JM, Eng DL, Black JA, Waxman SG, Kocsis JD (1992) Three types of sodium channels in adult rat dorsal root ganglion neurons. Brain Res 592: 283–297.

Chabal C, Jacobson L, Russell LC, Burchiel KJ (1989a) Pain responses to perineuronal injection of normal saline, gallamine, and lidocaine in humans. Pain 36: 321–325.

Chabal C, Russell LC, Burchiel KJ (1989b) The effect of intravenous lidocaine, tocainide, and mexiletine on spontaneously active fibers originating in rat sciatic neuromas. Pain 38: 333–338.

Chabal C, Jacobson L, Mariano A, Chaney E, Britell CW (1992) The use of oral mexiletine for the treatment of pain after peripheral nerve injury. Anesthesiology 76: 513–517.

Chahine M, George AL, Zhou M, Ji S, Sun W, Barchi RL, Horn R (1994) Sodium channel mutations in paramyotonia congenita uncouple inactivation from activation. Neuron 12: 281–294.

Devor M, Govrin-Lippmann R, Frank H, Raber P (1985) Proliferation of primary sensory neurons in adult rat dorsal root ganglion and the kinetics of retrograde cell loss after sciatic nerve section. Somatosens Res 3: 139–167.

Devor M, Wall PD, Catalan N (1992) Systemic lidocaine silences ectopic neuroma and DRG discharge without blocking nerve conduction. Pain 48: 261–268.

Dib-Hajj SD, Black JA, Felts P, Waxman SG (1996) Down-regulation of transcripts for Na channel a-SNS in spinal sensory neurons following axotomy. Proc Natl Acad Sci USA 93: 14950–14954.

Elliott AA, Elliott JR (1993) Characterization of TTX-sensitive and TTX-resistant sodium currents in small cells from adult rat dorsal root ganglia. J Physiol (Lond) 463: 39–56.

Fedulova SA, Kostyuk P, Veselovsky NS (1994) Comparative analysis of ionic currents in the somatic membrane of embryonic and newborn rat sensory neurons. Neuroscience 58: 341–346.

Galer BS, Miller KV, Rowbatham MC (1993) Response to intravenous lidocaine infusion differs based on clinical diagnosis and site of nervous system injury. Neurology 43: 1233–1235.

Gola M, Niel JP (1993) Electrical and integrative properties of rabbit sympathetic neurones re-evaluated by patch clamping non-dissociated cells. J Physiol (Lond) 460: 327–349.

Iwahashi Y, Furuyama T, Inagaki S, Morita Y, Takagi H (1994) Distinct regulation of sodium channel types I, II, and III following nerve transection. Mol Brain Res 22: 341–345.

Jeftinija S (1994) The role of tetrodotoxin-resistant sodium channels of small primary afferent fibers. Brain Res 639: 125–134.

Klugbauer N, Lacinova L, Flockerzi V, Hofmann F (1995) Structure and functional expression of a new member of the tetrodotoxin-sensitive voltage-activated sodium channel family from human neuroendocrine cells. EMBO J 14: 1084–1090.

Knutsdottir S (1993) Spinal cord injuries in Iceland, 1973–1989. A follow-up study. Paraplegia 31: 68–72.

Kostyuk PG, Veselovsky NS, Tsyndrenko AY (1981) Ionic currents in the somatic membrane of rat dorsal root ganglion neurons. I. Sodium currents. Neuroscience 6: 2423–2430.

Levi R, Hultling C, Nash MS, Seiger A (1995) The Stockholm spinal cord injury study. I. Medical problems in a regional SCI population. Paraplegia 33: 308–315.

Lisney SJW, Devor M (1987) Afterdischarge and interactions among fibers in damaged peripheral nerve in the rat. Brain Res 415: 122–136.

Matzner O, Devor M (1992) Na^+ conductance and the threshold for repetitive neuronal firing. Brain Res 597: 92–98.

Matzner O, Devor M (1994) Hyperexcitability at sites of nerve injury depends on voltage-sensitive Na^+ channels. J Neurophysiol 72: 349–359.

McLean MJ, Bennett PB, Thomas RM (1988) Subtypes of dorsal root ganglion neurons based on different inward currents as measured by whole-cell voltage clamp. Mol Cell Biochem 80: 95–107.

Nordin M, Nystrom B, Wallin U, Hagbarth KE (1984) Ectopic sensory discharges and paresthesiae in patients with disorders of peripheral nerves, dorsal roots, and dorsal columns. Pain 20: 231–245.

Nystrom B, Hagbarth KE (1981) Microelectrode recordings from transected nerves in amputees with phantom limb pain. Neurosci Lett 27: 211–216.

O'Donnell P, Grace AA (1995) Synaptic interactions among excitatory afferents to nucleus accumbens neurons: hippocampal gating of prefrontal cortical input. J Neurosci 15: 3622–3639.

Ogata N, Tatebayashi H (1992) Comparison of two types of Na^+ currents with low-voltage-activated T-type Ca^{2+} current in newborn rat dorsal root ganglia. Pflügers Arch 420: 590–594.

Ogata N, Tatebayashi H (1993) Kinetic analysis of two types of Na^+ channels in rat dorsal root ganglia. J Physiol (Lond) 466: 9–37.

Rizzo MA, Kocsis JD, Waxman SG (1994) Slow sodium conductances of dorsal root ganglion neurons: intraneuronal homogeneity and interneuronal heterogeneity. J Neurophysiol 72: 2796–2815.

Rizzo MA, Kocsis JD, Waxman SG (1995) Selective loss of slow and enhancement of fast Na^+ currents in cutaneous afferent dorsal root ganglion neurons following axotomy. Neurobiol Dis 2: 87–96.

Rizzo MA, Kocsis JD, Waxman SG (1996) Mechanisms of paraesthesiae, dysaesthesiae, and hyperaesthesiae: role of Na channel heterogeneity. Eur Neurol 36: 3–12.

Roy ML, Narahashi T (1992) Differential properties of tetrodotoxin-sensitive and tetrodotoxin-resistant sodium channels in rat dorsal root ganglion neurons. J Neurosci 12: 2104–2111.

Sangameswaran L, Delgado SG, Fish LM, Koch BD, Jakeman LB, Stewart GR, Sze P, Hunter JC, Eglen RM, Herman RC (1996) Structure and function of a novel voltage-gated tetrodotoxin-resistant sodium channel specific to sensory neurons. J Biol Chem 271: 5953–5956.

Schmued LC, Fallon JH (1986) Fluoro-gold: a new fluorescent retrograde axonal tracer with numerous unique properties. Brain Res 377: 147–154.

Study RE, Kral MG (1996) Spontaneous action potential activity in isolated dorsal root ganglion neurons from rats with a painful neuropathy. Pain 65: 235–249.

Stys PK, Ransom BR, Waxman SG (1992) Tertiary and quaternary local anesthetics protect CNS white matter from anoxic injury at concentrations that do not block excitability. J Neurophysiol 67: 236–240.

Stys PK, Sontheimer H, Ransom BR, Waxman SG (1993) Noninactivating, tetrodotoxin-sensitive Na^+ conductance in rat optic nerve axons. Proc Natl Acad Sci USA 90: 6976–6980.

Subbarao JV, Klopfstein J, Turpin R (1995) Prevalence and impact of wrist and shoulder pain in patients with spinal cord injury. J Spinal Cord Med 18: 9–13.

Wall PD, Gutnick M (1974) Ongoing activity in peripheral nerves: the physiology and pharmacology of impulses originating from a neuroma. Exp Neurol 43: 580–593.

Waxman SG, Kocsis JD, Black JA (1994) Type III sodium channel mRNA is expressed in embryonic, but not adult spinal sensory, neurons and is reexpressed following axotomy. J Neurophysiol 72: 466–470.

Yaari Y, Devor M (1985) Phenytoin suppresses spontaneous ectopic discharge in rat sciatic nerve neuromas. Neurosci Lett 58: 117–122.

Yang N, Ji S, Zhou M, Ptacek LJ, Barchi RL, Horn R, George AL (1994) Sodium channel mutations in paramyotonia congenita exhibit similar biophysical phenotypes in vitro. Proc Natl Acad Sci USA 91: 12785–12789.

Yip HK, Rich KM, Lampe PA, Johnson EM (1984) The effects of nerve growth factor and its antiserum on the postnatal development and survival after injury of sensory neurons in rat dorsal root ganglia. J Neurosci 4: 2986–2992.

29 Insertion of an SNS-Specific Tetrapeptide in S3–S4 Linker of D4 Accelerates Recovery from Inactivation of Skeletal Muscle Voltage-Gated Na Channel μ1 in HEK293 Cells

S. D. Dib-Hajj, K. Ishikawa, T. R. Cummins, S. G. Waxman

Abstract Na channel subunits αSNS (PN3) and αμ1 (SkM1) produce slowly inactivating/TTX-resistant and rapidly inactivating/TTX-sensitive currents, respectively. αSNS (PN3) current recovers from inactivation (reprimes) rapidly. Sequence alignment identified the tetrapeptide SLEN, in the S3–S4 linker of D4, as αSNS-specific. To determine whether SLEN endows Na channels with slow kinetics and/or rapid repriming, we analyzed the transient Na current produced by a chimera μ1SLEN in HEK293 cells. Neither kinetics nor voltage dependence of activation and inactivation was affected. However, repriming was twice as fast as in the wild type at −100 mV. This suggests that SLEN may contribute to the rapid repriming of TTX-resistant Na current.

1. Introduction

Voltage-gated sodium channels consist of a large, 260 kDa, pore-forming, α-subunit and one or more auxiliary β-subunits [1, 2]. The α-subunit polypeptide chain consists of four homologous domains (D1–4), each with six predicted transmembrane segments (S1–6) joined by cytoplasmic and extracellular loops [1]. Except for the loop joining domains III and IV (D3–4 linker), which contains the conserved inactivation particle [3, 4], the amino acid sequences of these loops and the N- and C-termini are less conserved than those of the transmembrane segments [5, 6]. The amphipathic S4 segment of each domain with its positively charged residues is thought to be the voltage sensor [1, 7, 8]. Two types of Na currents are produced by these α-subunits: slow inactivating, TTX-resistant (slow/TTX-R) and fast inactivating, TTX-sensitive (fast/TTX-S) [1]. The α-subunits from human and rat skeletal muscle, SkM1 and μ1, respectively, produce fast/TTX-S

Reprinted with permission from *FEBS Letters* 416: 11–14, 1997.

Na currents [9–12]. Recently, two groups have cloned an α-subunit SNS (PN3) which produces a slow/TTX-R Na current when expressed in *Xenopus* oocytes [13, 14]. Studies on dorsal root ganglion (DRG) neurons have provided strong evidence that SNS produces the slow/TTX-R current in these cells [15, 16].

A number of cDNAs encoding α-subunits have been cloned [6]. Amino acid residues that are proposed to play specific roles such as voltage sensors, inactivation particle, ion selectivity filters and toxin binding sites are conserved in these subunits [5, 6, 17]. In K channels, activation involves the movement of the N-terminal portion of S4 into the extracellular space from a position inside the membrane at rest [7]. The TTX-R current in C-type DRG neurons, which appears to be encoded by SNS [13, 18], is characterized by slow activation and inactivation kinetics [19–21] and by rapid recovery from inactivation (repriming) [16, 21]. We reasoned that sequence variation in or around the voltage sensor, S4, may contribute to the slow kinetics and rapid repriming of the SNS/PN3 current. Alignment of the amino acid sequence of the linker joining S3 and S4 of domain 4 (D4S3–S4) and D4S4 of SNS shows a non-conservative substitution of an invariant amino acid residue followed by a tripeptide insertion compared to the rest of the mammalian α-subunits. This difference is intriguing because this region appears to be crucial for coupling activation to fast inactivation [22, 23], slowing down inactivation and accelerating repriming of SkM1 [24, 25]. Therefore we constructed a chimera μ1 construct carrying the SNS-specific tetrapeptide at the analogous position in the D4S3–S4 linker and analyzed the Na current produced by this chimera in HEK293 cells.

2. Materials and Methods

2.1. Plasmid Construction

The plasmid µ1-RBG4 [10] was used to generate a chimera construct for this study. One wild type primer pair (F1 and R1) and one mutagenic pair (M1 and M2) were used to introduce the insertion into the S3–S4 linker. Wild type forward primer F1 (5′-CGGTGGTCAACAACAAGTCCG-3′) and reverse primer R1 (5′-ATGCCGAAGATC-GAGTAGATG-3′) correspond to nucleotides 4030–4050 and 4910–4930, respectively. Mutagenic primers M1 (5′-CACAAAGTTTTCC-AGTGATTTCTGTATCAAGTCAGAGAG-3′) and M2 (5′-CAGAAATCACTGGAAAACTT-TGTGTCACCCACGCTGTTC-3′) correspond to nucleotides 4725–4754 and 4740–4770, respectively, plus the extra 12 nucleotides (underlined). PCR was performed in 60 µl volume using 3 µM of each primer and 1.75 units of Expand Long Template DNA polymerase enzyme mixture in buffer 3 (Boehringer Mannheim). Amplification was carried out in two stages for a total of 30 cycles, as previously described [26], using a programmable thermal cycler (PTC-100, MJ Research, Cambridge, MA).

A PCR-based mutagenesis and cloning method [27] was used to produce µ1SLEN-RBG4 plasmid. Two separate PCR reactions were performed using 10 ng µ1-RBG4 as template and F1/M1 and M2/R1 primer pairs, respectively. The two PCR products were band isolated and used as a mixed template for PCR using primer pair F1/R1. The resulting PCR product, exchanged Y^{1433} with the tetrapeptide SLEN in the S3–S4 linker, was cloned using pCR-Script vector (Stratagene) to produce plasmid pSLEN. The insert in pSLEN was sequenced to confirm the nucleotide changes. Plasmid µ1SLEN-RBG4 was constructed by replacing the unique AccI/BspEI fragment, which corresponds to nucleotides 4067–4836, from the wild type construct µ1-RBG4 with that of the mutant construct pSLEN.

2.2. Expression System

The µ1-RBG4 and µ1SLEN-RBG4 constructs were cotransfected into HEK293 cells with a fluorescent reporter plasmid (pGreen Lantern-1 Gibco) using the calcium-phosphate precipitation technique [10]. HEK293 cells were grown in high-glucose DMEM (Gibco) supplemented with 10% fetal calf serum (FCS; Gibco). After 48 h, cells with green fluorescence were selected for recording.

2.3. Whole-Cell Recordings

Whole-cell patch-clamp recordings were conducted at room temperature (21 °C) using an EPC-9 amplifier. Data were acquired on a Macintosh Quadra 950 using the Pulse program (v. 7.52, HEKA, Germany). Fire-polished electrodes (0.8–1.5 MΩ) were fabricated from 1.65-mm capillary glass (WPI) using a Sutter P-87 puller. Cells were not considered for analysis if initial seal resistance was <5 GΩ, they had high leakage currents (holding current >0.1 nA at −80 mV), membrane blebs, or an access resistance >5 MΩ. Access resistance (3 ± 1 mV, mean ± S.D., $n = 42$) was monitored throughout the experiment and data were not used if resistance changes occurred. Voltage errors were minimized using 80% series resistance compensation and the capacitance artifact was cancelled using the amplifier computer-controlled. For comparisons of the voltage dependence of activation and inactivation, only cells with a maximum voltage error of <10 mV after compensation were used. The voltage error was 4 ± 3 mV for µ1-RBG4 ($n = 16$) and 5 ± 2 mV for µ1SLEN-RBG4 ($n = 14$). Linear leak subtraction was used for all voltage clamp recordings. Membrane currents were filtered at 5 kHz and sampled at 20 kHz. The pipette solution contained: 140 mM CsF, 2 mM $MgCl_2$, 1 mM EGTA, and 10 mM Na-HEPES (pH 7.3). The standard bathing solution was 140 mM NaCl, 3 mM KCl, 2 mM $MgCl_2$, 1 mM $CaCl_2$,

10 mM HEPES, and 10 mM glucose (pH 7.3). Data were not corrected for liquid junction potentials which were <5 mV. The osmolarity of all solutions was adjusted to 310 mOsm.

2.4. Data Analysis

Data were analyzed using Pulsefit (v. 7.52) or custom software developed by T. R. Cummins. Unpaired *t*-test analysis (using the Systat program) required $P < 0.05$ for significance. Analysis results are expressed as mean ± standard deviation. The curves in the figures are drawn to guide the eye unless otherwise noted.

3. Results and Discussion

All mammalian channels of subfamily 1 [28] including SNS (PN3) share a nearly identical D4S4 segment (figure 29.1), consistent with the role this segment plays as a voltage sensor [7, 8]. The exceptions are the three atypical sodium channels of subfamily 2 [28] whose current properties are not known since none has been successfully studied in an expression system [28–30]. The remarkable conservation of the S4 sequence, including all the charged residues (figure 29.1), suggests that this segment does not confer slow activation and inactivation and rapid repriming on the Na current produced by SNS.

The D4S3–S4 linker of SNS/PN3 is remarkably divergent from other subfamily 1 channels (figure 29.1). The linker is longer (13 amino acid residues instead of 10) and contains significant amino acid changes. Compared to channels other than muscle (cardiac and skeletal) and the atypical channels, a non-conservative change, glutamic acid (E) to leucine (L), occurs at position 1; the muscle and atypical channels have glutamine (Q) and glycine (G) residues, respectively. An invariant tyrosine (Y) residue at position 3 is replaced with serine (S) and the tripeptide leucine-glutamic acid-asparagine/serine

```
GSLLFSAILKSLENYFSPTLFRVIRLARIGRILRLIRAAKGIRTLL  rSNS
ASLLFSAILKSLESYFSPTFFRVIRLARIGRILRLIRAAKGIRTLL  mSNS
GTVLSDIIQKY---FFSPTLFRVIRLARIGRILRLIRGAKGIRTLL  rH1
GLALSDLIQKY---FVSPTLFRVIRLARIGRVLRLIRGAKGIRTLL  rμ1
GMFLAELIEKY---FVSPTLFRVIRLARIGRILRLIKGAKGIRTLL  rαI
GMFLAELIEKY---FVSPTLFRVIRLARIGRILRLIKGAKGIRTLL  rαII
GMFLAELIEKY---FVSPTLFRVIRLARIGRILRLIKGAKGIRTLL  rαIII
GMFLADIIEKY---FVSPTLFRVIRLARIGRILRLIKGAKGIRTLL  rαVI
GMFLAEMIEKY---FVSPTLFRVIRLARIGRILRLIKGAKGIRTLL  rPN1
GMFLAEMIETY---FVSPTLFRVIRLARIGRILRLIKGAKGIRTLL  NaS
GMFLADMIETY---FVSPTLFRVIRLARIGRILRLVKGAKGIRTLL  hNE
GLCLPMTVGSY---LVPPSLVQLILLSRIIHMLRLGKGPKVFHNLM  hNav2.1
GLLLPLTIGQY---FVPPSLVQLILLSRVIHILRPGKGPKVFHDLM  mNav2.3
GLLLPLSIGQY---FVPPSLVQLLLLSRIIHVLRPGKGPKVFHDLM  rNaG
■S3■■■■■       ■■■■■■■■S4■■■■■■■■■■■
GSLLFSAILKSLENYFSPTLFRVIRLARIGRILRLIRAAKGIRTLL  rSNS
GLALSDLIQKSLENFVSPTLFRVIRLARIGRVLRLIRGAKGIRTLL  rμ1SLEN
GLALSDLIQKY---FVSPTLFRVIRLARIGRVLRLIRGAKGIRTLL  rμ1
  *     123   45678910
```

Figure 29.1
Parsimonious alignment of select domain 4 sequences of mammalian *α*-subunits: S3 (terminal octatapeptide), S3–S4 linker and S4. Sequences of known mammalian *α*-subunit sequences were aligned to minimize number of gaps. The asterisk denotes L[1433] of huSkM1 whose mutation induces changes in inactivation and recovery from inactivation of the skeletal Na channel [24, 25]. The terminal octatapeptide of D4S3 and all of D4S4 are delineated by thick lines. The invariant Y residue at position 3 of the linker of rμ1 is changed to S followed by an insertion of the tripeptide LEN. Only one (rat) sequence is shown when the respective cognates from other species are identical or when the same subunit was reported by multiple groups. Accession numbers are: SNS: X92184 (rat); PN3: U53833 (rat, identical to SNS); mSNS: Y09108 (mouse); rH1: M27902 (rat); hSkM2: M77235 (human, rH1 cognate); rμ1: M26643 (rat); huSkM1: M26643 (human, rμ1 cognate); hoSkM1: U25990 (horse, rμ1 cognate); rαI: X03638 (rat); rαII: X03639 (rat); huαII: 476881 (human, rαII cognate); rαIII: Y00766 (rat); rαVI: L39018 (rat); mαVI: U26707 (mouse, rαVI); rPN1: U79568 (rat); hNE-Na: X82835 (human, rPN1 cognate); NaS: U35238 (rabbit, rPN1 cognate); hNav2.1: M91556 (human); mNav2.3: L36179 (mouse); NaG: M965778 (rat); and SCL-11: Y09164 (rat, full length NaG-like).

(LEN/S) insertion follows. Other more conservative changes, phenylalanine (F) to tyrosine (Y) and valine (V) to phenylalanine (F), occur at positions 4 and 5, respectively. The V to F substitution is also present in the cardiac channel (figure 29.1). We reasoned that this dramatic sequence difference in this linker may impact the kinetics of D4S4 and/or D4S3 conformational

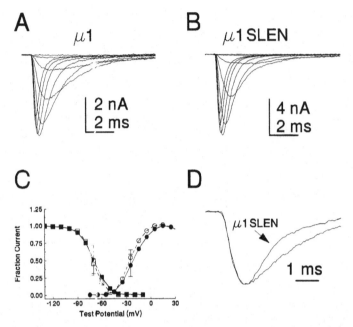

Figure 29.2
Comparison of μ1 and μ1SLEN currents in HEK293 cells. A, B: Family of traces from representative HEK293 cells expressing either μ1 (*A*) or μ1SLEN (*B*) channels. The currents were elicited by 40 ms test pulses to various potentials from −65 to 10 mV. Cells were held at −100 mV. (*C*) The activation (circles) and steady-state fast inactivation (squares) curves for μ1 (filled symbols; n = 16) and μ1SLEN (open symbols; n = 14) channels. Steady-state fast inactivation was measured with 500 ms inactivating prepulses. Cells were held at prepulse potentials over the range of −130 to +10 mV prior to a test pulse to −10 mV for 20 ms. Current is plotted as a fraction of peak current. (*D*) Representative traces from cells expressing μ1 and μ1SLEN channels. Cells were held at −100 mV and stepped to −35 mV for 20 ms. No difference was observed in the rate of activation, but the μ1SLEN current inactivated slightly faster than μ1 current.

transitions, hence the current properties. We tested the possibility that this difference may contribute to the slow kinetics and/or rapid re-priming of the SNS/PN3 current by characterizing the current properties of the μ1SLEN chimera in HEK293 cells.

Sodium currents were recorded from cells expressing either the μ1 (figure 29.2A) or the μ1SLEN channels (figure 29.2B). The peak current density was slightly larger in cells expressing μ1SLEN channels (728 ± 616 pA/pF, n = 20)

than in cells expressing μ1 channels (515 ± 517 pA/pF, n = 23).

In DRG neurons, the TTX-R current activates at potentials that are 10–15 mV more depolarized than the TTX-S current [16, 19, 21, 31]. Activation kinetics are also much slower for TTX-R currents than for TTX-S neuronal or skeletal muscle sodium currents. Kostyuk et al. [19] estimated that the time constant of activation is about 5–10 times slower for the TTX-R current than for TTX-S currents. The SLEN

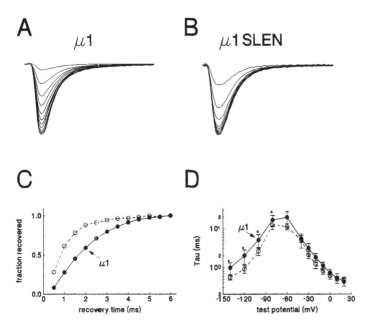

Figure 29.3
Recovery from fast inactivation is quicker for μ1SLEN currents than μ1 currents. (*A, B*) Family of traces from cells expressing μ1 (*A*) and μ1SLEN (*B*) currents showing the rate of recovery from inactivation. The cells were prepulsed to −10 mV for 20 ms to inactivate all of the current, then brought back to −120 mV for increasing recovery durations prior to the test pulse to 0 mV. The recovery time at −120 mV ranged from 0.5 ms to 6 ms in increments of 0.5 ms. (*C*) Recovery from inactivation time course for the μ1 (filled circles) and μ1SLEN (open circles) currents shown in (*A, B*). The μ1SLEN current recovers about twice as fast as the μ1 current. (*D*) Comparison of μ1 (n = 6) and μ1SLEN (n = 7) inactivation kinetics as a function of voltage. Time constants were measured from the rate of decay (test potentials between −50 and 20 mV) or from the time course for the recovery from fast inactivation (test potentials between −150 and −50 mV).

mutation, however, did not alter activation of μ1 channels. We found no difference in the voltage dependence of activation (figure 29.2C) or in the rate of activation (figure 29.2D). At −35 mV, the time constant for activation was 0.46 ± 0.05 ms (*n* = 11) for μ1 and 0.43 ± 0.07 ms (*n* = 15) for μ1SLEN currents.

TTX-R currents in DRG neurons also exhibit very different inactivation properties from TTX-S currents. The midpoint for steady-state inactivation (V_h) is near −35 mV, which is about 30 mV more depolarized than what is typically observed

for most TTX-S currents, including μ1. The V_h for recombinant SNS channels expressed in oocytes, which are TTX-R, is near −30 mV [13]. However, no difference was observed in the voltage dependence of steady-state inactivation of μ1SLEN and μ1 currents (figure 29.2C). The rate for the development of inactivation was, if anything, slightly faster for μ1SLEN than for μ1 currents (figure 29.2D). At −35 mV the time constant for fast inactivation was 3.5 ± 1.0 ms (*n* = 11) for μ1 and 2.7 ± 0.8 ms (*n* = 15) for μ1SLEN currents.

Repriming is much quicker for TTX-R currents in DRG neurons than for TTX-S currents [16, 21]. At −120 mV, µ1SLEN currents reprimed faster than did µ1 currents (figure 29.3A, B, C). The time constant for repriming was about twice as fast for µ1SLEN currents ($\tau = 0.9 \pm 0.2$ ms, $n = 11$) than for µ1 currents ($\tau = 2.0 \pm 0.8$ ms, $n = 9$), and this difference was highly significant ($P < 0.001$). The rate of repriming was faster for µ1SLEN currents at all voltages tested (figure 29.3D).

These data indicate that the D4S3–S4 linker is an important determinant of repriming in sodium channels. The accelerated rate of repriming may indicate a SLEN-induced destabilization of the closed-inactivated state of the channel, perhaps by affecting the conformational transition of D4S3 and/or D4S4. This is consistent with an earlier study [25] which concluded that D4S3 was an important determinant for repriming and suggested that repriming may be influenced by interaction between D4S3 and D4S4, such as sliding past each other. Notably, the SLEN insertion did not slow the onset of inactivation or shift steady-state inactivation to more depolarized potentials. Thus the alteration of an otherwise highly conserved D4S3–S4 linker appears to focally effect repriming. This observation may indicate a lower tolerance for substitution of residues within the membrane [25] compared to those within loop sequences.

Except for recovery from inactivation, the SLEN substitution did not seem to alter the properties of µ1 channels in HEK293 cells. A recent study suggested that the S3–S4 linker might be a determinant of activation kinetics of the potassium channel a-subunit [32]. Our data indicate that the D4S3–S4 linker does not play the same role in sodium channels. It remains unclear what causes the markedly slower kinetics in the TTX-R current and SNS recombinant channels. Because of the high degree of conservation of D4S1–S6 sequences, it is unlikely that these regions are responsible for the difference.

The D3–4 linker, which has been implicated as the inactivation particle, is also highly conserved between SNS and other sodium channel isoforms. It is possible that the SLEN sequence in the SNS subunit interacts with other sequences in the native channel to slow down the movement of S4 in the membrane, thus impacting the kinetic properties of the current. Although the SLEN substitution is not sufficient to induce the dramatic changes in gating kinetics or voltage dependence that are observed with SNS channels, it appears to contribute to rapid repriming in these channels.

Acknowledgments

This work was supported in part by grants from the National Multiple Sclerosis Society, the Medical Research Service, Department of Veterans Affairs. We thank B. R. Toftness for technical assistance.

References

[1] Hille, B. (1992) Ionic Channels of Excitable Membranes, Sinauer, Sunderland, MA.

[2] Isom, L. L., De Jongh, K. S. and Catterall. W. A. (1994) Neuron 12: 1183–1194.

[3] West, J. W., Patton, D. E., Scheuer, T., Wang, Y., Goldin, A. L. and Catterall, W. A. (1992) Proc. Natl. Acad. Sci. USA 89: 10910–10914.

[4] Eaholtz, G., Scheuer, T. and Catterall, W. A. (1994) Neuron 12: 1041–1048.

[5] Fozzard, H. A. and Hanck, D. A. (1996) Physiol. Rev. 76: 887–926.

[6] Goldin, A. L. (1995) in: Handbook of Receptors and Channels (North, R. A., Ed.), pp. 73–100, CRC press, Boca Raton, FL.

[7] Mannuzzu, L. M., Moronne, M. M. and Isacoff, E. Y. (1996) Science 271: 213–216.

[8] Yang, N., George Jr., A. L. and Horn, R. (1996) Neuron 16: 113–122.

[9] Trimmer, J. S. et al. (1989) Neuron 3: 33–49.

[10] Ukomadu, C., Zhou, J., Sigworth, F. J. and Agnew, W. S. (1992) Neuron 8: 663–676.

[11] George, A. L., Komisarof, R. G., Kallen, R. G. and Barchi, R. L. (1992) Ann. Neurol. 31: 131–137.

[12] Wang, D. W., George Jr., A. L. and Bennett, P. B. (1996) Biophys. J. 70: 238–245.

[13] Akopian, A. N., Sivilotti, L. and Wood, J. N. (1996) Nature 379: 257–262.

[14] Sangameswaran, L. et al. (1996) J. Biol. Chem. 271: 5953–5956.

[15] Dib-Hajj, S., Black, J. A., Felts, P. and Waxman, S. G. (1996) Proc. Natl. Acad. Sci. USA 93: 14950–14954.

[16] Cummins, T. R. and Waxman, S. G. (1997) J. Neurosci. 17: 3503–3514.

[17] Catterall, W. A. (1995) Annu. Rev. Biochem. 64: 493–531.

[18] Sangameswaran, L. et al. (1996) J. Biol. Chem. 271: 5953–5956.

[19] Kostyuk, P. G., Veselovsky, N. S. and Tsyndrenko, A. Y. (1981) Neuroscience 6: 2423–2430.

[20] Caffrey, J. M., Eng, D. L., Black, J. A., Waxman, S. G. and Kocsis, J. D. (1992) Brain Res. 592: 283–297.

[21] Elliott, A. A. and Elliott, J. R. (1993) J. Physiol. 463: 39–56.

[22] Chahine, M., George Jr., A. L., Zhou, M., Ji, S., Sun, W., Barchi, R. L. and Horn, R. (1994) Neuron 12: 281–294.

[23] Rogers, J. C., Qu, Y., Tanada, T. N., Scheuer, T. and Catterall, W. A. (1996) J. Biol. Chem. 271: 15950–15962.

[24] Yang, N., Ji, S., Zhou, M., Ptacek, L. J., Barchi, R. L., Horn, R. and George Jr., A. L. (1994) Proc. Natl. Acad. Sci. USA 91: 12785–12789.

[25] Ji, S., George Jr., A. L., Horn, R. and Barchi, R. L. (1996) J. Gen. Physiol. 107: 183–194.

[26] Dib-Hajj, S. D., Hinson, A. W., Black, J. A. and Waxman, S. G. (1996) FEBS Lett. 384: 78–82.

[27] Horton, R. M., Ho, S. N., Pullen, J. K., Hunt, H. D., Cai, Z. and Pease, L. R. (1993) Methods Enzymol. 217: 270–279.

[28] Felipe, A., Knittle, T. J., Doyle, K. L. and Tamkun, M. M. (1994) J. Biol. Chem. 269: 30125–30131.

[29] George Jr., A. L., Knittle, T. J. and Tamkun, M. M. (1992) Proc. Natl. Acad. Sci. USA 89: 4893–4897.

[30] Akopian, A. N., Souslova, V., Sivilotti, L. and Wood, J. N. (1997) FEBS Lett. 400: 183–187.

[31] Roy, M. L. and Narahashi, T. (1992) J. Neurosci. 12: 2104–2111.

[32] Mathur, R., Zheng, J., Yan, Y. and Sigworth, F. J. (1997) J. Gen. Physiol. 109: 191–199.

30 Sodium Channels and Pain

S. G. Waxman, S. Dib-Hajj, T. R. Cummins, and J. A. Black

Abstract Although it is well established that hyper-excitability and/or increased baseline sensitivity of primary sensory neurons can lead to abnormal burst activity associated with pain, the underlying molecular mechanisms are not fully understood. Early studies demonstrated that, after injury to their axons, neurons can display changes in excitability, suggesting increased sodium channel expression, and, in fact, abnormal sodium channel accumulation has been observed at the tips of injured axons. We have used an ensemble of molecular, electrophysiological, and pharmacological techniques to ask: what types of sodium channels underlie hyperexcitability of primary sensory neurons after injury? Our studies demonstrate that multiple sodium channels, with distinct electrophysiological properties, are encoded by distinct mRNAs within small dorsal root ganglion (DRG) neurons, which include nociceptive cells. Moreover, several DRG neuron-specific sodium channels now have been cloned and sequenced. After injury to the axons of DRG neurons, there is a dramatic change in sodium channel expression in these cells, with down-regulation of some sodium channel genes and up-regulation of another, previously silent sodium channel gene. This plasticity in sodium channel gene expression is accompanied by electrophysiological changes that poise these cells to fire spontaneously or at inappropriate high frequencies. Changes in sodium channel gene expression also are observed in experimental models of inflammatory pain. Thus, sodium channel expression in DRG neurons is dynamic, changing significantly after injury. Sodium channels within primary sensory neurons may play an important role in the pathophysiology of pain.

Pain pathways begin with primary sensory neurons [dorsal root ganglion (DRG) neurons; trigeminal neurons]. It is now clear that, in some pain syndromes, hyperexcitability and/or increased baseline sensitivity of these cells leads to abnormal bursting that can produce chronic pain (1–3). The pivotal position of primary sensory neu-

Reprinted with permission from *Proceedings of the National Academy of Sciences USA* 96: 7635–7639, 1999.

rons as distal sites of impulse generation along the nociceptive pathway, and the experimental and clinical accessibility of these neurons, has resulted in intense interest in mechanisms underlying action potential generation and transmission in them in disease states characterized by pain. Voltage-gated sodium channels, which produce the inward membrane current necessary for regenerative action potential production within the mammalian nervous system, are, of course, expressed in primary sensory neurons and have emerged as important targets in the study of the molecular pathophysiology of pain and in the search for new pain therapies. In this paper we focus on the potential role of sodium channels in the molecular pathophysiology of pain. We will emphasize, in particular, three motifs: first, that DRG neurons express a complex repertoire of multiple distinct sodium channels, encoded by different genes; second, that some of these sodium channels are sensory neuron specific; and third, that sodium channel expression in DRG neurons is highly dynamic, changing substantially not only during development, but also in various disease states, including some that are accompanied by pain.

Hyperexcitability in DRG Cells after Injury

Early studies (4, 5) demonstrated that, after injury to their axons, motor neurons display changes in excitability, suggesting increased sodium channel expression over the cell body and the dendrites, and similar changes were subsequently observed in sensory neurons (6, 7). Abnormal sodium channel accumulation at the tips of injured axons also has been observed (8–10), and both electrophysiological and computer simulation studies have suggested that abnormal increases in sodium conductance can lead to inappropriate, repetitive firing (11–13). Indeed, there is substantial evidence indicating that the abnormal excitability of DRG neurons, after axonal injury, is associated with an increased density of sodium channels (13, 14). These observations, together with experimental and clinical observations on partial efficacy of sodium channel-blocking agents in neuropathic pain (15–18), established a link between sodium channel activity and sensory neuron hyper-excitability producing pain. However, these studies did not examine the crucial question: what type(s) of sodium channels produce inappropriate sensory neuron discharge associated with pain?

Multiple Sodium Channels in Primary Sensory Neurons

Over the past decade, it has become clear that nearly a dozen, molecularly distinct voltage-gated sodium channels are encoded within mammals by different genes. DRG neurons, which had been known to display multiple, distinct sodium currents (19–22), express at least six sodium channel transcripts (23), as illustrated by the in situ hybridizations and reverse transcription–PCR shown in figures 30.1 and 30.2. These include high levels of expression of the a-I and Na6 channels, also expressed at high levels by other neuronal cell types within the central nervous system, which are known to support tetrodotoxin (TTX)-sensitive sodium currents. In addition, DRG neurons are unique in expressing four additional sodium channel transcripts that are not expressed at significant levels in other neuronal cell types: (i) PN1/hNE, which is expressed preferentially in DRG neurons (24), produces a fast, transient TTX-sensitive sodium current in response to sudden depolarizations and a persistent current elicited by slow depolarizations close to resting membrane potential (25); (ii) SNS/PN3, expressed preferentially in small DRG and trigeminal neurons, encodes a TTX-resistent sodium current (26, 27); (iii) NaN, expressed preferentially in small and trigeminal neurons, exhibits an amino acid sequence that, although only 47% similar to SNS-PN3, predicts that it encodes a TTX-resistant sodium channel (28); and (iv) NaG, another putative sodium channel that was originally cloned from astrocytes and at first thought to be glial specific (29), is also preferentially expressed at high levels within DRG neurons (23) and at low levels within other neurons of neural crest origin but not within other neuronal types (30).

Preferential expression of SNS/PN3 and NaN within small DRG neurons provides a molecular correlate for the observation (19–22, 32, 33) that these cells express several distinct sodium currents, including TTX-resistant sodium currents. A role for TTX-resistant sodium channels in action potential conduction along small diameter afferent fibers has been postulated (34), and TTX-resistant sodium potentials have, in fact, been recorded from unmyelinated C-fibers (35).

Preferential expression of SNS/PN3 and NaN in small DRG neurons, which include nociceptive cells, and the demonstration of a role of TTX-resistant sodium currents in conduction along their axons, have suggested that these channels may represent unique targets for the pharmacologic treatment of pain. PN1 and NaG also may represent useful molecular targets for the pharmacologic manipulation of DRG neurons because of their preferential expression in these cells.

Sodium Channel Gene Expression Is Altered after Injury to DRG Neurons

The first observations indicating that, in addition to production of excess channels, there is a switch in the type of channels produced after axonal injury were provided by Waxman et al. (36), who found a significant up-regulation of expression of the previously silent a-III sodium channel gene in DRG neurons after axotomy. This finding was followed by demonstration of down-regulation of the SNS/PN3 gene expres-

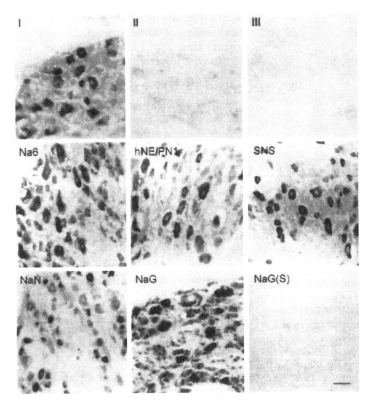

Figure 30.1
Sodium channel α-subunit mRNAs visualized in sections from adult rat DRG by in situ hybridization with subtype-specific antisense riboprobes. mRNAs for α-I, Na6, hNE/PN1, SNS, NaN, and NaG are present at moderate to high levels in DRG neurons. Hybridization signal is not present with sense riboprobes, e.g., for NaG (S). (Bar indicates 100 μm.)

sion, which can persist as long as 210 days after axotomy (37), and of down-regulation of the NaN gene (28). These changes are illustrated in figure 30.3.

Physiologic Changes Accompany Altered Sodium Gene Expression after DRG Neuron Injury

On the basis of the down-regulation of SNS/PN3 and NaN genes in DRG neurons after axonal transection, it would be expected that TTX-resistant sodium currents should be reduced in these cells after axotomy. Patch-clamp studies have demonstrated that, indeed, there is a loss of TTX-resistant sodium currents in DRG neurons after axonal transection (38); this down-regulation persists in small DRG neurons for at least 60 days (39), consistent with the long-lasting changes in gene expression that have been described (37) in these cells (figure 30.4). In addition, as shown in figure 30.5, there is a switch in the properties of the TTX-sensitive sodium

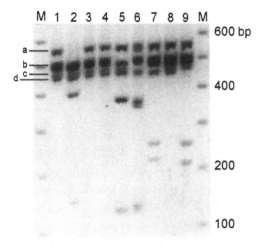

Figure 30.2
Restriction enzyme profile analysis of Na channel domain 1 reverse transcription–PCR products from DRG. M lanes contain 100-bp ladder marker. Lane 1 contains the amplification product from DRG cDNA. Lanes 2–9 show the result of cutting this DNA with *Eco*RV, *Eco*N1, *Ava*I, SphI, *Bam*HI, *Afl*II, *Xba*I, and *Eco*RI, which are specific to subunits *a*-I, -II, -III, Na6, PN1, SNS, NaG, and NaN, respectively. Reproduced with permission from ref. 28. (Copyright 1998, National Academy of Sciences, USA).

currents in these cells after axotomy, with the emergence of a rapidly repriming current (i.e., a current that recovers rapidly from inactivation) (39). Cummins and Waxman (39) have suggested that the type III sodium channel is responsible for the rapidly repriming sodium current, but this conjecture remains to be proven.

These changes may poise DRG neurons to fire spontaneously, or at inappropriately high frequencies, after injury. Increased sodium channel densities, in themselves, will tend to lower threshold (12). In addition, Rizzo et al. (40) have pointed out that the overlap between steady-state activation and inactivation curves, together with weak voltage dependence of TTX-resistant sodium channels may confer instability on the

neuronal membrane. Coexpression of abnormal combinations of several types of channels, whose window currents can bracket each other, would be expected to permit subthreshold oscillations in voltage, supported by TTX-resistant channels, to cross-activate other sodium channels, thereby producing spontaneous activity (40). Cummins and Waxman (39) noted that, because the TTX-sensitive sodium current in DRG neurons after axotomy reprimes relatively rapidly, injured neurons would be expected to sustain higher firing frequencies. Moreover, if persistent currents participate in setting the resting potential, as demonstrated in optic nerve axons (41), loss of TTX-resistant currents in DRG neurons after axotomy could produce a hyperpolarizing shift in resting potential, which, by relieving resting inactivation, might increase the amount of TTX-sensitive sodium current available for electrogenesis.

Neurotrophins Modulate Sodium Channel Expression in DRG Neurons

A number of studies have suggested that, in response to nerve or tissue injury, there are changes in synthesis or delivery of various neurotrophins to neurons. Early studies in culture demonstrated that nerve growth factor (NGF) can affect sodium channel expression in DRG neurons (42, 43). Black et al. (44) showed that NGF, delivered directly to DRG cell bodies, acts to down-regulate *a*-III mRNA and maintain high levels of SNS/PN3 mRNA expression in small DRG neurons in an in vitro model that mimics axotomy. Following up on these observations, Dib-Hajj et al. (45) studied small DRG neurons in vivo after axotomy and demonstrated that administration of exogenous NGF to the proximal nerve stump results in an up-regulation of TTX-resistant sodium current and of SNS/PN3 mRNA levels in small DRG neurons (figure 30.6). These observations suggest that at least some of the changes observed in DRG

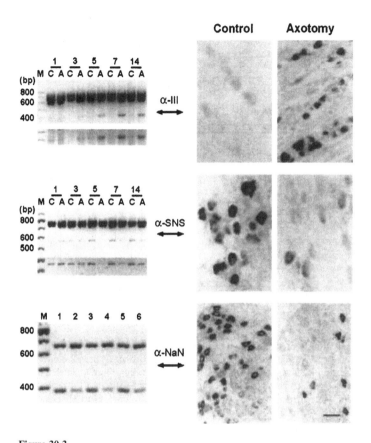

Figure 30.3

Transcripts for sodium channel *a*-III (*A*) are up-regulated, and transcripts for SNS (*B*) and NaN (*C*) are down-regulated, in DRG neurons after transection of their axons within the sciatic nerve. The micrographs (*Right*) shown in situ hybridizations in control DRG, and at 5–7 days postaxotomy. Reverse transcription–PCR (*Left*) shows products of coamplification of *a*-III (*A*) and SNS (*B*) together with *β*-actin transcripts in control (*C*) and axotomized (*A*) DRG (days postaxotomy indicated above gels in *A* and *B*), with computer-enhanced images of amplification products shown below gels. Coamplification of NaN (392 bp) and glyceraldehyde-3-phosphate dehydrogenase (GAPDH) (606 bp) (*C*) shows decreased expression of NaN mRNA at 7 days postaxotomy (lanes 2, 4, and 6) compared with controls (lanes 1, 3, and 5). (*A* and *B*) modified from ref. 37; *C* modified from ref. 28. (Copyright 1998, National Academy of Sciences, USA).

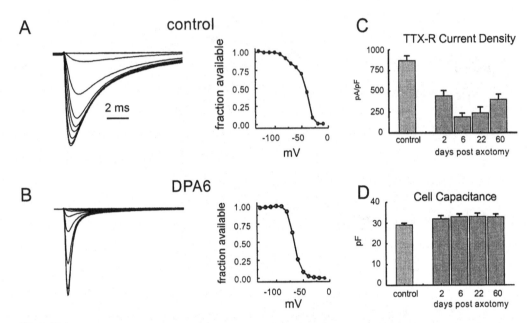

Figure 30.4
TTX-resistant sodium currents in small DRG neurons are down-regulated after axotomy. (*A* and *B*, *Left*) Whole-cell patch-clamp recordings from representative control (*A*) and axotomized (*B*, 6 days postaxotomy) DRG neurons. Note the loss of the TTX-resistant slowly inactivating component of sodium current after axotomy. Steady-state inactivation curves (*A* and *B*, *Right*) show loss of a component characteristic of TTX-resistant currents. (*C*) Attenuation of TTX-resistant current persists for at least 60 days postaxotomy. (*D*) Cell capacitance, which provides a measure of cell size, does not change significantly after axotomy (modified from ref. 39).

neurons after axotomy reflect loss of access to peripheral pools of neurotrophic factors.

Brain-derived growth factor has been studied and has been found not to alter sodium currents in DRG neurons, although it affects the expression of γ-aminobutyric acid receptor-mediated currents in these cells (46). Glial-derived growth factor has been found to modulate the expression of NaN in a subpopulation of small DRG neurons, which are known to express the ret receptor (53). Multiple neurotrophins and growth factors have effects on DRG neurons, and it is likely that sodium channel expression in these cells reflects combinatorial effects of multiple factors.

Sodium Channel Expression in Inflammatory Pain Models

Several studies have demonstrated that inflammatory molecules such as prostaglandins and serotonin can modulate TTX-resistant sodium currents in DRG neurons (47), possibly acting through a cyclic AMP-protein kinase A cascade (48). However, the question, of whether sodium channel gene expression is affected in inflammatory models of pain had not been addressed. To understand the role of sodium channels in inflammatory pain, we have carried out studies in the carageenan inflammatory pain model in the rat (49). In these studies, carried out before our

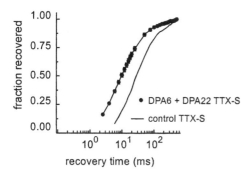

Figure 30.5
The kinetics of recovery from inactivation in TTX-sensitive sodium currents are different in axotomized DRG neurons. The graph shows recovery of TTX-sensitive sodium current from inactivation as a function of time in DRG neurons after axonal transection (6 and 22 days postaxotomy, results pooled) compared with uninjured controls. Note the leftward shift in the recovery curve. Modified from ref. 39.

cloning of NaN, we focused on SNS/PN3 because its expression was known to be labile. Based on our previous observation in which we detected peak changes in SNS/PN3 mRNA 5 days after axotomy (37), we studied rats in the subacute phase, 4 days after injection of carageenan into the hind paw. As shown in figure 30.7, these experiments demonstrated significantly increased SNS/PN3 mRNA expression in DRG neurons projecting to the inflamed limb, compared with DRG neurons from the contralateral side or naive (uninjected) controls. Moreover, our patch-clamp recordings demonstrated that the amplitude of the TTX-resistant sodium current in small DRG neurons projecting to the inflamed limb was significantly larger than on the contralateral side 4 days postinjection (31.7 ± 3.3 vs. 20.0 ± 2.1 nA). The TTX-resistant current density was also significantly increased in the carageenan-challenged DRG neurons. Consistent with these results, a persistent increase in sodium channel immunoreactivity is observed in DRG neurons within

24 hr of injection of complete Freund's adjuvant into their projection field and persists for at least 2 months (50). The mechanism responsible for this inflammation-associated change in sodium channel expression is not known. Interestingly, NGF normally is produced in peripheral target tissues by supporting cells that include fibroblasts, Schwann cells, and keratinocytes; NGF production is stimulated in immune cells, and increased NGF levels have been observed in the local area after treatment with inflammatory agents such as carageenan and Freund's adjuvant (51, 52), raising the possibility that inflammation may indirectly trigger changes in sodium channel gene expression via changes in neurotrophin levels.

Sodium Channels as Molecular Targets in Pain Research

Given what we have learned about sodium channels, where do we go next in the search for better treatments for pain syndromes? The answer to this question is not entirely clear at this time. We can, however, come to a number of conclusions. First, sodium channels are important participants in electrogenesis within primary sensory neurons, including DRG neurons. Second, a multiplicity of sodium channels are present within DRG neurons, where they probably subserve multiple functions (transduction, signal amplification, action potential electrogenesis, etc.) and interact in a complex manner. Third, DRG neurons express a number of sodium channel genes (SNS/PN3, NaN, PN1, and NaG) in a preferential manner, at levels much higher than in any other neuronal cell type. This observation may present a therapeutic opportunity for the selective manipulation of primary sensory neurons in general, or nociceptive neurons in particular. Fourth, sodium channel expression in DRG neurons is highly dynamic, with multiple sodium channel genes (including α-III, SNS/PN3, and NaN) exhibiting up- or down-regulation

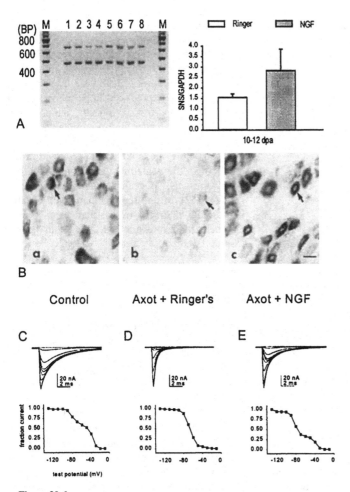

Figure 30.6
Reverse transcription–PCR (*A*), in situ hybridization (*B*), and patch-clamp recordings (*C*), showing partial rescue of
SNS mRNA and TTX-resistant sodium currents in axotomized DRG neurons after delivery of NGF to the proxi-
mal nerve stump. (*A*) Coamplification of SNS (479 bp) and glyceraldehyde-3-phosphate dehydrogenase (GAPDH)
(666 bp) products in Ringer's solution-treated axotomized DRG (lanes 1, 2, 5, and 6) and NGF-treated axotomized
DRG (lanes 3, 4, 7, and 8). The graph shows the increase in SNS amplification product in NGF-treated DRG. (*B*)
In situ hybridization showing down-regulation of SNS mRNA in DRG after axotomy (axotomy + Ringer's solution compared with control), and the partial rescue of SNS mRNA by NGF. (*C*) Representative patch-clamp
recordings showing partial rescue of slowly inactivating TTX-resistant sodium currents in axotomized DRG neurons after exposure to NGF. Corresponding steady-state inactivation curves are shown below the recordings.
Modified from ref. 45.

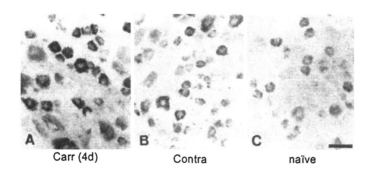

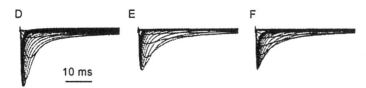

Figure 30.7
SNS mRNA levels and TTX-resistant sodium currents are increased 4 days after injection of carrageenan into the projection fields of DRG neurons. (*Upper*) In situ hybridization showing SNS mRNA in carrageenan-injected (*A*), contralateral control (*B*), and naive (*C*) DRG. Patch-clamp recordings (*D–F*) do not reveal any change in voltage dependence of activation or steady-state inactivation of TTX-resistant sodium currents after carrageenan injection, but demonstrate an increase in TTX-resistant current amplitude (*D*) and density. Modified from ref. 49.

after various injuries to these cells. Importantly, different injuries may trigger opposing changes of certain sodium channel genes (e.g., down-regulation of SNS/PN3 after axotomy vs. up-regulation in the carageenan inflammation model) in DRG neurons, so that it may be difficult to extrapolate from one model system to another. Nevertheless, we have learned, at a minimum, that sodium channel expression in DRG neurons is dynamic and can change significantly after injury, and that changes in sodium channel expression can substantially alter excitability in these cells.

Delineation of the precise role(s) of each sodium channel subtype in the physiology of DRG neurons and the pathophysiology of pain re-mains to be established, and the utility of selective blockade of each channel subtype as an approach to the treatment of pain will require further careful study. However, the stage has been set for these investigations. It is quite likely, in our opinion, that sodium channel blockade will emerge as a viable strategy for pharmacologic treatment of pain.

Acknowledgments

This work has been supported in part by grants from the National Multiple Sclerosis Society and the Paralyzed Veterans of America/Eastern Paralyzed Veterans Association, and by the Medical Research Service, Department of Veterans Affairs. T.R.C. was supported in part by a fellowship from the Spinal Cord Research Foundation.

References

1. Ochoa, J. and Torebjork, H. E. (1980) *Brain* 103: 835–854.

2. Nordin, M., Nystrom, B., Wallin, U. and Hagbarth, K.-E. (1984) *Pain* 20: 231–245.

3. Devor, M. (1994) in *Textbook of Pain,* eds. Wall, P. D. and Melzack, R. (Churchill Livingstone, Edinburgh), 2nd ed., pp. 79–101.

4. Eccles, J. C., Libet, B. and Young, R. R. (1958) *J. Physiol. (London)* 143: 11–40.

5. Kuno, M. and Llinas, R. (1970) *J. Physiol. (London)* 210: 807–821.

6. Gallego, R., Ivorra, I. and Morales, A. (1987) *J. Physiol. (London)* 391: 39–56.

7. Gurtu, S. and Smith, P. A. (1988) *J. Neurophysiol.* 59: 408–423.

8. Devor, M., Keller, C. H., Deerinck, T. J. and Ellisman, M. H. (1989) *Neurosci. Lett.* 102: 149–154.

9. England, J. D., Gamboni, F., Ferguson, M. A. and Levinson, S. R. (1994) *Muscle Nerve* 17: 593–598.

10. England, J. D., Happel, L. T., Kline, D. G., Gamboni, F., Thouron, C. L., Liu, Z. P. and Levinson, S. R. (1996) *Neurology* 47: 272–276.

11. Waxman, S. G. and Brill, M. H. (1978) *J. Neurol. Neurosurg. Psychiatr.* 41: 408–417.

12. Matzner, O. and Devor, M. (1992) *Brain Res.* 597: 92–98.

13. Matzner, O. and Devor, M. (1994) *J. Neurophysiol.* 72: 349–359.

14. Zhang, J.-M., Donnelly, D. F., Song, X.-J. and LaMotte, R. H. (1997) *J. Neurophysiol.* 78: 2790–2794.

15. Chabal, C., Russell, L. C. and Burchiel, K. J. (1989) *Pain* 38: 333–338.

16. Devor, M., Wall, P. D. and Catalan, N. (1992) *Pain* 48: 261–268.

17. Omana-Zapata, I., Khabbaz, M. A., Hunter, J. C. and Bley, K. R. (1997) *Brain Res.* 771: 228–237.

18. Rizzo, M. A. (1997) *J. Neurol. Sci.* 152: 103–106.

19. Kostyuk, P. G., Veselovsky, N. S. and Tsyandryenko, A. Y. (1981) *Neuroscience* 6: 2423–2430.

20. Roy, M. L. and Narahashi, T. (1992) *J. Neurosci.* 12: 2104–2111.

21. Caffrey, J. M., Eng, D. L., Black, J. A., Waxman, S. G. and Kocsis, J. D. (1992) *Brain Res.* 592: 283–297.

22. Elliott, A. A. and Elliott, J. R. (1993) *J. Physiol. (London)* 463: 39–56.

23. Black, J. A., Dib-Hajj, S., McNabola, K., Jeste, S., Rizzo, M. A., Kocsis, J. D. and Waxman, S. G. (1996) *Mol. Brain Res.* 43: 117–132.

24. Toledo-Aral, J. J., Moss, B. L., He, Z.-J., Koszowski, A. G., Whisenand, T., Levinson, S. R., Wolff, J. J., Silos-Santiago, I., Halegoua, S. and Mandel, G. (1997) *Proc. Natl. Acad. Sci. USA* 94: 1527–1532.

25. Cummins, T. R., Howe, J. R. and Waxman, S. G. (1999) *J. Neurosci.* 18: 9607–9619.

26. Akopian, A. N., Sivilotti, L. and Wood, J. N. (1996) *J. Biol. Chem.* 271: 5953–5956.

27. Sangameswaran. L., Delgado, S. G., Fish, L. M., Koch, B. D., Jakeman, L. B., Stewart, G. R., Sze, P., Hunter, J. C., Eglen, R. M. and Herman, R. C. (1996) *J. Biol. Chem.* 271: 5953–5956.

28. Dib-Hajj, S. D., Tyrrell, L., Black, J. A. and Waxman, S. G. (1998) *Proc. Natl. Acad. Sci. USA* 95: 8963–8969.

29. Gautron, S., Dos Santos, G., Pinto-Henrique, D., Koulkoff, A., Gros, F. and Berwald-Netter, Y. (1992) *Proc. Natl. Acad. Sci. USA* 89: 7272–7276.

30. Felts, P. A., Black, J. A., Dib-Hajj, S. D. and Waxman, S. G. (1997) *Glia* 21: 269–277.

31. Rizzo, M. A., Kocsis, J. D. and Waxman, S. G. (1995) *J. Neurophysiol.* 72: 2796–2816.

32. Rush, A. M., Brau, M. E., Elliott, A. A. and Elliott, J. R. (1998) *J. Physiol. (London)* 511: 771–789.

33. Scholz, A., Appel, N. and Vogel, W. (1998) *Eur. J. Neurosci.* 10: 2547–2556.

34. Jeftinija, S. (1994) *Brain Res.* 639: 125–134.

35. Quasthoff, S., Grosskreutz, J., Schroder, J. M., Schneider, U. and Grafe, P. (1995) *Neuroscience* 69: 955–965.

36. Waxman, S. G., Kocsis, J. K. and Black, J. A. (1994) *J. Neurophysiol.* 72: 466–471.

37. Dib-Hajj, S., Black, J. A., Felts, P. and Waxman, S. G. (1996) *Proc. Natl. Acad. Sci. USA* 93: 14950–14954.

38. Rizzo, M. A., Kocsis, J. D. and Waxman, S. G. (1995) *Neurobiol. Dis.* 2: 87–96.

39. Cummins, T. R. and Waxman, S. G. (1997) *J. Neurosci.* 17: 3503–3514.

40. Rizzo, M. A., Kocsis, J. D. and Waxman, S. G. (1996) *Eur. Neurol.* 36: 3–12.

41. Stys, P. K., Ransom, B. R. and Waxman, S. G. (1993) *Proc. Natl. Acad. Sci. USA* 90: 6976–6980.

42. Aguayo, L. G. and White, G. (1992) *Brain Res.* 570: 61–67.

43. Zur, K. B., Oh, Y., Waxman, S. G. and Black, J. A. (1995) *Mol. Brain Res.* 30: 97–103.

44. Black, J. A., Langworthy, K., Hinson, A. W., Dib-Hajj, S. D. and Waxman, S. G. (1997) *NeuroReport* 8: 2331–2335.

45. Dib-Hajj, S. D., Black, J. A., Cummins, T. R., Kenney, A. M., Kocsis, J. D. and Waxman, S. G. (1998) *J. Neurophysiol.* 79: 2668–2678.

46. Oyelese, A. A., Rizzo, M. A., Waxman, S. G. and Kocsis, J. D. (1997) *J. Neurophysiol.* 78: 31–42.

47. Gold, M. S., Reichling, D. B., Shuster, M. J. and Levine, J. D. (1996) *Proc. Natl. Acad. Sci. USA* 93: 1108–1112.

48. England, S., Bevan, S. and Docherty, R. J. (1996) *J. Physiol. (London)* 495: 429–440.

49. Tanaka, M., Cummins, T. R., Ishikawa, K., Dib-Hajj, S. D., Black, J. A. and Waxman, S. G. (1998) *NeuroReport* 9: 967–972.

50. Gould, H. J. III, England, J. D., Liu, Z. P. and Levinson, S. R. (1998) *Brain Res.* 802: 69–74.

51. Woolf, C. J., Safieh-Garabedian, B., Ma, Q.-P., Crilly, P. and Winter, J. (1994) *Neuroscience* 62: 327–331.

52. Weskamp, G. and Otten, U. (1987) *J. Neurochem.* 48: 1779–1786.

53. Fzell, J., Cummins, P. R., Dib-Hajj, S. D., Fried, K., Black, J. A. and Waxman, S. G. (1999) *Mol. Brain Res.* 67: 267–282.

XVII NEEDLE IN A HAYSTACK

If one were searching for more effective medications which would alleviate pain without side effects, one might begin by asking: "Are there any molecules that contribute to electrical bursting in pain-signaling neurons, which are not present in other types of nerve cells?" Molecules such as sodium channels that were *specific* to spinal sensory neurons, particularly pain-signaling neurons, might provide "therapeutic targets"; medications acting on these targets might be expected to dampen the barrages of nerve impulses carrying pain signals to the brain without interfering with other activities of the nervous system. We thus were especially interested in sodium channels specific to spinal sensory neurons, particularly the small C-type spinal sensory neurons which carry pain sensation.

SNS/PN3 had already been identified as one spinal sensory neuron-specific sodium channel (Akopian, Sivilotti, and Wood 1996; Sangameswaran et al. 1996). On the basis of our electrophysiological results we had a hunch that there might be an additional sensory neuron-specific sodium channel in pain-signaling neurons. Most sodium channels are blocked by a neurotoxin called tetrodotoxin, but our recordings suggested that the new channel, if present, might resist its blocking action.

Each nerve cell contains thousands of different types of protein molecules, and finding any one of them—particularly a previously unidentified one—is like searching for a needle in a haystack. How, then, can one identify a new channel? Sulayman Dib-Hajj began these experiments by designing a "molecular cloning" strategy that took advantage of the fact that spinal sensory neurons were likely to contain a message (mRNA) specifying the amino acid sequence of each channel they produced. For these experiments, this gifted molecular biologist constructed molecular primers, or chains of nucleotides, that would recognize and bind to the mRNAs for all sodium channels in these neurons, even previously unidentified channels, at highly conserved regions bordering a divergent core. He used a robotlike device (called a PCR, or polymerase chain reaction, machine) to amplify the sequences encoding these channels millions of times. He identified the mRNAs by their unique signatures, reflecting the presence of recognition sites for restriction enzymes which cleave them at specific regions. After measuring the sizes of the pieces of the mRNAs by determining how quickly they migrate in an electric field, one can tell whether they correspond to the fragments of previously identified messages. This type of analysis confirmed the presence of mRNAs encoding the previously known sodium channels in spinal sensory neurons. We were excited to see that it also revealed a novel mRNA fragment, suggesting that spinal sensory neurons produced a species of sodium channel that was not yet known.

Our cloning strategy called for a next step in which we would use the fragment of mRNA that we had found as a springboard, to design gene-specific primers that would permit us to amplify other, overlapping fragments of the mRNA. Once these were found, we could repeat the process, marching farther along the mRNA to map additional parts of it, then repeating the process until we had unraveled interesting parts, or even the full sequence. Even partial information about the nucleotide sequence could verify the existence of the new channel, and the complete sequence would tell us the identity of all of its amino acids.

Whether to completely sequence the new channel was not a trivial decision. This laborious process would require the diversion of significant manpower to the cloning effort and away from other projects. And there was no assurance that at the end of our search, we would find a new channel or that it would be important. Nonetheless, after a series of discussions we decided to move ahead. We tentatively named our target NaX (Na = sodium, X = unknown). We were joined shortly thereafter by Lynda Tyrrell, another superb molecular biologist who, together with Dib-Hajj, carried out the cloning. It took many months to complete. The results are shown in figure 2 of Dib-Hajj et al. (1998); NaN had a sequence of 1765 amino acids encoded by a series of 5,875 nucleotides. It included all of the relevant landmark sequences of sodium channels including S-4 segments in the four domains that make up these specialized molecules. As we had expected, the amino acid sequence of the channel predicted that it was tetrodotoxin-resistant. And it was, indeed, a new channel, sharing only 47 percent of its amino acid sequence with SNS/PN3. Joel Black did in situ hybridizations to visualize the mRNA for the new channel and these, together with northern blot analysis, showed us one additional important feature: the channel we had cloned was preferentially expressed in C-type spinal sensory and trigeminal neurons, which carry pain signals, and was present in these nociceptive neurons at much higher levels than in larger spinal sensory neurons which carry tactile and position sensation, or in other types of nerve cells. Because of this we changed its name to NaN (N = Nociceptive and New).

Our paper appeared in *Proceedings of the National Academy of Sciences* in July 1998. The strategic decision to divert resources to the cloning of NaN had led us to an important finding. But scientists do not work in a vacuum. Six months after our *PNAS* paper appeared, Tate et al. (1998) published the identical sequence in *Nature Neuroscience*; they called the channel SNS-2.[1]

The next step in studies of this type is usually to record the electrical currents produced by the new channel, to firmly establish its functional properties. Tate et al. included in their paper patch-clamp recordings of small currents in human kidney cells which they engineered in an attempt to express NaN; they interpreted these recordings as suggesting that NaN opened and closed relatively quickly and that it was, as we had proposed, tetrodotoxin-resistant. Members of our team, however, were concerned that the recordings of Tate et al. might not reflect the behavior of NaN channels, especially within their native environment within spinal sensory neurons (the reasons for this concern are outlined in the discussion and figure 4 of Cummins et al. 1999, which follows). The physiological properties of NaN, in our opinion, still required careful study and we took a number of approaches to this.

One of our strategies was to study "knock-out" mice, produced by John Wood and his coworkers at University College London, in which other tetrodotoxin-resistant channels (SNS/PN3) were absent (Akopian et al. 1999). Wood and his colleagues had not seen any residual tetrodotoxin-resistant sodium current in spinal sensory neurons from these mice. We were convinced, however, that the current should be there, and Wood was curious and generous enough to send us the knockouts. Ted Cummins, a biophysicist with an extraordinary grasp of channel physiology working in our group, suspected that the NaN current might be inactivated at the potentials at which cells were usually held for recording, but that it would be present at hyperpolarized potentials.

Because John Wood's knockout mice had been shipped from another country we had to wait for several months, after they arrived, for them to come out of quarantine. But when the quarantine was over we were able to proceed, and, as Cummins had predicted, when the knockout cells were held at a hyperpolarized potential a substantial tetrodotoxin-resistant sodium current was apparent in them. This current was quite different than the current reported by Tate et al., and it had several novel properties: the current was activated at a low threshold voltage, close to the "resting potential" where spinal sensory neurons normally sit when they are not active; it had a "window" of overlap of activation and steady-state inactivation indicating that it should generate current at resting potential; and the channel exhibited "persistent" activation, that is, it remained open without closing during a long stimulus (Cummins et al. 1999). A channel producing current with these properties would be expected to modulate the threshold and thus control the firing of neurons in which it was present. We had, in

---

1. The two names given to this channel (NaN and SNS2) and the two names given to another sodium channel (SNS and PN3) exemplify the fact that numerous laboratories are participants in the search for new channels, each assigning its own name to newly cloned molecules. It is likely that a standardized nomenclature will be adopted within the near future, and that these and other channels will be renamed to conform with it.

fact, seen the persistent sodium current two years previously in C-type spinal sensory neurons from normal rats (Cummins and Waxman 1997), but in these earlier experiments we could not tell which channel was responsible for it. Now we knew that it almost certainly represented the physiological signature of NaN.

We also demonstrated that NaN is present in humans (Dib-Hajj et al. 1999a). This was not easy, because spinal sensory neurons are usually obtained only at postmortem; and mRNAs usually degrade rapidly and cells often lose their ability to generate electrical activity in postmortem tissue. We were fortunate to be able to obtain spinal sensory ganglia from Patrick Wood, who had established a protocol for rapid postmortem retrieval of spinal cords at the University of Miami. Using this tissue, Dib-Hajj identified the amino acid sequence of NaN in human spinal sensory neurons and Cummins was able to demonstrate that a persistent sodium current, similar to that produced by NaN in mice, is present in these cells; the 15 millivolt hyperpolarizing shift in the voltage-dependence of human NaN, compared to mouse NaN, appeared to have a molecular basis in the presence of one additional charged amino acid residue in the S-4 region, which acts as a voltage sensor, in the human channel.

In parallel with these studies, we also learned about other aspects of NaN. Jenny Fjell, an M.D.-Ph.D. student from the Karolinska Institute in Stockholm working in our laboratory together with Joel Black, did a series of experiments to find out how the production of NaN is controlled. She found that glial cell-derived neurotrophic factor (GDNF), a "trophic" factor, modulates the expression of NaN in spinal sensory neurons (Fjell et al. 1999). We developed antibodies directed against NaN, and, using these, Fjell found that NaN molecules are localized along nonmyelinated nerve fibers and at the nodes of Ranvier in small diameter, thinly myelinated fibers in peripheral nerve, a pattern of localization that is consistent with a role of NaN in pain signaling (Fjell et al. 2000). And we localized the NaN gene to specific parts of chromosome 9 in mice and chromosome 3 in humans (Dib-Hajj et al. 1999b).

It is hard to know where these studies will lead. We have progressed from molecular cloning (the "genomic" phase of this project) to studies on the biology, physiology and pharmacology of NaN (the "postgenomic" phase). In a sense, having found the needle in the haystack, we must now learn how sharp it is and what it can do. This is an evolving story, and I have an exhilarating sense of forward motion. With hard work we may be able to learn more about how the molecular structure of NaN determines its behavior, about how NaN shapes the electrical activity in sensory neurons, and about how its activity can be altered. With luck we may even learn how to manipulate this molecular needle in a haystack. That would be really exciting. If we can reach that goal, perhaps we can help people in pain.

References

Akopian, A. N., Sivilotti, L., and Wood, J. N. A tetrodotoxin-resistant voltage-gated sodium channel expressed by sensory neurons. *Nature* 379: 257–262, 1996.

Akopian, A. N., Souslova, V., England, S., Okuse, K., Ogata, N., Ure, J., Smith, A., Kerr, B. J., McMahon, S. B., Boyce, S., Hill, R., Stanfa, L. C., Dickenson, A. H., and Wood, J. N. The tetrodotoxin-resistant sodium channel SNS has a specialized function in pain pathways. *Nature Neurosci.* 2: 541–548, 1999.

Cummins, T. R., Dib-Hajj, S. D., Black, J. A., Akopian, A. N., Wood, J. N., and Waxman, S. G. A novel persistent tetrodotoxin-resistant sodium current in SNS-null and wild-type small primary sensory neurons. *J. Neurosci.* 19: RC43(1–6), 1999.

Cummins, T. R., and Waxman, S. G. Down-regulation of tetrodotoxin-resistant sodium currents and up-regulation of a rapidly repriming tetrodotoxin-sensitive sodium current in small spinal sensory neurons following nerve injury. *J. Neurosci.* 17: 3503–3514, 1997.

Dib-Hajj, S. D., Tyrrell, L., Black, J. A., and Waxman, S. G. NaN, a novel voltage-gated Na channel preferentially expressed in peripheral sensory neurons and down-regulated following axotomy. *Proc. Natl. Acad. Sci. U.S.A.* 95: 8963–8968, 1998.

Dib-Hajj, S. D., Tyrrell, L., Cummins, T. R., Black, J. A., Wood, P. M., and Waxman, S. G. Two tetrodotoxin-resistant sodium channels in human dorsal root ganglion neurons. *FEBS Letts.* 462: 117–120, 1999a.

Dib-Hajj, S. D., Tyrrell, L., Escayg, A., Wood, P. M., Meisler, M. H., and Waxman, S. G. Coding sequence, genomic organization and conserved chromosomal localization of mouse Scn11a gene encoding the sodium channel NaN. *Genomics* 59: 309–318, 1999b.

Fjell, J., Cummins, T. R., Dib-Hajj, S. D., Fried, K., Black, J. A., and Waxman, S. G. Differential role of GDNF and NGF in the maintenance of two TTX-resistant sodium channels in adult DRG neurons. *Molec. Brain Res.* 67: 267–282, 1999.

Fjell, J., Hjelmstrom, P., Hormuzdiar, W., Milenkovic, M., Aglieco, F., Tyrrell, L., Dib-Hajj, S., Waxman, S. G., and Black, J. A. Localization of the tetrodotoxin-resistant sodium channel NaN in nociceptors. *NeuroReport* 11: 199–202, 2000.

Sangameswaran, L., Delgado, S. G., Fish, L. M., Koch, B. D., Jakeman, L. B., Stewart, G. R., Sze, P., Hunter, J. C., Eglen, R. M., and Herman, R. C. Structure and function of a novel voltage-gated, tetrodotoxin-resistant sodium channel specific to sensory neurons. *J. Biol. Chem.* 271: 5953–5956, 1996.

Tate, S., Benn, S., Hick, C., Trezise, D., John, V., Mannion, R. J., Costigan, M., Plumpton, C., Grose, D., Gladwell, Z., Kendall, G., Dale, K., Bountra, C., and Woolf, C. J. Two sodium channels contribute to the TTX-R sodium current in primary sensory neurons. *Nature Neurosci.* 1: 653–655, 1998.

31 NaN, a Novel Voltage-Gated Na Channel, Is Expressed Preferentially in Peripheral Sensory Neurons and Down-Regulated after Axotomy

S. D. Dib-Hajj, L. Tyrrell, J. A. Black, and S. G. Waxman

Abstract Although physiological and pharmacological evidence suggests the presence of multiple tetrodotoxin-resistant (TTX-R) Na channels in neurons of peripheral nervous system ganglia, only one, SNS/PN3, has been identified in these cells to date. We have identified and sequenced a novel Na channel a-subunit (NaN), predicted to be TTX-R and voltage-gated, that is expressed preferentially in sensory neurons within dorsal root ganglia (DRG) and trigeminal ganglia. The predicted amino acid sequence of NaN can be aligned with the predicted structure of known Na channel a-subunits; all relevant landmark sequences, including positively charged S4 and pore-lining SS1–SS2 segments, and the inactivation tripeptide IFM, are present at predicted positions. However, NaN exhibits only 42–53% similarity to other mammalian Na channels, including SNS/PN3, indicating that it is a novel channel, and suggesting that it may represent a third subfamily of Na channels. NaN transcript levels are reduced significantly 7 days post axotomy in DRG neurons, consistent with previous findings of a reduction in TTX-R Na currents. The preferential expression of NaN in DRG and trigeminal ganglia and the reduction of NaN mRNA levels in DRG after axonal injury suggest that NaN, together with SNS/PN3, may produce TTX-R currents in peripheral sensory neurons and may influence the generation of electrical activity in these cells.

Voltage-gated Na channels in rat brain are composed of three subunits: the pore-forming a-subunit (260 kDa), which is sufficient to generate Na current flow across the membrane, and two auxiliary subunits. $\beta1$ (36 kDa) and $\beta2$ (33 kDa), which can modulate the properties of the a-subunit (1, 2). Nine distinct a-subunits have been identified in the rat (ref. 3 and references therein, refs. 4–6), and homologues have been cloned from various mammalian species, including humans (3). Specific a-subunits are expressed in a tissue- and developmentally specific manner

Reprinted with permission from *Proceeding of the National Academy of Sciences USA* 95: 8963–8968, 1998.

(7). Aberrant expression patterns or mutations of voltage-gated sodium channel a-subunits underlie a number of human and animal disorders (1, 8–11).

Multiple voltage-gated Na currents, some tetrodotoxin-sensitive (TTX-S) and others TTX-resistant (TTX-R) (12–15), have been observed in dorsal root ganglia (DRG) neurons, which express multiple Na channel a-subunit mRNAs (16). The complex Na current profile in DRG neurons influences their excitability (13, 17–19) and may contribute to ectopic or spontaneous firing in these cells after injury to their axons (8, 20, 21).

Excitability and Na current density are altered in neurons after axonal injury (22–25). After axotomy, rat DRG neurons display dramatic changes in their TTX-R and TTX-S Na currents and in their Na channel mRNA profile; these changes include an attenuation of TTX-R and enhancement of TTX-S Na currents (21, 26), down-regulation of SNS/PN3 transcripts and up-regulation of aIII transcripts (20), and moderate elevation in the levels of aI and aII mRNAs (27). Inflammatory modulators also up-regulate TTX-R current (28–30) and SNS/PN3 transcripts (30) in C type DRG neurons. These results suggest that changes in the Na current profile may contribute to neuropathic and inflammation-evoked pain.

DRG neurons, particularly C type neurons, are unique in expressing high levels of TTX-R Na current (12–15, 21) but until recently, the identity of the channels that produce these currents was unknown. A recently identified Na channel a-subunit (SNS/PN3), which produces a slowly inactivating TTX-R current when expressed in *Xenopus* oocytes, is expressed preferentially in small peripheral sensory neurons, which include nociceptive (C type) neurons (4, 6). However, physiological and pharmacological evidence (15, 31, 32) suggests the presence of multiple TTX-R Na channels in DRG and nodose ganglia neurons. We report here the identification of a distinct Na channel a-subunit with limited homology to existing subunits, which we term NaN. NaN is predicted to produce a TTX-R current and is expressed preferentially in small-diameter peripheral nervous system neurons. Consistent with its predicted role as a TTX-R Na channel in sensory neurons, NaN is down-regulated after axotomy.

Materials and Methods

RNA Preparation and Reverse Transcription

Total cellular RNA was isolated from L4–L5 DRG dissected from adult Sprague–Dawley rats by the single-step guanidinium isothio-cyanate/ acid phenol procedure (33). Poly(A)$^+$ RNA was purified from about 300 μg (28 animals) of total DRG RNA (Promega). Half of the purified RNA was used for preparation of Marathon cDNA (CLONTECH) and the other half was used for Northern blot analysis (see below).

First-strand cDNA was synthesized from total RNA as described previously (34). Marathon first- and second-strand cDNA were synthesized by using poly(dT) primer (CLONTECH). The final cDNA product ligated to the adapter primers was diluted 1:250 in Tricine/EDTA buffer and used as template in 5' and 3' rapid amplification of cDNA ends (RACE).

PCR

For the initial identification of NaN-specific fragment, we used generic primers (F1–4; R1–3) designed against highly conserved sequences in domain 1 (D1) of a-subunits (35). NaN sequences 3'-terminal to this fragment were amplified by using NaN-specific and two degenerate generic reverse primers, R4 and R5. The sequence of R4 (5'-ACYTCCATRCANWCC-

CACAT-3'; Y = T or C, R = A or G; W = A or T, N = A, C, G, or T) and R5 (5'-AGRAAR-TCNAGCCARCACCA) primers was based on the amino acid sequence MWV/DCMEV, located just N-terminal to domain II S6, and AWCWLDFL, which forms the N-terminal portion of domain III S3 segment, respectively. Amplification was carried out in two stages by using a PTC-200 programmable thermal cycler (34).

Primary RACE amplification was performed in 50 μl final volume using 4 μl diluted DRG marathon cDNA template, 0.2 μM marathon AP-1 and NaN-specific primers, 3.5 units of Expand Long Template enzyme mixture in buffer 3, and 3.0 mM $MgCl_2$ (Boehringer Mannheim). Extension period was adjusted at 1 min/800 bp based on the expected product. 5' RACE amplification was performed by using Marathon AP-1 (5'-CCATCCTAATACGACTCACTAT-AGGGC-3')/NaN-specific R6 (5'-TCTGCTG-CCGAGCCAGGTA-3') primers; nested PCR amplification under similar conditions used marathon AP-2 (5'-ACTCACTATAGGGCTC-GAGCGGC-3')/NaN-specific R7 (5'-CTGAG-ATAACTGAAATCGCC-3') primers. 3' RACE was performed similarly by using NaN-specific F5 (5'-AACATAGTGCTGGAGTTCAGG-3')/ Marathon AP-1 primers; nested PCR was performed by using NaN-specific F6 (5'-GTGGC-CTTTGGATTCCGGAGG-3')/Marathon AP-2 primers. Amplification was via (i) initial denaturation at 92 °C for 2 min; (ii) 35 cycles of denaturation at 92 °C for 20 sec, annealing at 60 °C for 1 min, and elongation at 68 °C; and (iii) elongation at 68 °C for 5 min. Nested amplification under similar conditions used 2 μl of a 1/500 diluted primary product. Secondary RACE amplification products from five independent reactions were typically pooled, band-isolated, and used as templates for sequencing by primer walking, with analysis using LASERGENE (DNAstar, Madison, WI) and BLAST (National Library of Medicine) software.

Tissue Distribution

Tissue-specific expression of NaN was investigated by reverse transcription–PCR (RT-PCR) and Northern blot analysis. NaN-specific forward (5′-CCCTGCTGCGCTCGGTGAAGAA-3′) and reverse (5′-GACAAAGTAGATCCCA-GAGG-3′) primers, which amplify nucleotides 765-1156 (392 bp), were used for RT-PCR under cycling conditions described previously (34).

Approximately 1 μg of poly(A)$^+$ rat DRG RNA, digoxigenin (DIG)-labeled RNA molecular weight marker 11 (Boehringer Mannheim), and 0.24–9.5 kb RNA ladder (GIBCO) with ethidium bromide were electrophoresed in a 0.8% agarose/2.2 M formaldehyde gel and RNA was transferred overnight to positively charged nylon membrane (Boehringer Mannheim) by capillary action (33).

A rat multiple-tissue Northern blot (CLONTECH) of poly(A)$^+$ RNA from heart, brain, spleen, lung, liver, skeletal muscle, kidney, and testis was hybridized along with the DRG blot by using the DIG-labeled, NaN-specific antisense riboprobe, described below. Blots were prehybridized for 3 hr at 60 °C in Dig Easy Hyb solution (Boehringer Mannheim), hybridized overnight with probe (100 ng/ml) at 60 °C, and washed under stringent conditions, and the hybridization signal was detected by chemiluminescence using disodium 3-(4-methoxyspiro{1,2-dioxetane-3,2′-(5′-chloro)tricyclo[3.3.1.1^{3,7}]decan}-4-ylphenyl phosphate (CSPD) as substrate (Boehringer Mannheim). The blots then were washed immediately in prehybridization solution at room temperature for 30 min, prehybridized for 2 hr at 60 °C in fresh solution, and reprobed for β-actin mRNA by using a DIG-labeled riboprobe (100 ng/ml, Boehringer Mannheim) under similar conditions.

Axotomy

Adult Sprague–Dawley female rats were anaesthetized with ketamine (40 mg/kg) and xylazine (2.5 mg/kg) i.p. Sciatic nerves were exposed on the right side, ligated with 4-0 sutures proximal to the pyriform ligament, transected, and placed in a silicon cuff to prevent regeneration (20). Seven days post axotomy (dpa), the rats were anesthetized, and control (contralateral) and axotomized (ipsilateral) L4/5 DRG were processed for quantitative RT-PCR and in situ hybridization.

Quantitative RT-PCR

Total cellular RNA was isolated from pooled L4–L5 DRGs of 5 rats, from the respective sides, and reverse transcription and quantitation were performed as described previously (36). PCR conditions for the simultaneous linear amplification of NaN and GAPDH, which was used as an endogenous internal control to compensate for sample-to-sample variation, were determined empirically. To prevent inhibition of the amplification of NaN by excess glyceraldehyde-3-phosphate dehydrogenase (GAPDH) templates, we delayed addition of GAPDH primers (37) for five cycles. GAPDH and NaN primers were used at final concentrations of 0.75 and 3.75 μM, respectively. Control PCR with water or RNA template produced no amplification products (data not shown). Amplification conditions were (*i*) denaturation at 94 °C for 3 min, annealing at 60 °C for 2 min, and elongation at 72 °C for 2 min; (*ii*) four cycles of denaturation at 94 °C for 30 sec, annealing at 60 °C for 1 min, and elongation at 72 °C for 1 min, followed by pause at 20 °C to add GAPDH primers; (*iii*) 23 cycles of denaturation at 94 °C for 30 sec, annealing at 60 °C for 1 min, and elongation at 72 °C for 1 min; and (*iv*) elongation at 72 °C for 10 min.

In Situ Hybridization

DIG-labeled sense and antisense riboprobes recognizing NaN nucleotide sequences 1371–1751 (GenBank numbering) were prepared by in vitro transcription. Transcript yield and integrity were determined by comparison with a control DIG-labeled RNA (Boehringer Mannheim) on 2% agarose/2.2 M formaldehyde gel. Tissue section (14 μm) preparation, in situ hybridization conditions, and quantitation of cell diameter (calculated from area in cells displaying nuclear diameters >50% cell diameter) were as described previously (16, 20, 36). Four separate experiments were analyzed for the expression of NaN mRNA in control and axotomized DRG neurons, and statistical significance was determined by using Student's *t* test.

Results

Restriction Enzyme Analysis Predicts the Presence of an Additional Na Channel

Restriction enzyme profile analysis (35) of amplification products from domain 1 (D1) of voltage-gated Na channel subunits from DRG (figure 31.1) reveals multiple amplification products (lane 1); bands "a," "b," and "c" are consistent with the presence of αI (558 bp), αII, and αIII (561 bp; band a), Na6 and PN1 (507 and 501 bp, respectively; band b), and SNS/PN3 (479 bp; band c). The presence of band d was unexpected and suggested the amplification of a novel product. Lanes 2–7 show the result of cutting this DNA with *Eco*RV, *Eco*NI, *Ava*I, *Sph*I, *Bam*HI, and *Afl*II, respectively. As expected, αI product appears to constitute most of band a (lane 2). αII (lane 3) and αIII (lane 4) are not evident by this analysis; however, their very low level of expression was demonstrated previously upon individual amplification (16). Na6 and PN1 products (lanes 5 and 6) are in agreement with the predicted results (35). The doublet migrating faster than the 400-bp marker in lane 6 is from the presence of a restriction site for *Bam*HI in both PN1 and SNS/PN3. SNS/PN3 comprises band c, which is cleaved by *Afl*II (lane 7). NaG (SCL-11) is not detected in this assay (lane 8),

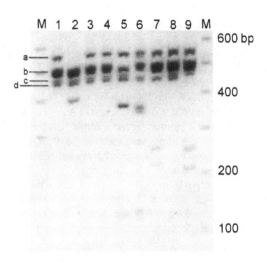

Figure 31.1
Restriction enzyme profile analysis of Na channel domain 1 RT-PCR products from DRG. "M" lanes contain the 100-bp ladder marker (Pharmacia). Lane 1 contains the amplification product from DRG cDNA. Lanes 2–9 show the result of cutting this DNA with *Eco*RV, *Eco*NI, *Ava*I, *Sph*I, *Bam*HI, *Afl*II, *Xba*I, and *Eco*RI, which are specific to subunits αI, -II, -III, Na6, PN1, SNS/PN3, NaG, and NaN, respectively. The image was digitized by using GELBASE 7500 system (Ultraviolet Products) and printed in black and white dye sublimation mode.

but was demonstrated when amplified individually (38).

Identification of NaN

The novel species "d" was amplified reproducibly by F1 and R3 primers (data not shown). The sequence of this PCR product defined a template that corresponds to nucleotides 608-1075 of NaN (GenBank numbering). Digestion by *Eco*RI was determined to be characteristic of NaN (figure 31.1, lane 9). Using NaN-specific and generic primers, the sequence was extended to DIIIS3. The remaining sequence was obtained from overlapping 5′ and 3′ RACE products.

```
MEERYYPVIFPDERNFRPFT SDSLAAIEKRIAIQKERKKS KDKAAAEPQPRPQLDLKASR    60
KLPKLYGDIPPELVAKPLED LDPFYKDHKTFMVLNKKRTI YRFSAKRALFILGPFNPLRS   120
LMIRISVHSVFSMFIICTVI INCMFMANSMERSFDNDIPE YVFIGIYILEAVIKILARGF   180
         DI-S1                                       DI-S2
IVDEFSFLRDPWNWLDFIVI GTAIATCFPGSQVNLSALRT FRVFRALKAISVISGLKVIV   240
                DI-S3                           DI-S4
GALLRSVKKLVDVMVLTLFC LSIFALVGQQLFMGILNQKC IKHNCGPNPASNKDCFEKEK   300
                 DI-S5
DSEDFIMCGTWLGSRPCPNG STCDKTTLNPDNNYTKFDNF GWSFLAMFRVMTQDSWERLY   360
                                      DI-SS1            DI-SS2
RQILRTSGIYFVFFFVVVIF LGSFYLLNLTLAVVTMAYEE QNRNVAAETEAKEKMFQEAQ   420
                  DI-S6
QLLREEKEALVAMGIDRSSL NSLQASSFSPKKRKFFGSKT RKSFFMRGSKTAQASASDSE   480
DDASKNPQLLEQTKRLSQNL PVDLFDEHVDPLHRQRALSA VSILTITMQEQEKFQEPCFP   540
CGKNLASKYLVWDCSPQWLC IKKVLRTIMTDPFTELAITI CIIINTVFLAVEHHNMDDNL   600
                            DII-S1
KTILKIGNWVFTGIFIAEMC LKIIALDPYHYFRHGWNVFD SIVALLSLADVLYNTLSDNN   660
    DII-S2                           DII-S3
RSFLASLRVLRVFKLAKSWP TLNTLIKIIGHSVGALGNLT VVLTIVVFIFSVVGMRLFGT   720
    DII-S4                                   DII-S5
KFNKTAYATQERPRRRWHMD NFYHSFLVVFRILCGEWIEN MWGCMQDMDGSPLCIIVFVL   780
                         DII-SS1      DII-SS2            DII-S6
IMVIGKLVVLNLFIALLLNS FSNEEKDGSLEGETRKTKVQ LALDRFRRAFSFMLHALQSF   840
CCKKCRRKNSPKPKETTESF AGENKDSILPDARPWKEYDT DMALYTGQAGAPLAPLAEVE   900
DDVEYCGEGGALPTSQHSAG VQAGDLPPETKQLTSPDDQG VEMEVFSEEDLHLSIQSPRK   960
KSDAVSMLSECSTIDLNDIF RNLQKTVSPKKQPDRCFPKG LSCHFLCHKTDKRKSPWVLW  1020
WNIRKTCYQIVKHSWFESFI IFVILLSSGALIFEDVNLPS RPQVEKLLRCTDNIFTFIFL  1080
       DIII-S1                                       DIII-S2
LEMILKWVAFGFRRYFTSAW CWLDFLIVVVSVLSLMNLPS LKSFRTLRALRPLRALSQFE  1140
                            DIII-S3                    DIII-S4
GMKVVVYALISAIPAILNVL LVCLIFWLVFCILGVNLFSG KFGRCINGTDINMYLDFTEV  1200
               DIII-S5
PNRSQCNISNYSWKVPQVNF DNVGNAYLALLQVATYKGWL EIMNAAVDSREKDEQPDFEA  1260
          DIII-SS1                 DIII-SS2
NLYAYLYFVVFIIFGSFFTL NLFIGVIIDNFNQQQKKLGG QDIFMTEEQKKYYNAMKKLG  1320
         DIII-S6
TKKPQKPIPRPLNKCQAFVF DLVTSHVFDVIILGLIVLNM IIMMAESADQPKDVKKTFDI  1380
                          DIV-S1
LNIAFVVIFTIECLIKVFAL RQHYFTNGWNLFDCVVVVLS IISTLVSRLEDSDISFPPTL  1440
    DIV-S2                           DIV-S3
FRVVRLARIGRILRLVRAAR GIRTLLFALMMSLPSLFNIG LLLFLVMFIYAIFGMSWFSK  1500
    DIV-S4                                   DIV-S5
VKKGSGIDDIFNFETFTGSM LCLFQITTSAGWDTLLNPML EAKEHCNSSSQDSCQQPQIA  1560
          DIV-SS1                 DIV-SS2
VVYFVSYIIISFLIVVNMYI AVILENFNTATEESEDPLGE DDFEIFYEVWEKFDPEASQF  1620
     DIV-S6
IQYSALSDFADALPEPLRVA KPNKFQFLVMDLPMVMGDRL HCMDVLFAFTTRVLGDSSGL  1680
DTMKTMMEEKFMEANPFKKL YEPIVTTTKRKEEEQGAAVI QRAYRKHMEKMVKLRLKDRS  1740
SSSHQVFCNGDLSSLDVAKV KVHND                                      1765
```

Figure 31.2
Predicted amino acid sequence of NaN. DI–DIV represent the four domains of Na channels, with the putative transmembrane segments underlined. The serine residue of DI-SS2 predicted to underline the TTX-R phenotype (S355), the PKC phosphorylation site in L3 (T1321), and the tripeptide IFM in L3 involved in fast inactivation (40) are in bold and larger type, and are underlined.

The final sequence of 5,875 bp predicts an ORF of 1,765 aa (figure 31.2), 40 bp and 536 bp of 5′ and 3′ untranslated sequences, respectively. A polyadenylation signal is present at position 5855, followed, 10 nt downstream, by a poly(A) tail. Northern analysis of DRG poly(A)+ RNA shows a single band corresponding to transcripts about 6.5-kb long (figure 31.3B), suggesting a much longer 5′ untranslated sequence. The first ATG codon matches the vertebrate consensus sequence at −3, +4 positions (39) and is pre-

dicted to initiate translation of NaN. Na channel subfamily 1 subunits meet this criterion; the initiator ATG of subfamily 2 members shows a suboptimal sequence at the +4 position. Unlike subfamily 1 members, and in common with subfamily 2 members, NaN does not have an out-of-frame ATG codon at positions −8 to −6.

The predicted amino acid sequence of NaN can be aligned with the predicted primary structures of all known Na channel *a*-subunits. All of the relevant landmark sequences of voltage-

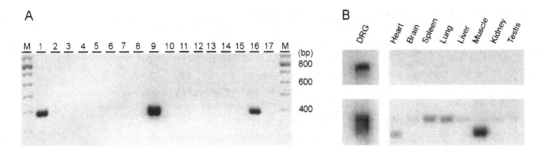

Figure 31.3
Tissue distribution of NaN in adult rat by RT-PCR (*A*) and Northern blot analysis (*B*). (*A*) "M" lanes contain the 100-bp ladder marker (Pharmacia). Amplification product from DRG (lanes 1 and 16), trigeminal ganglia (lane 9), cerebral hemispheres (lane 2), and retina (lane 4) are consistent with a predicted size of 392 bp. No detectable signal is seen in cerebellum (lane 3), optic nerve (lane 5), spinal cord (lane 6), sciatic nerve (lane 7), superior cervical ganglia (lane 8), skeletal muscle (lane 10), cardiac muscle (lane 11), adrenal gland (lane 12), uterus (lane 13), liver (lane 14), kidney (lane 15), or water (lane 17). (*B, upper*) An antisense riboprobe hybridized specifically to a single transcript (about 6.5 kb) in poly(A)$^+$ DRG RNA. No similar hybridization signal was seen in multiple-tissue Northern blot (CLONTECH) lanes containing poly(A)$^+$ RNA from heart, brain, spleen, lung, liver, muscle, kidney, and testis. (*B, lower*) β-actin (1.6 kb and 2.0 kb) hybridization signal. Heart and muscle lanes show an actin signal at 1.6 kb, consistent with hybridization to the α- or γ-actin forms in these tissues (Boehringer Mannheim).

gated Na channels, including the positively charged S4 and the putative pore-lining SS1–SS2 segments, are present at the predicted positions in each of the four domains, indicating that NaN is a member of the Na channel family. However, similarity to known rat Na channels is only 42–50% (table 31.1). Intracellular loop L3 shows the highest (51–91%) similarity. The inactivation tripeptide IFM (40) is conserved within L3 of NaN as is the consensus PKC phosphorylation site (T1301; S in all subfamily 1 channels). Intracellular loop L2 shows the lowest (13–20%) similarity compared with other channels, with only 18% similarity to SNS/PN3 (table 31.1). Multiple predicted phosphorylation sites also are present in the L1 and L2 loops of NaN. The S4 segments, the voltage sensors of Na channels (41), of NaN contain positively charged residues in the predicted pattern. The number and spacing of such charged residues in the S4 segments of domains I and IV are identical to those in subfamily 1; however, the S4 segments of NaN

domains II and III display an intermediate number compared with subfamilies 1 and 2.

NaN Is Expressed Preferentially in C Type DRG and Trigeminal Ganglia Neurons

Screening by RT-PCR (figure 31.3*A*) and Northern blot analysis (figure 31.3*B*) shows that NaN is expressed preferentially in DRG and trigeminal ganglia neurons. Lanes 1, 2, 4, 9, and 16 (figure 31.3*A*) show a single amplification product close to the 400-bp marker, in agreement with the predicted size of 392 bp. Abundant amplification products were obtained from DRG (lanes 1 and 16) and trigeminal ganglia (lane 9). Very faint bands are detectable in cerebral hemisphere and retina (lanes 2 and 4, respectively). NaN was not detected in cerebellum, optic nerve, spinal cord, sciatic nerve, superior cervical ganglia, skeletal muscle, cardiac muscle, adrenal gland, uterus, liver, or kidney (lanes 3, 5–8, and 10–15, respectively). The attenuated

Table 31.1
Amino acid similarity between NaN and rat Na channel α-subunits

Subunit	% amino acid similarity									
	Total	N	DI	L1	D2	L2	D3	L3	D4	C
αI	47	59	51	30	55	15	61	85	60	51
αII	47	59	51	26	55	18	63	85	60	54
αIII	48	58	52	24	57	16	63	85	60	53
Na6	47	54	50	20	57	14	61	87	59	52
PN1	47	55	56	29	56	17	62	85	59	53
μI	50	53	52	24	56	13	62	81	60	53
rH1	49	59	53	36	57	20	66	89	59	57
SNS	47	62	54	32	54	18	62	91	61	52
SCL-11	42	50	35	13	38	14	45	51	42	41

Percentage amino acid similarity was determined after aligning NaN and previously identified rat Na channels by using the CLUSTAL method (Megalign of LASERGENE software, DNAstar). DI–D4 represent the four domains of transmembrane segments and their linkers; L1–L3 represent the intracellular loops linking the four domains; N and C represent N and C termini, respectively. Pairwise alignment of NaN and these channels, using GAP software (GCG), produced higher identity, 39–55% (SNS/PN3, 54%; rH1, 55%), and similarity, 49–64% (SNS/PN3, 62%; rH1, 64%). By comparison, SNS/PN3 is 65% identical to rH1 (4). All subunit sequences are based on the Genbank database [accession nos. X03638 (αI), X03639 (αII), Y00766 (αIII), L3901S (Na6), U79568 (PN1), M26643 (μI), M27902 (rH1), X92184 (SNS), and Y09164 (SCL-11)].

NaN signal in cerebral hemisphere and retina, as well as the absence of this signal in the remaining tissues, is not a result of degraded RNA or of PCR inhibitors in the cDNA templates because GAPDH amplification products were obtained in parallel PCRs (data not shown). Northern blot analysis (figure 31.3B) shows a NaN hybridization signal only in DRG, and its absence from multiple other neuronal and nonneuronal samples. The absence of a signal in brain is not surprising given the weak amplification by PCR (figure 31.3A, lane 2).

In situ hybridization revealed intense ($\geq$5-fold above background levels) NaN hybridization signals in 82.9% ($n = 241$) of small (<30-μm diameter) neurons in DRG (figure 4b). In contrast, only 18.8% ($n = 64$) of larger (>30 μm) neurons displayed significant NaN mRNA hybridization signals. Trigeminal ganglion neurons also expressed high levels of NaN mRNA (figure

31.4a). No hybridization signal was detected in cerebellum (figure 31.4d), spinal cord, liver, heart, kidney, or adrenal gland (data not shown) or in DRG hybridized with NaN sense riboprobe (figure 31.4c).

NaN Transcript Levels Decrease After Axotomy of DRG Neurons

Because TTX-R Na currents are known to decrease in DRG neurons after axonal transection (21, 26), DRG neurons were axotomized via sciatic nerve transection, and NaN transcript levels were examined by quantitative RT-PCR and in situ hybridization at 7 dpa, a time when TTX-R Na currents are reduced substantially (21, 26).

Amplification products of NaN and GAPDH migrated in the gel consistent with their predicted sizes of 392 and 666 bp, respectively (figure 31.5a). A significant reduction in NaN

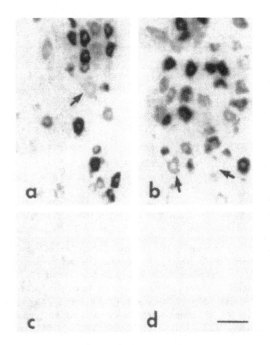

Figure 31.4
NaN mRNA expression in adult rat tissue by in situ hybridization. Strong hybridization signal for NaN mRNA is present in many small-diameter neurons within trigeminal ganglia (*a*) and DRG (*b*). Large-diameter neurons (arrow) generally lack NaN mRNA hybridization signal. DRG neurons hybridized with NaN sense riboprobe do not show signal above background (*c*). Hybridization signal for NaN mRNA is not present in cerebellum (*d*) or in liver, spinal cord, heart, kidney, and adrenal (not shown). (Bar = 50 μm.)

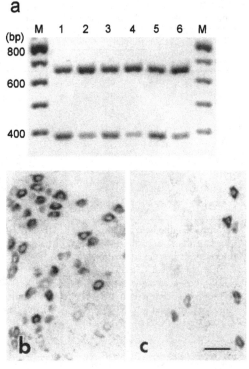

Figure 31.5
Analysis of NaN expression in control and axotomized DRG neurons by quantitative RT-PCR (*a*) and in situ hybridization (*b* and *c*). (*a*) A representative gel analysis of three independent coamplifications of NaN (392 bp) and GAPDH (666 bp) products from control (lanes 1, 3, and 5) and axotomized (lanes 2, 4, and 6) DRG. (*b*) NaN mRNA is expressed in many small neurons in control DRG. (*c*) At 7 dpa, NaN hybridization signal is attenuated, with only a few small neurons displaying hybridization signal. (Bar = 50 μm.)

amplification product is evident in the ipsilateral side after axotomy (figure 31.5*a*, lanes 2, 4, and 6). RT-PCR showed a decrease to approximately 40% of control NaN levels in axotomized DRG (mean ratios ± SD for NaN/GAPDH products, from seven independent amplifications, for uninjured and axotomized DRG neurons = 0.8200 ± 0.0857 and 0.3054 ± 0.0313, respectively; $P < 0.001$). Consistent with the RT-PCR results, the hybridization signal for NaN mRNA was attenuated (to approximately 60% of control levels)

in DRG neurons at 7 dpa (OD = 0.111 ± 0.032 ipsilateral, $n = 138$, vs. 0.183 ± 0.04 contralateral, $n = 240$; $P < 0.001$) (figure 31.5*b* and *c*). A few, small DRG neurons continued to display high levels of NaN mRNA; these are likely to represent those DRG neurons not axotomized by midthigh sciatic nerve transection.

Discussion

Our major findings are as follows. (*i*) We have identified and sequenced a previously unidentified Na channel, which we have termed NaN. (*ii*) Based on its predicted amino acid sequence, NaN is expected to produce a TTX-R current and may have altered voltage-dependent properties compared with SNS/PN3 channels. (*iii*) NaN is expressed preferentially in DRG and trigeminal ganglia neurons, particularly C type DRG neurons. (*iv*) NaN transcripts are down-regulated in DRG neurons after transection of their axons within the sciatic nerve.

Previously cloned Na channels, expressed within the nervous system, include αI, -II, -III (42–44), and Na6 (45); of these, αI, -II, and -III now have been characterized in heterologous expression systems (46–48) and are known to be TTX-S. NaG, originally thought to be glial-specific (49), also is expressed in sensory neurons of neural crest origin (38). PN1, cloned from PC-12 cells, is expressed preferentially in peripheral nervous system tissues (50). SNS/PN3, preferentially expressed in DRG and trigeminal neurons, produces a TTX-R current (4, 6).

NaN is distinct from all of the known rat Na channels, exhibiting ≤50% similarity with them (similarity highest to μI/SkM1; 50%) as determined by the CLUSTAL method. However, NaN's 1,765 aa can be aligned precisely with all known Na channels and contains all the relevant landmark sequences at the predicted positions. Surprisingly, NaN is only 47% similar to the other TTX-R channel expressed in DRG and trigeminal neurons (SNS/PN3) and 49% similar to the TTX-R cardiac muscle Na channel (rH1/SkM2). Indeed, NaN appears to be equally distant from all previously identified mammalian Na channels (data not shown). Coupled with the fact that NaN shares structural features characteristic of both subfamilies 1 and 2, this may suggest an ancestral relationship between NaN and these Na channels. Alternatively, NaN may represent a

third Na channel subfamily, with properties intermediate between the existing two subfamilies.

NaN demonstrates features in common with both subfamilies 1 and 2 (51). NaN transcripts lack the out-of-frame ATG at position −8 to −6 that is present in all previously cloned subfamily 1 cDNAs (data not shown), but is absent in transcripts of subfamily 2 members (5, 51). The inactivation IFM tripeptide (40) is present in NaN; the sequence of L3 including IFM is more like subfamily 1 than it is like subfamily 2. Notably, a serine residue is located in DI-SS2 of NaN at a position analogous to that of SNS/PN3 and to the cysteine residue in rH1 where they confer TTX-R phenotype (52, 53), which suggests that NaN encodes a TTX-R channel. The linker joining S3 and S4 of D4 of NaN is longer, as in SNS/PN3, than those of the other channels; site-directed mutagenesis suggests that this may contribute to faster recovery from inactivation (54).

NaN has distinct structural features, compared with SNS/PN3 and rH1, that suggest different properties and/or modulation. Because NaN has a reduced number [intermediate between that of subfamilies 1 and 2 (5, 51)] of positively charged residues in DII- and DIII-S4 segments, it is not unreasonable to predict that NaN may have altered voltage-dependence or kinetic properties compared with SNS/PN3 and rH1. The putative intracellular L1 and L2 loops of NaN show the least similarity to the other channels. L2 of NaN shows only 18% similarity to L2 of SNS/PN3. These loops contain predicted phosphorylation sites that have been shown to modulate Na currents (55, 56). The different sequence of these loops in NaN and SNS/PN3 suggests that NaN may be regulated/modulated differently than SNS/PN3 in vivo.

Our RT-PCR and Northern analysis results indicate that NaN is expressed preferentially in peripheral sensory ganglia, i.e., DRG and trigeminal ganglia, but is not detectable by these assays in other neural tissues, nor is it detectable in other nonneuronal tissues that possess excitable membranes. Very low levels of NaN expression were detected in the retina and cerebral hemisphere. Retinal ganglion neurons of the newt have been shown recently to produce a TTX-R current (57) that could arise from a NaN-like channel; rat retina lacks transcripts of SNS/PN3 and displays only very low levels of rH1, the two previously identified TTX-R channels, as determined by RT-PCR and in situ hybridization (35).

In situ hybridization confirms the results of RT-PCR and Northern blot analysis and indicates that NaN is expressed preferentially in small DRG neurons, which include C type nociceptive cells (58). Consistent with this result, small, C type DRG neurons preferentially express TTX-R currents (12–15, 21). The presence of transcripts of NaN, in addition to those of SNS/PN3 in these cells, suggests that they express two different TTX-R Na channels. Electrophysiological and pharmacological studies have demonstrated heterogeneity in the TTX-R currents in DRG and nodose ganglia neurons (15, 31) and, in fact, led Rush and Elliott (32) to suggest that there are at least two distinct TTX-R Na channels in these cells.

TTX-R Na currents contribute to the encoding and/or transmission of nociceptive information in DRG neurons and appear to participate in the generation of abnormal burst activity underlying paresthesias and chronic pain (18, 21, 26, 28, 30). Previous electrophysiological studies have shown that after transection of their axons within peripheral nerve, TTX-R currents are attenuated in DRG neurons (21, 26). The present observations, of a significant reduction in NaN transcripts in DRG neurons after axotomy, are consistent with the idea that NaN encodes a TTX-R Na channel in these cells.

In summary, the present results demonstrate the presence of a previously unidentified Na channel, NaN, which may represent a prototype of a third class of Na channels in C type DRG and trigeminal neurons. The preferential expression of NaN in these sensory neurons and the plasticity of NaN transcript levels after axotomy suggest that NaN produces TTX-R currents and influences the generation of electrical activity in these cells.

Acknowledgments

We thank B. R. Toftness for technical assistance. This work was supported in part by a grant from the National Multiple Sclerosis Society.

References

1. Barchi, R. L. (1995) *Annu. Rev. Physiol.* 57: 355–385.

2. Catterall, W. A. (1993) *Trends Neurosci.* 16: 500–506.

3. Goldin, A. L. (1995) in *Handbook of Receptors and Channels*, ed. North, R. A. (CRC, Boca Raton, FL), pp. 73–100.

4. Akopian, A. N., Sivilotti, L. and Wood, J. N. (1996) *Nature (London)* 379: 257–262.

5. Akopian, A. N., Souslova, V., Sivilotti, L. and Wood, J. N. (1997) *FEBS Lett.* 400: 183–187.

6. Sangameswaran, L., Delgado, S. G., Fish, L. M., Koch, B. D., Jakeman, L. B., Stewart, G. R., Sze, P., Hunter, J. C., Eglen, R. M. and Herman, R. C. (1996) *J. Biol. Chem.* 271: 5953–5956.

7. Beckh, S., Noda, M., Lubbert, H. and Numa, S. (1989) *EMBO J.* 8: 3611–3616.

8. Rizzo, M. A., Kocsis, J. D. and Waxman, S. G. (1996) *Eur. Neurol.* 36: 3–12.

9. Dumaine, R., Wang, Q., Keating, M. T., Hartmann, H. A., Schwartz, P. J., Brown, A. M. and Kirsch, G. E. (1996) *Circ. Res.* 78: 916–924.

10. Ptacek, L. J. (1997) *Neuromuscular Dis.* 7: 250–255.

11. Cannon, S. C. (1997) *Neuromuscular Dis.* 7: 241–249.

12. Roy, M. L. and Narahashi, T. (1992) *J. Neurosci.* 12: 2104–2111.

13. Elliott, A. A. and Elliott, J. R. (1993) *J. Physiol.* 463: 39–56.

14. Caffrey, J. M., Eng, D. L., Black, J. A., Waxman, S. G. and Kocsis, J. D. (1992) *Brain Res.* 592: 283–297.

15. Rizzo, M. A., Kocsis, J. D. and Waxman, S. G. (1994) *J. Neurophysiol.* 72: 2796–2815.

16. Black, J. A., Dib-Hajj, S., McNabola, K., Jeste, S., Rizzo, M. A., Kocsis, J. D. and Waxman, S. G. (1996) *Mol. Brain Res.* 43: 117–131.

17. Honmou, O., Utzschneider, D. A., Rizzo, M. A., Bowe, C. M., Waxman, S. G. and Kocsis, J. D. (1994) *J. Neurophysiol.* 71: 1627–1637.

18. Jeftinija, S. (1994) *Brain Res.* 639: 125–134.

19. Schild, J. H., Clark, J. W., Hay, M., Mendelowitz, D., Andresen, M. C. and Kunze, D. L. (1994) *J. Neurophysiol.* 71: 2338–2358.

20. Dib-Hajj, S., Black, J. A., Felts, P. and Waxman, S. G. (1996) *Proc. Natl. Acad. Sci. USA* 93: 14950–14954.

21. Cummins, T. R. and Waxman, S. G. (1997) *J. Neurosci.* 17: 3503–3514.

22. Gallego, R., Ivorra, I. and Morales, A. (1987) *J. Physiol. (London)* 391: 39–56.

23. Kuno, M. and Linas, R. (1970) *J. Physiol. (London)* 210: 807–821.

24. Titmus, M. J. and Faber, D. S. (1986) *J. Neurophysiol.* 55: 1440–1454.

25. Sernagor, E., Yarom, Y. and Werman, R. (1986) *Proc. Natl. Acad. Sci. USA* 83: 7966–7970.

26. Rizzo, M. A., Kocsis, J. D. and Waxman, S. G. (1995) *Neurobiol. Dis.* 2: 87–96.

27. Waxman, S. G., Kocsis, J. D. and Black, J. A. (1994) *J. Neurophysiol.* 72: 466–470.

28. Gold, M. S., Reichling, D. B., Shuster, M. J. and Levine, J. D. (1996) *Proc. Natl. Acad. Sci. USA* 93: 1108–1112.

29. England, S., Bevan, S. and Docherty, R. J. (1996) *J. Physiol. (London)* 495: 429–440.

30. Tanaka, M., Cummins, T. R., Ishikawa, K., Dib-Hajj, S. D., Black, J. A. and Waxman, S. G. (1998) *NeuroReport* 9: 967–972.

31. Schild, J. H. and Kunze, D. L. (1997) *J. Neurophysiol.* 78: 3198–3209.

32. Rush, A. M. and Elliott, J. R. (1997) *Neurosci. Lett.* 226: 95–98.

33. Ausubel, F. M., Brent, R., Kingston, R. E., Moore, D. D., Seidman, J. G., Smith, J. A. and Struhl,

K. (1994) in *Current Protocols*, ed. Janssen, K. (Wiley, New York).

34. Dib-Hajj, S. D., Hinson, A. W., Black, J. A. and Waxman, S. G. (1996) *FEBS Lett.* 384: 78–82.

35. Fjell, J., Dib-Hajj, S., Fried, K., Black, J. A. and Waxman, S. G. (1997) *Mol. Brain Res.* 50: 197–204.

36. Dib-Hajj, S. D., Black, J. A., Cummins. T. R., Kenney, A. M., Kocsis, J. D. and Waxman, S. G. (1998) *J. Neurophysiol.* 79: 2668–2676.

37. Kinoshita, T., Imamura, J., Nagai, H. and Shimotohno, K. (1992) *Anal. Biochem.* 206: 231–235.

38. Felts, P. A., Black, J. A., Dib-Hajj, S. D. and Waxman, S. G. (1997) *Glia* 21: 269–276.

39. Kozak, M. (1991) *J. Biol. Chem.* 266: 19867–19870.

40. West, J. W., Patton, D. E., Scheuer, T., Wang, Y., Goldin, A. L. and Catterall, W. A. (1992) *Proc. Natl. Acad. Sci. USA* 89: 10910–10914.

41. Yang, N., George, A. L., Jr. and Horn, R. (1996) *Neuron* 16: 113–122.

42. Noda, M., Ikeda, T., Kayano, T., Suzuki, H., Takeshima, H., Kurasaki, M., Takahashi, H. and Numa, S. (1986) *Nature (London)* 320: 188–192.

43. Auld, V. J., Goldin, A. L., Krafte, D. S., Marshall, J., Dunn, J. M., Catterall, W. A., Lester, H. A., Davidson, N. and Dunn, R. J. (1988) *Neuron* 1: 449–461.

44. Kayano, T., Noda, M., Flockerzi, V., Takahashi, H. and Numa, S. (1988) *FEBS Lett.* 228: 187–194.

45. Schaller, K. L., Krzemien, D. M., Yarowsky, P. J., Krueger, B. K. and Caldwell, J. H. (1995) *J. Neurosci.* 15: 3231–3242.

46. Noda, M., Ikeda, T., Suzuki, H., Takeshima, H., Takahashi, T., Kuno, M. and Numa, S. (1986) *Nature (London)* 322: 826–828.

47. Suzuki, H., Beckh, S., Kubo, H., Yahagi, N., Ishida, H., Kayano, T., Noda, M. and Numa, S. (1988) *FEBS Lett.* 228: 195–200.

48. Smith, R. D. and Goldin, A. L. (1998) *J. Neurosci.* 18: 811–820.

49. Gautron, S., Dos Santos, G., Pinto-Henrique, D., Koulakoff, A., Gros, F. and Berwald-Netter, Y. (1992) *Proc. Natl. Acad. Sci. USA* 89: 7272–7276.

50. Toledo-Aral, J. J., Moss, B. L., He, Z. J., Koszowski, A. G., Whisenand, T., Levinson, S. R., Wolf,

J. J., Silossantiago, I., Halegoua, S. and Mandel, G. (1997) *Proc. Natl. Acad. Sci. USA* 94: 1527–1532.

51. Felipe, A., Knittle, T. J., Doyle, K. L. and Tamkun, M. M. (1994) *J. Biol. Chem.* 269: 30125–30131.

52. Satin, J., Kyle, J. W., Chen, M., Bell, P., Cribbs, L. L., Fozzard, H. A. and Rogart, R. B. (1992) *Science* 256: 1202–1205.

53. Sivilotti, L., Okuse, K., Akopian, A. N., Moss, S. and Wood, J. N. (1997) *FEBS Lett.* 409: 49–52.

54. Dib-Hajj, S. D., Ishikawa, K., Cummins, T. R. and Waxman, S. G. (1997) *FEBS Lett.* 416: 11–14.

55. Li, M., West, J. W., Numann, R., Murphy, B. J., Scheuer, T. and Catterall, W. A. (1993) *Science* 261: 1439–1442.

56. Smith, R. D. and Goldin, A. L. (1997) *J. Neurosci.* 17: 6086–6093.

57. Kaneko, Y., Matsumoto, G. and Hanyu, Y. (1997) *Biochem. Biophys. Res. Commun.* 240: 651–656.

58. Harper, A. A. and Lawson, S. N. (1985) *J. Physiol. (London)* 359: 31–46.

32

A Novel Persistent Tetrodotoxin-Resistant Sodium Current in SNS-null and Wild-Type Small Primary Sensory Neurons

Theodore R. Cummins, Sulayman D. Dib-Hajj, Joel A. Black, Armen N. Akopian, John N. Wood, and Stephen G. Waxman

Abstract TTX-resistant (TTX-R) sodium currents are preferentially expressed in small C-type DRG neurons, which include nociceptive neurons. Two mRNAs that are predicted to encode TTX-R sodium channels, SNS and NaN, are preferentially expressed in C-type DRG cells. To determine whether there are multiple TTX-R currents in these cells, we used patch-clamp recordings to study sodium currents in SNS-null mice and found a novel persistent voltage-dependent sodium current in small DRG neurons of both SNS-null and wild-type mice. Like SNS currents, this current is highly resistant to TTX ($K_i = 39 \pm 9$ μM). In contrast to SNS currents, the threshold for activation of this current is near -70 mV, the midpoint of steady-state inactivation is -44 ± 1 mV and the time constant for inactivation is 43 ± 4 ms at -20 mV. The presence of this current in SNS-null and wild-type mice demonstrates that a distinct sodium channel isoform, which we suggest to be NaN, underlies this persistent TTX-R current. Importantly, the hyperpolarized voltage-dependence of this current, the substantial overlap of its activation and steady-state inactivation curves and its persistent nature suggest that this current is active near resting potential, where it may play an important role in regulating excitability of primary sensory neurons.

Introduction

Small dorsal root ganglion (DRG) neurons (which include nociceptive cells) are unusual in expressing tetrodotoxin-resistant (TTX-R) sodium currents, in addition to the TTX-sensitive (TTX-S) sodium currents that are present in many neurons (Kostyuk et al., 1981). Because of their preferential expression in nociceptive neurons, the channels responsible for these TTX-R currents are of special interest. One TTX-R channel that has been cloned from DRG neurons, SNS (Akopian et al., 1996; Sangameswaran et

Reprinted with permission from *Journal of Neuroscience* 19: RC43(1–6), 1999.

al., 1996), produces a slowly inactivating sodium current ($\tau_{inactivation} \sim 5$ ms for the peak current) with relatively depolarized voltage-dependence of activation and inactivation. A second sodium channel, NaN, with a sequence predicting a TTX-resistance similar to that of SNS is also preferentially expressed in small DRG neurons (Dib-Hajj et al., 1998, 1999; Tate et al., 1998).

A recent study on DRG neurons from SNS-null mutant mice demonstrated only TTX-S sodium currents (Akopian et al., 1999). These findings were unexpected in light of the presence of NaN transcript within these cells. The present study revisits this issue and shows that DRG neurons from SNS-null mice (Akopian et al., 1999) express a TTX-R sodium current with novel properties. We also demonstrate that this TTX-R current is present in small wild-type (WT) mouse DRG neurons. The relatively hyperpolarized voltage-dependence of activation and inactivation of this current, and its persistent nature, suggest that it contributes to setting the firing properties of small DRG neurons by modulating their resting potentials and/or thresholds.

Materials and Methods

Whole-Cell Patch-Clamp Recordings

DRG cultures from L4 and L5 ganglia of WT and SNS-null mice (Akopian et al., 1999) were established as previously described (Cummins and Waxman, 1997). Sodium currents were studied in small (18–27 μm diameter) DRG neurons after short-term culture (6–24 hrs); at this time in culture, neurites are not generally present. Whole-cell patch-clamp recordings were conducted at room temperature (~21 °C) using an EPC-9 amplifier and the Pulse program (v 7.89). Fire-polished electrodes (0.8–1.5 MΩ) were fabricated from 1.7-mm capillary glass using a Sutter P-97 puller. The average cell capacitance was 21 ± 1 pF (mean $\pm$ SE, n = 55) for WT and 23 ± 1 pF (n = 91) for SNS-null cells. The average access resistance was 2.1 ± 0.1 MΩ for WT and 2.0 ± 0.1 MΩ for SNS-null cells. Voltage errors were minimized using 80% series resistance compensation. The maximum theoretical voltage error was 2 ± 1 mV for TTX-R sodium currents in SNS-null neurons; this and the spherical nature of the cells provided nearly ideal recording conditions. Linear leak subtraction was used for all recordings. The pipette solution contained (in mM): 140 CsF, 1 EGTA, 10 NaCl and 10 HEPES, pH 7.3. The standard bathing solution was (in mM) 140 NaCl, 3 KCl, 1 MgCl$_2$, 1 CaCl$_2$, 0.1 CdCl$_2$ and 10 HEPES, pH 7.3. Cadmium was included to block calcium currents. The osmolarity of all solutions was adjusted to 310 mosM.

RT-PCR

Total cellular RNA was extracted from trigeminal ganglia of each animal whose DRG neurons were studied to confirm the SNS-null genotype and the presence of the expected NaN products (figure 32.3). First strand cDNA synthesis and PCR were performed as previously described (Dib-Hajj et al., 1998).

Results

Whole-cell patch-clamp recordings demonstrate the presence of fast and slow inactivating voltage-dependent inward currents from the cultured DRG neurons of WT and SNS-null mice with a holding potential of −120 mV (figure 32.1). In the presence of 250 nM TTX in the bathing solution, TTX-R inward currents were recorded from 77% of small WT neurons (24/31) and 74% of SNS-null neurons (37/50). However, the inward currents were strikingly different in the two

groups of cells. The majority of WT neurons (18/31) showed slowly inactivating TTX-R currents (which activated between −40 and −30 mV and resemble currents in heterologously expressed SNS channels; see Akopian et al., 1996) together with persistent TTX-R currents (which did not inactivate during the 100 ms depolarization at negative test potentials). Consistent with the conclusion that SNS encodes a slowly inactivating channel (Akopian et al., 1996; Sangameswaran et al., 1996), SNS-null neurons did not express the slowly inactivating TTX-R currents. However, a persistent TTX-R current was clearly present in these cells (figure 32.1d) and the amplitude was as large as 11 nA. This persistent current activated between −60 and −70 mV and peaked at about −20 mV (peak amplitude = 5.0 ± 0.6 nA; peak density = 235 ± 77 pA/pF; n = 22).

Because the persistent TTX-R current was recorded with cadmium in the bath and fluoride in the pipette solution, we suspected that it was a sodium current. Whole-cell recordings of SNS-null cells in the presence of low external calcium (10–50 μM) but high external sodium (140 mM) demonstrated large persistent inward currents in 15/25 cells. Increasing external calcium from 50 μM to 1 mM did not increase the size of the current (figure 32.2a; n = 4). Additionally, when the external medium contained high calcium (1 mM) but zero sodium we did not observe any inward currents activating at negative potentials (n = 15). We could often observe small inward currents that activated near −20 mV if cadmium was not included in the external solution, but these high voltage activated currents could be blocked with 50–100 μM cadmium and appear to be L-type calcium currents. However, in 4 out of 6 SNS-null cells tested, the low-voltage activated (LVA) persistent inward was revealed in the presence of cadmium when external sodium was increased from zero to 50 mM (figure 32.2b). Based on these experiments, we conclude that the LVA persistent current that we observe in SNS-null neurons is indeed a sodium current.

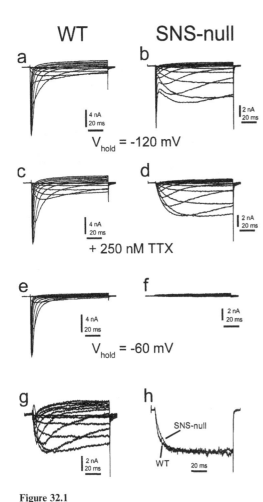

WT

SNS-null

a

b

V_{hold} = -120 mV

c

d

+ 250 nM TTX

e

f

V_{hold} = -60 mV

g

h

SNS-null

WT

Figure 32.1

Multiple sodium currents are expressed in small DRG neurons from WT and SNS-null mice. (*a, b*) Representative recordings from a holding potential of –120 mV. Calcium currents were blocked with 100 μM cadmium in the bath solution. (*c, d*) TTX (250 nM) blocks the fast-inactivating component. A persistent current is expressed in both the WT (*c*) and SNS-null (*d*) neurons, but the slowly inactivating component is seen only in the WT neuron. (*e, f*) When the neurons were held at –60 mV and a 100 ms step to –120 mV preceded the test pulses, the persistent current is not obvious in either WT (*e*) or SNS-null (*f*) neurons. (*g*) Subtraction of the slowly inactivating component (*e*)

The LVA persistent sodium current is only marginally inhibited by 1 μM TTX (6 ± 5%; n = 6) and as shown in figure 32.2c, 10 μM TTX inhibited this LVA sodium current in SNS-null neurons by ~20% (estimated K_i = 39 ± 9 μM, n = 5). Thus, the LVA current in DRG neurons is highly resistant to TTX, like SNS (K_i ~ 60 μM) (Akopian et al. 1996) and unlike the cardiac TTX-R isoform (K_i ~ 1 to 2 μM; Satin et al., 1992).

Although the TTX resistance of the current in SNS-null DRG neurons is similar to that reported for SNS, its voltage-dependence and kinetic properties are quite distinct. As seen in figure 32.1d, the TTX-R currents in SNS-null neurons had extremely slow kinetics, with $\tau_{inactivation}$ = 43 ± 4 ms at –20 mV (n = 18). These currents activated at hyperpolarized potentials, with a threshold around –70 mV and a midpoint of activation of –47 ± 1 mV (n = 17). The overshoot in the activation curve (figure 32.2d) could be due to the presence of multiple TTX-R channels in SNS-null neurons. Alternatively, it could be due to a TTX-R channel with complex behavior, such as one that has multiple open states or an inactivated state from which recovery is ultra-slow (ultra-slow recovery from inactivation is supported by data presented below). The voltage-dependence of steady-state inactivation was also fairly negative, with a midpoint of –44 ± 1 mV (n = 10). The considerable overlap between the activation and steady-state inactivation curves (figure 32.2d) should generate persistent window currents that are active near resting potential. Indeed, large persistent currents were observed in the region of overlap when the holding potential (V_{hold}) was

from the total TTX-R current (*c*) reveals the persistent current in WT neurons. (*h*) The persistent current derived by this subtraction process from WT neurons is similar to that recorded in SNS-null neurons. Test potential is –60 mV and traces are normalized for comparison.

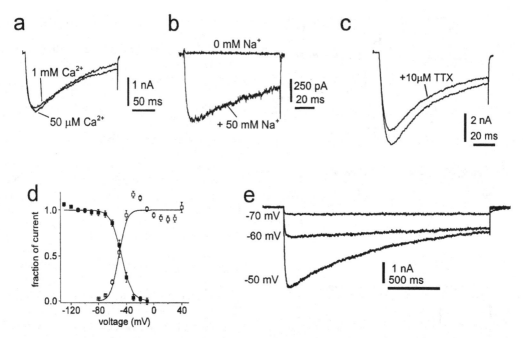

Figure 32.2
SNS-null neurons express a TTX-R sodium current. (*a*) The current recorded from a SNS-null neuron in low calcium (50 µM) was not altered by increasing calcium to 1 mM. $V_{test} = -30$ mV. (*b*) In zero sodium (160 mM TEA)
inward current is not elicited by a step depolarization to -30 mV. Addition of 50 mM sodium reveals the TTX-R
current. (*c*) The TTX-R current in SNS-null neurons is resistant to high concentrations of TTX (10 µM).
$V_{test} = -40$ mV. (*d*) Activation and steady-state inactivation curves exhibit significant overlap for the TTX-R current in SNS-null neurons. The inter-pulse interval was 5 s. Steady-state inactivation was measured with 500 ms
prepulses. $V_{test} = -10$ mV. (*e*) TTX-R persistent currents from a SNS-null neuron elicited with 2 s step depolarizations to the voltage indicated. All recordings were made with 250 nM TTX, 100 µM cadmium and $V_{hold} =$
-120 mV.

-120 mV (figure 32.2e). The amplitude of the
TTX-R persistent current measured at -60 mV
($V_{hold} = -120$ mV) was 1.6 ± 0.5 nA for WT
neurons (n = 17) and 1.7 ± 0.4 nA for SNS-null
neurons (n = 22).

Based on the midpoint of steady-state inactivation, it might be expected that large persistent
TTX-R currents would also be readily observed
from a V_{hold} of -60 mV; however, when the
neurons were held at -60 mV and currents
were elicited following a brief hyperpolarizing

prepulse (100 ms at -120 mV), the persistent
TTX-R current was not apparent in either WT
(figure 31.1e) or SNS-null (figure 31.1f) neurons.
Under these conditions, only the slowly inactivating TTX-R currents were observed in WT
neurons and, as previously reported by Akopian
et al. (1999) who studied cells with relatively
depolarized holding potentials, there was no
obvious TTX-R current in SNS-null neurons.
Consistent with this, we found a prominent
ultra-slow inactivation of the LVA channels

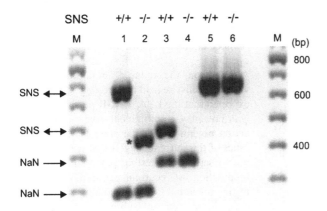

Figure 32.3
RT-PCR products from DRG of WT ($+/+$) and SNS-null ($-/-$) mutant mice. SNS and NaN products were co-amplified from WT (lanes 1 and 3), and SNS-null mutants (lanes 2 and 4). Two primer pairs, Pr1 and Pr2, for SNS were previously described (Pr1, lanes 1 and 2: Akopian et al., 1999; Pr2, lanes 3 and 4: F1/R2, Dib-Hajj et al., 1998). The sizes of SNS products from WT tissue using Pr1 and Pr2 are consistent with the predicted lengths of 673 bp (nt. 100–772) and 482 bp (nt. 594–1075), respectively. The smaller SNS product (denoted by an asterisk in lane 2; 450 bp) from SNS-null tissue is consistent with splicing exon 3 to exon 6 (Akopian et al., 1999), while lack of SNS signal in lane 4 is due to the replacement of F1-containing sequence by the PGK-neo cassette in the null allele. Primers for mouse NaN amplify nucleotides 708–995 (288 bp; lanes 1 and 2) and 626–995 (370 bp; lanes 3 and 4) (Dib-Hajj et al., 1999). Comparable levels of GAPDH were amplified from WT (lane 5) and SNS-null mutants (lane 6) using primers that were previously described (Dib-Hajj et al., 1998).

($\tau_{recovery} = 16 \pm 4$ s at -120 mV in SNS-null neurons; n = 5). For SNS-null neurons that expressed large TTX-R currents (peak amplitude $= 8.0 \pm 1.2$ nA with V_{hold} of -120 mV), the peak amplitude elicited following a 100 ms pre-pulse to -120 mV from a V_{hold} of -60 mV was only 260 ± 57 pA (n = 8), indicating that ~97% of the LVA TTX-R channels are ultra-slow inactivated at -60 mV. We observed a similar ultra-slow inactivation for the LVA TTX-R current in WT neurons.

Because of the ultra-slow inactivation of the LVA TTX-R currents, subtraction of the slowly inactivating current recorded with $V_{hold} = -60$ mV from total TTX-R current would be expected to yield the persistent current in WT neurons. In fact, a LVA TTX-R current could be derived in this way in WT neurons (figure 32.1g)

and closely matched the persistent current recorded in SNS-null DRG neurons (figure 32.1h). Thus we can isolate LVA TTX-R currents with similar properties in both WT and SNS-null DRG neurons.

The molecular identity of the novel persistent TTX-R current cannot be positively determined at this time. However, transcripts for NaN, which is predicted to encode a TTX-R channel, are present in WT and SNS-null trigeminal ganglia (figure 32.3; lanes 1–4) and DRG neurons (data not shown). Residual SNS transcript in SNS-null ganglia lacks the sequence encoded by exons 4 and 5 (figure 32.3, lanes 1–4), which truncates the protein due to a reading frame shift in exon 6 (Akopian et al., 1999). Therefore, we suggest that NaN underlies this novel TTX-R persistent current.

Discussion

In this study we have identified and characterized a novel persistent TTX-R sodium current in SNS-null and WT small diameter DRG neurons. Although previous studies have suggested the presence of multiple TTX-R currents in DRG neurons, these currents have been either slowly inactivating, with time constants of 3–8 ms (Rizzo et al. 1994; Rush et al., 1998), or rapidly inactivating (time constants < 2 ms; Scholz et al. 1998). TTX-R persistent currents have not been previously identified. The persistent currents that have been reported in large sensory neurons (Baker and Bostock, 1997) and other neuronal cell types, e.g. cortical (Crill, 1996) and thalamocortical neurons (Parri and Crunelli, 1998), are TTX-S. The persistent TTX-R current in small sensory neurons thus appears to be a distinct sodium current, not present in other types of neurons.

The kinetic properties of the LVA TTX-R persistent current that we describe here are different from those of SNS currents. In contrast to SNS currents, which activate around -30 mV, the TTX-R persistent current activated around resting potential (~ -70 to -60 mV). This may have important functional implications because there are few channels of any kind that are active near resting potential, so that even small persistent currents can have a significant influence on excitability (Crill, 1996). While the LVA persistent current in SNS-null neurons was quite large when elicited from hyperpolarized holding potentials, suggesting a relatively high density of channels, it was greatly reduced near normal resting potential (~ -60 mV for small DRG neurons) by an apparent ultra-slow inactivation. Ultra-slow inactivation decreased the amplitude of the LVA TTX-R persistent current by more than 95% with $V_{hold} = -60$ mV, and should result in a low probability of opening of any single channel around resting potential. One possible advantage is that a large number of channels

with a low open probability might produce a small yet more consistent current than a smaller number of channels with a higher probability of opening.

Based on the reduced amplitude observed when the cells are held near resting potential, it is expected that the LVA TTX-R persistent current will not play a prominent role in generating action potentials. On the other hand, the properties of this current suggest that it may contribute to setting the resting potential, and to the modulation of neuronal excitability close to resting potential. Persistent sodium currents have been implicated in subthreshold oscillations (Kapoor et al., 1997), in amplification of depolarizing inputs (Schwindt and Crill, 1995), and in impulse initiation (Stafstrom et al., 1982). The LVA TTX-R persistent current that we describe here might similarly be expected to have important consequences on subthreshold electrogenesis in small DRG neurons.

A previous study on SNS-null neurons (Akopian et al., 1999) did not observe the persistent TTX-R currents that we describe here. Two methodological differences may account for the failure of Akopian et al. to detect this current: (1) Akopian et al. used depolarized holding potentials, at which the LVA TTX-R persistent current is slow-inactivated and thus not detectable. (2) Akopian et al. studied SNS-null neurons after 1–5 days in culture. While we observed large TTX-R currents in SNS-null neurons studied after < 24 hrs in culture, these currents were greatly reduced in amplitude at longer times in culture (data not shown).

DRG neurons are known to express at least six sodium channel transcripts (Black et al., 1996; Dib-Hajj et al., 1998). Only two of these, SNS and NaN, are predicted to encode TTX-R currents. DRG neurons do not express mRNA for the TTX-R cardiac channel (Donahue, 1995; Black et al., 1998; Akopian et al., 1999) and SNS-null neurons do not express functional SNS channels. Since NaN transcript is present in SNS-null DRG (figure 32.3), and is expressed preferentially in small sensory neurons (Dib-Hajj et al., 1998), we suggest that the LVA TTX-R persistent current that we describe here is produced by channels encoded by NaN. Although the molecular identity of the channel that produces the LVA TTX-R persistent current cannot be definitively established at this time, the hypothesis that NaN underlies the LVA TTX-R current in small DRG neurons is supported by data showing that the loss of persistent currents in rat small DRG neurons following axotomy (Cummins and Waxman, 1997) is accompanied by a decrease in NaN mRNA levels (Dib-Hajj et al., 1998; Tate et al., 1998).

Patch-clamp studies on HEK293T cells transfected with recombinant NaN (also referred to as SNS2) channels demonstrated a TTX-R sodium current with considerably faster kinetics ($\tau_{inactivation} = 1.3$ ms at ~ -20 mV) and a greater TTX sensitivity ($K_i \sim 1$ μM) than SNS (Tate et al., 1998). This is surprising because sodium currents with a TTX K_i of 1 to 2 μM have never been described in DRG neurons. Both SNS and NaN have a serine in the position (S356 in SNS; S355 in NaN) that has been shown (Chen et al., 1992; Satin et al., 1992) to be crucial for TTX resistance, and thus these two channels would be expected to have similar K_i's for TTX. Sivilotti et al. (1997) have demonstrated that mutation of SNS S356 to phenylalanine changes the TTX K_i to 8 nM, suggesting that this serine residue alone confers the high TTX-resistance of SNS channels. Therefore, the high TTX-resistance of the LVA persistent current in SNS-null neurons is consistent with a channel isoform that has a serine at the TTX binding site.

The difference between the currents recorded in SNS-null DRG neurons (this paper) and the HEK293T current ascribed to NaN by Tate et al. (1998) raises several possibilities: (1) NaN could be differentially processed or modulated in DRG and HEK293T cells. Skeletal muscle sodium (SkM1) channels expressed in *Xenopus* oocytes can have different kinetic properties from native SkM1 channels (Trimmer et al., 1989), and thus differences between HEK293T cells and DRG neurons might account for kinetic differences. However, SkM1, cardiac and neuronal sodium channels (including SNS) have essentially the same TTX resistance in heterologous expression systems and native cells (Trimmer et al. 1989; Chen et al. 1992; Akopian et al. 1996). Therefore it seems unlikely that NaN will have a different TTX resistance in DRG neurons and HEK293 cells. (2) NaN might not underlie the LVA persistent TTX-R current that is recorded in SNS-null and WT DRG neurons. If this was the case, it would be expected that TTX-R currents such as those described by Tate et al. (1998) should also be observed in the majority of small DRG neurons of SNS-null mice, because NaN transcript and protein are observed in the majority of small DRG neurons (Dib-Hajj et al., 1998; Tate et al., 1998). However, currents like those described by Tate et al. (1998) are not observed in SNS-null neurons. (3) The small current recorded in NaN transfected HEK293T cells (Tate et al., 1998) might not be encoded by NaN but could be an endogenous TTX-R current that was observed in NaN transfected HEK293T cells. This possibility is supported by recordings showing small endogenous sodium currents in non-transfected HEK293 cells with the same properties as those ascribed to NaN channels by Tate et al. (figure 32.4). We observed small TTX-R currents in 4 out of 5 non-transfected HEK293 cells when $V_{hold} = -120$ mV (peak amplitude $= 505 \pm 111$ pA, $n = 4$). The properties of these endogenous HEK293 TTX-R currents are strikingly similar to those of cloned cardiac sodium channels (Chahine et al., 1996). Because currents with the properties described by Tate et al. (1998) for NaN are not present in SNS-null neurons but are present in non-transfected HEK293 cells, it is likely that the currents reported by Tate et al. are endogenous HEK293 currents.

Our observations show that: (1) a distinct TTX-R sodium current is expressed at high densities in small DRG neurons from SNS-

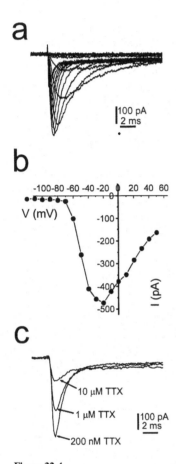

null mice; (2) this current has a hyperpolarized voltage-dependence compared to SNS; (3) this current is persistent at negative potentials close to resting potential; and (4) this current is present in the majority of small WT DRG neurons. These results provide strong evidence for the presence of a distinct TTX-R sodium channel in addition to SNS, which produces this persistent current in small DRG neurons. Irrespective of the identity of the channel that produces it, it is likely that the low threshold, persistent TTX-R sodium current that we have identified in SNS-null and WT neurons contributes to subthreshold electrogenesis in C-type primary sensory neurons, and affects the excitability of these neurons.

Acknowledgements

This work was supported in part by grants from the National Multiple Sclerosis Society; the Medical Research Service and Rehabilitation Research Service, Department of Veterans Affairs (SGW); and the Wellcome Trust and MRC (to JNW and ANA).

References

Akopian AN, Sivilotti L, Wood JN (1996) A tetrodotoxin-resistant voltage-gated sodium channel expressed by sensory neurons. Nature 379: 257–262.

Akopian AN, Souslova V, England S, Okuse K, Ogata N, Ure J, Smith A, Kerr BJ, McMahon SB, Boyce S, Hill R, Stanfa LC, Dickenson AH, Wood JN (1999) The tetrodotoxin-resistant sodium channel SNS has a specialized function in pain pathways. Nature Neurosci 2: 541–548.

Baker MD, Bostock H (1997) Low-threshold, persistent sodium current in rat large dorsal root ganglion neurons in culture. Neurophysiology 77: 1503–1513.

Black JA, Dib-Hajj S, Cohen S, Hinson AW, Waxman SG (1998) Glial cells have heart: rH1 Na+ channel mRNA and protein in spinal cord astrocytes. Glia 23: 200–208.

Figure 32.4
Non-transfected HEK293 cells exhibit an endogenous TTX-R current. (A) Representative TTX-R currents recorded from a non-transfected HEK293 cell (cell capacitance 24 pF; access resistance 1.1 MΩ). A single-exponential decay function fitted to the inactivation phase of the peak current estimated that $\tau_{inactivation} = 1.2$ ms. The bath solution contained 200 nM TTX. (B) Peak current-voltage relationship for the currents shown in (A). The midpoint of activation was -42.4 ± 3.2 mV and the midpoint of steady-state inactivation was -88.4 ± 1.9 mV for the endogenous TTX-R current in HEK293 cells (n = 4). Recordings were made 3–6 minutes after establishing the whole-cell configuration. (C) The endogenous TTX-R current in HEK293 cells is inhibited by TTX with a K_i of 1–2 µM.

Black JA, Dib-Hajj S, McNabola K, Jeste S, Rizzo MA, Kocsis JD, Waxman SG (1996) Spinal sensory neurons express multiple sodium channel a-subunit mRNAs. Molec. Brain Res 43: 117–132.

Chahine M, Deschene I, Chen LQ, Kallen RG. (1996) Electrophysiological characteristics of cloned skeletal and cardiac muscle sodium channels. Am J Physiol 271: H498–506.

Chen LQ, Chahine M, Kallen RG, Barchi RL, Horn R (1992) Chimeric study of sodium channels from rat skeletal and cardiac muscle. FEBS Lett 309: 253–257.

Crill, WE (1996) Persistent sodium currents in mammalian central neurons. Annu Rev Physiol 58: 349–362.

Cummins TR, Waxman SG (1997) Down-regulation of TTX-resistant sodium currents and upregulation of a rapidly repriming TTX-sensitive sodium current in small spinal sensory neurons after nerve injury. J Neurosci 17: 3503–3514.

Dib-Hajj SD, Tyrrell L, Black JA, Waxman SG (1998) NaN, a novel voltage-gated Na channel, is expressed preferentially in peripheral sensory neurons and downregulated after axotomy. Proc Natl Acad Sci 95: 8963–8968.

Dib-Hajj SD, Tyrrell L, Escayg A, Wood, PM, Meisler MH, Waxman SG. (1999) Coding sequence, genomic organization and conserved chromosomal localization of the mouse gene Scn11a encoding the sodium channel NaN. Genomics 59: 309–318.

Donahue LM (1995) The tetrodotoxin-insensitive sodium current in rat dorsal root ganglia is unlikely to involve the expression of the tetrodotoxin-resistant sodium channel, SkM2. Neurochem Res 20: 713–717.

Kapoor R, Li YG, Smith KJ (1997) Slow sodium-dependent potential oscillations contribute to ectopic firing in mammalian demyelinated axons. Brain 120: 647–652.

Kostyuk PG, Veselovsky NS, Tsyndrenko AY (1981) Ionic currents in the somatic membrane of rat dorsal root ganglion neurons – I. Sodium currents. Neuroscience 6: 2423–2430.

Parri HR, Crunelli V (1998) Sodium current in rat and cat thalamocortical neurons: role of a non-inactivating component in tonic and burst firing. J Neurosci 18: 854–867.

Rizzo MA, Kocsis JD, Waxman SG (1994) Slow sodium conductances of dorsal root ganglion neurons: intraneuronal homogeneity and interneuronal heterogeneity. J Neurophysiol 72: 2796–2815.

Rush AM, Brau ME, Elliott AA, Elliott JR (1998) Electrophysiological properties of sodium current subtypes in small cells from adult rat dorsal root ganglia. J Physiol (Lond) 511: 771–789.

Sangameswaran L, Delgado SG, Fish LM, Koch BD, Jakeman LB, Stewart GR, Sze P, Hunter JC, Eglen RM, Herman RC (1996) Structure and function of a novel voltage-gated tetrodotoxin-resistant sodium channel specific to sensory neurons. J Biol Chem 271: 5953–5956.

Satin J, Kyle JW, Chen M, Bell P, Cribbs LL, Fozzard HA, Rogart RB (1992) A mutant of TTX-resistant cardiac sodium channels with TTX-sensitive properties. Science 256: 1202–1205.

Scholz A, Appel N, Vogel W (1998) Two types of TTX-resistant and one TTX-sensitive Na+ channel in rat dorsal root ganglion neurons and their blockade by halothane. Eur J Neurosci 10: 2547–56.

Schwindt PC, Crill WE (1995) Amplification of synaptic current by persistent sodium conductance in apical dendrite of neocortical neurons. J Neurophysiol 74: 2220–2224.

Sivilotti L, Okuse K, Akopian AN, Moss S, Wood JN (1997) A single serine residue confers tetrodotoxin insensitivity on the rat sensory-neuron-specific sodium channel SNS. FEBS Lett 409: 49–52.

Stafstrom CE, Schwindt PC, Crill WE (1982) Negative slope conductance due to a persistent subthreshold sodium current in cat neocortical neurons in vitro. Brain Res 236: 221–226.

Tate S, Benn S, Hick C, Trezise D, John V, Mannion RJ, Costigan M, Plumpton C, Grose D, Gladwell Z, Kendall G, Dale K, Bountra C, Woolf CJ (1998) Two sodium channels contribute to the TTX-R sodium current in primary sensory neurons. Nat Neurosci 1: 653–555.

Trimmer JS, Cooperman SS, Tomiko SA, Zhou JY, Crean SM, Boyle MB, Kallen RG, Sheng ZH, Barchi RL, Sigworth FJ, Goodman RH, Agnew WS, Mandel G. (1989) Primary structure and functional expression of a mammalian skeletal muscle sodium channel. Neuron 3: 33–49.

XVIII REBUILDING THE BRAIN AND SPINAL CORD

Can the nervous system be rebuilt after it is injured? Doctors routinely rebuild other parts of the body by transplanting corneas, kidneys, even hearts. But what about brain or spinal cord transplants? Are they just a fantasy from futuristic novels? Put another way, is there any reality to the idea that neural tissue can be transplanted to replace injured cells in the brain or spinal cord after injury?

Studies on demyelinating diseases suggest that the answer may be yes. During normal development, Schwann cells and oligodendrocytes produce myelin to insulate axons within peripheral nerves and within the brain and spinal cord, respectively. In diseases characterized by demyelination, there is loss of the myelin insulation that surrounds nerve fibers, and the conduction of nerve impulses is impaired. In some experimental models where myelin is injured, endogenous oligodendrocytes can remyelinate axons, producing new myelin that improves impulse conduction in the brain and spinal cord; and Schwann cells can sometimes invade the demyelinated spinal cord, where they form myelin that enhances conduction.

These observations suggest that oligodendrocytes and Schwann cells might be good candidates for transplantation to the demyelinated brain and spinal cord. But success in the transplantation of myelin-forming cells requires answers to critical questions: What are the best methods for delivering cells to the brain and spinal cord? Will these transplanted cells survive? Do scarring cells in the brain and spinal cord present a barrier that will interfere with the survival or function of transplanted cells? Can transplanted cells migrate to find the correct axonal partners? If so, will they form myelin within the new terrain of the host? And, importantly, will the newly formed myelin enhance the conduction of nerve impulses within the injured brain or spinal cord?

Studies in laboratories around the world had addressed some of these questions, and demonstrated that Schwann cells and oligodendrocytes can be transplanted to the demyelinated central nervous system where they survive, find axons, and form new myelin sheaths (see, e.g., Blakemore and Franklin 1991; Duncan et al. 1988; Gout and Dubois-Dalcq 1993; Lachapelle et al. 1994; Yandava, Billinghurst, and Snyder 1999). But what about the effects of this transplantation-induced myelination on the *function* of the demyelinated nerve fibers, that is, on their ability to carry nerve impulses? In the mid 1990s Jeffery Kocsis, who pioneered methods for studying impulse conduction along nerve fibers in the spinal cord and brain, began to use these methods to examine the function of demyelinated spinal cord axons that had been remyelinated following cell transplantation. Our early studies focused on *myelin-deficient* rats (which lack myelin in the brain and spinal cord as a result of a mutation that affects their oligo-dendrocytes). These experiments showed that myelin, formed by exogenous, transplanted oligoden-drocytes within the *myelin-deficient* spinal cord, can enhance the conduction of nerve impulses. The speed of impulse conduction, which had been severely reduced in the *myelin-deficient* nerve fibers, approached normal after transplantation. And the ability of the nerve fibers to transmit high frequency series of impulses was improved (Utzschneider et al. 1994).

The paper by Honmou et al. (1996), which follows, extends this line of research and shows that transplantation of Schwann cells to the spinal cord also results in the formation of new myelin. It demonstrates, moreover, that this results in a striking enhancement of impulse conduction in adult rats harboring experimental demyelinating lesions. As with myelination by transplanted oligodendrocytes, the conduction velocity and the ability of nerve fibers to carry trains of impulses at high frequencies are restored to near-normal levels.

More recent experiments have demonstrated that cells that normally populate the nerve to the nose, called olfactory ensheathing cells, can also remyelinate axons within the demyelinated spinal cord, significantly enhancing their ability to conduct impulses (Imaizumi et al. 1998). Experiments in the

Kocsis laboratory have extended these observations to human olfactory ensheathing cells transplanted into the demyelinated rat spinal cord (Kato et al., 2000) and have also shown that olfactory ensheathing cells can myelinate regenerating axons within the transected rat spinal cord, improving the speed of impulse conduction along them (Imaizumi, Lankford, and Kocsis 2000).

Neuroscientists are now searching for cell types that are optimal for transplantation into the nervous system. Some of these cell types may make it possible to avoid the operational and ethical issues involved in the use of fetal tissue. The demonstration that various types of myelin-forming cells, not just oligodendrocytes, can be transplanted to the spinal cord, and that they can enhance impulse conduction, suggests an important degree of freedom: Schwann cells or olfactory ensheathing cells might, in principle, be removed from a human patient, leaving little functional deficit; the cell population could then proliferate in tissue culture prior to autotransplantation back into the same patient. "Engineered" cell lines that form myelin are also being developed; some of these are immunologically invisible so that they do not trigger rejection by the host. If these approaches are successful, there might be less need for the immunosuppression that makes postoperative care in most transplantation procedures so difficult.

There is much work to be done before injured brains and spinal cords can be repaired. Transplantation of myelin-forming cells to humans will require answers to many questions, including questions about the best cell types and long-term effects of cell transplantation, the stability of the transplanted cells and the new myelin, the possibility of overgrowth of cells following transplantation, and the most effective strategies for cell delivery. A network of investigators around the world is trying to answer these questions. If these researchers are successful, cell transplantation to the brain and spinal cord may, one day, no longer be an experimental technique. One can imagine that transplantation of neural cells might even become a routine clinical procedure—similar to cornea or kidney transplantation—which will permit repair of the injured spinal cord or brain.

References

Blakemore, W. F., and Franklin, R. J. Transplantation of glial cells into the CNS. *Trends Neurosci.* 14: 323–327, 1991.

Duncan, I. D., Hammang, J. P., Jackson, K. F., Wood, P. M., Bunge, R. P., and Langford, L. Transplantation of oligodendrocytes and Schwann cells into the spinal cord of the myelin-deficient rat. *J. Neurocytol.* 17: 351–360, 1988.

Gout, O., and Dubois-Dalcq, M. Directed migration of transplanted glial cells toward a spinal cord demyelinating lesion. *Int. J. Devel. Neurosci.* 11: 613–623, 1993.

Honmou, O., Felts, P. A., Waxman, S. G., and Kocsis, J. D. Restoration of normal conduction properties in demyelinated spinal cord axons in the adult rat by transplantation of exogenous Schwann cells. *J. Neurosci.* 16: 3199–3208, 1996.

Imaizumi, T., Lankford, K. L., and Kocsis, J. D. Transplantation of olfactory ensheathing cells or Schwann cells restores rapid and secure conduction across the transected spinal cord. *Brain Res.* 854: 70–78, 2000.

Imaizumi, T., Lankford, K. L., Waxman, S. G., Greer, C. A., and Kocsis, J. D. Transplanted olfactory ensheathing cells remyelinate and enhance axonal conduction in the demyelinated dorsal columns of the rat spinal cord. *J. Neurosci.* 18: 6176–6185, 1998.

Kato, T., Honmou, O., Uede, T., Hoshi, K., and Kocsis, J. D. Transplantation of human olfactory ensheathing cells elicits remyelination of demyelinated rat spinal cord. *Glia*, 30: 209–218, 2000.

Lachapelle, F., Duhamel-Clerin, E., Gansmuller A., Baron-Van Evercooren, A., Villarroya, H., and Gumpel, M. Transplanted transgenically marked oligodendrocytes survive, migrate and myelinate in the normal mouse brain as they do in the shiverer mouse brain. *Eur. J. Neurosci.* 6: 814–824, 1994.

Utzschneider, D. A., Archer, D. R., Kocsis, J. D., Waxman, S. G., and Duncan, I. D. Transplantation of glial cells enhances action potential conduction of amyelinated spinal cord axons in the myelin-deficient rat. *Proc. Natl. Acad. Sci. USA* 91: 53–57, 1994.

Yandava, B. D., Billinghurst, L. L., and Snyder, E. Y. "Global" cell replacement is feasible via neural stem cell transplantation: evidence from the dysmyelinated *shiverer* mouse brain. *Proc. Natl. Acad. Sci. USA* 96: 7029–7034, 1999.

33 Restoration of Normal Conduction Properties in Demyelinated Spinal Cord Axons in the Adult Rat by Transplantation of Exogenous Schwann Cells

Osamu Honmou, Paul A. Felts, Stephen G. Waxman, and Jeffery D. Kocsis

Abstract Although remyelination of demyelinated CNS axons is known to occur after transplantation of exogenous glial cells, previous studies have not determined whether cell transplantation can restore the conduction properties of demyelinated axons in the adult CNS. To examine this issue, the dorsal columns of the adult rat spinal cord were demyelinated by x-irradiation and intraspinal injections of ethidium bromide. Cell suspensions of cultured astrocytes and Schwann cells derived from neonatal rats transfected with the (β-galactosidase) reporter gene were injected into the glial-free lesion site. After 3–4 weeks nearly all of the demyelinated axons were remyelinated by the transplanted Schwann cells. The dorsal columns were removed and maintained in an in vitro recording chamber; conduction properties were studied using field potential and intra-axonal recording techniques. The demyelinated axons exhibited conduction slowing and block, and a reduction in their ability to follow high-frequency stimulation. Axons remyelinated by transplantation of cultured Schwann cells exhibited restoration of conduction through the lesion, with reestablishment of normal conduction velocity. The axons remyelinated after transplantation showed enhanced impulse recovery to paired-pulse stimulation and greater frequency-following capability as compared with both demyelinated and control axons. These results demonstrate the functional repair of demyelinated axons in the adult CNS by transplantation of cultured myelin-forming cells from the peripheral nervous system in combination with astrocytes.

Demyelination of axons in the CNS occurs in a number of neurological disorders including multiple sclerosis (MS) and contusive spinal cord injury (Blight, 1983; Byrne and Waxman, 1990; Bunge et al., 1993; McDonald, 1995). Even if the progression of MS were to be halted or slowed via immunotherapy, MS patients would continue to harbor demyelinating lesions that produce significant functional deficits. Cell transplantation has been suggested as a strategy for repair of demyelinated CNS axons (Blakemore and Crang, 1985; Groves et al., 1993; Vignais et al., 1993). In some experimental models of CNS demyelination, remyelination by *endogenous* oligodendrocytes (Gledhill et al., 1973; Gledhill and McDonald, 1977; Clifford-Jones et al., 1980) or by invasion of peripheral Schwann cells (Blakemore, 1976; Blakemore et al., 1977) occurs, with the reestablishment of relatively normal impulse conduction (Smith et al., 1979, 1981; Blight and Young, 1989; Felts and Smith, 1992), but permanent remyelination is very limited in humans (Ghatak et al., 1973; Prineas and Connell, 1979; Itoyama et al., 1985). Substantial anatomically defined myelination can also be induced by transplantation of *exogenous* cultured glial cells derived from fetal or neonatal as well as adult animals (Blakemore and Crang, 1985; Duncan et al., 1988; Rosenbluth et al., 1990; Gout and Dubois-Dalcq, 1993; Lachapelle et al., 1994). Moreover, human Schwann cells can produce compact myelin in an immunodeficient mouse mutant model (Levi and Bunge, 1994).

Oligodendrocyte remyelination subsequent to transplantation of CNS glial cell suspensions into the amyelinated immature *myelin-deficient* mutant rat spinal cord (5 d old) has been demonstrated to result in increased conduction velocity (Utzschneider et al., 1994). However, whereas it is known that compact myelin may be formed after transplantation of exogenous glial cells into demyelinated regions of adult CNS (Blakemore and Franklin, 1991), virtually no assessment of the electrophysiological properties of the remyelinated axons has been undertaken. Such studies are important because reliable impulse conduction in remyelinated axons requires not only the formation of compact myelin but also the establishment of appropriate myelin segment length (Huxley and Stämpfli, 1949; Waxman and Brill, 1978) and ion channel organization at the newly formed nodes of Ranvier

Reprinted with permission from *The Journal of Neuroscience* 16: 3199–3208, 1996.

(Ritchie and Rogart, 1977; Waxman, 1977; Moore et al., 1978; Hines and Shrager, 1991). It is not known whether remyelination by transplanted *exogenous* glial and Schwann cells, especially in the *adult* CNS, meets these criteria for the reestablishment of normal conduction.

To test directly whether cultured exogenous Schwann cells interact with axons in the adult CNS after transplantation so as to reestablish normal impulse conduction, we transplanted cultured neonatal Schwann cells, in some cases transfected with the *LacZ* reporter gene, and astrocytes derived from immature rats into the spinal cords of demyelinated adult rat spinal cord. We report restoration of nearly normal conduction properties in axons of the adult rat spinal cord after remyelination by transplanted, exogenously derived Schwann cells.

Materials and Methods

Demyelination Model (X-ray Irradiation and Ethidium Bromide Injection)

Rats were anesthetized with ketamine (75 mg/kg, i.p.) and xylazine (10 mg/kg, i.p.) and x-irradiated utilizing a method similar to that of Blakemore and Patterson (1978). Briefly, a 40 Grays surface dose of x-irradiation was delivered through a 2×4 cm opening in a lead shield (4 mm thick) to the spinal cord caudal to T10 using a Siemens Stabilipan radiotherapy machine (250 kV, 15 mA, 0.5 mm Cu, and 1.0 mm Al filters, SSD 28 cm, dose rate 220.9 cGy/min; Siemans AG, Erlangen, Germany). Three days after irradiation, rats were anesthetized as above and, using sterile technique, a laminectomy was performed at T11. The demyelinating lesion was induced by the direct injection of ethidium bromide (EB), a nucleic acid-chelating agent that induces primary demyelination by killing oligodendrocytes, into the dorsal columns via a drawn glass micropipette. Injections of 0.5 µl of 0.3 mg/ml EB in saline were made at depths of 0.7 and

0.4 mm at three longitudinal sites 2 mm apart for a total of six injections.

Primary Cell Culture, Transfection of LacZ Gene, and Cell Transplantation

Primary Schwann cell cultures were established from the sciatic nerve of neonatal rats (P1–P3) according to the method of Brockes et al. (1979). Briefly, the cell suspension resulting from enzymatically and mechanically dissociating sciatic nerves was plated onto 100 mm^2 poly-L-lysine-coated tissue culture plates at 8×10^5 cells per plate and cultured in DMEM supplemented with 10% (v/v) fetal calf serum (figure 33.1).

Primary astrocyte cell cultures were established from the neonatal rat optic nerve based on the method of McCarthy et al. (1980). After enzymatic and mechanical dissociation, cells were plated onto 100 mm^2 poly-L-lysine-coated tissue culture plates at 8×10^5 cells per plate and cultured in minimum essential media (MEM) supplemented with 15% (v/v) fetal calf serum.

A replication-defective retrovirus vector was used to transduce the bacterial β-galactosidase (β-gal) gene into primary cultures of Schwann cells. Schwann cells were transfected by the BAG retroviral vector (Price et al., 1987) contained in the $\Psi2$ packaging line (Mann et al., 1983). The BAG vector is constructed by cloning the β-gal gene into the pDOL vector derived from the Maloney murine leukemia virus (Mo-MuLV). The wild-type Mo-MuLV LTR provided the promoter for the β-gal gene. The simian virus 40 early promoter and the Tn5 neomycin-resistance gene, transmitting G418 resistance, are present downstream from the β-gal gene to permit selection of infected colonies. Supernatants from packaging cells were used, in the presence of polybrene (8 µg/ml), to infect cultured Schwann cells, which were rapidly proliferating under the influence of 2 µM forskolin and glial growth factor (Brockes et al., 1979). Before transfection, contaminating fibroblasts were eliminated by treatments with the antimitotic agent cytosine

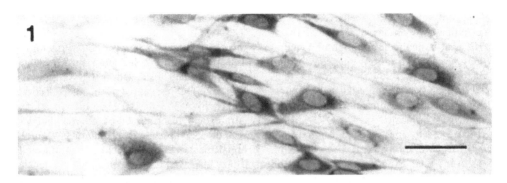

Figure 33.1
β-Gal gene products are detected as a blue color in neonatal sciatic nerve Schwann cells in vitro. Scale bar, 50 μm.

arabinoside (10 μM) and antibody-complement-mediated cell lysis using the monoclonal anti-Thy 1.1 antibody and rabbit complement (Porter et al., 1986). Transfected Schwann cells were then selected by incubation with neomycin analog G418 (400 μg/ml). Under ketamine/xylazine anesthesia, a suspension of 5×10^4 Schwann cells and astrocytes (~3/2) in 1 μl of DMEM was injected into the middle of the EB-X-induced lesion 3 d after the EB injection.

Histological Examination

The rats were deeply anesthetized with sodium pentobarbital (50 mg/kg, i.p.) and perfused through the heart, first with PBS at room temperature and then with a fixative solution containing 2% glutaraldehyde and 2% para-formaldehyde in 0.14 M Sorensen's phosphate buffer, pH 7.4. After in situ fixation for 10 min, the spinal cord was carefully excised, cut into 1 mm segments, and placed in fresh fixative. The tissue was washed several times in Sorensen's buffer, post-fixed with 1% OsO$_4$ for 2 hr at 25 °C, dehydrated in graded ethanol solutions, passed through propylene oxide, and embedded in Epon. After polymerization at 60 °C, thick sections (1 μm) were cut, counterstained with 0.5% methylene blue, 0.5% azure II in 0.5% bo-

rax, and examined with a light microscope. Thin sections were counterstained with uranyl and lead salts and examined with a Zeiss EM902A electron microscope operating at 80 kV.

Detection of β-gal Reaction Products in vitro and in vivo

β-Gal-expressing cells were detected in vitro by incubating the cultured Schwann cells with X-Gal to form a blue color within the cell (figure 33.1). Schwann cells were fixed in 0.05% gluta-raldehyde, washed with PBS, and then incubated with X-Gal to a final concentration of 1 mg/ml in X-Gal developer (35 mM K$_3$Fe(CN)$_6$/35 mM K$_4$Fe(CN)$_6$·^{3}H$_2$O/2 mM MgCl$_2$ in PBS). Cells were incubated at 37 °C overnight and examined by light microscopy for the presence of a blue reaction product. Over 99% of cells were marked by the *LacZ* gene. The presence of helper virus in the tissue culture medium was also assayed according to the method of Price et al. (1987); supernatants from transfected Schwann cells were not able to infect NIH3T3 cells.

Three weeks after transplantation, β-gal-expressing Schwann cells were detected in vivo. Spinal cords were removed and fixed in 0.5% glutaraldehyde in phosphate buffer for 1 hr. Sections (100 μm) were cut with a vibratome, and β-gal-expressing Schwann cells were detected by incubating the sections at 37°C overnight with X-Gal to a final concentration of 1 mg/ml in X-Gal developer to form a blue color within the cell. The slices were then fixed for an additional 3 hr in 3.6% (v/v) glutaraldehyde in phosphate buffer (0.14 M). Before embedding in epon, the tissue was osmicated in 1% OsO_4, dehydrated in a graded series of ethanols, and infiltrated briefly with propylene oxide. Ultrathin sections were then examined in the electron microscope without further staining.

Field Potential Recording

After induction of deep anesthesia (sodium pentobarbital 50 mg/kg, i.p.), the spinal cords of control, demyelinated, and transplanted rats were quickly removed and maintained in an in vitro submersion-type recording chamber with a modified Krebs' solution (containing 124 mM NaCl, 26 mM $NaHCO_3$, 3 mM KCl, 1.3 mM NaH_2PO_4, 2 mM $MgCl_2$, 10 mM dextrose, 2 mM $CaCl_2$; saturated with 95% O_2/5% CO_2). Field potential recordings of compound action potentials were obtained with glass microelectrodes (1–5 MΩ; 1 M NaCl) positioned in the dorsal columns (figure 33.4A), and signals were amplified with a high input impedance amplifier and stored on a digital oscilloscope. The axons were activated by electrical stimulation of the dorsal columns with bipolar Teflon-coated stainless steel electrodes cut flush and placed lightly on the dorsal surface of the spinal cord. Constant current stimulation pulses were delivered through stimulus isolation units, and the timing of the pulses was controlled by a digital timing device. The recorded field potentials were positive–negative–positive waves corresponding to source–sink–source currents associated with propagating axonal action potentials (Kocsis and Waxman, 1980); the negativity represents inward current associated with the depolarizing phase of the action potential.

Intra-axonal Recording

Intra-axonal recordings were obtained with borosilicate electrodes pulled on a Brown-Flaming P-80 puller and filled with 4 M KAc and 0.1 M KCl. The DC resistances of the microelectrodes ranged from 100 to 150 MΩ. Identification of intra-axonal recordings used criteria that have been discussed previously (Honmou et al., 1994). Impalements were considered to be intracellular if they displayed a resting potential greater than −50 mV with spike overshoot and if passage of a constant hyperpolarizing current caused an increase in action potential amplitude (Barrett and Barrett, 1982; Kocsis and Waxman, 1982; Blight and Someya, 1985; Kapoor et al., 1993). Dorsal column stimulation pulses were delivered through a bipolar. Teflon-coated, stainless steel stimulation electrode cut flush and placed directly on the dorsal column segment. Single axon stimulation pulses were delivered through the recording microelectrode and consisted of constant-current pulses (up to 0.5 nA) of up to 100 msec duration provided by the step current command of the recording amplifier and monitored on a separate channel. An active bridge circuit was used to compensate for electrode and preparation resistance.

Results

The dorsal columns of the normal adult rat consist largely of myelinated axons (figures 33.2A, B, 33.3A). The axons were demyelinated using the EB/x-irradiation (EB-X) lesion model; the axons in the lesion were virtually completely demyelinated, and the lesion site was largely glial-free (figures 33.2C, D, 33.3B). The demyelinated lesions were large and well circumscribed, encompassing 70–80% of the transverse extent of the dorsal column and measuring 7–8 mm longitudinally. There was no evidence of remyelination by either oligodendrocytes or Schwann

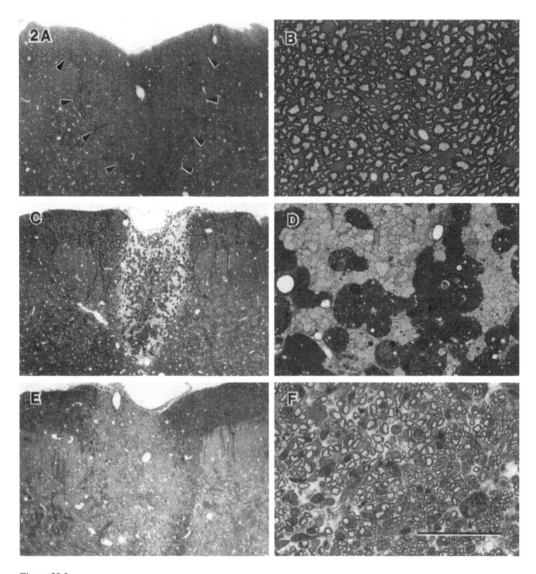

Figure 33.2
Low (*A*, *C*, *E*) and high (*B*, *D*, *F*) magnification light micrographs of transverse sections through the dorsal columns of normal (*A*, *B*), demyelinated but untransplanted (*C*, *D*; 25 d after EB injection), and transplanted (*E*, *F*; 24 d after EB injection) animals. In the absence of a transplant, the lesion (translucent region within the dorsal columns in *C*) is composed of naked, demyelinated axons and debris-filled phagocytes (*D*). Transplantation of cultured Schwann cells and astrocytes results in a large region (light blue area within the dorsal columns in *E*) of Schwann cell-remyelinated axons (*F*). For orientation at low magnification, the dorsal columns have been outlined with arrowheads in (*A*). Scale bar: (*A*, *C*, *E*) 500 μm; (*B*, *D*, *F*) 50 μm.

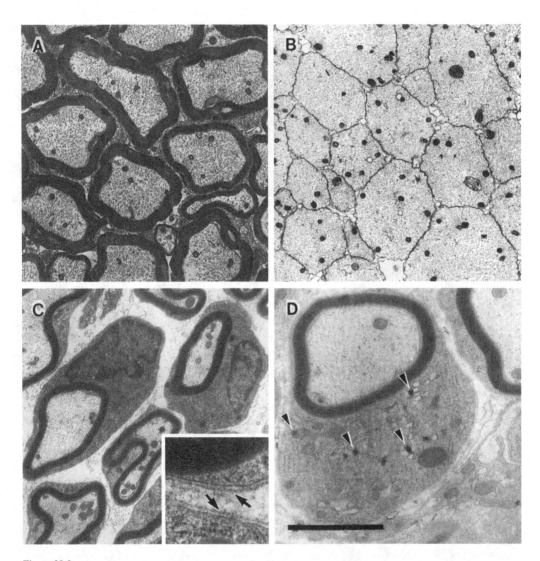

Figure 33.3

Electron micrographs showing normal (*A*) and demyelinated (*B*) axons in the dorsal columns. All demyelinated spinal cords that received cell injections showed clear evidence of remyelination (*C*) of the demyelinated axons. Examination at higher magnification (inset in *C*) showed the presence of a basal lamina (arrows) as well as extracellular collagen fibrils surrounding the individual fibers, indicative of Schwann cell myelination. (*D*) Schwann cells carrying the β-gal gene (reaction product indicated by arrowheads) could be detected in the lesion by treating the tissue with the substrate X-Gal. Scale bar: (*A–C*) 4 µm; *D*, 2 µm; inset in (*C*), 0.6 µm.

cells 1–6 weeks after lesion induction. The demyelinated axons within the lesion were clumped together, and macrophages filled with myelin debris were located between the naked axons. No axonal ensheathment was observed in the lesions. Unlike many experimentally induced demyelination models where endogenous remyelination commences within days of lesion induction, the glial-free zone remains intact for more than 5–6 weeks in the EB-X model. This offers experimental advantage in that transplanted cells can be introduced and remyelinate the demyelinated axons without competition from endogenous cells. Virtually all of the axons within the lesion zone were remyelinated by 3 weeks after Schwann cell and astrocyte transplantation (figures 33.2*E*, *F*, 33.3*C*), with the exception of the very finest caliber axons, which likely represent normally unmyelinated axons. In some experiments Schwann cells were transfected with the *LacZ* reporter gene to confirm that the remyelination was indeed produced by transplanted cells (figure 33.3*D*).

In normal dorsal columns the negativity of the field potential increased in latency and decreased in amplitude with increasing conduction distance (figure 33.4*B1*, *C*). After 5 mm of conduction in control dorsal columns, the amplitude of the response was reduced to $13.4 \pm 4.4\%$ (average $\pm$ SEM; $n = 5$) of the response recorded at 2 mm. In the demyelinated axons, the amplitude decreased precipitously with increasing conduction distance (figure 33.4*B2*, *C*), and virtually no impulse activity was observed at a distance of 5 mm from the stimulating electrode, indicating extensive conduction block in the demyelinated axons. In contrast, amplitude decrement with distance was indistinguishable from controls in transplanted dorsal columns (figure 33.4*B3*, *C*) indicating that conduction was similar to normal, with action potentials propagating for a greater distance into the lesion than observed in demyelinated axons.

Conduction velocity was considerably reduced in the demyelinated axons at both 26 and 36 °C,

and was restored to normal values at both temperatures after transplantation (figure 33.5); conduction velocity (at 36 °C) was 10.2 ± 0.9 m/sec ($n = 5$) in control and 0.9 ± 0.1 m/sec ($n = 5$) in the demyelinated dorsal columns. After transplant-induced remyelination, conduction velocity was restored to virtually the same values as in controls (11.4 ± 0.7 m/sec, $n = 5$). These results indicate that essentially normal conduction velocity is restored by remyelination induced by Schwann cell transplantation.

Conduction velocity was also studied in single axons that traversed the lesion site using intra-axonal recording techniques. Arrays of stimulating electrodes were placed on the spinal cord dorsum within the lesion and on the nondemyelinated dorsal column several millimeters away. Axons were then impaled at a site between the two arrays of stimulating electrodes within the nondemyelinated region, thus permitting study of conduction along segments of the same axon that included and excluded the lesion. In demyelinated spinal cords that had not received a transplant, the portion of the axon passing through the region of demyelination (figure 33.6*B2*) exhibited considerably longer latencies indicative of slower conduction velocity than the nondemyelinated part of the same axon (figure 33.6*B1*). In contrast, in spinal cords that had received transplants, conduction velocity was virtually the same for fibers remyelinated by transplanted Schwann cells (figure 33.6*C2*) as compared to conduction along their trajectory outside of the transplant region (figure 33.6*C1*). A plot of conduction velocity including the lesion versus conduction velocity excluding the lesion from each of the two experimental groups (demyelinated without transplant vs transplant-induced remyelinated) is shown in figure 33.6*D*. The remyelinated axons have a conduction velocity that is substantially greater than in the demyelinated axons. Moreover, action potentials evoked from stimulation within the transplant region propagated into the nondemyelinated portion of the spinal cord (figure 33.6*C2*), dem-

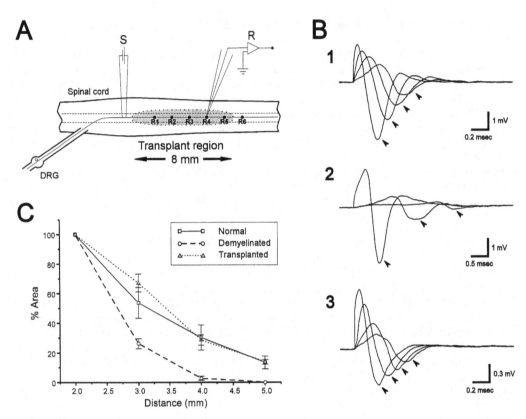

Figure 33.4
(*A*) Schematic showing the dorsal surface of spinal cord with the positions of the stimulating (*S*) and recording (*R*) electrodes. Shaded region indicates the area of demyelination or remyelination. (*B*) Compound action potentials recorded at 1 mm increments along the dorsal columns in control (*1*), EB-X-demyelinated (*2*), and transplant-induced remyelinated (*3*) axons. (*C*) Compound action potential area (*% Area*) plotted versus conduction distance for normal, demyelinated, and transplant-induced remyelinated dorsal columns (n = 5).

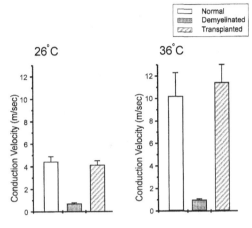

Figure 33.5
Conduction velocity for control, demyelinated, and remyelinated axons recorded at 26 and 36 °C. Error bars indicate SEM in this and subsequent figures.

onstrating that axonal conduction occurred through the zone of potential impedance mismatch between the remyelinated region and normal region of the host nervous system.

Recovery properties of the axons were studied using paired-pulse stimulation (figure 33.7). In normal dorsal columns (26 °C), impulse activity was blocked for ~2 msec after the conditioning stimulus, and recovery began at ~3 msec. Full recovery of field potential amplitude was attained at ~10 msec. The onset of recovery in the demyelinated axons was delayed as compared with control by ~1 msec, but the slope of recovery was similar to control at 26 °C (figure 33.7D). Axons remyelinated after transplantation had a more rapid recovery than control axons. The onset of recovery occurred sooner, and the slope of recovery was greater. At 36 °C, recovery for all three groups of axons occurred earlier than at 26 °C, but the relative difference between control and demyelinated axons was increased, and the difference between control and remyelinated axons was smaller (figure 33.7E), although at 36 °C the remyelinated

axons still displayed recovery that was faster than in controls.

Another difference in conduction in the remyelinated axons was their enhanced ability to follow high-frequency stimulation; the demyelinated axons showed considerable reduction in the ability to follow high-frequency stimulation (figure 33.8). At both 26 and 36 °C, the fiber volley amplitude of the demyelinated axons was reduced compared with controls for stimulus trains at 50 Hz and higher. Frequency–response properties in remyelinated axons after transplantation were enhanced. Remyelinated axons were able to follow high-frequency stimulation as well as controls but exhibited less amplitude decrement at high stimulus frequencies than the control axons.

Discussion

Functional repair of the CNS by cell transplantation has been considered as a potential therapeutic approach for a number of neurological disorders. Indeed, clinical studies introducing dopamine-producing cells into the caudate nucleus in humans have been underway for several years in patients with basal ganglia disorders (Lindvall et al., 1994). The prospect of introducing myelin-forming cells into patients with demyelinating disease has also been considered, but limited laboratory work in experimental animal models examining the electrophysiological or functional consequences of such interventions has been performed. Whereas cultured oligodendrocyte progenitor cells can remyelinate demyelinated CNS axons, Schwann cells are also capable of myelinating CNS axons (Blakemore and Crang, 1985; Duncan et al., 1988). A potential advantage in the use of Schwann cells for transplantation is that they are derived from peripheral tissues and potentially could be derived from the same animal or patient (e.g., via sural nerve biopsy) with minimal adverse effects, thereby obviating problems of cell rejection and

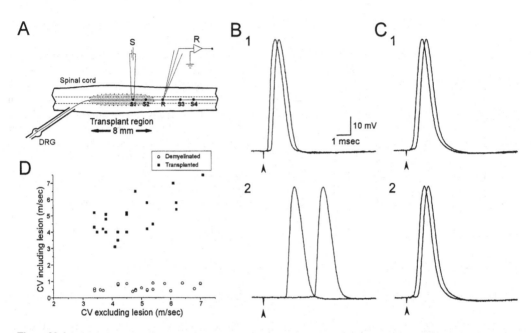

Figure 33.6

(*A*) Schematic showing arrangement of intra-axonal recording and extracellular stimulation sites. Intra-axonal recordings were obtained from dorsal column axons outside of the lesion where the axons were normally myelinated (*R*). Stimulating electrodes were positioned within (*S1–S2*) and outside (*S3–S4*) of the lesion zone to assess conduction velocity over both the demyelinated or the remyelinated axon segment, and a normally myelinated axon segment of the same axon. (*B*) Pairs of action potentials recorded from a spinal cord that did not receive a transplant at comparable conduction distances for a conduction path that either included (*2*) or excluded (*1*) the lesion. Note the increased latency for conduction over the axon trajectory that included the demyelinated region. (*C*) Similar stimulation-recording protocol as (*B*), but for transplant-induced remyelinated axons. The latencies for conduction through the remyelinated axon trajectory are similar to those of the axon segment outside of the lesion zone. (*D*) Plot of the conduction velocity of axon segments including the lesion versus conduction velocity of the axon segment outside of the lesion for demyelinated and transplant-induced remyelinated groups.

the necessity for immunosuppression. Moreover, Schwann cell remyelination of CNS axons in immunologically mediated CNS-demyelinating diseases may be resistant to further immunological attack.

In the model system used in the current study, introduction of Schwann cells alone into the EB-X lesion results in remyelination limited to a region near the injection site. However, as initially reported by Blakemore and colleagues (Blakemore et al., 1987; Franklin et al., 1992), when a

combination of Schwann cells and astrocytes is injected simultaneously, the Schwann cells displayed extensive migration and remyelinated virtually the entire demyelinated region. This suggests that some component of, or factor derived from, astrocytes is essential at the time of donor cell introduction into the host CNS to confer migratory and possibly myelinating potential to the Schwann cells (Blakemore and Crang, 1985). Future work to determine the molecular nature of the astrocytic influence on

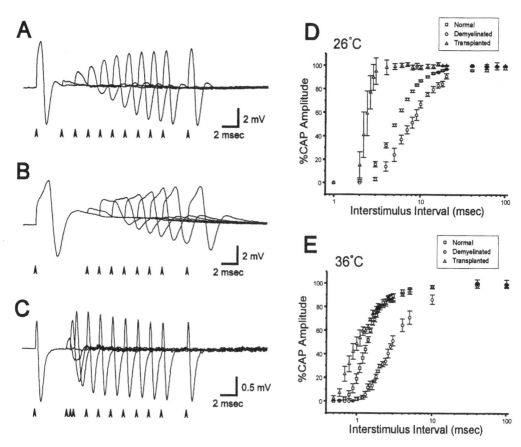

Figure 33.7
Paired-pulse stimuli at varying interstimulus intervals were applied to study the refractory period for transmission in normal (*A*), demyelinated (*B*), and transplant-induced (*C*) remyelinated axons. Compound action potentials resulting from the second of two paired stimuli were plotted at increasing interstimulus intervals for three groups at 26 °C (*D*) and 36 °C (*E*). Amplitude recovery was reduced in the demyelinated axons compared with normal axons, but transplant-induced remyelinated axons exhibited faster recovery properties than control axons.

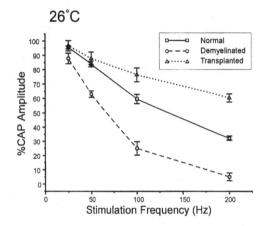

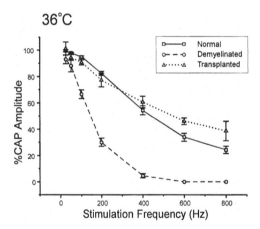

Figure 33.8
The compound action potential amplitudes of the last response of a train (1 sec, 26 °C; 0.5 sec, 36 °C), expressed as a percentage of the first response, were plotted at various frequencies. These frequency–response curves were plotted for normal, demyelinated, and transplant-induced remyelinated axons at 26 and 36 °C. The demyelinated axons showed reduced frequency–response properties. Transplantation-induced remyelinated axons showed less decrement in their frequency–response properties compared with those of the demyelinated axons; at higher frequencies, the remyelinated axons showed less amplitude decrement than controls.

the Schwann cell's migratory potential will be needed if monocellular transplant approaches, using only Schwann cells, are to be developed.

Whereas the presence of cultured astrocytes together with the donor Schwann cells is critical for the achievement of extensive myelination of the EB-X lesion which is glial-free, introduction of Schwann cells alone or in combination with astrocytes does not result in myelin formation that is as extensive as the remyelination in lesion models that contain resident astrocytes. For example, the *md* rat has virtually no endogenous CNS myelin, but the CNS is replete with astrocytes; introduction of Schwann cells and combinations of Schwann cells and astrocytes results in myelination of the *md* axons, but migration is more limited than in the glial-free environment of the EB-X lesion (Duncan et al., 1988). This suggests that resident astrocytes may impede the migration of Schwann cells. The most notable example of this is the glial limitans at the junction of spinal cord and PNS where an astrocytic layer prevents Schwann cell entry into the CNS (Sims et al., 1985). It is not clear whether extensive remyelination, as observed in the EB-X lesion, will occur in more naturally occurring demyelinating disorders, in which astrocytes are present.

The axon membrane of normal myelinated fibers has a heterogeneous distribution of Na^+ channels along the longitudinal axis of the axon. Na^+ channels cluster at the node of Ranvier with a density of $\sim 1000/\mu m^2$ as compared with the internodal axon membrane, which has a Na^+ channel density of $\sim 25/\mu m^2$ (Ritchie and Rogart, 1977; Shrager 1989; Waxman, 1997). The mechanism for the clustering of nodal Na^+ channels at the node is not known, but is associated with axo-glial contact and precedes myelination (Waxman and Foster, 1980; Wiley-Livingston and Ellisman, 1980). Although anatomical myelination occurs after transplantation of myelin-forming precursor cells into the EB-X lesion, one could not assume, *a priori*, that the transplanted cells would interact with axons in the glial-free microenvironment in a manner that permits Na$^+$ channel clustering at the newly formed nodes of Ranvier so that channel densities appropriate for secure conduction would be achieved. Moreover, internodal distances, myelin thickness, and axon diameter along axons after endogenous remyelination are altered compared with normal (Harrison and McDonald, 1977), and these changes can lead to impedance mismatch that produces conduction block (Koles and Rasminsky, 1972; Waxman and Brill, 1978). These complex structural changes in remyelinated axons make it difficult to predict, *a priori*, the physiological effects of remyelination by transplanted cells.

Our results indicate that demyelinated axons of the adult mammalian CNS, remyelinated by transplantation of exogenously derived Schwann cells, conduct action potentials in a manner similar to normal control myelinated axons. Conduction velocities of the transplant-induced remyelinated axons were similar to controls. This is consistent with observations that showed that the relationship between internode distance and conduction velocity is hyperbolic with a broad maximum (Huxley and Stampfli, 1949); reductions in internode distance of threefold or less, as observed in many remyelinated axons, would be expected to result in conduction velocities close to normal (Brill et al., 1977). The frequency–response properties of the remyelinated axons did, however, display enhanced frequency–response characteristics, compared with controls, over the same frequency range (figures 33.7, 8). The enhanced frequency–response properties after transplant-induced remyelination were unexpected. They may reflect differences in nodal geometry of Schwann cell- versus oligodendrocyte-myelinated axons (Peters, 1966; Berthold, 1995) or in altered ionic homeostasis mechanisms at nodes of Ranvier along Schwann cell-remyelinated CNS axons after cell transplantation. It is well-established that the extracellular concentration of K$^+$, which is regulated by glial cells, can influence axonal conduction properties in the CNS (Kocsis et al. 1983), and

changes in axo-glial organization could affect axonal frequency–response properties. Moreover, conduction extended for a much greater longitudinal distance into the transplant zone as compared with the demyelinated axons, suggesting the overcoming of conduction block, and impulses can propagate past the transition zone between remyelinated and normally myelinated axon segments. These results indicate that sufficient nodal clustering of Na$^+$ channels occurs and appropriate internodal lengths are established in the remyelinated axons to restore essentially normal conduction.

The restoration of conduction velocity and security of impulse conduction after remyelination by transplanted heterologous Schwann cells reported here indicates that an exogenous source of myelin-forming cells can elicit the formation of myelinated internodes and associated structures such as nodes of Ranvier that support secure impulse conduction in the host adult CNS. Thus, the present study indicates that the conduction properties of demyelinated axons in the adult mammalian spinal cord can be markedly improved after the transplantation of exogenous Schwann cells and astrocytes, indicating that demyelinated mammalian CNS white matter is amenable to not only anatomical, but also functional repair by transplantation of exogenous myelin-forming cells.

References

Barrett EF, Barrett JN (1982) Intracellular recording from vertebrate myelinated axons: mechanism of the depolarizing afterpotential. J Physiol (Lond) 323: 117–144.

Berthold C, Rydmark M (1995) Morphology of normal peripheral axons. In: The axon: structure, function and pathophysiology (Waxman SG, Kocsis JD, Stys PK, eds), pp 13–50. New York: Oxford UP.

Blakemore WF (1976) Invasion of Schwann cells into the spinal cord of the rat following local injections of lysolecithin. Neuropathol Appl Neurobiol 2: 21–39.

Blakemore WF, Crang AJ (1985) The use of cultured autologous Schwann cells to remyelinate areas of persistent demyelination in the central nervous system. J Neurol Sci 70: 207–223.

Blakemore WF, Franklin RJ (1991) Transplantation of glial cells into the CNS. Trends Neurosci 14: 323–327.

Blakemore WF, Patterson RC (1978) Suppression of remyelination in the CNS by x irradiation. Acta Neuropathol (Berl) 42: 105–113.

Blakemore WF, Eames RA, Smith KJ, McDonald WI (1977) Remyelination in the spinal cord of the cat following intraspinal injections of lysolecithin. J Neurol Sci 33: 31–43.

Blakemore WF, Crang AJ, Patterson RC (1987) Schwann cell remyelination of CNS axons following injection of cultures of CNS cells into areas of persistent demyelination. Neurosci Lett 77: 20–24.

Blight AR (1983) Axonal physiology of chronic spinal cord injury in the cat: intracellular recording in vitro. Neuroscience 10: 1471–1486.

Blight AR, Someya S (1985) Depolarizing afterpotentials in myelinated axons of mammalian spinal cord. Neuroscience 15: 1–12.

Blight AR, Young W (1989) Central axons in injured cat spinal cord recover electro-physiological function following remyelination by Schwann cells. J Neurol Sci 91: 15–34.

Brill MH, Waxman SG, Moore JW, Joyner RW (1977) Conduction velocity and spike configuration in myelinated fibres: computed dependence on internode distance. J Neurol Neurosurg Psychiatry 40: 769–774.

Brockes JP, Fields KL, Raff MC (1979) Studies on cultured rat Schwann cells. I. Establishment of purified populations from cultures of peripheral nerve. Brain Res 165: 105–118.

Bunge RP, Puckett WR, Becerra JL, Marcillo A, Quencer RM (1993) Observations on the pathology of human spinal cord injury. A review and classification of 22 new cases with details from a case of chronic cord compression with extensive focal demyelination. In: Advances in neurology: neural injury and regeneration. Vol 59 (Seil FJ, ed), pp 75–89. New York: Raven.

Byrne TN, Waxman SG (1990) Spinal cord compression. Philadelphia: Davis.

Clifford-Jones RE, Landon DN, McDonald WI (1980) Remyelination during optic nerve compression. J Neurol Sci 46: 239–243.

Duncan ID, Hammang JP, Jackson KF, Wood PM, Bunge RP, Langford L (1988) Transplantation of oligodendrocytes and Schwann cells into the spinal cord of the myelin-deficient rat. J Neurocytol 17: 351–360.

Felts PA, Smith KJ (1992) Conduction properties of central nerve fibers remyelinated by Schwann cells. Brain Res 574: 178–192.

Franklin RJM, Crang AJ, Blakemore WF (1992) Type-1 astrocytes fail to inhibit Schwann cell remyelination of CNS axons in the absence of cells of the O-2A lineage. Dev Neurosci 14: 85–92.

Ghatak NR, Hirano A, Doron Y, Zimmerman HM (1973) Remyelination in multiple sclerosis with peripheral type myelin. Arch Neurol 29: 262–267.

Gledhill RF, McDonald WI (1977) Morphological characteristics of central demyelination and remyelination: a single-fiber study. Ann Neurol 522–560.

Gledhill RF, Harrison BM, McDonald WI (1973) Pattern of remyelination in the CNS. Nature 244: 443–444.

Gout O, Dubois-Dalcq M (1993) Directed migration of transplanted glial cells toward a spinal cord demyelinating lesion. Int J Dev Neurosci. 11: 613–623.

Groves AK, Barnett SC, Franklin RJ, Crang AJ, Mayer M, Blakemore WF, Noble M (1993) Repair of demyelinated lesions by transplantation of purified O-2A progenitor cells. Nature 362: 453–455.

Harrison BM, McDonald WI (1977) Remyelination after transient experimental compression of the spinal cord. Ann Neurol 1: 542–551.

Hines M, Shrager P (1991) A computational test of the requirements for conduction in demyelinated axons. Rest Neurol Neurosci 3: 81–93.

Honmou O, Utzschneider DA, Rizzo MA, Bowe CM, Waxman SG, Kocsis JD (1994) Delayed depolarization and slow sodium currents in cutaneous afferents. J Neurophysiol 71: 1627–1637.

Huxley AF, Stämpfli R (1949) Evidence for saltatory conduction in peripheral myelinated nerve fibers. J Physiol (Lond) 108: 315–339.

Itoyama Y, Ohnishi A, Tateishi J, Kuroiwa Y, Webster HD (1985) Spinal cord multiple sclerosis lesions in Japanese patients: Schwann cell remyelination occurs in areas that lack glial fibrillary acidic protein (GFAP) Acta Neuropathol (Berl) 65: 217–223.

Kapoor R, Smith KJ, Felts PA, Davies M (1993) Internodal potassium currents can generate ectopic impulses in mammalian myelinated axon. Brain Res 611: 165–169.

Kocsis JD, Waxman SG (1980) Absence of potassium conductance in central myelinated axons. Nature 287: 348–349.

Kocsis JD, Waxman SG (1982) Intra-axonal recordings in rat dorsal column axons: membrane hyperpolarization and decreased excitability precede the primary afferent depolarization. Brain Res 238: 222–227.

Kocsis JD, Malenka RC, Waxman SG (1983) Effects of extracellular potassium concentration of the excitability of the parallel fibres of the rat cerebellum. J Physiol (Lond) 334: 225–244.

Koles ZJ, Rasminsky M (1972) A computer simulation of conduction in demyelinated nerve fibres. J Physiol (Lond) 227: 351–364.

Lachapelle F, Duhamel-Clerin E, Gansmuller A, Baron-Van Evercooren A. Villarroya H, Gumpel M (1994) Transplanted transgenically marked oligodendrocytes survive, migrate and myelinate in the normal mouse brain as they do in the shiverer mouse brain. Eur J Neurosci 6: 814–824.

Levi AD, Bunge RP (1994) Studies of myelin formation after transplantation of human Schwann cells into the severe combined immunodeficient mouse. Exp Neurol 130: 41–52.

Lindvall O, Sawle G, Widner H, Rothwell JC, Bjorklund A, Brooks D, Brundin P, Frackowiak R, Marsden CD, Odin P, Rehncrona S (1994). Evidence for long-term survival and function of dopaminergic grafts in progressive Parkinson's disease. Ann Neurol 35: 172–180.

Mann R, Mulligan RC, Baltimore D (1983) Construction of a retrovirus packaging mutant and its use to produce helper-free defective retrovirus. Cell 33: 153–159.

McCarthy KD, de Vellis J (1980) Preparation of separate astroglial and oligodendroglial cell cultures from rat cerebral tissue. J Cell Biol. 85: 890 902.

McDonald WI (1995) Overview of clinical aspects of multiple sclerosis including cognitive deficit. In: The axon: structure, function and patho-physiology (Waxman SG, Kocsis JD, Stys PK, eds), pp 661–668. New York: Oxford UP.

Moore JW, Joyner RW, Brill MH, Waxman SG, Najar-Joa M (1978) Simulations of conduction in uniform myelinated fibres: relative sensitivity of changes in nodal and internodal parameters. Biophys J 21: 147–161.

Peters A (1966) The node of Ranvier in the central nervous system. Q Exp Physiol Cogn Med Sci 51: 229–236.

Porter S, Blairclark M, Glaser L, Bunge RP (1986) Schwann cells stimulated to proliferate in the absence of neurons retain full functional capability. J Neurol Sci 6: 3070–3078.

Price J, Turner D, Cepko C (1987) Lineage analysis in the vertebrate nervous system by retrovirus-mediated gene transfer. Proc Natl Acad. Sci USA 84: 156–160.

Prineas J, Connell F (1979) Remyelination in multiple sclerosis. Am Neurol 5: 22–31.

Ritchie JM, Rogart RB (1977) Density of sodium channels in mammalian myelinated nerve fibers and nature of the axonal membrane under the myelin sheath. Proc Natl Acad Sci USA 74: 211–215.

Rosenbluth J, Hasegawa M. Shirasaki N, Rosen CL, Liu Z (1990) Myelin formation following transplantation of normal fetal glia into myelin-deficient rat spinal cord. J Neurocytol 19: 718–730.

Shrager P (1989) Sodium channels in single demyelinated mammalian axons. Brain Res 483: 149–154.

Sims TJ, Gilmore SA, Waxman SG, Klinge E (1985) Dorsal-ventral differences in the glia limitans of the spinal cord: an ultrastructural study in developing normal and irradiated rats. J Neuropathol Exp Neurol 44: 415–429.

Smith KJ, Blakemore WF, McDonald WI (1979) Central remyelination restores secure conduction. Nature 280: 395–396.

Smith KJ, Blakemore WF, McDonald WI (1981) The restoration of conduction by central remyelination. Brain 104: 383–404.

Utzschneider DA, Archer DR, Kocsis JD, Waxman SG, Duncan ID (1994) Transplantation of glial cells enhances action potential conduction of amyelinated spinal cord axons in the myelin-deficient rat. Proc Natl Acad Sci USA 91: 53–57.

Vignais L, Nait Oumesmar B, Mellouk F, Gout O, Labourdette G, Baron-Van Evercooren A, Gumpel M (1993) Transplantation of oligodendrocyte precursors in the adult demyelinated spinal cord: migration and remyelination. Int J Dev Neurosci 11: 603–612.

Waxman SG (1977) Conduction in myelinated, unmyelinated, and demyelinated fibers. Arch Neurol 34: 585–589.

Waxman SG, Brill MH (1978) Conduction through demyelinated plaques in multiple sclerosis: computer simulations of facilitation by short internodes. J Neurol Neurosurg Psychiatry 41: 408–417.

Waxman SG, Foster RE (1980) Development of the axon membrane during differentiation of myelinated fibres in spinal nerve roots. Proc R Soc Lond [Biol] 209: 441–446.

Wiley-Livingston C, Ellisman MH (1980) Development of axonal membrane specializations defines nodes of Ranvier and precedes Schwann cell myelin elaboration. Dev Biol 79: 334–355.

XIX YOU CAN'T STEP IN THE SAME RIVER TWICE

The ten billion neurons within the brain and spinal cord form a computer that is more complex and flexible than any device produced thus far by man. They are "electrogenic" and communicate with each other by generating sequences of brief "all-or-none" electrical impulses, called action potentials, that last about a millisecond. Each action potential, according to classical neurophysiological doctrine, is the same. In encoding information for transmission to other neurons, a neuron uses its all-or-none impulses as basic coinage, like the dots in morse code. Changes in the rate and pattern of action potentials convey each neuron's message, but the action potentials do not vary. Because of this, research on plasticity in the nervous system—the structural and molecular basis for adaptive changes that include learning and memory—has not focused on the action potential-producing machinery.

Synapses, in contrast, have classically been considered as an important source of neuronal plasticity. In deciding whether or not to generate an action potential at any given moment, the neuron assesses information which has been transmitted to it from other neurons at synapses, which can be excitatory or inhibitory. The neuron integrates incoming synaptic signals by a process similar to algebraic summation: in a crude sense, it adds up the excitatory (positive) and inhibitory (negative) synaptic signals. If the sum reaches a critical value, called the threshold, the neuron generates an action potential. If threshold is not reached, the neuron remains silent. Synaptic strength—the size of the signal produced by the synapse—has long been known to be modifiable by experience. Synapses can become stronger or weaker, depending on the context in which they are activated, and this "synaptic plasticity" can strengthen or weaken neuronal circuits as a result of experience, thereby contributing to learning and memory.

Might the electrogenic machinery, which produces action potentials, also be modifiable? The generation of action potentials depends on sodium channels, which, as discussed in part XV, are the molecular batteries of the nervous system. Over the past few years we have learned that nearly a dozen genes encode different sodium channels with different molecular properties. At least eight of these are expressed, alone or in various combinations, within various types of neurons. The different sodium channels open and close at different rates. They also require different degrees of stimulation to generate their electrical currents. That is, they have different thresholds.

A given neuron does not always transmit the same message—if it did, it would not convey much information. A neuron may be in a quiescent state (generating action potentials at low frequencies, for example, 1–2 impulses per second) at some times, and in a bursting state (generating impulses at a higher frequency of, say, 20–30 per second) at other times. It had long been recognized that, when neurons pass from a quiescent state to a bursting state, they utilize their repertoire of preexisting sodium channels in different ways, opening and closing them at various times to generate a series of action potentials with different rates and patterns. But do neurons deploy a new and different ensemble of sodium channels as they move from one activity state to another? The answer might tell us whether, in addition to synaptic plasticity, functional remodeling of the neuron itself—changes within its electrogenic apparatus—can contribute to plasticity in neuronal circuits.

We knew that there are changes in the production of sodium channels within neurons during development of the brain and spinal cord, and we had previously shown that some of these developmental changes were activity-dependent, requiring sensory input (Sashihara et al. 1996, 1997). Now, however, we wanted to look for changes in sodium channel expression in the adult nervous system. In choosing a model system we were influenced by Masaki Tanaka, an expert on the hypothalamus from Kyoto, who was spending a year on sabbatical in our laboratory. Tanaka lobbied for a cluster of neurons (called magnocellular neurosecretory neurons) that is located within the supraoptic nucleus of the hypothalamus. The supraoptic nucleus acts as a thirst center within the brain. In its basal state, the magnocellular neurons are relatively quiescent, firing irregularly at low frequencies (fewer than three impulses per second). However, when there is a need for more water in the body, these neurons generate bursts of action potentials at much higher frequencies, signaling the need to drink. This provided a model in which we could manipulate the environment and then study the effects on the expression of sodium channels. We hypothesized that as these neurons adapt to meet the need for more water by moving from a quiescent to a bursting state, they rebuild their electrogenic membranes by deploying a new repertoire of sodium channels with lower thresholds (Tanaka et al. 1999). To test this hypothesis, we studied magnocellular neurons under normal conditions and following salt-loading of rats (by feeding them salt water), a manipulation that causes these animals to become thirsty.

As a first step we studied sodium channel gene expression by measuring the mRNAs which encode sodium channels within the magnocellular neurons. In these experiments we used in situ hybridization to visualize the mRNAs for various sodium channels. These experiments showed us that there is an up-regulation of the genes encoding two sodium channels (called a-II and Na6) after salt-loading. This suggested that the neurons might be deploying new sodium channels as they adapted to increased salt loads. A next step was to learn whether the increased activity of these genes was accompanied by an increase in production of sodium channel protein. To do this, we used antibodies directed against sodium channels so that we could visualize them. These experiments taught us that the increase in sodium channel gene expression resulted in an increase in the amount of sodium channel protein in magnocellular neurons.

We had learned that activity of two sodium channel genes was up-regulated, resulting in the production of increased amounts of sodium-channel protein, as the magnocellular neurons made the transition to the bursting state. We now wanted to know whether these molecular changes altered the function of the neurons. To address this we asked whether the channels were inserted into the membranes of the magnocellular neurons, and, if so, whether they became functional so that they could alter the thresholds or firing patterns of these cells. For these experiments we used patch-clamp recording to eavesdrop on the tiny electrical currents produced by the two different sodium channels (a-II and Na6) in these cells. The currents produced by these two channels have different molecular signatures, much like the different footprints left by different people. The a-II sodium channel is fast, and it opens during the nerve impulse itself. The Na6 sodium channel, in contrast, is slow, and it is opened by smaller stimuli. Because of its low threshold, the Na6 channel can respond to relatively subtle stimuli in resting neurons, and serves as a booster, amplifying various inputs (such as inputs signaling changes in salt concentration). Our patch-clamp recordings showed us that there was, indeed, an increase in the number of sodium channels in the membranes of salt-loaded magnocellular neurons. But they also revealed another aspect of the molecular remodeling that had gone on in these cells: The number of fast sodium channels in the membranes of the salt-loaded magnocellular neurons was increased by 20 percent; but in contrast, the number of slow channels was increased by 50 percent. As the magnocellular neurons entered the bursting state, they thus expressed a different mixture of sodium channels. The larger proportion of slow channels in salt-loaded neurons would be expected to increase the sensitivity of these cells, so that they generate more action potentials in response to a given stimulus. These neurons thus had rebuilt themselves at the molecular and functional levels, retuning their electrogenic membranes as they made the transition to a bursting state.

We do not yet know whether changes in sodium channel expression, similar to those in magnocellular neurons, contribute to processes such as learning and memory, but the available data provide some hints suggesting that this may occur (Waxman 1999a, 1999b; Desai, Rutherford, and Turrigiano 1999). It has been suggested, on the basis of computer modeling, that neurons may adjust their own ion channel expression in an ongoing way, so as to constantly maximize the information that they can encode (Stemmler and Koch 1999).

Irrespective of whether changes in ion channel deployment contribute to learning and memory at the level of the organism, we are learning that the plasticity of the brain extends even to the electrogenic molecules—such as sodium channels that generate nerve impulses—that make it special. We are again reminded of the nervous system's complexity and richness: The cells and molecules of the brain and spinal cord are subject to constant change. Clearly, you can't step in the same river twice.

References

Desai, N. S., Rutherford, L. C., and Turrigiano, G. G. Plasticity in the intrinsic excitability of cortical pyramidal neurons. *Nature Neurosci.* 2: 515–520, 1999.

Sashihara, S., Greer, C. A., Oh, Y., and Waxman, S. G. Cell specific differential expression of Na^+ channel $\beta 1$ subunit mRNA in the olfactory system during postnatal development and following denervation. *J. Neurosci.* 16: 702–714, 1996.

Sashihara, S., Waxman, S. G., and Greer, C. A. Down-regulation of Na^+ channel mRNA following sensory deprivation of tufted cells in the neonatal rat olfactory bulb. *NeuroReport* 8: 1289–1293, 1997.

Stemmler, M., and Koch, C. How voltage-dependent conductances can adapt to maximize the information encoded by neuronal firing rate. *Nature Neurosci.* 2: 521–527, 1999.

Tanaka, M., Cummins, T. R., Ishikawa, K., Black, J. A., Ibata, Y., and Waxman, S. G. Molecular and functional remodeling of electrogenic membrane of hypothalamic neurons in response to changes in their input. *Proc. Natl. Acad. Sci. USA* 96: 1088–1093, 1999.

Waxman, S. G. The neuron as a dynamic electrogenic machine: modulation of sodium channel expression as a basis for functional plasticity in neurons. *Phil. Trans. Roy. Soc. B.*, 1999a.

Waxman, S. G. The molecular basis for electrogenic computation in the brain: you can't step in the same river twice. *Molec. Psychiatry* 4: 222–228, 1999b.

34 Molecular and Functional Remodeling of Electrogenic Membrane of Hypothalamic Neurons in Response to Changes in Their Input

M. Tanaka, T. R. Cummins, K. Ishikawa, J. A. Black, Y. Ibata, and S. G. Waxman

Abstract Neurons respond to stimuli by integrating generator and synaptic potentials and generating action potentials. However, whether the underlying electrogenic machinery within neurons itself changes, in response to alterations in input, is not known. To determine whether there are changes in Na^+ channel expression and function within neurons in response to altered input, we exposed magnocellular neurosecretory cells (MNCs) in the rat supraoptic nucleus to different osmotic milieus by salt-loading and studied Na^+ channel mRNA and protein, and Na^+ currents, in these cells. In situ hybridization demonstrated significantly increased mRNA levels for α-II, Na6, β1 and β2 Na^+ channel subunits, and immunohistochemistry/immunoblotting showed increased Na^+ channel protein after salt-loading. Using patch-clamp recordings to examine the deployment of functional Na^+ channels in the membranes of MNCs, we observed an increase in the amplitude of the transient Na^+ current after salt-loading and an even greater increase in amplitude and density of the persistent Na^+ current evoked at subthreshold potentials by slow ramp depolarizations. These results demonstrate that MNCs respond to salt-loading by selectively synthesizing additional, functional Na^+ channel subtypes whose deployment in the membrane changes its electrogenic properties. Thus, neurons may respond to changes in their input not only by producing different patterns of electrical activity, but also by remodeling the electrogenic machinery that underlies this activity.

The nervous system responds to environmental stimuli with altered patterns of electrical activity that trigger physiological responses and behaviors that tend to protect the organism and/or help it adapt to its environment. The molecular and cellular mechanisms underlying these altered patterns of neuronal activity are not fully understood. They depend, in part, on the integration of generator potentials and excitatory and inhibitory postsynaptic potentials that impinge on

Reprinted with permission from *Proceedings of the National Academy of Sciences USA* 96: 1088–1093; 1999.

neurons within the circuit under study. Whether the electrogenic machinery responsible for this signal integration within these neurons itself changes, however, in response to environmental changes is not well understood.

A model for studying the neuronal response to environmental changes is provided by the magnocellular neurosecretory cells (MNCs) in the supraoptic nucleus (SON), which send axons to the neurohypophysis and fire in bursts so as to release vasopressin in response to increases in plasma osmolality. Vasopressin release is a function of action potential frequency in these cells (1, 2) and firing frequency, in turn, is modulated by osmotic stimuli (3–5). Action potential activity in these cells is Na^+ dependent and tetrodotoxin (TTX) sensitive, indicating that it is mediated by Na^+ channels (6–9). While it is known that eight types of Na^+ channels, encoded by distinct genes, are expressed in neurons (10–17), the identity of the Na^+ channels in supraoptic MNCs is not known. Moreover, the basic mechanisms that lead to these environmentally triggered changes in firing pattern in supraoptic neurons have been only partially delineated. It is known that MNCs possess an intrinsic regenerative mechanism (6, 18, 19), which can be triggered by endogenous osmosensitivity mediated by mechanosensitive channels (20), providing an electrogenic cascade that can respond to changes in the environment. There is also evidence for synaptic activation of MNCs, which leads to their firing and release of vasopressin, after exposure of circumventricular neurons to osmotic stimulation (21). In the present report we demonstrate an additional, previously undescribed, response of these cells to changes in their input: molecular and functional remodeling by means of the increased expression of specific Na^+ channel α- and β-subunit genes and addition of additional functional Na^+ channels that alter the electrogenic properties of the cell membrane.

Materials and Methods

Salt-Loading

Adult male Sprague–Dawley rats (200–220 g), housed under a 12-h–12-h dark–light cycle, were salt-loaded with 2% NaCl (ad libitum) in their drinking water and unlimited access to food, and they were sacrificed after 7 days. All experiments were approved by the institutional animal use and care committee. To confirm the extent of salt-loading, plasma osmotic pressure was measured (vapor pressure osmometer model 5500; Wescor, Logan, UT), demonstrating a significant ($P < 0.01$) increase in salt-loaded rats (321.5 ± 4.48 milliosmolar) compared with controls (292.4 ± 0.79 milliosmolar). Body weights were significantly ($P < 0.01$) lower in salted-loaded (194.3 ± 11.9 g) compared with control (248.4 ± 7.11 g) rats. Ten animals (five control and five salt-loading) each were used for in situ hybridization, SP20 immunocytochemistry, and immunoblot analysis. Six control and six salt-loaded rats were used for patch-clamp studies.

In Situ Hybridization

Rats were anesthetized with ketamine/xylazine (40/2.5 mg/kg, i.p.) and perfused with 4% paraformaldehyde in 0.14 M phosphate buffer. Brains were postfixed overnight at 4 °C and cryoprotected, and serial coronal sections (30 μm) of hypothalamus were cut and collected in 4× SSC. Sections, including the SON from the level of the preoptic area rostrally to the retrochiasmatic area caudally, were divided into six groups for detection of Na$^+$ channel mRNAs. Sections from control and salt-loaded groups were hybridized in the same chamber by a free-floating method (22). Sections were deproteinized with proteinase K (2.5 μg/ml) acetylated with 0.25% acetic anhydride and 0.1 M triethanolamine and were incubated in hybridization buffer (50% formamide/10% dextran sulfate/20 mM Tris·HCl,

pH 7.5/5 mM EDTA/0.3 M NaCl/0.2% SDS/ 500 μg/ml yeast tRNA/1× Denhardt's solution/ 10 mM DTT), containing digoxigenin (DIG)-UTP-labeled Na$^+$ channel riboprobe (0.25 ng/μl) for 12 h at 60 °C. After rinsing in 2× SSC/50% formamide and RNase solution in 0.5× SSC, sections were transferred into buffer 1 (100 mM Tris·HCl, pH 7.5/150 mM NaCl), incubated in alkaline phosphatase-labeled anti-DIG antibody (dilution, 1:500 in buffer 1) overnight at 4 °C, and reacted in a chromogen solution containing 4-nitroblue tetrazolium chloride (NBT) and 5-bromo-4-chloro-3-indolyl phosphate (BCIP) in buffer (100 mM Tris·HCl, pH 9.5/10 mM NaCl/ 50 mM MgCl$_2$) for 4 h at room temperature.

DIG-labeled antisense and sense riboprobes for Na$^+$ channel α-subunits α-I (nucleotides 7385–7820, GenBank numbering), α-II (nucleotides 6807–7302), α-III (nucleotides 6325–6822), Na6 (nucleotides 6461–6761), and β-subunit β1 (nucleotides 457–790) and β2 (nucleotides 140–669) were synthesized from each cDNA as previously described by reverse transcription–PCR (11). Transcription was carried out with 120 units of appropriate RNA polymerase and 1 μg of linearized template in a reaction mixture containing buffer (1×), 0.35 mM DIG-11-UTP, 1 mM GTP, ATP, and CTP, 0.65 mM UTP, 10 mM DTT, and 10 units of RNase inhibitor (Boehringer Mannheim). Sense riboprobes yielded no signals on in situ hybridization.

For quantitation of hybridization signal, images were captured with a ComputerEyes/ 1024, version 1.07, capture board. Optical densities (ODs) of the circumscribed SON were obtained within the linear calibration range by using the NIH IMAGE program, calibrated with neutral density filters of 0.1, 0.3, and 0.6 OD, and fitted to a straight line. Background OD, measured in the lateral hypothalamic area surrounding the SON in each section, was subtracted from all signals.

For colocalization of vasopressin and oxytocin peptide and α Na6 mRNA (figure 34.1), control

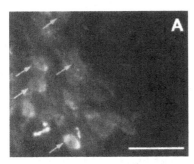

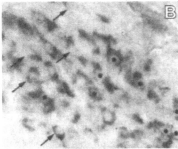

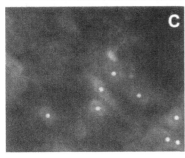

Figure 34.1

In situ hybridization together with double immuno-fluorescence labeling demonstrates that mRNA for the Na6 sodium channel α-subunit (*B*) is present in both vasopressin-containing MNCs (*A*; same cells marked with arrows in *B*) and oxytocin-containing MNCs (*C*; same cells marked with asterisks in *B*) within the SON. (Bar = 50 μm.)

rats were perfused and fixed as described above. Coronal cryostat sections (10 μm) were incubated overnight at 4 °C with a mixture of guinea pig anti-vasopressin (1:1500; Peninsula Lab Inc., USA) and rabbit anti-oxytocin (1:1000; Peninsula Laboratories) in 0.1 M phosphate-buffered saline (PBS), treated with diethyl pyrocarbonate to protect from RNase. Sections were rinsed twice in PBS and incubated with fluorescein isothiocyanate (FITC)-labeled goat anti-guinea pig IgG (1:250; Vector Laboratories) and Texas red-labeled goat anti-rabbit IgG (1:250; Vector Laboratories) in PBS for 3 h at room temperature. After rinsing in 0.1 M PBS, sections were mounted on poly(L-lysine)-coated slides coverslipped with Vectashield (Vector Laboratories), and examined and photographed with an epifluorescence microscope equipped with a double filter for FITC and Texas red fluorescence. Sections were subsequently processed for in situ hybridization as described above, using a DIG-labeled probe that recognizes Na⁺ channel α-subunit Na6. In control experiments. FITC-positive neurons after incubation with anti-oxytocin serum and Texas red-positive neurons after incubation with anti-vasopressin serum were not detected.

Immunocytochemistry and Immunoblotting

Antibody SP20 was generated against a conserved region of rat brain sodium channel (residues 1106–1126 of sodium channel II (23). The affinity purification and specificity of SP20 have been previously described (23).

Rats were perfused with 4% paraformaldehyde, and the brain and pituitary were removed and postfixed for 3 h. After immersion in 20% sucrose in 0.1 M PBS for 24 h, cryosections (25 μm) containing SON, median eminence, and pituitary neural lobe were cut. Sections were incubated in blocking solution (PBS containing 5% normal goat serum and 1% BSA) containing 0.1% Triton X-100 twice for 15 min at room temperature, incubated with antibody SP20

(1:50) in blocking solution overnight at 4°C, washed twice in PBS, and incubated overnight at 4°C with biotinylated anti-rabbit serum (1:1000, Vector Laboratories). Sections were then incubated in avidin-biotin-peroxidase complex (ABC) (1:1000, Vector Laboratories) for 2 h, exposed for 10 min to 0.015% 3,3'-diaminobenzidine·4HCl in 0.05 M Tris·HCl buffer containing 0.005% H_2O_2. Control experiments in which the primary antibody or secondary antibody was omitted showed no staining.

Immunoblotting was carried out on samples derived from the SON of single rats and from the pooled posterior pituitary lobes of two rats. Equal volumes of membrane protein from each group ($\approx$10–40 µg) were added to reducing SDS sample buffer, incubated at 37°C for 30 min, separated by SDS/6% polyacrylamide gel electrophoresis, and electrotransferred onto poly-(vinylidene difluoride) (PVDF) membrane. Membranes were blocked with 10% nonfat dry milk in Tris-buffered saline (100 mM Tris, pH 8.0/0.9% NaCl) containing 0.1% Tween-20, and then incubated overnight at 4°C with SP20 (1:100). Membranes were washed and incubated with alkaline phosphatase-conjugated goat anti-rabbit IgG secondary antibody (1:1000) for 2 h at room temperature. After a brief wash, immunoreactive bands were visualized with 0.38% 4-nitroblue tetrazolium chloride/0.19% 5-bromo-4-chloro-3-indolyl phosphate.

Membrane Preparations

SON and posterior lobe of the pituitary from control and salt-loading rats were quickly microdissected after decapitation, and crude lysed membrane fractions were prepared (24). In brief, 10- to 40-mg tissue samples were homogenized in 5 mM Tris·HCl, pH 7.4/0.3 M sucrose containing protease inhibitors (1 mM phenylmethanesulfonyl fluoride, 1 µg/ml leupeptin, and 2 µg/ml aprotinin), and nuclei and other debris were pelleted twice at 1,000 × g for 10 min. Supernatants were centrifuged at 350,000 × g for 5 min and resuspended in homogenization buffer. To obtain solubilized membrane fractions, 12.5% Triton X-100, 100 mM EDTA, and 2 M KCl were added to final concentrations of 2.5%, 2.5 mM, and 100 mM, and supernatants were incubated at 4°C for 1 h and then centrifuged at 16,000 × g for 10 min. Supernatants were used for protein quantitative analysis and immunoblot analysis. Protein was determined by using the D_c protein assay (Bio-Rad) with BSA as a standard.

Whole-Cell Patch Clamp

MNCs in the SON from adult male rats were dissociated as previously described (25) with modification. SON were dissected with iridectomy scissors in ice-chilled Ringer's solution without Ca^{2+}. They were transferred into complete saline solution (CSS; 137 mM NaCl/ 5.3 mM KCl/1 mM $MgCl_2$/25 mM sorbitol/ 10 mM Hepes, pH 7.2) supplemented with proteases X and XIV (1 mg/ml, Sigma), for 45 min at 23°C under oxygen bubbling and gentle stirring, rinsed in CSS for 15 min at 23°C under oxygen bubbling, and dissociated by mechanical trituration with graduated polished pipettes and placed on laminin-coated cover glasses in 35-mm Petri dishes. SON neurons were recorded in the whole-cell patch-clamp configuration within 2 h after dissociation. All recordings were made with an EPC-9 amplifier (v 7.52, HEKA Electronics. Lambrecht/Pfalz, Germany). Recording electrodes were 1-2 MΩ, and 80% series resistance compensation was used. The pipette solution contained 140 mM CsF, 2 mM $MgCl_2$, 1 mM EGTA, and 10 mM NaHepes, pH 7.3, and the extracellular solution contained 140 mM NaCl, 3 mM KCl, 2 mM $MgCl_2$, 1 mM $CaCl_2$, and 10 mM Hepes, pH 7.3. All recordings were conducted at room temperature ($\approx$21°C).

Results

We first investigated expression of mRNA encoding Na^+ channel α (I, II, III, Na6) and β (β1 and β2) subunits known to be present in

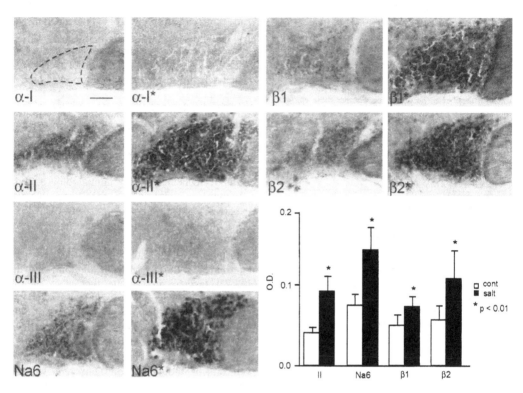

Figure 34.2

In situ hybridization with subtype-specific riboprobes for Na^+ channel subunits α-I, α-II, α-III, Na6, β1, and β2 in the SON. α-I and α-III mRNA are not detectable. Low levels of α-II, Na6, β1, and β2 mRNA are present in the control SON (no asterisks), and there is a distinct up-regulation of each of these transcripts after salt-loading (asterisks). The fields shown were scanned from micrographs and digitally enhanced to illustrate the up-regulation of specific transcripts, but they do not illustrate the quantitative magnitudes of the changes. Optical densities from unenhanced micrographs (histogram, *lower right*) provide a quantitative measure of mRNA levels and show significant changes for α-II, Na6, β1, and β2 transcripts in salt-loaded rats. (Bar = 100 μm.)

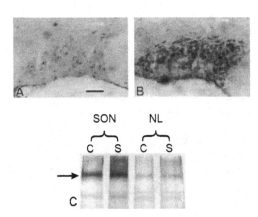

Figure 34.3
Sodium channel immunoreactivity with SP20 antibody is increased in the SON of salt-loaded rats (*B*) compared with controls (*A*). Immunoblotting (*C*) shows a 230-kDa band (arrow) that is denser in the salt-loaded (S) SON than in the control (C) SON. There is a less pronounced increase in density of this band in the salt-loaded pituitary neural lobe (NL). (Bar = 100 μm.)

the brain by in situ hybridization using isoform-specific riboprobes in adult rats under normal conditions and after chronic salt-loading, which exposes SON neurons to elevated extracellular osmolality (26–28).

Almost all MNCs in the SON displayed moderate levels of α-II and Na6 mRNA in control rats. Combining in situ hybridization with double immunofluorescence labeling, we observed that both vasopressin and oxytocin-containing MNCs of the SON express Na6 mRNA (figure 34.1). Significant levels of α-I and α-III mRNA could not be detected in MNCs. mRNAs for both Na$^+$ channel β subunits are present in MNCs, β1 at low-to-moderate levels and β2 at moderate levels (figure 34.2).

There was distinct up-regulation of α-II, Na6, β1, and β2 mRNA levels, but not of α-I or α-III mRNA, in salt-loaded rats (figure 34.2), which was reflected by significant increases in optical density (histogram in figure 34.2). In addition to an increase in optical density, there was a signif-

icant increase in the area of SON expressing each of these transcripts (figure 34.2), because of increased cell sizes, as previously reported (29) in salt-loaded rats. Thus expression of specific Na$^+$ channel transcripts in MNCs was increased by salt-loading.

To determine whether the changes in Na$^+$ channel mRNA in the salt-loaded SON were paralleled by increases in Na$^+$ channel protein, we used SP20 antibody, which recognizes a conserved region in Na$^+$ channels (23), for immunocytochemistry and immunoblot analysis. Immunoreactivity in the SON was distinctly increased in salt-loaded rats (figure 34.3*A* and *B*). In contrast, we did not detect differences in immunoreactivity of the median eminence or posterior pituitary, the sites of the axons and terminals of the SON MNCs (data not shown).

To further substantiate the effect of salt-loading on Na$^+$ channel expression, we performed Western blot analysis with SP20 antibody, using membrane preparations from the SON and from the site of termination of MNC axons, the posterior pituitary (figure 34.3*C*). In all lanes, a band of about 230 kDa, consistent with that previously reported (23), was present. Additional minor bands at ≈170 kDa may represent channel precursors or breakdown products. The 230-kDa immunoreactive band was stained more densely in the salt-loaded SON than in the control SON. The 230-kDa band from salt-loaded posterior pituitary gland was also denser than the control, but the difference was less pronounced. These immunoblots confirm and extend the results of SP20 immunocytochemistry in showing an increase in Na$^+$ channel protein in the salt-loaded SON and posterior pituitary.

These results show that the transcription of Na$^+$ channel mRNA is up-regulated in the salt-loaded SON and suggest that this up-regulation results in increased synthesis of Na$^+$ channel protein in these cells. To determine whether these changes result in increased incorporation of functional Na$^+$ channels in the membranes of these cells, we dissociated MNCs and carried out

Table 34.1
Properties of Na$^+$ channels

Measurement	Control	Salt-loaded	P
Cell capacitance, pF	16.2 ± 0.4	21.5 ± 0.8	<0.001
Transient current			
Peak amplitude, nA	15.8 ± 1.1	25.3 ± 2.1	<0.001
Density, pA/pF	989 ± 70	1206 ± 95	0.09
	$n = 44$	$n = 45$	
$V_{1/2}$ activation, mV	-28.5 ± 1.4	-34.4 ± 1.2	<0.005
$V_{1/2}$ inactivation, mV	-62.9 ± 1.3	-68.6 ± 1.4	<0.01
	$n = 17$	$n = 17$	
Inactivation kinetics			
Recovery at -80 mV, ms	13.6 ± 0.7	19.6 ± 1.7	<0.005
Development at -80 mV, ms	28.8 ± 2.2	37.7 ± 3.6	<0.05
	$n = 33$	$n = 30$	
Ramp current			
Amplitude, pA	190.3 ± 17	396.2 ± 50	<0.001
Density, pA/pF	12.0 ± 1.0	19.5 ± 2.3	<0.005
	$n = 34$	$n = 29$	

patch-clamp studies. MNC neurons were rapidly isolated from control rats ($n = 6$) and salt-loaded rats ($n = 6$). Both groups (table 34.1) expressed fast, TTX-sensitive, sodium currents, but the peak sodium current amplitude (measured at 0 mV from a -130 mV holding potential) was 60% larger for MNC neurons isolated from the salt-loaded SON neurons (figure 34.4A; 15.8 ± 1.1 nA for control, $n = 44$; 25.3 ± 2.1 nA for salt-loaded, $n = 45$; $P < 0.001$). However, because the MNC neurons also exhibited a significant increase in soma size (measured by cell capacitance; 16.2 ± 0.4 pF control, 21.5 ± 0.8 pF salt-loaded; $P < 0.001$), peak current density (peak current amplitude divided by cell capacitance) was only 20% larger in freshly isolated salt-loaded MNC neurons. The voltage dependence of activation and steady-state inactivation were shifted about -6 mV for salt-loaded neurons compared with control neurons (figure 34.4B).

Because persistent sodium currents might contribute to the intrinsic burst activity of MNC neurons, we also examined sodium currents elicited with slow ramp depolarizations (0.23 mV/ ms) in control and salt-loaded neurons. While TTX-sensitive sodium currents that activated near threshold (i.e., at potentials from -65 to -55 mV) were recorded in both groups, the salt-loaded neurons exhibited significantly ($P < 0.005$) larger threshold ramp currents (figure 34.4C). Because slow closed-state inactivation of sodium channels can underlie ramp currents (30), we examined the kinetics of inactivation at -80 mV. Both the development of inactivation and recovery from inactivation were significantly slower in salt-loaded neurons (table 34.1), suggesting that the increased ramp currents in salt-loaded neurons arise at least in part from an increase in sodium channels with slow closed-state inactivation. The maximum ramp current amplitude was doubled (table 34.1) and

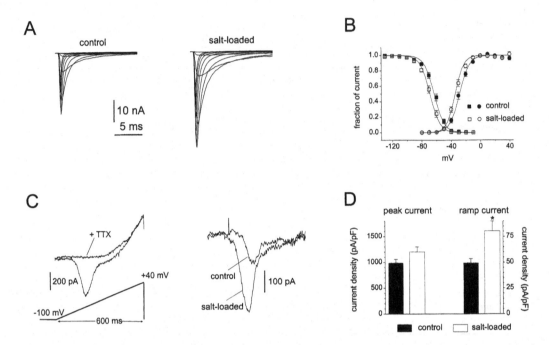

Figure 34.4

Comparison of Na$^+$ currents in control and salt-loaded SON neurons. (*A*) Family of traces from representative SON neurons freshly isolated from control (*left*) or salt-loaded (*right*) rats. The currents were elicited by 40-ms test pulses to various potentials from −60 to 30 mV. Cells were held at −100 mV. (*B*) Normalized activation (circles) and steady-state inactivation (squares) data for control (filled symbols; $n = 17$) and salt-loaded (open symbols; $n = 17$) neurons. Curves through the points are fits to Boltzmann functions. For activation the $V_{1/2}$ and k values were −28.5 ± 1.4 and 6.7 ± 0.3 mV for control MNCs and −34.4 ± 1.2 and 5.8 ± 0.2 mV for salt-loaded MNCs. For inactivation the $V_{1/2}$ and k values were −62.9 ± 1.3 and 6.6 ± 0.2 mV for control MNCs and −68.6 ± 1.4 and 6.5 ± 0.2 mV for salt-loaded MNCs. Steady-state inactivation was measured with 500-ms inactivating prepulses. Cells were held at prepulse potentials over the range of −130 to −10 mV prior to a test pulse to 0 mV for 20 ms. Error bars indicate SE. (*C*) Ramp currents are elicited in MNCs by slow voltage ramps (600-ms voltage ramp extending from −100 to +40 mV). *Left* shows the ramp current in a salt-loaded MNC before and after the addition of 250 nM TTX to the extracellular solution. TTX blocks the ramp current. *Right* shows the TTX-sensitive ramp currents in representative control and salt-loaded MNCs. Leak currents recorded after application of 250 nM TTX were subtracted. (*D*) The peak and ramp current densities (estimated by dividing the maximum currents by the cell capacitance) are larger in salt-loaded neurons (n = 29) than in control neurons (n = 34); note that the increase is proportionately greater for the ramp currents. Error bars indicate SE, and the ∗ indicates P < 0.005.

the ramp current density was ≈50% larger in the salt-loaded neurons (figure 34.4D). Thus, the peak and ramp currents were both increased after salt-loading, but to significantly different degrees. These results show that the functional properties of the sodium currents in salt-loaded SON neurons differ from those in control neurons in several ways. Because ramp currents activate at potentials close to threshold, these changes are expected to have an impact on the excitability of MNCs.

Discussion

Our observations indicate that two Na^+ channel α subunits, α-II and Na6, are coexpressed in most MNCs in the SON. Two separable components of the Na^+ current have been identified in these cells, with transient and persistent kinetics (9, 25). In cerebellar Purkinje cells, which also express two Na^+ channel transcripts, Na6 appears to produce a persistent sodium current and α-I appears to produce a transient current (31). Ramp currents in Purkinje cells, similar to those that we evoked in MNCs, are produced by Na6 channels (32).

Our results demonstrate an up-regulation of mRNA for two Na^+ channel α subunits (α-II and Na6) and both β subunits (β1 and β2), and show increased levels of Na^+ channel protein and Na^+ current, in MNCs in the SON of salt-loaded rats. These results suggest that MNCs insert additional Na^+ channels, including auxiliary β subunits (33–35) in their membranes in response to osmotic changes. Peak sodium current amplitudes in salt-loaded MNCs were increased from 15.8 ± 1.1 nA to 25.3 ± 2.3 nA, while peak sodium current densities were increased by a smaller fraction ($1{,}206 \pm 95$ pA/pF, salt-loaded; 989 ± 70 pA/pF, controls). This is probably due to the increase in cell size within the SON that occurs in salt-loaded animals (29). The increase in SP20 immunoreactivity within

the salt-loaded SON, in the context of the relatively small increase in sodium current density (which provides a measure of average sodium channel density over the cell body, assuming a relatively uniform distribution of channels), might be interpreted as suggesting that additional Na^+ channels may have been added in a nonuniform pattern, clustered close to action potential trigger zones or other critical regions. Increased SP20 immunoreactivity within the salt-loaded SON, however, is also consistent with the alternative possibility of an increased pool of intracellular channels or channel precursors. This intracellular pool could serve to maintain Na^+ channel densities, possibly in the context of activity-related turnover of channels (36–38), so as to maintain an appropriate level of electrogenic tuning. The increase in the ramp currents (figure 34.4C and D), however, was greater than that of peak transient Na^+ current. This difference may be functionally important because non-inactivating and slowly inactivating Na^+ channels, which produce ramp currents, can amplify generator and postsynaptic potentials and can contribute to the generation of tonic and phasic burst patterns in neurons (39–44).

Insertion of Na^+ channels in the membrane of MNCs may poise them to respond to changes in their input. MNCs release vasopressin [and oxytocin (45, 46)] from their terminals in response to osmotic stimulation. This neuropeptide release is related to the frequency of action potentials, which are known to be Na^+ dependent and TTX sensitive (6, 9) in these cells. Thus the expression of Na^+ channels may effect the burst threshold and contribute to the synaptically driven (21) as well as the endogenous component of the response to osmotic changes in these cells. Interestingly, there is a continued increase in the firing rate within bursts, from day to day, that is observed in phasic SON MNCs during a 5-day period of water deprivation (47).

Our results may have implications for neuronal cell types other than hypothalamic neurons.

Persistent Na^+ channels contribute to oscillatory bursting behavior in a number of types of neurons (48–53). Electrical activity, cAMP, and cytosolic calcium levels regulate Na^+ channel α subunit expression in muscle (54) and neural cells (55–57). There is evidence for plasticity in expression of other ion channels, including K^+ and Ca^{2+} channels that also contribute to neuronal excitability (58, 59). It is thus possible that expression of voltage-sensitive channels contributing to excitability is altered in neuronal cell types outside of the hypothalamus in response to changes in their input.

We have demonstrated that, in response to external stimuli, SON neurons respond not only by altering their firing patterns but also by selectively activating specific Na^+ channel genes and deploying additional functional channels so as to change the electrogenic properties of their membrane. Thus, these cells not only integrate incoming signals (generator potentials, post-synaptic potentials) so as to produce different patterns of electrical activity in response to changes in their environment but also rebuild the electrogenic machinery that integrates these signals and generates electrical activity. This molecular and functional remodeling may provide a novel mechanism that underlies state-dependent changes in the input-output functions of neurons.

Acknowledgments

We thank W. A. Catterall and R. Westenbroek for the gift of SP-20 antibody. This work was supported, in part, by the Medical Research Service, Department of Veterans Affairs, and by Grant RG-1912 from the National Multiple Sclerosis Society. M.T. was supported by Kyoto Prefectural University of Medicine. T.R.C. was supported by a fellowship from the Spinal Cord Research Foundation. K.I. was supported by a Multiple Sclerosis Research Fellowship from the Eastern Paralyzed Veterans Association.

References

1. Dreifuss, J. J., Kalnins, I., Kelly, J. S. and Ruf, K. B. (1971) *J. Physiol. (London)* 215: 805–817.

2. Dyball, R. E. J. and Pountney, P. S. (1973) *J. Endocrinol.* 56: 91–98.

3. Walters, J. K. and Hatton, G. I. (1974) *Physiol. Behav.* 13: 661–667.

4. Arnauld, E., Dufy, B. and Vincent, J.-D. (1975) *Brain Res.* 100: 315–325.

5. Mason, W. T. (1980) *Nature (London)* 287: 154–157.

6. Andrew, R. D. and Dudek, F. E. (1983) *Science* 221: 1050–1052.

7. Cobbett, P. and Mason, W. T. (1987) *Brain Res.* 409: 175–180.

8. Inenaga, K., Nagatomo, T., Kannan, H. and Yamashita, H. (1993) *J. Physiol. (London)* 465: 289–301.

9. Li, Z. and Hatton, G. I. (1996) *J. Physiol. (London)* 496: 379–394.

10. Akopian, A. N., Sivilotti, L., and Wood, J. N. (1996) *Nature (London)* 379: 258–262.

11. Black, J. A., Dib-Hajj, S., McNabola, K., Jeste, J. Rizzo, M. A., Kocsis, J. D. and Waxman, S. G. (1996) *Mol. Brain Res.* 43: 117–131.

12. Kayano, T., Noda, M., Flockerzi, V., Takahashi, H. and Numa, S. (1988) *FEBS Lett.* 228: 187–194.

13. Noda, M., Ikeda, T., Kayano, T., Suzuki, H., Takeshima, I. I., Kurasaki, M. and Numa, S. (1986) *Nature (London)* 320: 188–192.

14. Sangameswaran, L., Delgado, S. G., Fish, L. M., Koch, B. D., Jakeman, L. B., Stewart, G. R., Sze, P., Hunter, J. C., Eglen, R. M. and Herman, R. C. (1996) *J. Biol. Chem.* 271: 5953–5956.

15. Schaller, K. L., Krzemien, D. M., Yarowsky, P. J., Krueger, B. K. and Caldwell, J. H. (1995) *J. Neurosci.* 15: 3231–3242.

16. Toledo-Aral, J. J., Moss, B. L., He, Z.-J., Koszowski, A. G., Whisenand, T., Levinson, S. R., Wolf, J. J., Silos-Santiago, I., Halegoua, S. and Mandel, G. (1997) *Proc. Natl. Acad. Sci. USA* 94: 1527–1532.

17. Dib-Hajj, S. D., Tyrrell, L., Black J. A. and Waxman, S. G. (1998) *Proc. Natl. Acad. Sci. USA* 95: 8963–8968.

18. Hatton, G. I. (1982) *J. Physiol. (London)* 327: 273–284.

19. Andrew, R. D. and Dudek, F. E. (1984) *J. Neurophysiol.* 51: 552–566.

20. Ollet, S. H. R. and Bourque, C. W. (1993) *Nature (London)* 364: 341–343.

21. Richard, D., and Bourque, C. W. (1992) *Neuroendocrinology* 55: 609–611.

22. Tanaka, M., Matsuda, T., Shigeyoshi, Y., Ibata, Y. and Okamura, H. (1997) *J. Histochem. Cytochem.* 45: 1231–1237.

23. Westenbroek, R. E., Merrick, D. K. and Catterall, W. A. (1989) *Neuron* 3: 695–704.

24. Hartshorne, R. P. and Catterall, W. A. (1984) *J. Biol. Chem.* 259: 1667–1675.

25. Widmer, H., Amerdeil, H., Fontanaud, P. and Desarmenien, M. G. (1997) *J. Neurophysiol.* 77: 260–271.

26. Jones, C. W. and Pickering, B. T. (1969) *J. Physiol. (London)* 203: 449–458.

27. Balment, R. J., Brimble, M. J. and Forsling, M. L. (1980) *J. Physiol. (London)* 308: 439–449.

28. Dogterom, J., Van Wimersma Greidanus, B. and Swaab, D. F. (1977) *Neuroendocrinology* 24: 108–118.

29. Hatton, G. I. and Walters, J. K. (1973) *Brain Res.* 59: 137–154.

30. Cummins, T. R., Howe, J. R. and Waxman, S. G. (1998) *J. Neurosci.* 18: 9607–9619.

31. Vega-Saenz de Miera, E., Rudy, B., Sugimori, M. and Llinás, R. (1997) *Proc. Natl. Acad. Sci. USA* 94: 7059–7064.

32. Raman, I. M., Sprunger, L. K., Meisler, M. K. and Bean, B. P. (1997) *Neuron* 19: 881–891.

33. Isom, L. L., De Jongh, K. S., Patton, D. E., Reber, B. F. X., Offord, J., Charbonneau, H., Walsh, K., Goldin, A. L. and Catterall, W. A. (1992) *Science* 256: 839–842.

34. Isom, L. L., Ragsdale, D. S., De Jongh, K. S., Westenbroek, R. E., Reber, B. F. X., Scheuer, T. and Catterall, W. A. (1995) *Cell* 83: 433–442.

35. Isom, L. L., De Jongh, K. S. and Catterall, W. A. (1994) *Neuron* 12: 1183–1194.

36. Waxman, S. G. (1997) *Adv. Neurol.* 73: 109–121.

37. Dargent, B., Paillart, C., Carlier, E., Alcaraz, G., Martin-Eauclaire, M. F. and Couraud, F. (1994) *Neuron* 13: 683–690.

38. Wonderlin, W. F. and French, R. J. (1991) *Proc. Natl. Acad. Sci. USA* 88: 4391–4395.

39. Stafstrom, C. E., Schwindt, P. C., Flatman, J. A. and Crill, W. E. (1984) *J. Neurophysiol.* 52: 244–263.

40. Huguenand, J. R., Hammill, O. P. and Prince, D. A. (1989) *Proc. Natl. Acad. Sci. USA* 86: 2473–2477.

41. Matzner, O. and Devor, M. (1992) *Brain Res.* 597: 92–98.

42. Lipowsky, R., Gillessen, T. and Alzheimer, C. (1996) *J. Neurophysiol.* 76: 2181–2191.

43. Stuart, G. and Sakmann, B. (1995) *Neuron* 15: 1065–1076.

44. Pennartz, C. M., Bierlaagh, M. A. and Geurtsen, A. M. S. (1997) *J. Neurophysiol.* 78: 1811–1825.

45. Franco-Bourland, R. E. and Fernstrom, J. D. (1981) *Endocrinology* 109: 1097–1102.

46. Van Tol, H. H. M., Voorhuis, O. T. A. M. and Burbach, J. P. H. (1987) *Endocrinology* 120: 71–76.

47. Walters, H. K. and Hatton, G. I. (1974) *Physiol. Behav.* 13: 661–667.

48. Alonso, A., and Llinas, R. R. (1989) *Nature (London)* 342: 175–177.

49. Llinás, R. R., Grace, A. A. and Yarom, Y. (1991) *Proc. Natl. Acad. Sci. USA* 88: 897–901.

50. Fleidervish, I. A., Friedman, A. and Gutnick, M. J. (1996) *J. Physiol. (London)* 493: 83–97.

51. Jahnsen, H. and Llinas, R. (1984) *J. Physiol. (London)* 349: 227–247.

52. Parri, H. and Crunelli, V. (1998) *J. Neurosci.* 18: 854–867.

53. Stafstrom, C. E., Schwindt, P. C., Chubb, M. C. and Crill, W. E. (1985) *J. Neurophysiol.* 53: 153–170.

54. Offord, J. and Catterall, W. A. (1989) *Neuron* 2: 1447–1452.

55. Hirsh, J. K. and Quandt, F. N. (1996) *Brain Res.* 706: 343–346.

56. Sashihara, S., Waxman, S. G. and Greer, C. A. (1997) *NeuroReport* 8: 1289–1293.

57. Oh, Y., Lee, Y.-J. and Waxman, S. G. (1997) *Neurosci. Lett.* 234: 107–110.

58. Wu, R.-L. and Barish, M. E. (1994) *J. Neurosci.* 14: 1677–1687.

59. O'Dowd, D. K., Ribera, A. B. and Spitzer, N. C. (1988) *J. Neurosci.* 8: 792–805.

Index

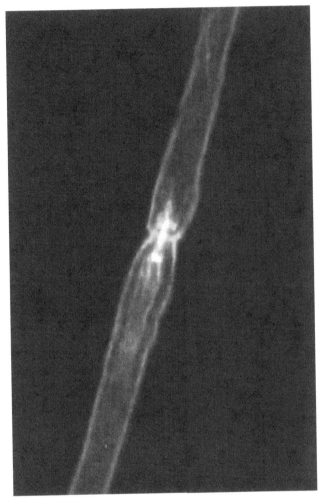

This micrograph was produced by an M.D., Ph.D. student, Jenny Fjell and a colleague, Joel Black, nearly a century after Cajal drew the figure in the frontispiece. It illustrates the complex and elegant molecular architecture of the myelinated nerve fiber. As a result of binding with antibodies that can be visualized by computer-enhanced fluorescence microscopy, clusters of NaN sodium channels within the nerve fiber appear yellow or green (see part XVII), while other molecules (called Kv1.2 potassium channels) appear red.

The richness of this image reminds us that the brain, spinal cord, and nerves have begun to reveal their secrets. The intricacies—even of a single nerve fiber—that are shown in this micrograph also hint at the many mysteries of the nervous system that remain unsolved. These mysteries will fascinate neuroscientists for many years to come.

Printed in the United States
by Baker & Taylor Publisher Services